T3-BNO-492

# Nutrition Management
# of the
# Cancer
# Patient

Edited by
**Abby S. Bloch, MS, RD**
Director, Clinical Nutrition Support
Memorial Sloan-Kettering Cancer Center
New York, New York

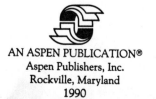

AN ASPEN PUBLICATION®
Aspen Publishers, Inc.
Rockville, Maryland
1990

BRESCIA COLLEGE
LIBRARY
59632

Library of Congress Cataloging-in-Publication Data

Nutrition management of the cancer patient / edited by Abby S. Bloch.
p. cm.

"An Aspen publication"
Includes bibliographical references.
ISBN: 0-8342-0132-1
1. Cancer--Nutritional aspects. 2. Cancer--Diet therapy.
I. Bloch, Abby S.
[DNLM: 1. Neoplasms--diet therapy
QZ 266 N9754]
RC268.45.N88    1990
616.99'40654--dc20
DNLM/DLC
for Library of Congress
89-18410
CIP

Copyright © 1990 by Aspen Publishers, Inc.
All rights reserved.

Aspen Publishers, Inc., grants permission for photocopying for limited personal or
internal use. This consent does not extend to other kinds of copying, such as copying for
general distribution, for advertising or promotional purposes, for creating new collective
works, or for resale. For information, address Aspen Publishers, Inc., Permissions
Department, 1600 Research Boulevard, Rockville, Maryland 20850.

Aspen Publishers, Inc., is not affiliated with the American Society of Parenteral and
Enteral Nutrition

Editorial Services: Lisa J. McCullough

Library of Congress Catalog Card Number: 89-18410
ISBN: 0-8342-0132-1

*Printed in the United States of America*

1 2 3 4 5

# Table of Contents

# Contributors

**SAUNDRA N. AKER, RD, CD**
Director, Clinical Nutrition Program
Division of Clinical Research
Fred Hutchinson Cancer Research Center
Clinical Instructor, School of Nursing
University of Washington
Seattle, Washington

**PAUL AKERMAN, MD**
Research Fellow, Nutrition Support Service
New England Deaconess Hospital
Boston, Massachusetts

**RACHEL BARCIA-MORSE**
Clinical Diet/Nutrition Specialist
Memorial Sloan Kettering Cancer Center
New York, New York

**STACEY J. BELL, MS, RD**
Nutrition Support Dietitian
Nutrition Metabolism Lab, CRI
New England Deaconess Hospital
Boston, Massachusetts

**GEORGE L. BLACKBURN, MD, PhD**
Chief, Nutrition Metabolism Laboratory
Cancer Research Institute
Associate Professor of Surgery
Harvard Medical School
Boston, Massachusetts

**DIANA FULLEN BOWERS, MS, RD, LD**
Clinical Dietitian, Medical Intensive Care

Department of Nutrition and Dietetics
The Ohio State University Hospitals
Clinical Instructor, School of Allied Medical
  Professions
The Ohio State University
Columbus, Ohio

**KATHRYN LEE BRADFORD, RD**
Market Manager
Johnson and Johnson Professional Marketing
New Brunswick, New Jersey

**AMY AUSTIN BREWER, MS, RD**
Director, Nutrition Intervention
Department of Preventive Medicine
University of Tennessee Center for Health
  Sciences
  *formerly of St. Jude Children's Research
  Hospital*
Memphis, Tennessee

**JULIENE B. BURGESS, MS, RD**
Nutritionist/Partner
Dinners a la Heart
  *formerly of St. Jude Children's Research
  Hospital*
Memphis, Tennessee

**KAREN MUELLER BUZBY, RD, CNSD**
Nutrition Consultant
Bala Cynwyd, Pennsylvania

**SHEILA M. CAMPBELL, MS, RD**
Clinical Research Associate
Medical Nutritional Education
Ross Laboratories
Columbus, Ohio

**NANCY COSTLOW, RD, PA-C**
Pediatric Oncology
The Johns Hopkins Oncology Center
Baltimore, Maryland

**ANN M. COULSTON, MS, RD**
Research Dietitian, General Clinical Research
   Center
Stanford University Medical Center
Stanford, California

**JEANNE A. DARBINIAN, MS, RD, CNSD**
Pediatric Nutritionist
Department of Nutrition and Dietetics
The Medical Center at the University of
   California, San Francisco
San Francisco, California

**CAROL FRANKMANN, MS, RD, LD**
Associate Director, Clinical Nutrition
Department of Nutrition and Food Service
M.D. Anderson Cancer Center
The University of Texas
Houston, Texas

**MONIQUE D. GELINAS, PhD, DtP,
CNSD**
Associate Professor, Department of Nutrition
Faculty of Medicine
University of Montreal
Montreal, Quebec
Canada

**SUZANNE P. GEERTS, MS, RD**
Adjunct Instructor
Jefferson State Community College
Birmingham, Alabama

**MINDY HERMANN-ZAIDINS, MBA,
   RD**
Clinical Diet/Nutrition Specialist
Memorial Sloan-Kettering Cancer Center

New York, New York
President, The Hermann Group, Inc.
Mt. Kisco, New York

**URSULA G. KYLE, MS, RD, LD**
Consulting Dietitian
Geneva, Switzerland
   formerly, Clinical Dietitian
Department of Nutrition and Food Service
M.D. Anderson Cancer Center
The University of Texas
Houston, Texas

**JULIE O'SULLIVAN MAILLET, PhD, RD**
Director, Dietetic Internship and Associate
   Professor
Department of Primary Care
School of Health Related Professions
University of Medicine and Dentistry of New
   Jersey
Newark, New Jersey

**IRA MILNER, RD**
Nutrition Agent
Cornell Cooperative Extension of Rockland
   County
Thiells, New York

**GAILE L. MOE, RD**
Coordinator of Food Services
Clinical Nutrition Program
Division of Clinical Research
Fred Hutchinson Cancer Research Center
Seattle, Washington

**MARCIA L. NAHIKIAN-NELMS, MEd,
   RD, LD**
Clinical Dietitian, Bone Marrow Transplant
   Program
Department of Nutrition and Dietetics
The Ohio State University Hospitals
Clinical Instructor, School of Allied Medical
   Professions
Ohio State University
Columbus, Ohio

**L. CHARNETTE NORTON, MS, RD, LD**
Partner, The Norton Group
Houston, Texas

**BONNIE TERRILL ROSS, MS, RD**
Radiation Oncology Dietitian
Methodist Hospital of Indiana, Inc.
Radiation Oncology Department
Methodist Hospital Cancer Center
Indianapolis, Indiana

**JACALYN SEE, MS, RD**
Clinical Dietitian
Mayo Comprehensive Cancer Center
Mayo Clinic
Rochester, Minnesota

**MAURICE E. SHILS, ScD, MD**
Adjunct Professor of Medicine and Public
    Health Sciences (Nutrition)
Bowman Gray School of Medicine
Winston-Salem, North Carolina
Professor Emeritus of Medicine
Cornell University Medical College
New York, New York

**DEBBIE ZIBELL-FRISK, MS, RD, CNSD**
Metabolic Support Dietitian
Metabolic Support Service
Providence Hospital
Southfield, Michigan

# Foreword

Remember grandmother's nutrition remedy to feed a cold and starve a fever—or was it the other way around? That is about the level of sophistication that was applied to nutrition problems of patients with cancer not so many years ago. What did it matter? Wouldn't these patients die anyway? Fortunately, a number of developments have changed all that for the better. The advent of super-radical head and neck surgery and abdominal surgery in the past quarter-century required special attention to general and specific problems of nutrition just to carry the patient through a prolonged period of wound healing. Aggressive chemotherapy, as for patients with acute leukemia or breast or ovarian cancer, caused severe problems of nausea, vomiting, fluid and electrolyte balance (i.e., hypokalemic alkalosis), and protein and mineral depletion due to cancer cachexia as well as cancer therapy. Measures had to be taken to deal with these problems, and research has been very successful in finding answers.

Planning aggressive chemotherapy had to take into account nutrition factors. A malnourished patient had a much poorer prognosis of surviving a course of chemotherapy or surgery than an adequately nourished patient: delaying treatment until these circumstances were at least partially reversed would often tip the balance toward a more favorable outcome, one with lower morbidity and mortality. As a result more patients were surviving their treatments and, by living longer in remission, uncovering unique nutrition conditions that needed resolution.

More than anything, emergence of the specialties within oncology encouraged medical, nursing, and nutrition specialists who became excellent care givers in these neglected areas; they also became advocates for those measures that could improve the quality of life of their patients.

We are at a point in the evolution of oncology that a critical mass of information exists about the management of common conditions. Abby Bloch and her contributing authors have consolidated and synthesized a remarkable body of information for health professionals who care for cancer patients in hospitals and at home. Patient needs do vary, of course, as a function of type and stage of cancer, type of treatment, and comorbid conditions. Needs also vary according to the preferences and attitudes of patient, family, and staff. There is a great deal of misinformation out there about cancer and nutrition, especially in the area of prevention but certainly not limited to that. The ability to apply a body of knowledge to individual circumstances is what leads to a satisfactory result for the patient and satisfaction for the care giver.

A famous rabbi was once taunted by a smart-alecky pupil that he should teach him the Bible while the student stood on one foot. The rabbi replied "Do unto others as you would have them do unto you. That is the essence of the Bible—all the rest is commentary. Now go and learn." Although no book about cancer is the medical equivalent of the Bible, this book will give us the tools to go out and learn, and to serve.

*John Laszlo, MD*
Senior Vice President for Research
American Cancer Society National Office
June 26, 1989

# Preface

In 1989, about 1 million people will be diagnosed as having cancer. More cancer patients are being treated and more are living longer; four of ten patients will be alive 5 years after their diagnosis. These changes create increased demands on health professionals.

Interest in the interrelationships among diet, nutrition, and cancer has intensified since the report by the National Cancer Institute's Committee on Diet, Nutrition, and Cancer was released in 1982. With cancer being the second leading cause of death in Americans, books providing nutrition guidelines and management techniques for cancer patients are needed. This book was written for health professionals who work with cancer patients and their families by some of America's most knowledgeable dietitians, nutritionists, and physicians. Each contributor has seen first-hand the problems, frustrations, and difficulties in managing the nutrition needs of cancer patients during and after treatment. The skills and techniques acquired by these experts through years of experience with patients are offered to other professionals who have not had the same exposure to this specialized patient population. Similar problems recur in many areas of cancer management; therefore, some duplication of ideas and suggestions appears throughout the book. Nevertheless, each contributor applies his or her personal perspective to each problem.

We have endeavored to create a practical resource in the care and management of patients who already have cancer and are struggling with the dietary and nutrition demands resulting from their cancer treatment. The book focuses on the patient who has specific nutrition problems rather than on the population concerned with prevention. The chapters encompass a broad spectrum of topics and issues. Altogether, the book is intended to provide the health community with the important elements of the care and management of this specialized group, which is so in need of nutrition support.

*Abby S. Bloch*

# Part I

# Introduction: Identification and General Feeding

# Chapter 1

# Nutrition Needs of Cancer Patients

*Maurice E. Shils*

## A LOOK BACKWARD AND FORWARD

When one compares experiences 30 odd years ago of an intern on a pioneering adult chemotherapy unit with what one sees today in a hospital with a high-grade nutrition team, the difference is monumental. Then, malnutrition was the usual situation in patients with advanced cancer or experiencing the deleterious effects of its various treatments. Little, if anything, was done about their nutrition state other than correcting fluid and electrolyte abnormalities. Phase I, II, and III drug testing was being performed on such patients, and one wondered how their outcomes were affected by the profound undernutrition that often was present. Today, advances in treatments of cancer have been matched by progress in nutrition management.

The importance attributed to nutrition support will increase as more effective therapeutic regimens for the cure and palliation of cancer develop. Until effective, highly specific, antitumor treatment modalities are developed against a wide variety of malignancies, it is likely that physicians will have to contend with serious and long-term modalities that depress nutrition for many reasons. At the same time, there will be better nutrition support because of advances in understanding of nutrient requirements during chemotherapy, radiation therapy, and other therapies; improved substrates to meet those needs; better control of anorexia and nausea; and increased concern on the part of physicians about the nutrition status of their patients. Certain vitamins such as A and D, which cause differentiation of neoplastic cells, as well as more specific essential nutrient antimetabolites, may come to play roles in therapy. Compassion through understanding must be the motivating force in nutrition support.

The other area in which continuing progress is being made is basic nutrition research and its application in cancer prevention. Understanding in this area is still a long way behind; for example, knowledge of the relation of certain dietary and metabolic factors in coronary artery disease is lacking. That gap can only be closed by research involving physicians and dietitians in basic science, clinical medicine, and epidemiology. The future for research-based, clinically applied nutrition support of cancer patients (preferably through clinical nutrition teams) seems to be as promising as the past three decades have been in this area.

## OVERVIEW OF NUTRITION AND CANCER RELATIONSHIPS

The term cancer embraces a large number of complex neoplastic diseases. They not only differ in significant ways among each other, but each type may also have different biologic effects on individual patients depending on a number of factors. They may be rather slow growing or aggressive, depending on their specific characteristics and on the defenses of the host. Some, for example, may induce little or no anorexia and weight loss until the patient's disease is advanced, whereas others may induce severe anorexia at an early stage even though the tumor may not be widespread. Effective treatments differ for various kinds of neoplasms and also in relation to the stage of a particular tumor and its resistance to previous therapies.

As malignancies are diagnosed earlier and as the palliative effects of treatments become more effective, cancer patients tend to have significantly increased life expectancies. The diseases therefore become chronic. Even when the disease appears to be eradicated, the affected individual often remains uncertain about this for a period of years and has to live with the possibility of recurrence. Hence for many patients psychologic stress is added to the various other problems induced by the tumors and the therapies.

As is indicated below, a significant proportion of patients with cancer tend to develop one or more nutrition problems; often the etiologies are different. It is essential that the underlying causes for the nutrition problems that occur or are likely to occur are understood by the physician and dietitian so that a rational and effective nutrition support program may be developed for the individual concerned. Failure to understand the nature of the actual problems may lead to incorrect therapies. For the dietitian as for the physician, the ancient precept *primum non nocere* (of primary importance, do not injure) must always be remembered.

## SYSTEMIC AND LOCALIZED EFFECTS OF NEOPLASTIC DISEASES

### Systemic Effects

Systemic effects are multiple and vary with different kinds of neoplasms, manifesting themselves with different intensities in different individuals (Exhibit 1-1). Their presence and severity can be identified, in large part, from the history and physical examination of the patient together with appropriate laboratory and other work-up.

Although anorexia is not unique to cancer, its incidence and duration and the consequent weight loss are often sufficiently great to make it of special concern. Its etiologies remain uncertain. Recent animal experiments support a widely held but still unproven belief that secretion into the systemic circulation of a substance or substances produced or induced in other cells by a malignancy may play a significant role in its development. It is well established that various biologically active amines and peptides can stimulate or depress appetite in experimental animals and in humans. To date, studies with laboratory animals on the effects of serotonin and cholecystokinin, for example, have thus far produced no firm evidence for hormone roles in tumor-related depressed appetite. Recently, there has been much interest in relation to cancer of the effects of cytokines, which are produced from macrophages and lymphocytes, and of growth factors (Theologides, 1986; Abeloff, 1987; Klasing, 1988). The cytokines interleukin-1 and cachetin ($\alpha$ tumor necrosis factor) induce anorexia as part of their catabolic effects, but their roles in cancer anorexia are still unproven. A number of these and other metabolic effects of cancer have been reviewed recently (Shils, 1988; Kern & Norton, 1988).

Insulin has been studied as an antianorexigenic agent. In rats insulin improved food intake, but the doses required induced significant hypoglycemia, and survival was not improved (Kern & Norton, 1988). Another agent that has also received renewed attention is hydrazine sulfate, which inhibits gluconeogenic enzymes; in a clinical trial in patients with advanced cancer and cachexia, there were some improvements in glucose metabolism but none in survival (Kern & Norton, 1988).

Improved appetite and weight gain have been observed in patients with prostate (Bonomi et al., 1985) and breast cancer (Aisner, Tchekmedyian, Moody, & Tait, 1987) and in an initial

**Exhibit 1-1** Nutrition Problems Associated with the Presence of Neoplastic Disease

1. Anorexia with progressive weight loss and undernutrition
2. Taste changes causing depressed or altered food intake
3. Alterations in protein, carbohydrate, and fat metabolism
4. Hypermetabolism (in a variable number of patients)
5. Impaired food intake and malnutrition secondary to bowel obstruction at any level
6. Malabsorption associated with

   - deficiency or inactivation of pancreatic enzymes
   - deficiency or inactivation of bile salts
   - failure of food to mix with digestive enzymes (e.g., enzyme dilution, pancreaticocibarian asynchrony)
   - fistulous bypass of small bowel
   - infiltration of small bowel wall or lymphatics and mesentery by malignant cells
   - blind loop occurring with depressed gastric secretion or partial upper small bowel obstruction leading to bacterial overgrowth
   - malnutrition-induced villous hypoplasia
7. Protein-losing enteropathy with various malignancies
8. Hormonal abnormalities induced by tumors

   - hypercalcemia induced by increased serum calcitriol, other hormones, and osteoclastic processes
   - osteomalacia with hypophosphatemia often associated with depressed serum calcitriol
   - hypoglycemia of insulin-secreting tumors
   - hyperglycemia, for example, with insulinoma, glucagonoma, or somatostatinoma
9. Anemia of chronic blood loss
10. Electrolyte and fluid problems with

    - persistent vomiting with intestinal obstruction or intracranial tumors
    - intestinal fluid losses through fistulas or diarrhea
    - intestinal secretory abnormalities with hormone-secreting tumors (e.g., carcinoid syndrome, Zollinger-Ellison syndrome [gastrinoma], Verner-Morrison syndrome [pancreatic cholera], increased calcitonin, villous adenoma)
    - inappropriate antidiuretic hormone secretion associated with certain tumors (e.g., lung carcinomas)
    - hyperadrenalism with tumors producing corticotropin or corticosteroids
11. Miscellaneous organ dysfunction with implications for nutrition (e.g., intractable gastric ulcers with gastrinomas, Fanconi's syndrome with light-chain disease, coma with brain tumors)

*Source:* From *Modern Nutrition in Health and Disease*, 7th ed. by M.E. Shils and V.R. Young (Eds.), 1988, Philadelphia: Lea & Febiger. Copyright 1988 by Lea & Febiger. Reprinted by permission.

report of anorectic patients with acquired immunodeficiency syndrome given megestrol acetate (Megace) (Von Roenn, Murphy, Weber, Williams, & Weitzman, 1988). This is a synthetic, orally active progestational agent with antineoplastic and corticosteroid activities. At conventional doses of 160 mg/day, approximately 30% of patients were noted to have gained weight. At 6 weeks all but one of 35 patients taking 1,600 mg/day gained weight; the median gain was 5.2 kg, with a range of −0.1 to 22.3 kg. Body composition studies were not performed, but it was believed that the weight gain was not attributable to edema even though about 26% of the patients had some fluid accumulation. The weight gain was consistent regardless of whether the patients were underweight, of normal weight, or overweight and regardless of the site of disease involvement (Aisner et al., 1987).

Even though anorectic cancer patients may have normal or even low metabolic rates (Knox et al., 1983), they often behave as though they are hypermetabolic (Knox et al., 1983; Cohen et al., 1981; Shaw & Wolfe, 1987). For example, during a period of inadequate caloric intake the patient may not mobilize fat normally and hence not spare lean body mass. Compared with non–tumor-bearing patients, cancer patients are found not to have significant reductions in their fat stores until weight loss exceeds 10%; during this period, there is increased muscle catabolism (Cohen et al., 1981). Basal rates of glucose turnover have been found to be similar in normal volunteers and in patients with early colon cancer. Such rates were significantly higher in those with advanced gastrointestinal malignancies, however. The infusion of glucose led to less suppression of endogenous glucose production in both early and late cancer patients compared to controls, and glucose oxidation rates increased progressively in proportion to tumor burden (Shaw & Wolfe, 1987). Some, but not all, cancer patients have been shown to have protein kinetic changes similar to those of patients in the catabolic phases of severe trauma, sepsis, or chronic infection. When the catabolic rate persistently exceeded the synthetic rate, depletion of body protein occurred in accordance with the degree of the discrepancy. On the other hand, there have been studies in which protein kinetic changes were similar in malnourished cancer patients and those with nonmalignant diseases (Shils, 1988). It is obvious that a patient with a combination of systemic factors, such as anorexia, hypermetabolism, sepsis, and malabsorption, will undergo a much more rapid decline in weight than a patient who has a similar degree of anorexia but is hypometabolic and has normal absorption.

A multitude of ectopic hormones have been documented in human tumors (Abeloff, 1987; Creutzfeldt, 1980). The effects of their unregulated production may induce various clinical problems, many of which have deleterious nutritional effects.

### Localized Effects

Localized tumor effects are usually those associated with malabsorption, obstruction, diarrhea, and vomiting that result in inadequate nutrition and electrolyte and fluid imbalances. Depending on the rate at which such changes have occurred, patients may become rapidly or slowly depleted.

Hypoalbuminemia is frequently noted in advanced cancer. Depressed albumin levels may be attributable to an inability to produce sufficient albumin secondary to serious protein-calorie deficiency or liver damage. There may be losses of albumin from the body in excess of synthetic ability (i.e., in protein-losing enteropathy or nephrotic syndrome); there also may be dilution of albumin into abnormally large extracellular compartments associated with ascites or edema, or there may be a metabolic effect of the malignancy and of cytokines (i.e., inhibition of protein synthesis).

Anemia is also frequently noted in advanced cancer. This is usually normochromic and normocytic and usually does not respond to nutrition factors. There may be anemias of either microcytic or macrocytic type, however, which may be caused by iron depletion secondary to blood loss or to folate or vitamin $B_{12}$ deficiency secondary to persistent malabsorption.

As a result of impaired intake or altered physiology, concentrations of a number of micronutrients may be abnormal, and these have been documented. A high incidence of depressed serum zinc has been noted both in malnourished children and in adults with cancer. On the other hand, copper is usually elevated in cancer patients, presumably secondary to increased levels of circulating ceruloplasmin.

## NUTRITION PROBLEMS ARISING FROM THE TREATMENTS OF CANCER

One cause of undernutrition in cancer patients is the specific treatment of the cancer. The factors involved may also be complex and require the physician and dietitian caring for such patients to be aware of the various changes that may occur (Exhibit 1-2). As is often the case in modern antitumor protocols, the treatments are frequently multidisciplinary. Some protocols include surgery, radiation therapy, and chemotherapy in increasing association with immunotherapy, or surgery may precede by some time either radiation therapy or chemotherapy; the added effects may severely affect the

**Exhibit 1-2** Consequences of Cancer Treatment Predisposing to Nutrition Problems

1. Radiation treatment
   - Radiation of oropharyngeal area
       destruction of sense of taste
       xerostomia and odynophagia
       loss of teeth
   - Radiation to lower back and mediastinum
       esophagitis with dysphagia
       fibrosis with esophageal stricture
   - Radiation of abdomen and pelvis
       bowel damage, acute and chronic, with diarrhea, malabsorption, stenosis and obstruction, fistulization
2. Surgical treatment
   - Radical resection of oropharyngeal area
       chewing and swallowing difficulties
   - Esophagectomy
       gastric stasis and hypochlorhydria secondary to vagotomy
       steatorrhea secondary to vagotomy
       diarrhea secondary to vagotomy
       early satiety
       regurgitation
   - Gastrectomy (high subtotal or total)
       dumping syndrome
       malabsorption
       achlorhydria and lack of intrinsic factor and R protein
       hypoglycemia
       early satiety
   - Intestinal resection
       jejunum: decreased efficiency of absorption of many nutrients
       ileum: vitamin $B_{12}$ deficiency, bile salt losses with diarrhea or steatorrhea, hyperoxaluria and renal stones, calcium and magnesium depletion, fat-soluble vitamin depletion
       massive bowel resection: life-threatening malabsorption, malnutrition, metabolic acidosis, dehydration
       ileostomy and colostomy: complications of salt and water balance
   - Blind-loop syndrome
       vitamin $B_{12}$ malabsorption
   - Pancreatectomy
       malabsorption
       diabetes mellitus
3. Drug treatment
   - Corticosteroids
       fluid and electrolyte problems
       nitrogen and calcium losses
       hyperglycemia
   - Sex hormone analogs
       may induce nausea and vomiting
   - Immunotherapy (interleukin-2)
       azotemia
       hypotension
       fluid retention
   - Antimetabolites, alkylating agents, and other drugs
       side effects (see Table 64-3 in Kern & Norton [1988])

*Source:* From *Modern Nutrition in Health and Disease*, 7th ed. by M.E. Shils and V.R. Young (Eds.), 1988, Philadelphia: Lea & Febiger. Copyright 1988 by Lea & Febiger. Reprinted by permission.

patient's nutrition status. Surgery may be required when intestinal radiation damage has resulted in fistulas or obstruction and a consequent additional decrease in remaining absorbing surfaces.

Cancer research is now in a period of active investigations and trials of new therapeutic modalities. These include genetically engineered molecules with various cell growth factors and cytokines, combinations of tumor-infiltrating activated lymphocytes with interleukin-2 promotion, interleukin-2–activated killer cells, and other mitogens and immune system–stimulating agents. When effective, these may be given in combination with more traditional types of chemotherapy as well as with new agents and dosages plus radiation and surgery. It is known that large doses of interleukin-2 are associated with common side effects, including fever, nausea, hepatotoxicity and nephrotoxicity, and skin rash (Kradin et al., 1989).

Awareness on the part of the dietitian of proposed therapeutic protocols before they are given to patients and of their possible side effects should permit appropriate decisions to be made concerning the need for early involvement of nutrition support. The purpose of the nutrition support is to provide essential nutrients and energy sources to meet the patient's needs when voluntary intake is significantly impaired and an impending or actual serious nutrition problem has developed. In addition to the classic nutrients and amino acids, other substrates have been tested or are being tested in an attempt to improve utilization of substrates for various cellular processes under specific circumstances. These new substrates, whether designed for use in oral, enteral, or intravenous feeding, merit research and evaluation by physicians and dietitians in clinical trials.

## THE EFFECTIVENESS OF NUTRITION SUPPORT IN THE CANCER PATIENT

It is still important to stress the fact that nutrition intervention for the cancer patient is primarily a form of support for that patient; it serves the same general purpose as antibiotics given to a cancer patient with an infection or hemodialysis to support a patient who has developed acute nephrotoxicity.

There have been series of studies by oncologists comparing survival of cancer patients (usually those with poorly responding types of advanced solid tumors) with and without parenteral nutrition support. In many such reports it was concluded that nutrition support did not usually extend survival and, on occasion, may even have decreased it (e.g., American College of Physicians, 1989). Such types of research were, in effect, testing the hypothesis that improved nutrition could synergistically improve the therapeutic effectiveness of drugs that were relatively ineffective by themselves. In addition to the apparent improbability of this thesis, the approach utilized was often flawed. On examination of the protocols of almost all these studies, it is apparent that the aggressive nutrition support of the patients was discontinued during the periods when they were at home. Hence these patients were getting intermittent nutrition support, usually for relatively short periods in hospital, compared to the total time on chemotherapy and nutrition support in hospital and no support at home. This procedure may have seriously compromised the value of nutrition support over a long-term period for those patients for whom adequate and continuous nutrition support might have made a difference in life expectancy for nutrition reasons alone.

Other types of controlled studies in both adults and children have effectively repudiated earlier claims from the uncontrolled studies that nutrition support reduced toxicity or other side effects of certain antitumor treatments. They indicate that nutrition support during aggressive cancer chemotherapy (e.g., Evans et al., 1987) and during chemotherapy combined with radiation (e.g., Ghavimi, Shils, Scott, Brown, & Tamaroff, 1982) will not significantly protect against the toxic effects of the therapy on the bone marrow and the intestinal tract. In children receiving total parenteral nutrition, weight was maintained or improved (Ghavimi et al., 1982); oral support was minimally effective in terms of weight in adults (Evans et al., 1987). Another lesson that was learned from these controlled studies, particularly with children (Ghavimi et al., 1982), was that when children were started on antitumor treatments early in the course of disease (when they were in good nutritional condition) their responses to the therapy varied quite widely. Some of the patients tolerated chemotherapy and radiation well and continued to eat reasonably well throughout the study; others were devastated by the chemotherapy and were anorectic in association with frequent nausea and vomiting.

Additionally, there are studies indicating that some patients benefit by preoperative nutrition support (Shils, 1988). Malnourished patients with localized tumors, such as in the esophagus, have been shown to derive nutrition benefit from their feeding programs. A complicating factor is the catabolic influence of chemotherapy and radiation. For example, patients with untreated advanced testicular cancer given parenteral nutrition were able to maintain normal protein kinetics as well as nitrogen balance before undergoing chemotherapy; as soon as they were given drugs (e.g., vinblastine, cisplatin, and bleomycin), however, they developed a negative nitrogen balance and their protein turnover (synthesis and catabolism) decreased despite continuing intravenous nutrition support (Shils, 1988). The variability among cancer patients is well demonstrated in a study in which body composition was measured initially and after 2 weeks of intravenous feeding in 17 malnourished cancer patients; the results indicated that 8 had appreciably improved body cell mass and decreased extracellular volume, whereas those patients who did not improve had advanced neoplastic disease or sepsis or both (Shils, 1988). A well-documented study comparing malnourished cancer patients with malnourished noncancer subjects before and after a period of enteral feeding found that both groups responded well, showing weight gain and restored energy and nitrogen balance (Shils, 1988).

## NUTRITION SUPPORT RECOMMENDATIONS

Despite the metabolic problems, complications, and uncertainties about response and survival that often occur in cancer patients, the physician must decide whether to initiate some form of nutrition support, particularly in those patients who are becoming undernourished for the various reasons noted above. Although some patients do respond to adequate nutrition support and show subjective and objective improvement, others do not. Furthermore, there are no diagnostic tests that will indicate objectively which patients may respond and which may not; consequently, physicians frequently have to make decisions that are not based on solid data in hopes of benefitting the patient.

A factor that often plays a role in decision making concerns the attitudes of both patients and family members about diet and nutrition. Progressive weight loss, increasing weakness, and debilitation are undesirable prognostic signs in terms of the outcome of the disease. Often the patient and family members are as aware of this as the physician; such changes create much anxiety and feelings of hopelessness, leading to demands to the physician and dietitian to "do something," usually in the form of nutrition support. The issue of "doing something" for a particular patient requires careful consideration. The following guidelines are offered.

1. For the seriously anorectic patient who is no longer a candidate for further antitumor therapy of any kind, who has a functioning alimentary tract, and whose quality of life is reasonably acceptable and likely to be maintained or improved by enteral feeding, this method of feeding should be used if desired by the patient and family.
2. For the patient with intestinal obstruction due to active abdominal disease and for whom all therapy has failed, a rapid downhill course out of hospital is common. This situation presents difficult emotional problems, particularly if prior use of total parenteral nutrition had improved physical

capacity and weight and consideration is being given to its cessation. All too frequently, the physician is pressured to continue total parenteral nutrition in hospital or at home despite the clear statement that it has no antitumor benefit and may have its own complications. The attending physician must present the options, with their benefits and drawbacks (including the financial cost), of home parenteral nutrition to the patient and family. The mentally competent patient must then make the decision. If the patient is deemed incompetent, the issues become more complicated in that family members must make the decisions with information provided by the physician; they may wish to consult with the hospital ethics committee before reaching a decision.

## REFERENCES

Abeloff, M.D. (1987). Paraneoplastic syndromes: A window on the biology of cancer. *New England Journal of Medicine, 317,* 1598–1600.

Aisner, J., Tchekmedyian, N.S., Moody, M., & Tait, N. (1987). High-dose megastrol acetate for the treatment of advanced breast cancer: Dose and toxicities. *Seminars in Hematology, 24*(Suppl. 1), 48–55.

American College of Physicians. (1989). Position paper: Parenteral nutrition in patients receiving cancer chemotherapy. *Annals of Internal Medicine, 110,* 734–736.

Bonomi, P., Pessis, O., Bunting, N., Block, M., Anderson, K., Wolter, J., Rossof, A., Slayton, R., & Harris, J. (1985). Megestrol acetate used as primary hormonal therapy in stage D prostate cancer. *Seminars in Oncology, 12*(Suppl. 1), 36–39.

Cohen, S.H., Gartenhaus, W., Vartsky, D., Sawitsky, A., Zanzi, I., Vaswani, A., Yasumura, S., & Rai, K. (1981). Body composition and dietary intake in neoplastic disease. *American Journal of Clinical Nutrition, 34,* 1997–2004.

Creutzfeldt, W. (Ed.). (1980). Gastrointestinal hormones. *Clinical Gastroenterology, 9,* 483–803.

Evans, W.K., Nixon, D.W., Daly, J.M., Ellenberg, S.S., Gardner, L., Wolfe, E., Shepherd, R.A., Feld, R., & Gralla, R. (1987). A randomized study of oral nutritional support versus ad lib nutritional intake during chemotherapy for advanced colorectal and non–small-cell lung cancer. *Journal of Clinical Oncology, 5,* 113–124.

Ghavimi, F., Shils, M.E., Scott, B.F., Brown, M., & Tamaroff, M. (1982). Comparison of morbidity in children requiring abdominal radiation and chemotherapy, with and without total parenteral nutrition. *Journal of Pediatrics, 4,* 530–537.

Kern, K.A., & Norton, J.A. (1988). Cancer cachexia. *Journal of Enteral and Parenteral Nutrition, 12,* 286–296.

Klasing, K.C. (1988). Nutritional aspects of leukocytic cytokines. *Journal of Nutrition, 118,* 1436–1446.

Knox, L.S., Crosby, L.O., Feurer, I.D., Buzby, G.P., Miller, C.L., & Mullen, J.L. (1983). Energy expenditure in malnourished cancer patients. *Annals of Surgery, 197,* 152–162.

Kradin, R.L., Kurnick, J., Lazarus, D.S., Preffer, F.I., Dubinett, S.M., Pinto, C.E., Gifford, J., Davidson, E., Grove, B., Callahan, R.J., & Strauss, H.W. (1989). Tumour-infiltrating lymphocytes and interleukin-2 in treatment of advanced cancer. *Lancet, 1,* 577–580.

Shaw, J.H., & Wolfe, R.R. (1987). Glucose and urea kinetics in patients with early and advanced gastrointestinal cancer: The response to glucose infusion, parenteral feeding and surgical resection. *Surgery, 101,* 181–191.

Shils, M.E. (1988). Nutrition and diet in cancer. In M.E. Shils & V.R. Young (Eds.), *Modern nutrition in health and disease* (7th ed., pp. 1380–1422). Philadelphia: Lea & Febiger.

Theologides, A. (1986). Anorexins, asthenins, and cachectins in cancer. *American Journal of Medicine, 81,* 696–698.

Von Roenn, J.H., Murphy, R.L., Weber, K.M., Williams, L.M., & Weitzman, S.A. (1988). Megestrol acetate for treatment of cachexia associated with human immunodeficiency virus (HIV) infection. *Annals of Internal Medicine, 109,* 840–841.

# Chapter 2

# Cancer's Impact on the Nutrition Status of Patients

*Bonnie Terrill Ross*

Malnutrition is the most common secondary diagnosis in cancer patients. A malignancy can affect a patient's nutrition status in various ways. Nutrition may be compromised because of the anatomic location of the cancer, resulting in mechanical barriers to eating. Poor nutrition intake may be secondary to impaired chewing or swallowing or to partial gastrointestinal obstruction. Esophageal cancers, for example, tend to be constricting tumors that impair swallowing.

Another way in which malignancies affect nutrition status is from cancer therapies. Major surgery, chemotherapy, and radiation therapy treatments often compromise a cancer patient's ability and desire to eat. The emotional stress from a cancer diagnosis and from the cancer therapies can often suppress appetite, leading to inadequate intake.

A major contributor to the poor nutrition status of cancer patients is the systemic effects of the neoplasm. Many investigators have attempted to unravel the complex interrelationships among tumor growth, host malnutrition, and metabolic abnormalities. Anorexia and altered metabolism in cancer are poorly understood, and widely differing opinions and experimental results have been expressed in the literature (Copeland, Daly, & Dudrick, 1977).

## CACHEXIA AND ANOREXIA

Cachexia is a complicated physiologic state seen in most patients with advanced metastatic cancer. It can also affect patients with localized disease. The etiology of the cachectic state is not entirely clear.

The cachectic state features anorexia, premature satiety, weight loss, muscle wasting, increased basal metabolic rate and energy expenditure, electrolyte abnormalities, impaired organ function, and immunosuppression. The severity of cachexia is not entirely related to the type of cancer, site, or bulk of disease. In cachectic patients with progressive weight loss, there is deterioration of performance status and increased morbidity and mortality. Ideally, before or during the early stages of anorexia there should be dietary intervention in the hope of delaying, minimizing, or even preventing the debilitating progression of cachexia.

Decreased food intake does not entirely account for weight loss in cancer patients. Weight loss can sometimes occur in the presence of normal or even supranormal intake. To some extent, there is tumor competition for host nutrients. The tumor can parasitize the host and thus add to the patient's malnutrition.

Anorexia is a monumental barrier to nutrition. Many cancer patients are in a paradoxic dilemma: an increased need for nourishment with a decreased desire for eating. Anorexia is unquestionably one of the prime causes of weight loss and cachexia. Postulated etiologies for cancer anorexia include increased lactic acid levels, hyperglycemia, appetite-suppressing toxins produced by the cancer cells, increased circulation of free fatty acids, alterations in smell or taste perception, and psychologic factors. Anorexia and taste abnormalities can develop early in a cancer patient. They may be one of the symptoms that prompt the patient to seek medical attention.

## ALTERED METABOLISM

Derangements in metabolism contribute greatly to the malnutrition seen in many cancer patients. Again, the mechanisms are not clearly understood. It is important to understand that metabolism varies significantly among patients. The metabolism in a particular patient is not always static but depends on the course of the disease and its treatment. Cancer is actually a term for more than 200 different diseases that can vary in degree of malignancy. Therefore, the inconsistent metabolic peculiarities of a specific cancer do not allow for simple explanations and necessitate individualized assessment and management.

## ENERGY EXPENDITURE

Many malnourished cancer patients display inefficient energy expenditure. With simple starvation in healthy individuals, the metabolic rate is known to decrease. In cancer patients, however, metabolic rate may increase despite decreased caloric intake. Oxygen consumption and carbohydrate production may be inappropriately high in the cancer patient.

Energy-wasting pathways of metabolism are to blame for the inefficient energy expenditure seen in some cancer patients. This may be due to the body's reaction and attempt to meet the energy needs of the tumor. It is a known fact that

the patient can be wasting while the tumor is actually growing. This is because the tumor can successfully compete for nutrients.

## CARBOHYDRATE METABOLISM

Individuals with cancer often display derangements in carbohydrate metabolism. An increased turnover in glucose is a major contributor to the high energy expenditure observed in cancer patients. It is believed that the tumor's energy is primarily derived from anaerobic glycolysis. Anaerobic glycolysis is far less efficient in energy production than normal aerobic metabolism of glucose.

One of the end products of anaerobic glycolysis is lactic acid. The high levels of lactic acid common in cancer patients significantly contribute to anorexia. The lactic acid produced by anaerobic glycolysis is recruited back into glucose production, resulting in an increased rate of gluconeogenesis. This cycle of glucose to lactic acid and back to glucose is called the Cori cycle. The Cori cycle is an energy-wasting process (Groenwald, 1987). Because the energy required for the accelerated gluconeogenesis cannot be provided by lactic acid alone, there is a net energy deficit. The result is depletion of host reserves, leading to malnutrition.

Another deviation of carbohydrate metabolism seen in individuals with cancer is impaired glucose tolerance and insulin resistance.

## PROTEIN METABOLISM

There is decreased protein synthesis with a decrease in circulating proteins in some cancer patients. Cancer patients can also exhibit a high protein turnover and impaired muscle protein synthesis. Loss of skeletal mass is a common finding in malnourished cancer patients. This can be observed even if the diet is adequate in calories and protein.

Some tumors act as a nitrogen trap or take up circulating proteins, growing at the expense of the host. Some protein is known to be lost secondary to the increased gluconeogenesis seen in cancer patients. Progressive malnutrition may alter the intestinal mucosa, resulting in protein-losing enteropathy.

## FAT METABOLISM

Cancer patients also tend to exhibit abnormal lipid metabolism. Serum free fatty acids are often elevated. Fats stores can be rapidly depleted. Fatty acids may be preferentially used for energy because of the alteration in carbohydrate metabolism. Fat wasting may be due to the high energy expenditure and possibly from lipolytic substance production by the tumor.

## CONCLUSION

There is a wide margin of variability in the nature and degree of metabolic aberrations that can present in a cancer patient. Despite the lack of clarity in the understanding of the precise mechanisms of the metabolic abnormalities, some basic assumptions can be made. Cancer patients usually have increased nutrient needs, particularly for energy and protein. Cancer patient care should be individualized on the basis of an initial nutrition assessment and evaluation of presenting symptoms. The patient should have ongoing nutrition care and repeat assessments to evaluate the appropriateness of the nutrition care provided.

## REFERENCES

Copeland, E.M., Daly, J.M., & Dudrick, S.J. (1977). Nutrition as an adjunct to cancer treatment in the adult. *Cancer Research, 37,* 2451–2456.

Groenwald, S.L. (1987). Nutritional disorders. In S.L. Groenwald (Ed.), *Cancer nursing principles and practice* (pp. 141–170). Boston: Jones & Bartlett.

# Chapter 3

# Overview: Screening, Assessing, and Monitoring

*Karen Mueller Buzby*

Severe malnutrition is a clinical reality in many cancer patients. Cancer cachexia, a syndrome characterized by anorexia, early satiety, weight loss, anemia, and marked asthenia, has long been recognized as a major source of morbidity and mortality in cancer patients. The syndrome of cancer cachexia is thought to result from a combination of factors that affect nutrient intake, absorption, metabolism, and requirements and perhaps act synergistically to create a generalized state of catabolism and host depletion (Buzby & Steinberg, 1981). Although anorexia and wasting are often thought to be hallmarks of advanced and disseminated disease, the incidence and severity of cachexia cannot be correlated with tumor type, size, site, extent, or stage of disease (Waterhouse, 1963).

Significant malnutrition in the patient with cancer is a poor prognostic sign. A clear relationship has been demonstrated between the occurrence of complications and death and the presence of malnutrition in cancer patients undergoing surgery (Buzby, Mullen, Matthews, Hobbs, & Rosato, 1980; Smale, Mullen, Buzby, & Rosato, 1981).

The incidence of malnutrition and its impact on morbidity and mortality provide ample justification for early nutrition assessment, intervention to prevent nutrition deterioration, and long-term nutrition follow-up in patients undergoing antineoplastic therapy. To prevent and correct malnutrition, all cancer patients admitted to the hospital should be carefully evaluated and fed appropriately. A three-stage approach to nutrition assessment can be employed to achieve this goal:

1. completion of a nutrition screen for all patients admitted to the hospital
2. performance of a comprehensive nutrition assessment for patients found to be malnourished or at risk of malnutrition
3. serial monitoring of the patient's nutrition status and response to nutrition therapy

By focusing on the assessment of nutrition status and nutrition intervention strategies, this chapter will help the practitioner recognize and treat the signs, symptoms, and factors that contribute to malnutrition in the cancer patient.

## NUTRITION SCREEN

The purposes of the nutrition screen are to prioritize nutrition care and to facilitate the early identification and treatment of malnourished patients. The data collected are used to assign each patient to an acuity or risk level. Three categories are usually used to classify patients according to risk of malnutrition: high risk, intermediate or moderate risk, and low risk or not compromised. The nutrition care plan is determined by the risk category to which the patient is assigned. Standards of care, which reflect the optimal level of care to be achieved, should be developed for each risk category and disease state. The standards should be consistent with the institution's philosophy, nutrition care policies and procedures, and professional standards of practice.

The nutrition screen is based on clinically applicable measures of nutrition status (Exhibit 3-1). A limited nutrition history should be conducted to obtain dietary and weight history information that will be helpful in assessing the patient's past and present intake and caloric balance. Pertinent facts to be obtained during the initial patient contact are previous dietary modifications; recent appetite or dietary changes; presence of oral ulcerations; difficulty with chewing, swallowing, or digestion of food; incidence of nausea and vomiting; food allergies and general food intake patterns; and occurrence of altered bowel habits.

In addition to the dietary history, the patient's age, height, weight, usual body weight, diet order, serum albumin level, other pertinent laboratory parameters and diagnoses should be collected. These data are generally readily available and can be obtained from past medical records, the admission medical or nursing history, patient or family interview, and routine laboratory tests.

The screening criteria used to assess the likelihood of malnutrition are outlined in Exhibit 3-2. On the basis of these criteria, the patient's nutrition status is assessed as high risk,

---

**Exhibit 3-1** Nutrition Screening Parameters

Subjective data
  Recent appetite changes (difficulty chewing or swallowing; nausea or vomiting)
  Diarrhea or constipation (food allergies and intolerances)
  Previous dietary modifications
  Usual body weight

Objective data
  Diagnosis
  Age
  Height
  Current weight (verify reported usual body weight)
  Serum albumin
  Prealbumin or total lymphocyte count (if available)
  Diet order and duration
  Current or previous use of nutrition support

*Source:* From "Nutrition Screening and Assessment in a University Hospital" by S. DeHoog, 1988, in *Nutrition Screening and Assessment as Components of Hospital Admission: Report of the Eighth Ross Roundtable on Medical Issues* (pp. 2–8). Copyright 1988 by Ross Laboratories, Columbus, OH.

---

**Exhibit 3-2** Screening Criteria Used To Evaluate the Likelihood of Malnutrition in Cancer Patients

High-risk criteria*
  Recent weight loss ($\geq$ 5% loss of usual body weight in 1 month or $\geq$ 10% loss of usual body weight in 6 months)
  Serum albumin $\leq$ 3.0 g/dL
  Prealbumin $\leq$ 10 mg/dL
  Total lymphocyte count $\leq$ 1,200/mm$^3$
  Patient receiving nothing by mouth for 5 days or maintained on 5% dextrose solution or clear liquids for $\geq$ 5 days
  Current use of parenteral or enteral nutrition

Moderate-risk criteria
  Recent involuntary weight loss (< 5% loss of usual body weight in 1 month or < 10% loss of usual body weight in 6 months)
  Serum albumin 3.0 to 3.4 g/dL
  Transitional feeding
  Select dietary modification

Low-risk criteria (not compromised)
  Weight stable
  Serum albumin $\geq$ 3.5 g/dL
  No indications for dietary modification

*If more than one high-risk criterion is observed, a comprehensive nutrition assessment should be performed.

*Source:* From "Identifying Patients at Nutritional Risk and Determining Clinical Productivity: Essentials for an Effective Nutrition Care Program" by S. DeHoog, 1985, *Journal of the American Dietetic Association, 85,* pp. 1620–1622. Copyright 1985 by the American Dietetic Association.

moderate risk, or not compromised. If one or more of the high-risk screening criteria are observed, an in-depth nutrition assessment is indicated to determine the etiology and extent of depletion. To avoid overlooking patients with subtle findings, it is preferable that the screening criteria have a low threshold for subjecting a patient to a thorough assessment (Buzby & Mullen, 1984).

Patients who are identified to be at moderate risk for malnutrition should be provided with appropriate nutrition services and monitored on a recurring basis, such as every 3, 5, or 7 days. Patients who are not compromised should receive the basic nutrition services and be reevaluated if their length of stay exceeds the average (DeHoog, 1988). If the patient's ability to consume an adequate diet is in question, a calorie count can be initiated to document oral macronutrient intake. In addition, the screening criteria can be used to monitor the patient's course. Any trend toward decline in nutrition status should be recorded so that adequate follow-up can be implemented.

Many institutions have instituted a routine nutrition screening program. Therefore, all cancer patients should be identified during the screening process. To be effective in facilitating the early identification of patients requiring nutrition intervention, screening should be performed within 48 to 72 hours of admission. Depending on institutional resources and personnel, data can be collected by a registered dietetic technician, a trained dietetic services employee, or a nurse; in some cases the patient can complete a nutrition questionnaire. If hospitalwide screening is not being performed in a particular institution, the development of a limited screening program directed toward the inpatient units with a high census of oncology patients can be undertaken. This may facilitate the early identification of cancer patients requiring a comprehensive nutrition assessment and active nutrition intervention.

Traditionally, oncology patients receiving chemotherapy have been discharged within 48 hours of treatment. For this patient subset, screening is not an effective means of evaluating or monitoring nutrition status because patients may be discharged before screening is completed. In addition, the increased use of short-stay units for the administration of chemotherapy on an outpatient basis and home chemotherapy programs highlights the need for the development and implementation of an outpatient nutrition screening, assessment, and monitoring program.

## NUTRITION ASSESSMENT

Patients at risk of protein-calorie malnutrition should undergo evaluation to confirm the presence of this entity, to determine its severity, and to ascertain the type of malnutrition that is present. There is no general agreement as to which studies most accurately characterize protein-calorie malnutrition. Because there are many potential measures of nutrition status, the clinician must select a subset to be used in a routine nutrition assessment battery. The ideal assessment method should be objective, reliable, clinically practical, noninvasive, simple to perform, and inexpensive. The most frequently used assessment parameters are outlined in Exhibit 3-3.

## MEDICAL HISTORY

Many clinical variables can affect nutrient intake, digestion, or absorption in the cancer patient. Determination of the nature and duration of the illness as well as current and planned therapies (chemotherapy, radiation therapy, or surgery) facilitates the identification of potential nutrition-related problems. The presence or suspicion of digestive or absorptive abnormalities resulting from the cancer or previous therapy (e.g., radiation-induced enteritis or surgical resection of the gastrointestinal tract) should be evaluated.

Potential drug-nutrient interactions can be identified by a review of the medication profile. Methotrexate may cause folate and calcium deficiency, and cisplatin may cause magnesium deficiency. In addition, the use of chemotherapeutic

**Exhibit 3-3** Nutrition Assessment Parameters for Cancer Patients

Medical history
   Tumor location
   Distant metastases that may affect nutrient assimilation
   Medications; drug-nutrient interactions
   Previous gastrointestinal surgery
   Ongoing treatment modalities and planned antineoplastic therapies
   Concomitant acute or chronic disease processes

Nutrition history
   Macronutrient intake, (kilocalories per day) and protein intake (grams per kilogram of body weight per day)
   Comparison of intake to needs
   Restrictions on fluid intake
   Constraints on nutrient delivery
   Weight history

Anthropometric measurements
   Weight, height
   Ideal body weight
   Midarm circumference (centimeters)
   Midarm muscle circumference (centimeters, percentile)
   Triceps skin fold (millimeters, percentile)

Expanded clinical laboratory profile
   Albumin (grams per deciliter)
   Transferrin (milligrams per deciliter)
   Prealbumin (milligrams per deciliter)
   Retinol-binding protein (milligrams per deciliter)
   Total lymphocyte count (per cubic millimeter)

Determination of nutrient requirements
   Energy expenditure (EE)
   • estimated by predictive equations
   • measured by indirect calorimetry
   Nutrition and metabolic goals
   • weight gain (EE × 1.5); weight maintenance (EE × 1.15 to 1.3)
   • weight loss (EE × 0.5 to 1.0)
   • protein repletion (1.5 to 2.0 g/kg)
   • protein maintenance (0.8 to 1.4 g/kg)

agents can result in a number of gastrointestinal side effects, including anorexia, nausea, diarrhea, esophagitis, mucositis, abdominal pain, constipation, and intestinal ulceration (Shils, 1988).

The presence of other acute or chronic diseases may affect nutrition status and influence nutrition intervention strategies. Patients may present with preexisting cardiac, pancreatic, renal, or hepatic disease. Social risk factors, such as alcohol or drug abuse, can also influence nutrition status and should be treated appropriately.

## NUTRITION HISTORY

A detailed dietary history is performed to evaluate the patient's food habits and eating patterns and to identify any factors resulting in diminished nutrient intake. Recent changes in tolerance to food, aversions, and taste changes should be documented. Because some cancer patients may try unorthodox medical or nutrition therapies, the dietitian should inquire about the use of megavitamins and "fad" diets to evaluate for possible nutrient deficiencies or toxicities.

Past and present calorie and protein intake should be measured. Current nutrient intake should be compared to predicted requirements to determine the extent of macronutrient deficiencies. Special dietary needs and disease-specific constraints on nutrient delivery must be evaluated before the institution of nutrition support.

## ANTHROPOMETRIC MEASUREMENTS

Comparisons of current weight to usual weight and ideal body weight are used to estimate the severity of nutrition depletion and to define caloric goals. Weight loss must be described in relation to its duration for the value to be meaningful. Short-term weight changes, within the 4 to 6 weeks before admission, should be evaluated. Comparing current weight to usual weight (premorbid weight) determines the extent of weight loss from a previously stable weight. To gain additional insight into the patterns of weight change, it may be helpful to identify the patient's maximum body weight and lowest adult body weight (by age). To minimize inaccuracies in patient recall, the medical records, if available, can be reviewed to verify weight data. Generally, a loss of more than 5% of the usual body weight in 1 month or more than 10% over 6 months is a positive historical indicator of malnutrition and merits review of other parameters.

Comparison of current weight to ideal body weight can be used as a basis for establishing caloric goals (e.g., weight gain is indicated if the current weight is less than 90% of the ideal body weight, and weight loss is indicated if the current weight is more than 130% of the ideal body weight). Evaluation of ideal body weight also provides comparative figures for estimating normal weight in patients who cannot provide accurate information about weight loss or usual weight. The standards for ideal body weight that are most commonly used are the 1983 Metropolitan Life Insurance Company height and weight tables (Metropolitan Life Insurance Company, 1983).

The limitations of body weight as an index of malnutrition must be considered. Conditions associated with an increase in total body water mask the patient's true body weight. A patient may be malnourished without showing significant weight loss. Also, the extent of weight loss does not necessarily correlate with the degree of malnutrition. Standards of ideal body weight, although they are associated with the lowest mortality for a healthy population, may not necessarily be associated with minimal morbidity, clinical outcome, or incidence of disease. The percentage weight loss does not provide any information about the nature of the tissue loss (fat or muscle).

The primary methods for estimating body fat and muscle mass in the clinical setting are upper arm anthropometric measures of triceps skin fold and midarm muscle circumference. Standardized equipment and measurement procedures must be used to ensure accurate and reproducible results. The patient's baseline measurements are compared to standards developed from a healthy reference group (Frisancho, 1981). Small changes in body composition are not identified accurately by these anthropometric measurements. Serial evaluation during a long course of nutrition support provides a useful record of body composition changes, however, especially

when large changes in fat and muscle mass occur.

## LABORATORY ASSESSMENTS

All laboratory parameters that deviate from normal should be evaluated in terms of their nutrition relevance, the impact on nutrition status, and the nutrition management of the patient. No single biochemical marker can identify all states of malnutrition. The visceral and hepatic transport proteins used to evaluate protein nutriture are albumin, transferrin, thyroxine-binding prealbumin, and retinol-binding protein. When a visceral protein (or proteins) is selected for use as a routine assessment parameter, consideration should be given to its half-life, the clinical parameters influencing its concentration, the test availability, and the test cost. Total lymphocyte count is an indicator of immune function and reflects the number of B cells and T cells. Leukopenia in the cancer patient may be a result of radiation therapy or chemotherapy rather than poor nutrition, however. Therefore, this parameter needs to be interpreted with caution in the cancer patient.

## DETERMINATION OF NUTRIENT REQUIREMENTS

Because the effects of malignancy on host metabolism are only partially understood, a degree of uncertainty remains in determining the nutrition needs of the cancer patient. Abnormalities in resting energy expenditure (REE), hypermetabolism, and hypometabolism have been observed in a large number of cancer patients (Knox, Crosby, Feurer, Buzby, & Mullen, 1983; Dempsey et al., 1984; Dempsey et al., 1986). Therefore, the best guide to determining nonprotein energy requirements is to measure energy expenditure when possible. The factors influencing metabolic rate include nutrition status, effects of therapy, body size, and disease (tumor type and burden). The REE measured by indirect calorimetry is a composite of the effect of these parameters. To determine the total nonprotein calories needed, the EE is multiplied by a factor of 1.15 to 1.3 for weight maintenance or a factor of 1.5 if a weight gain regimen is indicated (Dempsey & Mullen, 1985).

Although it is recognized that measurement of energy expenditure is the preferred method to predict daily energy requirements, in the absence of an indirect calorimeter the following general guidelines can be used. The patient's basal energy expenditure (BEE), a measurement that reflects the caloric needs in the resting, fasting, and unstressed state, can be derived from the equation of Harris and Benedict (1919). These equations (Exhibit 3-4) take into account the physiologic factors that influence energy requirements, namely sex, age, and body size. To determine the total nonprotein caloric requirements, the factors described for the EE are applied to the BEE (1.15 to 1.3 times BEE for weight maintenance and 1.5 times BEE for weight gain). Because the patient's actual needs may vary considerably from this estimated value, the response to the nutrition regimen must be monitored and changes made in the caloric goals if indicated.

The protein requirement for healthy adults established by the Food and Nutrition Board of the National Research Council (1980) is 0.8 g/kg/day. Injury and illness produce a marked increase in endogenous urinary nitrogen excretion secondary to inefficient utilization of amino acids. Cancer and antineoplastic therapy may represent a similar metabolic stress. In general, positive nitrogen balance may be achieved by providing 1.5 g of protein per kilogram of body weight unless the patient is severely stressed, in which case 2.0 g/kg may be required (Dempsey & Mullen, 1985).

It cannot yet be stated what combination of exogenous energy sources would promote efficient energy utilization in the cancer patient. Administration of adequate carbohydrate and lipid calories, or nonprotein calories, is extremely important for efficient utilization of dietary amino acids for protein synthesis. The criteria used to evaluate the adequacy of calorie and protein intake are weight gain and nitrogen retention in the malnourished patient and weight maintenance with nitrogen equilibrium in the adequately nourished patient.

## MONITORING NUTRITION STATUS

Follow-up is an essential component of optimal nutrition management. Serial evaluations must be performed to monitor the patient's nutrition status and response to therapy. Clinical progress, changes in treatment-related symptoms, and changes in anthropometric and laboratory data should be monitored at regular intervals. On the basis of findings on reevaluation, changes in the patient's nutrition care plan should be implemented.

---

**Exhibit 3-4** Equations for Predicting Caloric Requirements

In males
$$BEE \text{ (kcal/day)} = 66(13.7 \times W) + (5 \times H) - (6.8 \times A)$$

In females
$$BEE \text{ (kcal/day)} = 665(9.6 \times W) + (1.7 \times H) - (4.7 \times A)$$

where
  $W$ = weight (kilograms)
  $H$ = height (centimeters)
  $A$ = age (years)

*Source:* From *A Biometric Study of Basal Metabolism in Man* by J.A. Harris and F.G. Benedict, 1919, Washington D.C.: Carnegie Institute of Washington.

## NUTRITION INTERVENTION STRATEGIES

On the basis of the evaluation of the nutrition data, a nutrition care plan should be developed and recommendations made for nutrition support indicating the type of support to be given and its delivery system. Nutrition intervention in the cancer patient can be categorized as (1) supportive, in which nutrition support is instituted to prevent nutrition deterioration in the adequately nourished patient or to rehabilitate the depleted patient before definitive therapy; (2) adjunctive, in which nutrition support plays an integral role in the therapeutic plan; and (3) definitive, in which aggressive nutrition support is required for the patient's existence. The routes for providing nutrition support include an oral diet, tube feeding, and peripheral or total parenteral nutrition.

## DIETARY MANAGEMENT

In the patient in whom oral intake is not contraindicated, the optimal and preferred method is to induce the patient to ingest voluntarily an adequate diet. This is a formidable task and may be difficult to accomplish in many patients. Nevertheless, with effective dietary planning and counseling, methods can be devised to increase the likelihood of patients' meeting their nutrition needs by the oral route.

Many cancer patients not requiring specific dietary modifications are placed on a regular house diet without consideration being given to their unique food and palatability problems. It is of primary importance that patients be offered foods that appeal to them. The following simple dietary modifications may stimulate appetite and favor increased consumption:

1. Change the consistency of the diet; soft or pureed food may be better tolerated.
2. Cold foods may be more acceptable than hot.
3. Avoid serving foods that the patient may find offensive; some foods may cause nausea, or alternating changes in taste may decrease the palatability of certain foods. Many patients express strong aversion for meats and sweet or salty foods, whereas bitter or sour foods, fruits and vegetables, and dairy products are acceptable.
4. Six small feedings may be indicated if the patient complains of early satiety.

A thorough dietary history and a periodic check on the patient's food preferences while he or she is undergoing therapy will provide the dietitian with the necessary information to institute appropriate changes.

Some patients may require a high-calorie, high-protein diet. In those patients who are unable to consume or tolerate the volume of food required for optimum intake, the protein and calorie content of many foods can be manipulated to achieve an increased density. The protein content of foods can be increased by the addition of skim milk powder to recipes containing milk or to cereals, eggs, soups, and ground meats; the use of milk or half-and-half instead of water in the preparation of foods; and the addition of diced or ground meat or grated cheese to soups and casseroles. The calorie content of foods can be increased by the use of high-fat foods such as butter or margarine, sour cream, mayonnaise, peanut butter, or whipped cream; the use of high-carbohydrate foods; or the use of commercially available powder or liquid carbohydrate supplements. Improvement in calorie and nutrient intake can be accomplished by substituting palatable supplement formulas for low-calorie drinks. These supplements can be kept at the patient's bedside in ice so that they are readily available throughout the day. Various high-calorie formulas are available for use. Evaluation of patient acceptability and tolerance and the occurrence of taste fatigue with long-term use of these products is important for successful use.

In many instances, the cancer patient may require a special therapeutic diet in addition to a high-calorie, high-protein regimen. Patients may present with preexisting medical disorders such as diabetes, gastrointestinal disease, kidney disease, or malabsorption due to specific organ impairment by tumor or secondary to radiation therapy, surgical resection, or chemotherapy. In each case, appropriate dietary modifications must be instituted to accomplish the therapeutic goals.

## PARENTERAL AND ENTERAL NUTRITION

An alternate to oral feeding is tube feeding by means of nasogastric, nasoduodenal, esophagostomy, gastrostomy, or jejunostomy tubes. The general requisites for enteral nutrition include the following: (1) the patient is unable to ingest an adequate amount of nutrients by mouth, and (2) the gastrointestinal tract can be used safely and effectively (American Society for Parenteral and Enteral Nutrition [ASPEN], 1987). The use of tube feeding for either partial or total nutrient supply is indicated in patients with severe dysphagia, patients with protein-calorie malnutrition demonstrating inadequate intake for the previous 5 days, patients with normal nutrition status demonstrating less than 50% of the required nutrient intake for the previous 6 to 10 days, and patients with low-output (<500 mL/day) gastrointestinal fistulas (ASPEN, 1987). Tube feeding may be helpful in patients receiving radiation therapy and mild chemotherapy (ASPEN, 1987). The type of tube, method of delivery (intermittent, gravity, continuous, or nocturnal), and formula composition depend on the functional state of the gastrointestinal tract. The patient's nutrient requirements also influence formula selection. Many nutritionally complete, commercially prepared formulas are readily available, and comparative analytical data on their composition have been published (Shils, 1988).

When enteral feeding into the gastrointestinal tract is contraindicated, the next alternative is total parenteral nutrition. Use of a central venous catheter permits the infusion of concentrated dextrose solutions together with appropriate amino acids, lipids, vitamins, minerals, and electrolytes. The routine use of total parenteral nutrition is suggested for patients who are unable to absorb nutrients from the gastrointestinal tract

(e.g., those with massive small bowel resections, radiation enteritis, severe diarrhea, or intractable vomiting); patients undergoing high-dose chemotherapy, radiation therapy, and bone marrow transplantation; and patients with severe protein-calorie malnutrition and a nonfunctional gastrointestinal tract (ASPEN, 1986). There are also other conditions in which total parenteral nutrition may be helpful, including major surgery, moderate stress, and enterocutaneous fistula and during intensive cancer chemotherapy (ASPEN, 1986). In all cases, the patient's clinical condition and nutrition status should be reviewed by a team of professionals before the institution of active nutrition intervention.

Numerous reports have documented the beneficial effects of parenteral and enteral nutrition in patients with neoplastic disease. It is beyond the scope of this chapter to review these studies, but several generalizations can be made. Nutrition support, either enteral or parenteral, is well tolerated in the cancer patient. Aggressive nutrition support is effective in improving nutrition status. A definitive statement regarding the effect of nutrition support on either tolerance of or response to antineoplastic therapy or survival cannot be made.

## COUNSELING

In all instances, an essential component in nutrition care is patient education. The side effects of antineoplastic therapy can be anticipated, and the patient and family can be made aware of the potential impact on the patient's ability to eat. It is the role of the clinical dietitian to counsel the patient and family in potential food and eating problems. This allows the patient and family the opportunity to voice concerns, questions, and fears about nutrition before the onset of therapy. General eating and food problems can be discussed and suggestions for dealing with the difficulties of eating given.

Establishing realistic goals for food intake with the patient and family is essential. Suggestions about how to modify eating behavior should be given to the patient and family.

Encouragement to eat, concern for the patient's food preferences, and attention to the most pleasant social setting for serving meals can have a positive impact on the patient's eating behavior. The potential benefits of early dietary counseling are many. While the patient is being monitored in the hospital, feedback can be given to reinforce good eating habits.

All too often, the patient who has experienced nutritional improvement in the hospital is discharged without appropriate consideration being given to nutrition follow-up. Three-day dietary records and home dietary diaries can be used on an outpatient basis to evaluate home food intake, and suggestions for improvement can be made to the patient and family on the basis of these records.

The incidence and severity of malnutrition in cancer patients confirm the need for long-term nutrition care of those undergoing antineoplastic therapy and suggest a need for postdischarge outpatient dietary counseling and nutrition assessment on a routine basis.

## REFERENCES

American Society for Parenteral and Enteral Nutrition, Board of Directors. (1986). Guidelines for the use of total parenteral nutrition in the hospitalized adult patient. *Journal of Parenteral and Enteral Nutrition, 10*, 441–445.

American Society for Parenteral and Enteral Nutrition, Board of Directors. (1987). Guidelines for the use of enteral nutrition in the adult patient. *Journal of Parenteral and Enteral Nutrition, 11*, 435–439.

Buzby, G.P., & Mullen, J.L. (1984). Nutrition assessment. In J.L. Rombeau & M.D. Caldwell (Eds.), *Enteral nutrition and tube feeding* (pp. 127–147). Philadelphia: Saunders.

Buzby, G.P., Mullen, J.L., Matthews, D.L., Hobbs, C.L., & Rosato, E.F. (1980). Prognostic nutritional index in gastrointestinal surgery. *American Journal of Surgery, 139*, 160–167.

Buzby, G.P., & Steinberg, J.J. (1981). Nutrition in cancer patients. *Surgical Clinics of North America, 61*, 691–700.

DeHoog, S. (1988). Nutrition screening and assessment in a university hospital. In *Nutrition screening and assessment as components of hospital admission, report of the eighth Ross roundtable on medical issues* (pp. 2–8). Columbus, OH: Ross Laboratories.

Dempsey, D.T., Feurer, I.D., Crosby, L.O., Knox, L.S., Buzby, G.P., & Mullen J.L. (1984). Energy expenditure in malnourished gastrointestinal cancer patients. *Cancer, 53*, 1265–1273.

Dempsey, D.T., Knox, L.S., Mullen, J.L., Miller, C., Feurer, I.D., & Buzby, G.P. (1986). Energy expenditure in malnourished patients with colorectal cancer. *Archives of Surgery, 121*, 789–795.

Dempsey, D.T., & Mullen, J.L. (1985). Macronutrient requirements in the malnourished cancer patient. *Cancer, 55*, 290–294.

Food and Nutrition Board, National Research Council. (1980). *Recommended dietary allowances* (9th rev. ed.). Washington, DC: National Academy of Sciences.

Frisancho, A.R. (1981). New norms of upper limb fat and muscle areas for assessment of nutritional status. *American Journal of Clinical Nutrition, 34*, 2540–2545.

Harris, J.A., & Benedict, F.G. (1919). *A biometric study of basal metabolism in man* (Publication no. 279). Washington, DC: Carnegie Institute of Washington.

Knox, L.S., Crosby, L.O., Feurer, I.D., Buzby, G.P., & Mullen, J.L. (1983). Energy expenditure in malnourished cancer patients. *Annals of Surgery, 197*, 30–40.

Metropolitan Life Insurance Company. (1983). *Metropolitan Life Insurance Company Statistical Bulletin* (Vol. 64, p. 1). New York: Author.

Shils, M.E. (1988). Nutrition and diet in cancer. In M.E. Shils & V.R. Young (Eds.), *Modern nutrition in health and disease* (7th ed., pp. 1380–1422, 1607–1628). Philadelphia: Lea & Febiger.

Smale, B.F., Mullen, J.L., Buzby, G.P., & Rosato, E.F. (1981). The efficacy of nutritional assessment and support in cancer surgery. *Cancer, 47*, 2375–2381.

Waterhouse, C. (1963) Nutritional disorders in neoplastic disease. *Journal of Chronic Diseases, 16*, 637–644.

# Chapter 4

# Assessment

*Suzanne P. Geerts*

There are many challenges for the registered dietitian or nutritionist in the identification of nutrition problems and needs of the cancer patient. Nutrition problems are frequently found among this population (Shils, 1980). Also, cancer patients are known to be a diverse group with multiple types of cancers, therapies, and complications. The nutritionist often encounters variations in patient acuity level, ranging from the healthy, active patient who is in the hospital for medical follow-up to the critically ill patient requiring intensive care. Some of these variations lead to difficulties when the nutritionist tries to use traditional nutrition screening and assessment parameters to determine a patient's nutrition status. These assessment challenges can best be met by the following strategy:

1. Nutritionists must acquaint themselves with basic facts about clients with cancer and about the disease variations and changing health care environment.
2. Nutritionists must attain a working knowledge of cancer therapies and their common effects on nutrition screening and assessment parameters.
3. Nutritionists must recognize the frequent complications and treatments that occur in cancer patients that influence the validity of traditional assessment parameters. These parameters must often be repeated as medical conditions change.
4. Nutritionists must keep abreast of new chemotherapy agents and investigational cancer protocols.
5. Nutritionists must develop proper monitoring and recordkeeping systems that are equal in importance to nutrition screening and assessments.
6. Nutritionists must use patient-oriented and cost-effective counseling techniques for cancer patients.

This chapter deals with the general information that a nutritionist needs to complete a nutrition screen or assessment and to provide counseling to cancer patients.

## SELECTED FACTS ABOUT CANCER PATIENTS AND THE HEALTH CARE ENVIRONMENT THAT MAY INFLUENCE NUTRITION SCREENING AND ASSESSMENT PROCEDURES

Some initial considerations in determining cancer patients' nutrition needs are their diagnosis, their prognosis, and the setting in which they will receive treatment. Among cancer populations there are many types of cancers, and their disease courses can vary widely.

Generally, cancers are referred to as solid tumors, which are those occurring in a localized tissue or organ, and liquid tumors, which comprise hematologic abnormalities such as leukemias, myelomas, or lymphomas. Hematology patients often receive lengthy, aggressive chemotherapy treatments that can result in severe and prolonged problems such as decreased nutrient intake and prolonged or repeat hospital stays. Some solid tumors metastasize to other parts of the body and may result in compromised functions of vital organs or organ systems.

There are curable and terminal types of cancers. Some tumors may go into remission for various lengths of time. The anticipated disease outcome and life expectancy may influence how aggressively nutrition support will be pursued.

The nutritionist must realize that not all cancer patients are or will become malnourished (Shils, 1979). Some types of cancer, because of their site of origin (e.g., gastric cancer) or degree of severity (e.g., advanced pancreatic cancer), are more likely than others to render the patient at nutritional risk. Other diseases, such as early detected breast cancer, may pose no threat to nutrient intake.

Often, decreased food intake is not the direct result of the tumor type but a result of prolonged side effects or complications of cancer treatment. Also, many patients decrease their nutrient intake as they begin to deal with the psychologic and social dilemmas that arise after the diagnosis of cancer has been made.

The patient's psychologic status and the presence of a strong support system are often the determining factors in how he or she will tolerate cancer therapy and maintain his or her nutrition status. There are remarkable stories of patients who are cured despite medical evidence of "terminal" disease and those who live much longer than their projected medical prognosis. Most cancer centers have trained psychologic, religious, and social support persons available to assist clients with the emotional aspects of the disease and the problems that the disease can cause among the family. The nutritionist should make referrals when appropriate.

The care and treatment of cancer patients is changing from traditional in-hospital treatment to outpatient and home environments. The elements of each setting can vary according to the level of patient acuity and the medical data available. The nutritionist must individualize the work strategy for the type of patient encountered and the institution or agency used before nutrition care can begin.

Dwyer (1979) presents some basic criteria that are used to screen and complete nutrition assessments in an outpatient oncology setting. Initial criteria used to identify patients with nutrition problems include a review of the patient's current weight and height and significant changes from usual or preillness weight and between clinic visits, analysis of the patient's appetite and food intake and reported eating problems, and evaluation of current or planned therapy for the patient. If the patient demonstrates two or more high-risk criteria, additional assessment criteria such as 24-hour recalls or food records, anthropometrics, and biochemical, medical, dental, and social factors are evaluated to define nutrition problems and to develop a nutrition care plan.

Dwyer (1979) also discusses some common obstacles that complicate nutrition support in an outpatient setting. The atmosphere is often a busy and hurried one for both the patient and the health care team. There may not be a complete health care team to address complicated patient issues brought up by the disease. The health care professionals may not recognize the pressing need for aggressive nutrition support because the patient is not hospitalized. Also, third-party reimbursement may not apply to nutrition services and necessary nutrition supplements. These and other complicating factors must be evaluated before a successful nutrition program can begin.

Many of these facts about cancer patients that influence nutrition care are included in one of the first phases of the nutrition screen or assessment, the review of the medical history. Exhibit 4-1 summarizes the information to be evaluated in the medical history review. If any of the data are not available, the nutritionist may have to

**Exhibit 4-1** Review of the Medical History of a Cancer
Patient

---

Chief complaint
Diagnosis and stage of disease
Time since onset of disease
Presence of metastases or complications
Antitumor therapy (past, present, or future);
  concurrent modes of therapy
Performance and psychologic status
Prognosis
Presence of psychologic, dermatologic, and
  nutrition effects of drug regimen or protocol
Personal medical history
Medication profile
Presence of parenteral access equipment

---

request the information from other members of
the health care team.

## CANCER THERAPIES AND THEIR SIDE EFFECTS—A BASIC COMPONENT OF THE NUTRITION SCREENING AND ASSESSMENT PROCESS FOR CANCER PATIENTS

After evaluating the cancer patient's medical
history, the nutritionist must take an in-depth
look at what therapy the patient has previously
received and what plans are being made for
current therapy. Drug or therapy and nutrient
interactions have a direct impact on the evaluation of the nutrition needs of the cancer patient.
Before the clinician starts the screening and
assessment process, it is advisable for him or her
to study the cancer therapies commonly used and
to develop a working knowledge of the therapies
and of the available resources for this information.

In general, there are four common forms of
cancer therapy: surgery, chemotherapy, radiation therapy, and immunotherapy. Frequently
one cancer therapy is followed by another
adjunct therapy to improve outcome. When
evaluating the cancer patient's therapy, the
nutritionist will become aware that there are
established cancer protocols for most radiation

therapy and chemotherapy regimens. With
chemotherapy protocols, one should note what
drugs are used, the side effects that are common
and that may influence nutrition parameters and
intake, and the expected duration of therapy.
Often, aggressive and prolonged therapy can
result in long-term decreases in nutrient intake.
Abbreviations are frequently used in the medical
chart to describe chemotherapy protocols (e.g.,
CAV indicates cytoxan, adriamycin, and vincristine, which are used in the treatment of oat
cell carcinoma of the lung). Becoming familiar
with these abbreviations hastens the screening
and assessment process.

Along with evaluating chemotherapy agents,
the nutritionist should note the availability of
access sites and equipment in the event that
parenteral nutrition is required during therapy.
Hematology patients usually have surgically
implanted access devices such as double- or
triple-lumen Hickman catheters; these are readily available if nutrition support is needed. With
cancer patients with solid tumors, vascular sites
for peripheral parenteral nutrition often are limited as a result of sclerosed veins from previous
chemotherapy treatments. To avoid this problem, some surgically implanted devices such as
catheters and ports are now being used with these
patients.

In cancer centers and hospitals, several valuable resources are available to gather the complex information required to complete nutrition
screening and assessment. Members of the
health care team, such as the physician, the
oncology fellows, nurses, and pharmacists, are
available to provide information about the
patient's medical status, therapy protocols, and
medication profile. Often they can provide
essential literature. An additional valuable hospital resource person is the chemotherapy nurse
or oncology nurse specialist. These persons keep
a written record of the patient's protocol and
prognosis, and they are often personally familiar
with access sites if peripheral or parenteral nutrition support is indicated. Much of this essential
information is discussed during patient rounds or
in health care team conferences, so that attend-
ance by the nutritionist at least two or three times
per week is beneficial.

## TRADITIONAL NUTRITION SCREENING AND ASSESSMENT PARAMETERS USED FOR CANCER PATIENTS, AND FREQUENT CHEMOTHERAPY AND DISEASE COMPLICATIONS THAT ARE THOUGHT TO INFLUENCE THE VALIDITY OF THE PARAMETERS

The concept of a nutrition assessment became widespread in the 1970s. Since that time, there have been numerous clinical observations and studies regarding the validity of these parameters in various patient groups. Bozzetti (1987) and Weisberg (1983) take a critical look at many of the traditional assessment parameters. Nutritionists must be able to apply these principles to patient care.

For cancer patients Shils (1979) recommends basic nutrition screen techniques, and many of these principles remain in use today. The screening process consists of four phases:

1. brief diet history
2. assessment of weight and metabolic status
3. detailed review of the medical history and treatment plan
4. evaluation of laboratory data such as

   - hemoglobin
   - mean cell volume
   - white blood cell count
   - platelet count
   - blood urea nitrogen level
   - creatinine level
   - serum sodium and potassium levels
   - carbon dioxide level
   - chloride level
   - serum glucose level
   - total iron-binding capacity
   - bilirubin level
   - serum albumin level
   - serum glutamic-oxaloacetic transaminase (SGOT)

A similar assessment protocol for cancer patients is presented by Blackburn and Bothe (1980).

The nutrition assessment protocol used by nutritionists at the Johns Hopkins Oncology Center is described by Gildea, Motz, Costlow, Markley, and Pratt (1982). Layton, Gallucci, and Aker (1981) and Black, Gallucci, and Katakkar (1983) use some of these nutrition assessment criteria to assess the nutrition status of patients receiving chemotherapy and bone marrow transplants. In these studies, the investigators commented that the nutrition evaluation was often complicated by the disease itself or by the treatment modalities used.

Some difficulties in assessing nutrition status are frequently seen in the oncology unit. Disease and chemotherapy effects necessitate the use of caution in evaluating the results of anthropometric, biochemical, and physical examinations in nutrition assessment. Geerts (1985) has reviewed basic factors that influence nutrition parameters in the oncology patient. Table 4-1 summarizes common factors that are thought to influence the validity of these parameters. Many of these assessment complications parallel those reported in the nutrition support of trauma or organ failure patients. The nutritionist must be aware of these factors and use good clinical judgment when assessing nutrition status and designing nutrition therapy.

Chemotherapy is commonly used in cancer treatment and is known to have a number of effects on nutrition parameters. In general, the nutritionist must keep in mind that the potential side effects of chemotherapy are drug, dose, and patient specific (Geerts, 1985). Therefore, it is difficult to predict to what extent the agents will influence biochemical data. Each patient must be evaluated on an individual basis. Nutrition systems that are most affected by chemotherapy agents include the alimentary tract and the hematopoietic compartment (Ohnuma & Holland, 1977). Hematopoietic dysfunction or bone marrow depression can result in leukopenia or immunosuppression, thrombocytopenia, and various anemias. Gastrointestinal toxicities frequently include nausea, vomiting, abnormal peristalsis, and poor nutrient absorption. Control and treatment of the above side effects involve the routine use of antibiotics, antiemetics, and antidiarrheal and analgesic agents and the trans-

**Table 4-1** Assessment Parameters and Common Factors That Are Thought To Influence Their Validity in the Oncology Patient

| Assessment Parameter | Influencing Factors |
|---|---|
| **Anthropometrics** | |
| Weight | Hydration and volume status; ascites, edema (Shils, 1979) |
| Skin fold measurements (Weisberg, 1983, pp. 97–99) | Ascites, edema; accuracy of methodology; activity level (measurements may decrease as a result of inactivity) |
| **Biochemical parameters** | |
| Serum albumin level (Weisberg, 1983, pp. 100–101) | Defect in serum albumin metabolism (Bozzetti, 1987); hydration and volume status; hepatic metastasis or toxicity (Dorr & Fritz, 1980, chap. 6); renal metastasis or toxicity (Dorr & Fritz, 1980, chap. 6); sepsis (Beisel, 1983); recent blood transfusions |
| Total lymphocyte count | Hematopoietic defect or toxicity (Ohnuma & Holland, 1977); corticosteroid therapy (Dorr & Fritz, 1980, pp. 39–40) |
| Red blood cell profile (hemoglobin, packed cell volume, mean corpuscular volume, mean corpuscular hemoglobin) | Hematopoietic toxicity or defect (Ohnuma & Holland, 1977); recent transfusions |
| Renal function (blood urea nitrogen, creatinine, sodium, potassium levels; creatinine-height index) | Renal metastasis or toxicity (Dorr & Fritz, 1980, chap. 6); hydration status |
| Liver function (serum alkaline phosphatase, SGOT, total serum bilirubin levels) | Hepatic metastasis or toxicity (Dorr & Fritz, 1980, chap. 6) |
| Skin testing | Anergy secondary to hematopoietic toxicity (Ohnuma & Holland, 1977); tumor burden; previous antigen testing (Black et al., 1983) |
| Physical examination | Drug-induced alopecia; physiologic, dermatologic, drug side effects (can mimic nutrition deficiency symptoms) |

fusion of blood products as needed. The nutritionist must be aware of the patient's specific drug regimen, potential side effects, and when abative treatment agents are used because these can directly influence nutrition care.

Some chemotherapy agents are known to induce electrolyte abnormalities (Muller, 1984). One chemotherapy agent, cisplatin, causes hypokalemia, hypocalcemia, hypomagnesemia, and hyperuricemia. Muller (1984) summarizes electrolyte disturbances caused by nine antineoplastic agents. Efforts are made to control such electrolyte disturbances with proper hydration and replacement therapy, but these effects must be considered during nutrition screening, assessment, and monitoring.

Electrolyte balance and organ systems can also be influenced by antibiotic therapy, which is frequently used as a supportive measure when septic complications arise. Electrolyte abnormalities can result from commonly used antibiotics such as tobramycin and amphotericin. These abnormalities are drug and dose related but may influence electrolyte requirements. Flombaum (1984) describes parenteral requirements that are influenced by common antibiotics used with cancer patients. Some antibiotics can also cause renal or hepatic toxicities, which may alter the validity of nutrition assessment parameters as well as those commonly used to monitor parenteral nutrition.

As the nutritionist continues the nutrition screening and assessment process, anthropometric measures are evaluated. Shils (1979) emphasizes that the weight of oncology patients is frequently influenced by the presence of edema and ascites. Clinical experience with oncology patients indicates that volume status is frequently altered by dehydration, overhydration, prolonged vomiting or diarrhea, and blood transfusions as well as by edema and ascites. The nutritionist should always assess the hydration state of patients on hospital admission or during a clinic visit. When dehydration is present, the nutritionist should wait until hydration therapy is completed and then request that the patient be weighed again to establish a current weight. The nutritionist may also rely on previous records of usual body weight for the patient, if available. In the presence of edema or ascites, it is beneficial to establish a dry weight or to monitor changes in abdominal girth (or both) when evaluating changes in weight status.

Additional anthropometrics to evaluate fat reserves and somatic protein status in cancer patients have been widely used in clinical and research settings. Gildea et al. (1982, p. 26) recommend the inclusion of triceps skin fold, fat area, midarm circumference, and arm muscle area as nutrition assessment parameters. These measurements are given as percentiles on the basis of the Hanes Survey of the U.S. population. Shils (1979) excludes such anthropometric measures (except height and weight) in the initial assessment process but indicates that they may be of value as monitoring devices in evaluating long-term progress with nutrition support. In general, there is still much debate about the usefulness and reliability of such anthropometric measures and standards. Weisberg (1983, pp. 97–99) reviews some of these controversial issues. Also, clinical experience demonstrates that some cancer patients have poor performance status for prolonged periods. This can result in atrophy of lean body mass independent of that occurring solely with malnutrition. Often with debilitated cancer patients, the loss of lean body mass is due to the combination of inactivity and malnutrition. Edema is often present in cancer patients as well (Shils, 1979). The common occurrence of loss of lean body mass together with edema may influence the validity of anthropometric measurements and standards.

The next vital component of nutrition screening and assessment is the evaluation of biochemical parameters. Many of the traditional biochemical indexes used are influenced by changes in volume status, disease complications, and side effects of cancer therapy. In general, biochemical indexes expressed in terms of serum concentrations (such as albumin, hemoglobin, creatinine, and the like) may be influenced by changes in fluid status. Again, changes in volume status in cancer patients are commonly caused by dehydration, overhydration, blood transfusions, prolonged vomiting, diarrhea, and edema or ascites. Layton et al. (1981) question the reliability of such parameters as serum albumin level and creatinine-height index as nutrition parameters because of radical changes in hydration status for eight bone marrow transplant recipients whom they studied. These eight patients also required repeated blood transfusions after intensive chemotherapy and total body irradiation.

Many cancer patients receive blood or blood product transfusions when bone marrow depression is present as a result of disease or a side effect of chemotherapy. As indicated above, the quantities and frequencies of blood transfusions can alter several nutrition parameters, so that the nutritionist must be aware of when and what type of transfusions are given during treatment.

Septic conditions are also common among oncology patients, and infectious processes are known to cause various metabolic and nutrition aberrations (Beisel, 1983). In general, severe or chronic infections induce loss of body weight, nitrogen, and electrolytes such as potassium, magnesium, zinc, and sulfur. Also, sepsis increases the requirement for energy, amino acids, and vitamins as new antigenic substances are anabolized. The goal of nutrition therapy during sepsis is to reduce the absolute loss of body nutrients. The nutritionist must monitor the patient's medical condition on an ongoing basis; if septic complications arise, metabolic and nutrient requirements need to be evaluated accordingly.

Nutrition parameters are also influenced by the presence of hepatic or renal metastasis and drug toxicities. The liver is a frequent site of metastasis in solid tumors. Significant hepatic dysfunction decreases synthesis of serum albumin, which traditionally is a protein status indicator. With hypoalbuminemia, ascites and anascara can result. In cases of hypoalbuminemia in which low serum albumin levels are thought to be due to disease or drug complications in cancer patients, the nutritionist should provide accurate diet history and intake information to help diagnose the origin of the problem. Often poor intake and malnutrition accompany liver and renal abnormalities.

Dorr and Fritz (1980, chap. 6) report that some chemotherapy agents are known to have a toxic effect on liver or renal function. These investigators discuss other organs or systems (such as cardiovascular and pulmonary systems) that also may be affected by chemotherapy agents. Hepatic or renal toxicities may result in acute or chronic organ failure or insufficiency syndromes, electrolyte disturbances, or edema. It is desirable for the nutritionist to evaluate and monitor liver and renal function tests during nutrition screening and assessment and throughout the patient's treatment. Again, dehydration is commonly seen in cancer patients on hospital admission; these cases should be noted and liver and renal function evaluated as rehydration therapy is completed.

Bozzetti (1987) reports that there is some evidence suggesting that serum albumin level is not an accurate nutrition parameter for evaluation of nutrition status in cancer patients. Serum albumin levels can be decreased by a number of factors (such as chronic liver and renal disease, surgery, sepsis, and changes in hydration status) that are common in the cancer population but in some cases are independent of poor nutrient intake. Bozzetti (1987, pp. 117S–118S) cites four studies that attribute the hypoalbuminemia

of cancer patients to probable physiologic defects in serum albumin synthesis, degradation of transcapillary escape, and vascular compartment ratios. Two of the studies included were done on tumor-bearing rats, so that a direct comparison to humans may not be appropriate. Brennan and Lowry (1985) comment that the use of serum albumin level as a biochemical index of malnutrition does have some limitations but that it is helpful in diagnosing chronic malnutrition.

Bozzetti (1987, p. 118S) also cites four studies in which the use of both enteral and parenteral nutrition support in cancer patients did not increase serum albumin levels. One of these studies examined the change in serum albumin concentration in 139 cancer patients receiving total parenteral nutrition for 14 to 100 days (McCauley & Brennan, 1983). The results showed that albumin levels did not increase unless exogenous albumin was given. The investigators suggested that serum albumin level appeared to be a poor index of nutrition response in cancer patients receiving total parenteral nutrition (McCauley & Brennan, 1983). The nutritionist should keep abreast of the continuing controversy regarding the use of serum albumin level as a diagnostic and monitoring tool and use good clinical judgment in evaluating a patient's nutrition status and in developing nutrition care plans.

Lymphopenia and anergy on skin testing are two additional parameters traditionally assessed to determine protein status. In their evaluation of 14 patients receiving chemotherapy for solid tumors, Black et al. (1983) performed modified assessments excluding total lymphocyte count and skin testing. They held that these parameters were influenced by tumor burden and previous oncologic therapy as well as by nutrition status. Layton et al. (1981) also questioned the reliability of lymphocyte count and anergic skin testing in their evaluation of eight bone marrow transplant recipients.

It is recognized that some tumor types, particularly the liquid tumors, are characterized by depression of normal bone marrow function. As mentioned earlier, bone marrow depression may result in leukopenia, thrombocytopenia, and various anemias. Radiation and chemotherapy agents are known to cause hematopoietic toxicity. Large doses of steroids are frequently used in chemotherapy regimens and can cause similar decreases in lymphocyte counts (Dorr & Fritz, 1980, pp. 39–40.) The result of these immunosuppressive reactions is that lymphocyte count and skin testing may not be good indicators of protein status in cancer patients.

Thrombocytopenia or anemia due to disease- or drug-induced bone marrow depression may mimic the symptoms of iron- and folate-deficiency anemias. Normally, nutrient deficiencies are ruled out early in the hematologic work-up. Nutritionists must use caution when evaluating the red blood cell profile of oncology patients and present objective diet history and intake data if they believe that nutrient deficiencies such as iron and folate are also present.

Another biochemical and anthropometric parameter used to assess somatic protein status is the creatinine-height index (Bistrian, Blackburn, Sherman, & Scrimshaw, 1975). In cases of protein-calorie malnutrition muscle is catabolized, and excretion of creatinine decreases. A 24-hour urine creatinine excretion study is performed and the results compared to standard values. In a survey of the nutrition states of 53 hospitalized cancer patients, Nixon et al. (1980) found a 24-hour creatinine-height index to be the most sensitive indicator of protein-calorie malnutrition. Mullen and Torosian (1981) reported some limitations of analysis of creatinine excretion because there are changes in the quantities excreted by the same individual from day to day as well as changes that are due to the individual's variable protein intake. They suggest that serial measurements may provide a more accurate assessment.

After biochemical nutrition parameters are evaluated, a physical examination to detect any clinical evidence of malnutrition is a routine component of a nutrition assessment. Again, in many instances the disease or treatment side effects may interfere with this process (Geerts, 1985). For example, both radiation therapy and chemotherapy can induce hair loss. Therefore, one may not be able to use hair pluckability as one indicator of protein deficiency. Hematologic diseases such as leukemia often present as diffuse petechiae or abnormal bleeding tendencies such as bleeding gums. Both are also symptoms of ascorbic acid deficiency. Fingernails and toenails are often brittle and ridged; this is most often caused by drug effects on these tissues, which undergo rapid proliferation, and not by protein deficiency. Some chemotherapy agents such as vincristine can cause peripheral neuropathies that may mimic thiamine, vitamin $B_{12}$, or pyridoxine deficiencies.

When carrying out the steps of the physical examination, the nutritionist must be aware of how the disease and drug effects can manifest themselves to complete an accurate evaluation for malnutrition. If a vitamin or mineral deficiency is suspected, a thorough diet and intake history should be made available and a vitamin and mineral level or screen be requested to confirm a diagnosis. Also during the physical examination, the nutritionist should take an overall look at the patient for evidence of chronic poor nutrient intake such as adipose or muscle tissue wastage, lethargy, edemas, and so forth. Such symptoms should be included in the documentation of the examination.

## FINAL EVALUATION OF NUTRITION ASSESSMENT PARAMETERS

The nutritionist may find that a review of the screening and assessment parameters often yields information or questions that must be discussed with the health care team. It is the responsibility of the nutritionist to secure accurate diet history and intake information and to bring this, along with basic nutrition parameters of anthropometrics and biochemistry, for the team to discuss. Even though the validity of some traditional assessment parameters can be influenced by cancer disease complications and therapies, the collective laboratory results should be interpreted along with the patient's compromised medical status and inadequate nutrient intake to assess his or her nutrition status

(Weinsier & Butterworth, 1981). Bozzetti (1987, p. 118S) summarizes this concept by noting that, when nutrition assessment parameters are being used to plan nutrition support, one must use objective measurements and clinical judgment. The health care team should discuss the patient's medical and nutrition status. Then, goals and acceptable modes of nutrition support can be established.

## SUGGESTED TIME FRAME FOR THE NUTRITION SCREENING AND ASSESSMENT OF THE HOSPITALIZED CANCER PATIENT

Qualified dietary personnel should visit the patient or family for a brief nutrition history 24 to 48 hours after the patient's admission. The history should focus on any adverse changes in appetite, nutrient intake, usual body weight, stool habits, or dentition. Any food intolerances should be recorded if a select menu is not available or if the patient or family is unable to select meals. Any patients considered at nutrition risk or having multiple food intolerances should be immediately referred to the clinical nutritionist.

Within 48 to 72 hours of the patient's admission, the nutritionist should complete a basic nutrition screen. The nutrition screen should include evaluation of the patient's diet history, personal medical history (see Exhibit 4-1), and appropriate biochemical parameters. If disease or drug complications exist that may invalidate the biochemical parameters (such as dehydration), the nutritionist should request new data from the medical staff when appropriate.

If the patient is found to be malnourished or at risk (Weinsier & Butterworth, 1981) for developing malnutrition or if prolonged, aggressive therapy is anticipated, the nutritionist should request all additional biochemical parameters that are needed and complete a formal nutrition assessment within 3 to 5 days of the patient's admission. When the data are difficult to interpret because of disease or drug complications, the nutritionist should discuss the issues with other members of the health care team and formalize a nutrition care plan. The nutrition assessment and nutrition care plan information should then be documented in the patient's medical record.

## MONITORING THE CANCER PATIENT'S NUTRITION STATUS

Of equal importance to the initial nutrition assessment is monitoring of the cancer patient's nutrition status on a regular basis. Nutrition parameters vary depending on the patient's medical status and what indexes are available at the institution. Nutritionists at the Johns Hopkins Oncology Center recommend nutrition assessment on admission and biweekly (Gildea et al., 1982, p. 24).

Generally for a hospitalized patient receiving aggressive, lengthy therapy, changes in weight status over time need to be documented. For nutrition monitoring, the patient's weight should be checked on admission and at least once a week and should be compared to nutrient intake information to assess the adequacy of the kilocalorie intake. A more accurate estimate of kilocalorie needs can be made if indirect calorimetry methods are available. If disease or drug complications exist (such as ascites or overhydration), caution must be used when interpreting changes in weight status.

Nutrient intake measurements or calorie counts frequently must be done on a daily basis for an extended period if nutrient intake is poor. The calculation process can be expedited if the patient or family is able to list between-meal feedings for the nutrition personnel and if computer assistance is available. The health care team usually finds calorie count information to be valuable if it reflects a 3- to 5-day average and if it is compared to recent weight changes.

The choice of which parameters to use in monitoring changes in a patient's protein status remains controversial. Weisberg (1983) and Brennan and Lowry (1985) review some of the basic controversies regarding the use of serum transport proteins as indicators of visceral protein anabolism. As stated earlier, Bozzetti (1987) suggests that there is evidence to support changes in protein metabolism and compartmentalization in cancer patients. Also, in this population, it is recognized that serum albumin levels may be altered by a number of factors other than nutritional status (see Table 4-1). Because of these limitations, there has been increased interest in the use of calculated or measured serum transferrin and prealbumin levels as more sensitive but short-term indicators of protein concentrations. Tuten, Wogt, Dasse, and Leider (1985) demonstrated in 16 patients (4 of whom were cancer patients) that after 7 days of nutrition support there was a significant increase in both transferrin and prealbumin levels. They also state that a measured prealbumin level is a simpler and more cost-effective parameter to use because serum transferrin concentration is also dependent on iron status, so that iron concentration must also be evaluated.

Carpentier and Ingenbleek (1986) report that prealbumin level is also influenced by age, sex, pregnancy, severe metabolic stress, and inflammation. Because some of these factors are variables in cancer patients, the nutritionist must keep in mind the limitations of these indexes and always evaluate the patient's medical condition when using such parameters.

Brennan and Lowry (1985) report that estimated nitrogen balance is a gross but useful parameter to measure protein requirements in cancer patients. In clinical practice with hospitalized cancer patients, the investigators most often requested an estimated nitrogen balance to be calculated for patients with normal renal function who were critically ill or had advanced malnutrition. To optimize the accuracy of the test, nursing assisted with the urine collection and repeated the test in approximately 3 days to be sure that the patient was in positive nitrogen balance (Weinsier & Butterworth, 1981, p. 32).

Baseline nutrition assessment data should be maintained by the nutritionist for patients who will have repeated hospital admissions for therapy. The information can be stored on diet cardex cards or nutrition assessment forms or by computer. Data should be communicated to the outpatient clinic as patients are discharged from

the hospital. It is advisable to monitor the information for a period of 1 to 2 years. Most cancer treatment centers have records available of those clients who die so that their files can be deleted from the system.

Any dramatic change in weight or protein status between admissions or clinic visits should be brought to the immediate attention of the health care team. Having this information readily available is particularly advantageous in teaching institutions, where there are frequent rotations of the medical staff.

## COUNSELING THE CANCER PATIENT AND FAMILY

In developing a nutrition care plan, four important considerations are (1) the patient's diagnosis, (2) the anticipated duration and aggressiveness of therapy, (3) the patient's and family's personal goals for nutrition support, and (4) cost-effective methods of supplementation. The health care team should discuss the patient's prognosis and the intensity of therapy planned. These factors frequently affect the aggressiveness of all therapies, including nutrition support. When possible, the patient and family should be allowed to participate in this decision-making process along with the health care team. There have been cases of terminal patients who requested enteral feedings to maintain or improve the quality of their lives and of families who chose home enteral feedings to avoid repeated hospital admissions to treat dehydration.

Another element of nutrition care to be established is an estimate of kilocalorie and protein needs based on the cancer patient's metabolic needs and activity level and the availability of the gastrointestinal tract. Gildea et al. (1982) describe methods used to determine caloric and protein needs at the Johns Hopkins Oncology Center. Caloric needs are estimated by determining the patient's basal energy expenditure by the method of Harris and Benedict (1919) and multiplying this factor by a stress or disease factor determined by the patient's febrile status and the goal and route of nutrition support desired. Protein needs of cancer patients are estimated to be 1½ to 2½ times greater than the protein requirement for normal adults of the same age group. Protein intake is adjusted according to the results of nitrogen balance tests. Oncologists at Johns Hopkins generally try to achieve a nonprotein:calorie:nitrogen ratio of 1:120:180. Each patient is carefully monitored, and the necessary adjustments are made.

Dempsey and Mullen (1985) also discuss general macronutrient requirements and the factors that influence the nutrient needs of cancer patients. They stress that energy requirements have been found to be abnormal and variable in this population and that, if possible, measured resting energy expenditure (REE) should be used to determine energy needs. If maintenance of nutrition status is the goal, then 115% to 130% of the REE should be provided; if nutrition repletion is indicated, up to 150% of the measured REE may be needed. A number of factors are known to increase the nitrogen requirements of the cancer patient. Dempsey and Mullen (1985) recommend 0.25 to 0.35 g of nitrogen per kilogram of body weight per day for patients receiving nutrition support. These investigators have also reviewed and summarized current research on glucose and lipid metabolism in the cancer population (Dempsey & Mullen, 1985). Malnourished cancer patients demonstrate an increase in glucose and fatty acid oxidation, and most can metabolize exogenous lipid. On the basis of these observations, Dempsey and Mullen recommend nutrition supplements of mixed caloric substrates, with lipids accounting for 30% to 50% of the total nonprotein calories.

Brennan and Lowry (1985) recommend that the basis for nutrition therapy be an assessment of metabolic rate by measurement of oxygen consumption, if available, coupled with clinical judgment of the patient's depleted nutrition status and stress level. Protein requirements should take into consideration the appropriate restrictions imposed by hepatic or renal metastases or drug toxicities that may be present. Efforts should be made to correct existing fluid, electrolyte, fiber, and vitamin and mineral deficiencies. The health care team should also encourage

exercise as tolerated by the individual to help maintain or improve performance status and sense of well-being. Appropriate referrals should be made to psychologic, social, and physical therapy personnel.

Cancer patients who are to receive prolonged or aggressive therapy should receive diet education as therapy is initiated. Patients and their families should be counseled about the importance of maintaining good nutrition status and weight throughout treatment. If the cancer treatments result in serious side effects that decrease nutrient intake, patients should be counseled about eating habits to improve intake. Nutrition education tools can often be obtained free of charge by contacting local cancer information services or pharmaceutical companies. If the nutritionist finds that supplements are needed to boost the patient's nutrition intake, it is important that a variety of foods and beverages be recommended to avoid monotony. Economical recipes for high-protein, high-calorie foods should be made available. The need for a vitamin and mineral supplement should be evaluated on an individual basis. If commercial supplements or enteral tube feedings are indicated, the nutrition care plan should be tailored to the family's income and appropriate referrals made to help secure financial assistance or insurance reimbursement for such feedings. The patient's nutrition status and intake should be evaluated while therapy proceeds on both an inpatient and an outpatient basis. When the nutrition care plan is established, the hospital nutritionist should make appropriate referrals to outpatient facilities or to other health agencies to ensure continuity of care. There should be an open line of communication between the inpatient and outpatient nutritionists so that the patient's nutrition status can be monitored as therapy progresses and the care plan can be altered as needed. Often referrals need to be made to outside health care agencies for nursing visits or physical therapy if the patient lives outside the area of the cancer center, limiting follow-up visits. The nutritionist should also provide nutrition care plan information when the patient is referred to a hospice program so that appropriate goals for nutrition support can be established at that time.

## REFERENCES

Beisel, W.R. (1983). Infectious diseases. In H.A. Schneider, C.E. Anderson, & D.B. Coursin (Eds.), *Nutritional support of medical practice* (2nd ed., chap. 26). Philadelphia: Harper & Row.

Bistrian, B.R., Blackburn, G.L., Sherman, M., & Scrimshaw, N.S. (1975). Therapeutic index of nutritional depletion in hospitalized patients. *Surgery, Gynecology and Obstetrics, 141*, 512–516.

Black, M.L., Gallucci, B.B., & Katakkar, S.B. (1983). The nutritional assessment of patients receiving cancer chemotherapy. *Oncology Nursing Forum, 10*(2), 53–58.

Blackburn, G.L., & Bothe, A. (1980). Assessment of malnutrition in cancer patients. *Cancer Bulletin, 30*(3), 89–91.

Bozzetti, F. (1987). Nutritional assessment from the perspective of a clinician. *Journal of Parenteral and Enteral Nutrition, 11*(5), 115S–121S.

Brennan, M.F., & Lowry, S.F. (1985). Nutritional support in the cancer patient. In W.S. Howland & G.C. Carlon (Eds.), *Critical care of cancer patients* (chap. 15). Chicago: Year Book Medical.

Carpentier, Y.A., & Ingenbleek, Y. (1986). Utilization of prealbumin as a nutritional parameter [Letter to the editor]. *Journal of Parenteral and Enteral Nutrition, 10*(4), 435–436.

Dempsey, D.T., & Mullen, J.L. (1985). Macronutrient requirements in the malnourished cancer patient—How much of what and why? *Cancer, 55*, 290–294.

Dorr, R.T., & Fritz, W.L. (1980). *Cancer Chemotherapy*. New York: Elsevier.

Dwyer, J.T. (1979). Dietetic assessment of ambulatory cancer patients with special attention to problems of patients suffering from head-neck cancers undergoing radiation therapy. *Cancer, 43*, 2077–2086.

Flombaum, C.D. (1984). Influences on mineral and electrolyte requirements in TPN (with emphasis on the cancer patient). *Nutrition Support Services, 4*(2), 39–40.

Geerts, S.P. (1985). Nutritional screening of oncology patients. *Dietitians in Critical Care Newsletter, 7*(5), 3.

Gildea, J.L., Motz, K., Costlow, N., Markley, E., & Pratt, G. (1982). A systematic approach to providing nutritional care to cancer patients. *Nutritional Support Services, 2*(9), 24–27.

Harris, J.A., & Benedict, F.G. (1919). *A biometric study of basal metabolism in man* (Publication no. 279). Washington, DC: Carnegie Institute of Washington.

Layton, P.B., Gallucci, B.B., & Aker, S.N. (1981). Nutritional assessment of allogenic bone marrow recipients. *Career Nursing, 4*(2), 127–135.

McCauley, R.L., & Brennan, M.F. (1983). Serum albumin levels in cancer patients receiving total parenteral nutrition. *Annals of Surgery, 197*(3), 305–309.

Mullen, J.L., & Torosian, M.H. (1981). Biochemical testing in nutritional assessment. In G.R. Newell & N.M. Ellison (Eds.), *Progress in cancer research and therapy, nutrition and cancer: Etiology and treatment* (pp. 152–153). New York: Raven.

Muller, R.J. (1984). Nutrition and cancer part 2: Nutritional support of the cancer patient. *LymphoMed Nutritional Newsletter, 4*(2), 4.

Nixon, D.W., Heymsfield, S.B., Cohen, A.E., Kutner, M.H., Ansley, J., Lawson, D.H., & Rudman, D. (1980). Protein-calorie undernutrition in hospitalized cancer patients. *American Journal of Medicine, 68*, 613–619.

Ohnuma, T., & Holland, J.F. (1977). Nutritional consequences of cancer chemotherapy and immunotherapy. *Cancer Research, 37*, 2395–2403.

Shils, M.E. (1979). Principles of nutritional therapy. *Cancer, 43*, 2093–2102.

Shils, M.E. (1980). Nutrition and neoplasia. In R.S. Goodhart & M.E. Shils (Eds.), *Modern nutrition in health and disease* (6th ed., chap. 38). Philadelphia: Lea & Febiger.

Tuten, M.B., Wogt, S., Dasse, F., and Leider, Z. (1985). Utilization of prealbumin as a nutritional parameter. *Journal of Parenteral and Enteral Nutrition, 9*(6), 709–711.

Weinsier, R.L., & Butterworth, C.E. (1981). *Handbook of Clinical Nutrition* (chaps. 1 & 2). St. Louis, MO: Mosby.

Weisberg, H.F. (1983). Evaluation of nutritional status. *Annals of Clinical and Laboratory Science, 13*(2), 95–103.

# Chapter 5

# Counseling

*Bonnie Terrill Ross*

The desire to help others by addressing nutrition problems is universal among dietetic interns who pursue careers in clinical dietetics. This ideal, however, is not realized in many of the traditional areas of clinical dietetics. This is especially true in the stubbornly prevalent last-minute diet instruction orders for patients who are ready to be discharged, which do not provide an opportunity for follow-up counseling.

Oncology nutrition care is truly a helping profession that many interns regard highly. There are many attractive aspects to oncology dietetics. Oncologists tend to be especially open to dietitian assistance in contributing to the care of their patients than other types of physicians. Oncology clinics tend to use thoroughly the team approach to holistic, comprehensive care. Most oncology nutrition counseling focuses on creative, normal nutrition provided with an immensely caring spirit. Most cancer patients who are undergoing treatments absorb and greatly appreciate such counseling.

Of all diseases, cancer is one of the most feared. It is understandable that many dietitians feel unequipped to handle the raw, sensitive emotions that cancer patients experience. There is indeed an emotional risk in caring for cancer patients that can be inhibiting to those contemplating oncology careers. Nevertheless, most caretakers quickly discover that the satisfaction is enormous and that positive feedback can be abundant. Cancer care tends to tap the human desire to help others in a way that provides hope and maximizes the quality of life.

## PSYCHOLOGIC ASPECTS

Understanding the psychologic aspects of cancer as a disease state can enhance the efficacy of nutrition counseling. A cancer diagnosis elicits powerful emotions such as fear and grief. Cancer can have a shattering effect on a patient's self-image. This is particularly true for patients who have had any type of disfiguring surgery such as mastectomy, radical head and neck surgery, craniotomy, ostomy, or orchiectomy. Patients who have experienced alopecia likewise experience altered self-image.

A common feeling among cancer patients is the loss of control of life's events and anxiety over the incompleteness of their lives. Many patients experience guilt over their cancer. This guilt may be remorse over their past or present lifestyle, such as tobacco use, alcohol abuse, careless sun exposure, and poor eating habits. A cancer diagnosis often initiates painful reflection on life's experiences. Many patients focus on failed or strained relationships and failure to accomplish goals.

There are also dreadful fears surrounding cancer, such as fear of abandonment, fear of pain, fear of physical and mental disability, fear of disfigurement, and fear of dependency upon others. Cancer can often burden families with financial strains, time away from work, and drastic changes in family structure and roles.

The emotions that burden cancer patients often manifest themselves in eating disorders. Sometimes such emotions can cause overeating, but more often than not these emotions dampen the appetite. It is also well known that fear and anxiety can cause somatic symptomatology that often mimics cancer symptoms and treatment side effects. Combined with the many metabolic changes that result from cancer, this puts most patients at high risk for malnutrition. The complex physiologic and psychologic milieu that compromises eating requires that nutrition guidance be instituted at all levels of cancer care.

## REALISTIC GOALS

Before the nutrition counseling process begins, goals have to be determined. These goals must be matched with the patient's ability to achieve them. Goals cannot be rigid given the vast range of symptoms, cancers, and treatments plus the variable metabolic presentations seen in cancer patients. Patients who are not able to meet the goals should not be made out as failures.

## UNDERSTANDING THE PATIENT

When the dietitian first meets the patient, there is a complex overlay of emotions that must be worked through before reasonable give-and-take dialog can occur. Patients have been through a plethora of diagnostic studies culminating in a life-threatening or life-ending diagnosis. Next, the patient is faced with possible treatment decisions and choices. Treatment explanations are usually laden with a litany of side effects, and the treatments themselves are often difficult to understand. Radiation therapy, for example, is administered with large, highly sophisticated machinery and an invisible beam.

The patient's fears can be overwhelming. It takes time to break through these fears to an understanding that can give the patient the best view of his or her disease and the most balance in dealing with it.

Although loss of control is a frightening, consuming feeling of cancer patients, nutrition is one aspect of their care that they have some control over. Giving patients a feeling that they can help with their own well-being is important in and of itself.

Families of cancer patients likewise may feel impotent. They can be brought into the cancer care of their loved one by being included in the nutrition counseling setting. Family members should take part in reinforcing nutrition principles and encouraging improved eating. Family members should be cautioned not be too overbearing, however. There is often a fine line between nagging, which is counterproductive, and encouragement.

## SUCCESSFUL COUNSELING

There is no set formula for successful counseling that is appropriate for every cancer patient. Personalities, coping mechanisms, disease presentation, and response to treatment can all vary greatly among patients. The result is a boundless set of patient needs. Nevertheless, there are some basic counseling tools that are helpful in achieving patient goals.

### Listening

A significant portion of the time involved in nutrition counseling should be spent in listening. Listening attentively is one of the greatest compliments that one person can pay another. By concentrating wholly on what the patient is saying, the nutrition counselor conveys respect in the most convincing way possible. A high level of trust can be established, which in turn enables the patient to risk a greater degree of self-revelation and permits a greater degree of receptivity to the information and the emotional support being offered (Curry-Bartley, 1986).

Eye contact with the patient and family members also conveys attention, interest, and respect. Empathetic listening skills should be used when gathering data from the patient. This is important because many patients may feel defensive or embarrassed when reporting their eating habits.

Caring is a potent mediator in oncology nutrition counseling. Many times a warm, simple human gesture can express genuine concern and can break down fears and barriers to communication. This may be a soft touch on a patient's shoulder or even a gentle hand squeeze.

## Motivation

Grief and anxiety are multidimensional. Patients do adjust and adapt to their situations. Dietitians attending to the nutrition needs of cancer patients serve a far greater purpose than merely prescribing and overseeing nutrition plans. Cancer care providers can help patients deal with physical and psychologic stresses.

Food, food preparation, and eating with loved ones are quite symbolic in our society. When a loved one rejects food, the family may also feel rejected at some level. Patients and families need explanations that show that various eating problems are real and common with cancer.

Patients feel some degree of comfort when they understand that their eating problems are not unique. Dietary modifications may be more acceptable to a patient when presented as tips that have been used successfully by other patients who were having a similar problem. Another method in counseling cancer patients is literally to brainstorm together with them about foods that sound appealing. Even in the anorectic patient, there are usually a few foods that are acceptable. These acceptable foods should be a starting point in encouraging improved intake.

Goal setting is often a successful approach in directing patients toward improving their nutrition. The essential element in goal setting is making sure that the goals are realistically achievable within specific time frames. It is important for the nutrition counselor to acknowledge and praise a patient's efforts toward better nutrition. Every time a patient achieves a goal, it fosters confidence in his or her ability to improve nutrition and positively contributes to the cancer care.

## Ongoing Care

Even in the best of situations, patients do not retain a significant portion of the information provided during the initial consultation. This fact alone necessitates follow-up counseling sessions. Follow-up sessions allow questions to be asked, nutrition principles to be reviewed, the patient's nutrition status to be reassessed, symptoms and symptom management to be updated, and encouragement and additional information to be offered.

The cancer patient under treatment is indeed emotionally taxed. It is certainly understandable that there are days when patients are not receptive to discussion about nutrition. With each counseling session, the patient's ability and readiness to learn must be assessed. Nutrition success revolves around giving patients close attention and accurate information. Integrity will be demonstrated through thoroughness in following up on patients' requests and concerns.

Follow-up counseling sessions not only reinforce nutrition principles but also lessen the likelihood of patient involvement in unorthodox practices. Almost every cancer patient is confronted with opportunities to experiment in some form of unfounded cancer treatment or practice that is touted as an "all-natural" or "miracle" cancer treatment. These can range from sensationalized benefits of vitamins and minerals to such "detoxifying" procedures as coffee enemas. A cancer care program that integrates continuous nutrition counseling usually evolves into a trusting relationship. The dietitian and cancer care professionals will then be accessible to correct, clarify, and dispel the seduction of quack regimes.

Informing patients that good nutrition will complement their cancer care goes a long way in motivating them. The nutrition counselor can tap a patient's longing to recover. Patients respond positively to encouragement and guidance on ways to overcome barriers to eating. A cancer patient's courage and determination to survive are often reflected in his or her efforts to eat well despite symptoms.

## TERMINAL CARE

Patients who are dying need support, kindness, and tenderness for the remainder of their lives. A patient who has an incurable cancer is not necessarily no longer treatable. There are many patients who can go through the dying process mostly as outpatients in an independent manner. Likewise, many incurable patients who are receiving palliative treatment can live for months or years with good support systems.

Palliative nutrition counseling should be ongoing. It should focus on providing adequate calories so that the patient can be independent for as long as possible. One of the greatest fears that terminally ill patients have is the fear of being deserted. Nutrition attention is comforting and can lessen their loneliness and desperation. Nonabandonment is a fundamental principle of nutrition support of terminally ill patients.

REFERENCE

Curry-Bartley, K.R. (1986). The art and science of listening. *Topics in Clinical Nutrition, 1*(1), 14–24.

# Chapter 6

# General Feeding Problems

*Marcia L. Nahikian-Nelms*

For clinicians caring for cancer patients, it quickly becomes obvious that there are problems in maintaining adequate oral intake to meet nutrition requirements. The most difficult job for the clinician is to ascertain the exact etiology behind the symptom observed. The cancer patient may or may not initially recognize a change in appetite. More likely than not patients will state that they get full more quickly than before, or a family member will note that meal portions are not quite as large as they had been. Often what is observed clinically is an unexplained weight loss. This weight loss is often the first symptom of an occult malignancy.

Many variables, some of which cannot be controlled, affect the ability of cancer patients to maintain their nutrition status (Fig. 6-1). The direct effect of the tumor burden is one such variable, but there are others, particularly the specific feeding problems that are commonly recognized in the cancer patient. All these problems tend to inhibit optimal oral intake and thereby affect the overall nutrition status of the patient. It is often only after a patient's initiation of therapy that the clinician is faced with the progression of these now obvious problems. It is difficult to address each problem separately because in the cancer patient undergoing systemic or localized antineoplastic therapy the symptoms are interrelated and often affect one

another. Still, they must be addressed; the overall impact of these symptoms can affect the clinical course of the patient.

## ANOREXIA

Anorexia is defined as a loss of appetite. The etiology of anorexia is difficult to understand and remains controversial. Several concurrent variables in the tumor or the host as well as the effects of treatment may influence the progression of anorexia. Obviously, if decreased appetite and weight loss are the initial symptoms of the malignancy, it is most probable that they are a direct result of the tumor. These symptoms do not appear to be related in any way to the size of the tumor or the type of cancer, but anorexia does increase in frequency and severity in advanced stages of disease. This initial development of anorexia is different from the anorexia that may occur late in the disease, which is probably a result of several interrelated problems such as the physiologic effects of increased tumor burden, side effects of treatment, and generalized debility.

To begin to understand the loss of appetite, it is helpful to review the theories regarding normal food controls. There are many factors that control appetite and food intake as part of a

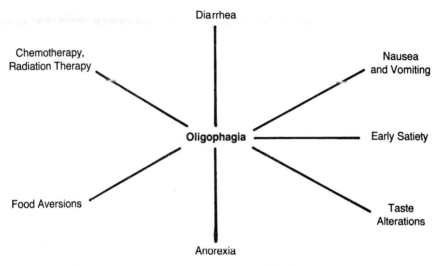

**Figure 6-1** Variables Affecting Cancer Patients' Ability To Maintain Nutrition Status

highly complex and integrated system that is not completely understood. Factors that control this system include thermostatic, glucostatic, lipostatic, and hormonal regulation and digestive tract functions (DeWys, 1979). The thermostatic control of appetite involves the innate response of mammals to increase food intake in the event of a decrease in environmental temperature. The glucostatic monitor of appetite is based on the rate of glucose utilization. Satiety results when there is an increased rate of glucose utilization. Oral intake is also affected by the concentrations of free fatty acids, glycerol, and body lipids. In hormonal regulation, hormones such as glucagon, epinephrine, enterogastrone, and cholecystokinin decrease appetite, whereas increased blood levels of insulin may stimulate oral intake (Norton, Peacock, & Morrison, 1987). The presence of malignancy has the potential to alter these control factors. The significance and extent of alterations in each of these control systems in the cancer patient has not been fully determined.

Davis and Levine (1977) provide a model that integrates central nervous system (CNS) mechanisms for stimulating appetite with the gastrointestinal physiologic response to the accumulation of food. The chemoreceptors in the mouth and nose send excitatory signals to the CNS for the initiation of the hunger response. When food has accumulated, the gastrointestinal tract coun-teracts the excitatory effect of taste and smell and thus inhibits oral intake. It is clear that a tumor may have a direct effect on appetite by inducing taste and smell abnormalities. Taste and smell changes are a well-established occurrence in the cancer patient. It is not certain that taste and smell actually control food intake, but they can definitely influence the CNS control center for eating. Also, a decrease in saliva production can lead to decreased stimulation of gastrointestinal secretions as well as cause difficulty with food ingestion.

Atrophic changes have been noted to occur in the mucosa of the small intestine in cancer patients (Barry, 1974). Gut atrophy may result in increased transit time and consequent delayed digestion. Metabolic abnormalities may cause wasting of the muscle in the stomach wall. In experimental animals, such muscle loss has corresponded to the loss of skeletal muscle (Kisner & DeWys, 1981), which affects visceral sensing. All these effects on the gastrointestinal tract may delay digestion and provide subsequent continuous stimuli to the satiety center. This is often the basis for the symptom of early satiety. Evidence of these effects can be noted in patient interviews when patients relate that breakfast is their best meal and that by the evening meal they are so full that it cannot be eaten. Such a description actually may be physiologically correct; digestion may truly be slowed down, and the accumulation of food taken throughout the day may remain in the stomach or small intestine.

Hormonal abnormalities in the cancer patient have been frequently documented. A decrease in insulin production or peripheral resistance (or both) has been observed. A postprandial elevation of blood glucose levels secondary to abnormal insulin performance may then suppress appetite (Lundholm, Holm, & Schersten, 1978).

Experimental evidence has also shown that the catecholaminergic system is involved in the regulation of feeding by means of the hypothalamus (Fanelli et al., 1986). Increased levels of plasma tryptophan have been documented in cancer patients. Because tryptophan is the precursor of serotonin, increased levels of tryptophan may increase the production of serotonin, resulting in continued satiety. Physiologically, 90% of tryptophan is bound to albumin. Increased levels of nonessential fatty acids as well as a number of drugs may displace tryptophan from albumin by competing for the same binding sites, thus increasing the amount of free tryptophan in the plasma (Fanelli et al., 1986).

Many metabolic abnormalities have been identified in the cancer patient. These in turn may affect the development of anorexia. Increases in lactic acid secondary to increased Cori cycle activity as well as imbalances in plasma amino acid levels may be anorexigenic. An increase in fatty acid mobilization may also stimulate the satiety center (Costa, 1977). In the cancer patient who is actively being treated with chemotherapy or radiation therapy there exists the potential for therapy-induced anorexia. The well-documented nutrition side effects of antineoplastic therapy can increase the severity of a baseline anorexia.

Another source of therapy-induced anorexia is the medications that are routinely prescribed for the cancer patient. Most clinicians participating in the care of the cancer patient may be tempted to blame nutrition complaints on antineoplastic therapy and ignore anorexigenic potential of the multitude of other drugs that the patient is receiving. It is not uncommon for the patient to be receiving numerous drugs, all of which may decrease nutrient intake. At Ohio State University Hospitals, for example, the medications of 100 patients were evaluated for nutrition side effects (Nahikian-Nelms & Baumann, 1988). The most common groups of medications found to result in nutrition side effects were antibiotic and antifungal agents and narcotics. Side effects included generalized anorexia, nausea, vomiting, diarrhea, and constipation.

In addition, the effect of pain on appetite should not be underestimated. The presence of uncontrolled pain undoubtedly has a significant effect on appetite and oral intake. Chronic cancer pain has been related to symptoms of anorexia, malaise, nausea, and vomiting (McCaffery, 1979; Foley, 1985). Various treatment methods exist, including the use of relaxation and imaging techniques (McCaffery, 1979; Barber, 1978), the use of nerve blockage, and the prescription of analgesics and narcotics. An appropriate pain control program can result in improved appetite and nutrient intake.

Finally, the emotional and psychologic effects of cancer on a patient can be tremendous. These usually manifest as depression and anxiety (Cushman, 1986). In turn, these symptoms can contribute to anorexia. DeWys (1974) postulates that a pleasant taste may be interpreted negatively in the depressed patient. Indeed, the stress of depression may cause a release of catecholamines, which depress stimulation to the hypothalamus and thereby decrease the desire to eat.

The practical management of anorexia may present a difficult challenge to the care giver. Each patient presents a unique set of symptoms, which necessitates an individualized approach to mediation. Various kinds of interventions—psychologic, environmental, medical, and nutrition—can be used.

Early education regarding the role of nutrition is an excellent starting place. Consistent encouragement of the patient to view eating as an essential part of treatment often motivates the patient to continue eating even when appetite is absent. It is often necessary to place the patient on a schedule for meals and supplements to ensure adequate intake.

Encouraging the patient to think of meals as an enjoyable social occasion will probably encourage a failing appetite. The clinical dietitian can do things to create just such an atmosphere. Providing an attractive table with china, tablecloth, and candles is one way. At Ohio State University Hospitals, a catered restaurant meal is often sent to a patient and his or her family. Serving favorite foods on fine china has often made the difference in patients' nutrition care during a hospital stay.

The registered dietitian may suggest a change in the timing of meals and perhaps an increase in their frequency along with a decrease in serving sizes. In addition, using nutrient-dense foods and high-calorie, high-protein supplements helps make every mouthful of food "count" nutritionally. Encouraging patients not to drink liquids until 20 to 30 minutes after a meal can also be of assistance.

It is not uncommon for physicians to prescribe a low dose of corticosteroids to assist with appetite stimulation. One study showed that 40% of patients so treated appeared to have an increase in appetite (Hanks, Trueman, & Twycross, 1983). Willox, Corr, and Shaw (1984) indicated in their study that prednisolone reduced anorexia. Twycross and Lack (1986) recommended treatment with prednisolone (10 mg two or three times a day) or dexamethasone (2 to 4 mg) on a trial basis for 7 to 10 days; if no improvement is seen, then the medication should be stopped.

The use of exogenous insulin as an appetite stimulant has been suggested (DeWys, 1979). This, of course, is not without significant risk of hypoglycemia. This mode of treatment is used only rarely in the typical clinical setting.

It is often suggested that alcohol, such as in a cocktail or a glass of wine, stimulates the appetite. This intervention tends to be helpful if the patient's meal plan normally includes such items at home. On the other hand, social and religious stigmas may prevent the use of this treatment; these factors must be taken into consideration.

## NAUSEA AND VOMITING

The presence of nausea and vomiting can severely debilitate the cancer patient. Twycross

and Lack (1986) estimate that 40% of all patients admitted to their hospice facility in London complain of nausea and vomiting. Welch (1980) reports that 79% of her patients who are receiving radiation therapy experience symptoms of nausea and vomiting. Most clinicians agree that there is a high incidence of this problem.

Nausea is defined as a sensation that often leads to the urge to vomit. Vomiting expels the contents of the stomach through the esophagus and out the mouth. The physiologic response of nausea and vomiting is an intricate process, so that it is easily understandable why these symptoms are difficult to suppress. Successful treatment depends on defining the specific factors that cause the problem (Twycross & Lack, 1986).

The causes of nausea and vomiting are also complex (Exhibit 6-1). More than one factor at a time may cause nausea and vomiting. Patients may also experience nausea without vomiting as well as vomiting that is not associated with nausea. It is also important for the clinician to establish that the patient is actually experiencing vomiting. The patient's description may only indicate regurgitation or reflux. For instance, periods of coughing can cause simple regurgitation without nausea and vomiting.

Bruera, Catz, Hooper, Lentle, and MacDonald (1987) established that gastroparesis was the cause of chronic nausea and vomiting in their patients. Gastroparesis is defined as a slight degree of paralysis of the musculature of the stomach wall. The mean gastric emptying time

---

**Exhibit 6-1** Causes of Nausea and Vomiting in the Cancer Patient

Irritation of upper gastrointestinal tract secondary to chemotherapy and radiation therapy
Use of chemotherapeutic drugs
Gastrointestinal obstruction
Delayed gastric emptying
Increased intracranial pressure
Hypercalcemia
Uremia
Use of antibiotics, antifungal agents, narcotics
Psychologic factors

was 190 ± 83 minutes for the patients under study compared to 65 ± 6 minutes for the controls. Clinically observed chronic nausea, vomiting, and early satiety may be due in part to some degree of gastroparesis.

Increased intracranial pressure, hypercalcemia, and uremia may also be causes of nausea and vomiting. These are generally encountered in patients with advanced disease. Increased intracranial pressure usually results from a primary brain tumor or metastatic disease to the brain. Vomiting presents as one of the initial symptoms and tends to be motion related.

Of patients with hypercalcemia, 20% to 40% have the diagnosis of breast or lung cancer or multiple myeloma (Twycross & Lack, 1986). The severity of vomiting associated with hypercalcemia tends to vary among individuals. It can be fairly well controlled with antiemetics and dissipates as the serum calcium level normalizes.

Antibiotics, antifungal agents, and narcotics can also produce the symptoms of nausea and vomiting. If a patient is experiencing toxic side effects from a specific drug, he or she should be evaluated for appropriate substitutions if possible. It is often not possible to change medications, however. For example, 21% of patients receiving miconazole experience severe nausea and vomiting (Brass, 1983). Frequently, an extended treatment period with this drug results in negligible oral intake, so that alternate nutrition support methods must be initiated.

Anticipatory nausea and vomiting is often a psychologic response to cancer and its treatment. Love, Nerenz, and Levanthal (1982) concluded from their research that two factors condition anticipatory nausea and vomiting: taste and smell, and anxiety. Anticipatory nausea and vomiting is common. Fetting et al. (1983) state that 31% of the 123 patients whom they surveyed had experienced nausea and vomiting before treatment. Morrow (1982) reported that 21% of 225 patients surveyed experienced nausea and vomiting. When these patients were questioned about why they experienced nausea and vomiting, they usually gave psychologic reasons such as nervousness, anxiety, and tension.

Generally, antiemetics tend to be the most successful treatment for nausea and vomiting (Kennedy, Packard, Grant, & Padilla, 1981). Prophylactic treatment appears to be most successful when given in regularly scheduled doses. Oral antiemetics may be effective, but often nausea and vomiting are so severe that oral drugs cannot be kept down. Suppositories and parenteral routes are often then required.

A wide range of medications are used as antiemetics. An antiemetic regimen may require several trials before optimum control is reached. Glass, Bechtel, and Leiby (1986) have documented recommendations for several antiemetic regimens that have been successful (Table 6-1).

Clinicians must realize that dietary management of nausea and vomiting rarely eliminates the problem. Nevertheless, manipulation of the patient's oral intake can often successfully reduce the severity of the symptoms. Assisting patients with appropriate food choices can decrease the likelihood of emesis. Foods that are low in fat, low in residue, and without odor are best tolerated. Temperatures of foods may also make a difference. Mixing of hot and cold foods has been known to initiate vomiting in the patient who is nauseated. The patient should be encouraged to eat slowly in small amounts and to avoid lying down after eating. Physical activity should also be limited before meals.

Behavioral strategies have also been employed to treat nausea and vomiting. Such strategies are particularly helpful if the problem appears to be psychologically induced. Hypnosis, guided imagery, and muscle relaxation training combined with relaxation and imaging are all examples of behavior techniques that can be used in this regard (Morrow, 1982; Lyles, Burish, Krozely, & Oldham, 1982). These strategies may also be combined with antiemetic therapy for improved results.

## TASTE ABNORMALITIES

One patient may describe food as being absolutely tasteless while another relates that she used to drink six cups of coffee every day but

**Table 6-1** Antiemetic Options and Dosages for Use with Cancer Patients Receiving Chemotherapy

| Drug | Dosage |
| --- | --- |
| *For severe emetogenesis* | |
| Dexamethasone (Decadron) | 10 to 20 mg intravenously (IV) 30 minutes before therapy |
| Diphenhydramine (Benadryl), plus | 50 mg IV 30 minutes before therapy |
| Metoclopramide (Reglan) | 1 to 3 mg/kg IV every 2 hours up to two doses |
| *OR* | |
| Lorazepam (Ativan) | 2 mg IV 30 minutes before therapy |
| Dexamethasone | 20 mg IV 30 minutes before therapy |
| Metoclopramide | 1 to 3 mg/kg IV 30 minutes before and 90 minutes after therapy |
| Lorazepam | 1 to 2 mg IV every 4 hours up to four doses as side effects permit |
| *OR* | |
| Dexamethasone | 12 mg orally the night before or the morning of therapy |
| Dexamethasone | 10 mg IV 30 minutes before therapy |
| Lorazepam | 2 mg IV 30 minutes before therapy |
| Dexamethasone | 4 to 8 mg IV or orally every 4 to 6 hours for 48 hours after therapy |
| Lorazepam | 2 mg IV every 4 hours up to four doses as side effects permit |
| *For moderate emetogenesis* | |
| Prochlorperazine (Compazine) | 10 mg orally 1 hour before therapy |
| Dexamethasone | 10 mg orally or IV 1 hour before therapy |
| Prochlorperazine | 10 mg orally or 25 mg to the far point of accommodation (PR) every 6 hours |
| *OR* | |
| Prochlorperazine | 10 mg orally 1 hour before therapy |
| Dexamethasone | 10 mg orally 1 hour before therapy or IV 30 minutes before therapy |
| Lorazepam | 2 mg IV 30 minutes before therapy |
| Prochlorperazine | 10 mg orally or 25 mg PR every 6 hours |
| *OR* | |
| Droperidol (Inapsine) | 2.5 mg IV 30 minutes before therapy, 1 to 2 mg IV every 4 to 6 hours up to four doses |
| *OR* | |
| Lorazepam | 2 mg IV 30 minutes before therapy, 2 mg orally or IV every 4 to 6 hours up to four doses as side effects permit |
| Prochlorperazine | 10 mg orally 1 hour before therapy and every 4 hours or 25 mg PR every 4 to 6 hours |
| *OR* | |
| Haloperidol (Haldol) | 2 mg orally or intramuscularly (IM) 1 hour before therapy and every 4 to 6 hours or 25 mg PR every 4 to 6 hours |
| *OR* | |
| Trimethobenzamide (Tigan) | 200 mg orally or IM 1 hour before therapy and every 4 to 6 hours |

*Source:* Courtesy of E. Glass, T. Bechtel, and J. Leiby, 1986, The Ohio State University Hospitals. Adapted by permission.

that now the smell of coffee nauseates her. Yet other patients may state that foods have a metallic taste or that favorite desserts seem to be too sweet. Such comments are commonly encountered by the clinician working with cancer patients. They all relate to the prominent feeding problem of dysgeusia or ageusia. Ageusia is defined as taste blindness, and dysgeusia is defined as abnormalities of taste. The etiology of dysgeusia is unknown but, as with most problems in the oncology patient, appears to be multifactoral.

It is important to examine the pathophysiology involved in the inability to taste. Twycross and Lack (1986) describe the location of taste buds in the lips, cheeks, tongue, and all other parts of the buccal cavity. Each bud has approximately 50 cells arranged to form a pear-shaped organ. The human distinguishes salty, sweet, sour, bitter, metallic, and soapy tastes. The tongue is most sensitive to salty and sweet tastes, and the palate is most sensitive to sour and bitter tastes. As with most cells of the gastrointestinal tract, the cells of the taste bud have a frequent turnover rate with an average life span of about 10 days. As Twycross and Lack (1986) summarize, many factors, including radiation therapy, chemotherapy, nutrition status, hormones, and various drugs, have potential to affect the cell turnover rate. The CNS is involved in taste sensation. Tumor involvement of the fifth, seventh, ninth, and tenth cranial nerves can affect taste as well.

Trant (1986) reviews the numerous studies that have been done on taste abnormalities in the cancer patient. There have been many difficulties in these studies; problems have included a lack of statistical comparison and a grouping together of many tumor types. In addition, taste threshold measurements have not utilized normal food media, which makes extrapolation of the findings to other scenarios difficult. Despite these research problems, it is evident to any practicing clinician that taste abnormalities do exist and can dramatically affect the cancer patient's ability to eat. Because symptoms are highly individualized, one must be careful not to make unwarranted generalizations because they often prove to be faulty.

Nevertheless, taste changes appear to occur during periods of tumor growth. They may be related to a possible release of a tumor by-product that may decrease taste sensitivity or stimulate the bitter taste sensation that is frequently described (DeWys & Walters, 1975).

Also, radiation therapy to the head and neck region can effectively result in ageusia. This is primarily related to actual tissue damage. The degree of taste loss, of course, is dependent on the site and dose of radiation (Donaldson, 1981). A decrease in saliva production during radiation therapy to the head and neck may also contribute to the development of ageusia. Food must be in solution to be tasted.

Chemotherapy may also affect the ability to taste. Certain drugs, such as methotrexate or cyclophosphamide (Cytoxan) may cause an abnormal metallic taste. Chemotherapy may also result in mucositis or enhance candidiasis, which alters the environment of the mouth. This results in a decreased sensitivity to tastes. Without good mouth care, there may be a covering over of the taste buds. Also, there may be a chronic bad taste in the mouth from decaying material or a build-up of bacterial products that interferes with flavor distinction (Twycross & Lack, 1986).

There have been many reports of drug-related taste abnormalities not induced by chemotherapy agents. Most of these have found a general decrease in taste sensitivity or the development of a metallic taste. These reports have tended to be anecdotal, but they do point out once again that each cancer patient is an individual and may experience a wide range of symptoms arising from many different sources.

There is no single means to eliminate taste alterations for the patient. Patients should be allowed to eliminate the distasteful food from their diet for the period of intolerance. Appropriate substitutions of nutrition-equivalent foods can be suggested. If, for example, meats taste bitter, protein needs can be met by dairy products, nuts, legumes, and whole grains. It is frequently suggested that tart substances such as lemon juice enhance flavors. Patients often attempt to compensate for a taste alteration by adding more of the needed taste. One patient who was experiencing a lowered sweet threshold, for example, began adding eight packets of sugar to one bowl of cereal. Such attempts at compensation are rarely, if ever, successful.

Because a dry mouth or decreased salivation also contributes to taste abnormalities, encouraging the intake of moist foods and frequent intake of liquids can help. Artificial salivas may assist some patients, but many complain that the products are too sticky and do not last long. A spray bottle of water can be just as helpful.

Taste changes are real for the cancer patient, and it is often difficult for the clinician to empathize with them when the clinician's taste sensitivity is normal. Also, it may be frustrating to the clinician when there is no easy resolution to a patient's difficulties. Consistent support, encouragement, and education to maintain adequate oral intake are required.

## LEARNED FOOD AVERSIONS

Learned food aversion (LFA) is defined as aversions to specific foods or tastes that result from the association of those foods with unpleasant internal symptoms such as malaise, illness, nausea, and vomiting (Twycross & Lack, 1986). The incidence of LFA in the general (healthy) population has been estimated to be from 38% to 65% (Garb & Stunkard, 1974; Logue, Logue, & Strauss, 1983), but because these aversions only affect the ingestion of one or two foods they do not appear to jeopardize the person's nutrition status.

Nevertheless, cancer patients' LFA, combined with other feeding problems, can result in serious weight loss (Neilson, Theologides, & Vickers, 1980). Several reasons may exist for this problem (Mattes, Arnold, & Boraas, 1987). Chemotherapy is often accompanied by nausea and vomiting, which increases the risk of forming food aversions. Further, the cancer patient may have many difficulties eating, so that his or her nutrition status is often adversely affected. The elimination of any food that was tolerated before the initiation of therapy may have a significant effect on the quality of the patient's diet.

Until recently, there were no successful interventions for LFA. Most clinicians simply advised patients to refrain from eating large amounts of food before therapy that involved a drug known to result in nausea and vomiting. Recent studies, however, have indicated that food aversions may form at any time during the 48 hours before or after the first therapy (Mattes et al., 1987). Patients cannot be told to refrain from eating for 4 days.

The most promising intervention appears to be the use of a "scapegoat"—a food or beverage that is intentionally introduced before the treatment period that blocks the formation of an aversion toward a usual dietary item. Mattes et al. (1987) observed the development of LFA in only 11.1% of their study patients during a 6-month follow-up period after the introduction of such a scapegoat. In contrast, 48.4% of patients not receiving a scapegoat formed food aversions to usual dietary items. Other studies have shown similar results (Bernstein, Webster, & Bernstein, 1982).

These studies seem to hold promise for those patients who are likely to experience LFA, but there is another problem that seems to contribute to the situation. Many patients have already formed LFA before they even begin therapy. This situation has been cited in animal studies that showed that tumor growth alone may serve as an ample stimulus for LFA formation (Cannon et al., 1985; Bernstein, Treneer, Goehler, & Murowehick, 1985; Bernstein & Fenner, 1983). It has been postulated that products secreted by the tumor may have a toxic effect on the body, leading to the formation of LFA (Bernstein, 1986). In addition, tumor fuel utilization may lead to a nutrient deficiency resulting in the host's rejection of specific foods (Lawson, Richmond, & Rudman, 1982). It is possible that both mechanisms may be present and that the specific tumor determines the mechanism involved.

Food aversions seem to be a topic of mystery in the care of the cancer patient, but recent research has begun to gather specific information about the formation of LFA and for the development of strategies to prevent it. Although in short-term studies LFA did not appear to affect a patient's weight or treatment outcome, they clearly showed the potential of LFA to affect negatively a cancer patient's nutrition status and quality of life. If a scapegoat method or other treatment can be perfected, then nutrient-dense and highly preferred foods may be found that will continue to be acceptable to cancer patients.

## REFERENCES

Barber, J. (1978). Hypnosis as a psychological technique in the management of cancer pain. *Cancer Nursing, 1,* 361–363.

Barry, R.E. (1974). Malignancy, weight loss, and the small intestine mucosa. *Gut, 15,* 562–570.

Bernstein, I.L. (1986). Etiology of anorexia in cancer. *Cancer, 58,* 1881–1886.

Bernstein, I.L., & Fenner, D.P. (1983). Learned food aversions: Heterogeneity of animal models of tumor-induced anorexia. *Appetite, 4,* 79–86.

Bernstein, I.L., Treneer, C.M., Goehler, L.E., & Murowehick, E. (1985). Interfering with taste aversion learning in rats: The role of associative interference. *Behavioral Neuroscience, 99,* 818–830.

Bernstein, I.L., Webster, M.M., & Bernstein, I.D. (1982). Food aversions in children receiving chemotherapy for cancer. *Cancer, 50,* 2961–2963.

Brass, C. (1983). Fungal infections in the immuno-compromised host. In D.J. Higby (Ed.), *Supportive care in the cancer patient* (pp. 17–18). Boston: Martinus Nijhoff.

Bruera, E., Catz, Z., Hooper, R., Lentle, B., & MacDonald, N. (1987). Chronic nausea and anorexia in advanced cancer patients: A possible role for autonomic dysfunction. *Journal of Pain and Symptom Management, 2,* 19–21.

Cannon, D.S., Best, M.R., Batson, J.D., Brown, E.R., Rubenstein, J.A., & Carrell, L.E. (1985). Interfering with taste aversion learning in rats: The role of associative interference. *Appetite, 6,* 1–19.

Costa, G. (1977). Cachexia, the metabolic component of neoplastic disease. *Cancer Research, 37,* 2327–2388.

Cushman, K. (1986). Symptom management: A comprehensive approach to increasing nutritional status in the cancer patient. *Seminars in Oncology Nursing, 2,* 30–35.

Davis, J.D., & Levine, M.W. (1977). A model for the control of ingestion. *Psychology Review, 84,* 379–412.

DeWys, W.D. (1974). Abnormalities of taste as a remote effect of neoplasm. *Annals of the New York Academy of Science, 230,* 427–434.

DeWys, W.D. (1979). Anorexia as a general effect of cancer. *Cancer, 43,* 2013–2019.

DeWys, W.D., & Walters, K. (1975). Abnormalities of taste sensation in cancer patients. *Cancer, 36,* 188–196.

Donaldson, S. (1981). Nutritional problems associated with radiation therapy. In G.R. Newell & N.M. Ellison (Eds.), *Nutrition and cancer: Etiology and treatment* (pp. 319–327). New York: Raven.

Fanelli, F., Cangiano, C., Ceci, F., Cellerino, R., Franchi, E., Muscaritoli, M., & Cascino, A. (1986). Plasma tryptophan and anorexia in human cancer. *European Journal of Cancer and Clinical Oncology, 22,* 89–95.

Fetting, J.H., Wilcox, P.M., Iwata, B.A., Criswell, E.L., Bosmajian, L.S., & Sheilder, V.R. (1983). Anticipatory nausea and vomiting in an ambulatory medical oncology population. *Cancer Treatment Reports, 67,* 1093–1098.

Foley, K.M. (1985). The treatment of cancer pain. *New England Journal of Medicine, 313,* 84–95.

Garb, J.L., & Stunkard, A.J. (1974). Taste aversions in man. *American Journal of Psychiatry, 131,* 1204–1207.

Glass, E., Bechtel, T., & Leiby, J. (1986). *Antiemetic options for use with cancer chemotherapy.* Columbus, OH: Ohio State University Hospitals.

Hanks, G.W., Trueman, T., & Twycross, R.G. (1983). Corticosteroids in terminal cancer—A prospective analysis of current practice. *Postgraduate Medical Journal, 59,* 702–706.

Kennedy, M., Packard, R., Grant, M., & Padilla, G.V. (1981). Chemotherapy-related nausea and vomiting: A survey to identify problems and interventions. *Oncology Nursing Forum, 8,* 19–22.

Kisner, D.L., & DeWys, W.D. (1981). Anorexia and cachexia in malignant disease. In G.R. Newell & N.M. Ellison (Eds.), *Nutrition and cancer: Etiology and treatment.* New York: Raven.

Lawson, D.H., Richmond, A., & Rudman, D. (1982). Metabolic approaches to cancer cachexia. *Annual Review of Nutrition, 2,* 277–301.

Logue, A.W., Logue, R.R., & Strauss, K.E. (1983). The acquisition of taste aversions in humans with eating and drinking disorders. *Behavioral Research and Therapy, 21,* 275–289.

Love, R.R., Nerenz, D.R., & Levanthal, H. (1982). The development of anticipatory nausea and vomiting during cancer chemotherapy. *Proceedings of the American Society of Clinical Oncologists, 23,* 47.

Lundholm, K., Holm, G., & Schersten, J. (1978). Insulin resistance in patients with cancer. *Cancer Research, 38,* 4665–4670.

Lyles, J.N., Burish, T.G., Krozely, M.G., & Oldham, R.K. (1982). Efficacy of relaxation training and guided imagery in reducing the aversiveness of cancer chemotherapy. *Journal of Consulting and Clinical Psychology, 50,* 509–524.

Mattes, R.D., Arnold, C., & Boraas, M. (1987). Management of learned food aversions in cancer patients receiving chemotherapy. *Cancer Treatment Reports, 71,* 1071–1078.

McCaffery, M. (1979). *Nursing management of the patient in pain* (2nd ed.). Philadelphia: Lippincott.

Morrow, G.R. (1982). Prevalence and correlates of anticipatory nausea and vomiting in chemotherapy patients. *Journal of the National Cancer Institute, 68,* 575–588.

Nahikian-Nelms, M., & Baumann, C. (1988). *A taxonomy of medications routinely prescribed to a hematology-oncology population*. Abstract presented at the American Dietetic Association Conference, San Francisco, CA, October 6, 1988.

Neilson, S.S., Theologides, A., & Vickers, Z.M. (1980). Influence of food odors on food aversions and preferences in patients with cancer. *American Journal of Clinical Nutrition, 33*, 2253–2261.

Norton, J.L., Peacock, J.L., & Morrison, S.D. (1987). Cancer cachexia. *CRC Critical Reviews in Oncology/Hematology, 7*, 289–327.

Trant, A.S. (1986). Taste and anorexia in cancer patients: A review. *Topics in Clinical Nutrition, 1*, 17–25.

Twycross, R.G., & Lack, S.A. (1986). *Control of alimentary symptoms in far advanced cancer*. New York: Churchill Livingstone.

Welch, D.A. (1980). Assessment of nausea and vomiting in cancer patients undergoing external beam radiotherapy. *Cancer Nursing, 3*, 365–371.

Willox, J.C., Corr, J., & Shaw, J. (1984). Prednisolone as an appetite stimulant in patients with cancer. *British Medical Journal, 288*, 27.

# Part II

# Specific Patient Populations

# Chapter 7

# The Patient with Head and Neck Cancer

*Ursula G. Kyle*

Head and neck cancers constitute only 5% of all cancers. Nevertheless, significant functional deficits and cosmetic deformities heighten their relative importance. In the United States, approximately 26,000 new cases of head and neck cancer are diagnosed each year (Zagars & Norante, 1983). This means that 26,000 individuals are at risk for its potential complications, which include an inability to speak, chew, swallow, smell, taste, or see.

A multidisciplinary approach to management that involves head and neck surgeons, oral surgeons, radiation oncologists, plastic surgeons, medical oncologists, pathologists, dentists and prosthodontists, dietitians, speech pathologists, nurses, and social workers is essential for continued improvements in the diagnosis and treatment of head and neck cancer (Zagars & Norante, 1983). The dietitian must be knowledgeable about existing and potential disease- and treatment-related impairments to provide adequate care for this patient population. Intervention should be early and aggressive to minimize deterioration of nutrition status.

## ETIOLOGY AND EPIDEMIOLOGY

Cancer of the upper aerodigestive tract includes neoplasms of the oral cavity, nasopharynx, oropharynx, hypopharynx, larynx, paranasal sinuses, salivary gland, and thyroid. Of all head and neck cancers (except skin), 75% are associated with smoking and alcohol consumption. Although alcohol is not considered a carcinogen, it is thought to be a cofactor or cocarcinogen. Other causes of head and neck cancer are Epstein-Barr virus (associated with nasopharyngeal cancer); occupational exposure to asbestos, dust, mineral oils, and mustard gas (cancer of the larynx and nasopharynx); and radiation treatment for acne and sun exposure (skin cancer) (Cann, Fried, & Rothman, 1985).

A number of nutrient deficiencies appear to be implicated in cancer of the head and neck. Deficiencies of vitamins A and C, riboflavin, niacin, zinc, and magnesium appear to increase the risk for head and neck cancer (Cann et al., 1985). At present it is not clear whether specific nutrient deficiencies or the overall poor nutrition status associated with alcoholism increases the risk for cancer.

Most cancers of the head and neck occur in the fifth and sixth decades of life and are more common in men than in women. Nasopharyngeal cancer is frequently seen in young patients, possibly because of its viral etiology.

## NUTRITION ASSESSMENT

The initial assessment includes a nutrition history, height and weight profile, medical history, treatment plan, and biochemical parameters. A number of disease-related problems (Exhibit 7-1) interfere with food intake (Kyle, 1988a). Many patients avoid medical attention until weight loss becomes severe (as much as 10%). Those patients with severe weight loss and decreased serum albumin levels are at nutrition risk and require early intervention. Severity of weight loss is evaluated at the University of Texas M.D. Anderson Cancer Center according to the weight change table of Blackburn, Bistrian, Maini, Schlamm, and Smith (1977). Weight loss of 1% to 2% in 1 week, more than 5% in 1 month, more than 7.5% in 3 months, and more than 10% in more than 6 months is considered severe. Weight loss at the time of diagnosis appears to be an adverse prognostic indicator for response to chemotherapy (Rich, 1987). The Eastern Cooperative Oncology Group (1980) found that chemotherapy patients who experienced weight loss had shorter survival times than patients without weight loss. Weight loss before treatment appears to presage poor response to chemotherapy (Rich, 1987) and suggests advanced disease.

The serum albumin level can be used to determine patients' visceral protein status on admission. It does not detect early protein deficiency, however because albumin levels fall and recover slowly with changes in nutrition. A number of nonnutrition factors also affect serum albumin levels. Liver disease, which alters synthesis, and sepsis and trauma, which alter intravascular and extravascular distribution of albumin, may result in decreased serum albumin levels. Furthermore, renal disease, cancer, increases in catabolic hormone levels, and poor hydration status can also decrease albumin levels (Bistrian, 1986; Grant & DeHoog, 1985). Caution must be used when interpreting laboratory values in the presence of these diseases. Decreased tube feeding tolerance has been reported with serum albumin levels less than 2.5 g/dL (Brinson & Kolts, 1987). Serum albumin levels of 2.5 to 3.0 mg/dL suggest moderate depletion of visceral protein, and levels less than 2.5 mg/dL suggest severe depletion.

Many patients with head and neck cancer are alcoholics (Zagars & Norante, 1983). Alco-

**Exhibit 7-1** Disease-Related Problems Interfering with Food Intake

Pharyngitis
Aglutition
Ulceration with bleeding of the mouth and pharynx
Oropharyngeal pain
Dysphagia
Trismus (inability to open the mouth)

*Source:* From "Nutritional Considerations in Head and Neck Cancer" by U.G. Kyle, 1988, *Dietitians in Nutrition Support Newsletter, 10*(5). Copyright 1988 by American Dietetic Association. Reprinted by permission.

holism can result in a number of malnutrition-induced deficiencies or abnormalities. Malnutrition due to inadequate nutrient intake is probable when alcohol replaces food in the diet. Inflammation of the gastrointestinal tract secondary to alcohol abuse can lead to nutrient malabsorption—specifically of thiamin, $B_{12}$, folic acid, and ascorbic acid—and to secondary malnutrition. Abnormal metabolism of vitamin D, thiamin, and folic acid has been reported (Krause & Mahan, 1984). B vitamin and magnesium needs may also be increased. Zinc deficiency has been reported (Krause & Mahan, 1984). The nutrition assessment of the patient with head and neck cancer should therefore include questions about alcohol consumption to determine whether dietary intake of these nutrients is adequate or inadequate in relation to possible increased needs.

A number of metabolic abnormalities secondary to alcoholism also can result. The increased vascular resistance in the liver secondary to cirrhosis leads to impaired lymphatic flow and the development of ascites (Hiyama & Fischer, 1988). Elevated bilirubin, alkaline phosphatase, lactic dehydrogenase, ammonia, and serum glutamic oxaloacetic and serum glutamic pyruvic transaminase levels have been noted. Glucose intolerance secondary to pancreatic inflammation or injury is common in alcoholics. In addition, severe liver disease affects the validity and interpretation of nutrition-related laboratory values.

The psychologic impact of cancer is considerable for head and neck cancer patients. The patient with head and neck cancer has to deal with the awareness that he or she has cancer and with concerns about how the cancer will affect his or her ability to function as a family member, an employee, and a member of society. The patient may also have to deal with significant functional loss and cosmetic disfigurement. Fear of cancer and the treatment consequences may be one reason why many patients with symptoms do not seek treatment until the disease is advanced. Those patients with family support tend to adjust better and to be more willing to comply with nutrition treatment than those without such support. The alcoholic patient who has no family support may agree to treatment but be noncompliant with treatment plans (e.g., continue tobacco and alcohol consumption, disregard nutrition counseling). Patients who express their feelings and have a strong self-image before treatment are more likely to return to work and to survive longer than those with a poor self-image (Henrichs & Schmale, 1983). In addition, patients with head and neck cancer experience variable degrees of organic brain syndromes (Adams, Larson, & Goepfert, 1984).

The health care professional must be aware of the feelings of guilt, anger, anxiety, depression, denial, resignation, and hope that the patient may experience and make note of them in the health care plan. Treatment goals must be realistic to be useful to the patient.

## TREATMENT AND MANAGEMENT OF SIDE EFFECTS

The goals of treatment in head and neck cancer are to eradicate the cancer, to maintain adequate physiologic function, and to achieve a socially acceptable appearance. Surgery and radiation therapy are curative modalities. Chemotherapy and immunotherapy may be effective as adjunctive treatments. Treatment-related problems (Exhibit 7-2) (Kyle, 1988a) may be transient or long term. Kelly (1986) discusses the management of treatment side effects, including nausea, vomiting, and diarrhea. The overall nutrition status of the patient at the time of admission determines the need for aggressive

**Exhibit 7-2** Treatment-Related Problems in Head and Neck Cancer

Surgery
  Negative nitrogen balance
  Inability to chew
  Aglutition (inability to swallow)
  Dysphagia
  Communication impairment
  Aspiration

Radiation
  Mucositis, sore mouth
  Xerostomia (dry mouth)
  Odynophagia (pain on swallowing)
  Ageusia, dysgeusia (loss of taste, distorted taste)
  Dysosmia (distorted odor perception)
  Dental caries associated with xerostomia
  Osteonecrosis

Chemotherapy
  Nausea
  Vomiting
  Diarrhea
  Cheilosis, glossitis
  Pharyngitis
  Esophagitis
  Anorexia

Immunotherapy
  Anorexia
  Diarrhea
  Flulike syndrome

*Source:* From "Nutritional Consideration in Head and Neck Cancer" by U.G. Kyle, 1988, *Dietitians in Nutrition Support Newsletter, 10*(5). Copyright 1988 by American Dietetic Association. Reprinted by permission.

intervention. Additional counseling and intervention are provided as needed.

### Surgery

Surgery in head and neck cancer is the primary curative treatment. Advantages of surgery are that it eradicates the primary tumor, permits accurate histologic assessment of affected tissues, and enables subsequent reconstruction of the defect resulting from the tumor or primary surgery. Disadvantages of surgery are that microscopic extension of cancer cells at the periphery may not be detected and that the physiologic loss of function and cosmetic deformities may be extensive. Wide resection margins are necessary but often unattainable. Inadequate or positive margins require postoperative radiotherapy (Zagars & Norante, 1983). Plastic surgery may minimize loss of function and deformities, and current techniques eliminate the need for the multistage surgery that was used in the past.

Surgery-related problems can be devastating. They can affect the patient's appearance and ability to eat, see, smell, and hear. An early, thorough nutrition assessment is necessary and aggressive intervention justified to minimize the impact of a prolonged postoperative period of receiving nothing by mouth and consequent negative nitrogen balance. Oral intake, which may be limited when the patient is on a liquid-only or pureed diet, should include nutrition supplements to meet 100% of the macronutrient and micronutrient requirements. At the University of Texas M.D. Anderson Cancer Center, all head and neck cancer patients for whom it is not anticipated that oral intake will be resumed within 3 to 5 days of surgery have a nasogastric tube placed at the time of surgery. The patient usually resumes an oral diet once the surgical incision is healed. Total parenteral nutrition may be indicated if unanticipated postoperative complications arise.

A total laryngectomy, which is often necessary in patients with cancer of the hypopharynx or larynx, disconnects the trachea from the larynx. This eliminates the chance for aspiration. The patient is no longer able to speak normally, however, and must undergo speech therapy to learn tracheoesophageal speech or to speak with an artificial speech device. The patient is allowed to eat as soon as the incision is completely healed.

A partial or supraglottic laryngectomy does not completely sever the trachea from the larynx, so that normal speech is possible. The risk of aspiration increases, however. Dysphagia and aspiration may be due to temporary postoperative swelling. Deglutition abnormalities can be evaluated by speech pathologists, who may initiate necessary therapy.

A glossectomy (tongue excision) disrupts the oral preparatory and oral phase of swallowing. Patients can eat by mouth once swallowing

rehabilitation takes place. The consistency of the diet is dictated by the amount of tongue resected. The use of a syringe and pureed or semisolid foods may facilitate the intake of food. A palatal prosthesis, which provides tongue-to-palate contact, is helpful for many patients with glossectomies. Nevertheless, many patients depend on supplemental tube feedings until oral intake is adequate.

A maxillectomy removes the soft and hard palate and leaves an opening between the mouth and the nasal cavity. Parts of the mandible may also be removed. The patient is able to eat and speak with an obturator, which is a prosthesis that fits into the defect and closes the opening between the oral and nasal cavities. A temporary obturator is fitted at the time of surgery. An adequate seal around the obturator is essential to prevent reflux into the nasal cavity. The patient is permitted a liquid or pureed diet once the packing is removed (at approximately postoperative day 2 to 5). Oral intake is limited in the early postoperative phase until the obturator fits properly. Patients' chewing ability is frequently limited by rocking of the obturator, especially if several teeth were extracted. Adequate oral intake depends on the motivation of the patient and his or her ability to chew. Liquid-only and pureed diets are tolerated without problems by maxillectomy patients.

Jejunal interposition used in hypopharyngeal reconstruction requires that the patient receive nothing by mouth during the early postoperative phase and can result in dysphagia once oral intake is resumed. The jejunal section lacks normal peristaltic movement and depends on gravity for passage of food. The patient may experience frustration with the slow process of swallowing. Eating semisolid foods and drinking liquids after each bite can decrease the amount of time required for eating. Oral intake may be inadequate to promote healing and to maintain weight while swallowing rehabilitation proceeds. Supplemental, usually jejunal, nocturnal tube feeding should therefore be continued until nutrition needs are met.

A gastric pull-up procedure may be used to replace tissue excised in the hypopharyngeal and cervical esophagus. The gastric pull-up results in a change in stomach configuration from a balloon shape to a small stomach reservoir. Postoperative jejunostomy feedings can be started 1 to 4 days after surgery because small bowel function returns by then. If possible, jejunostomy tube feeding tolerance should be established before oral intake begins. The change in the shape of the stomach can cause nausea, vomiting, cramping, and diarrhea. Nausea and vomiting are secondary to the distention of the stomach, and cramping and diarrhea are the result of dumping syndrome. The patient is probably experiencing dumping syndrome if no signs of intolerance occur with the jejunostomy tube feeding but begin after the initiation of oral intake. A postgastrectomy diet (Exhibit 7-3) may help decrease patient discomfort and dumping symptoms. The postgastrectomy diet can be liberalized as the dumping symptoms decrease.

Full-mouth dental extractions are performed if necessary before radiation therapy and chemotherapy to minimize local and systemic infections from carious teeth and periodontal disease. Food texture modification is necessary after surgery as a result of limited chewing ability. Discharge instructions should include techniques for chopping and pureeing food as well as recipes for milk shakes and suggestions for increasing protein and calorie intake.

A neck dissection without intraoral or intrapharyngeal incision generally does not prevent food intake for more than 3 to 5 days.

Orbital exenteration (surgery to remove orbital contents) and rhinectomy (nose excision) do not directly interfere with oral intake. The psychologic stress associated with these surgeries, however, can lead to depression and may result in reduced intake and consequent weight loss.

## Radiation Therapy

Radiation therapy is a curative treatment modality in early head and neck cancer lesions and is used as an adjunctive treatment in advanced-stage head and neck cancer. Exposing muscles, nerve, bones, and major blood vessels to minimal doses of radiation preserves function and appearance (Zagars & Norante, 1983). Advantages of radiation are that a relatively large area can be treated, subclinical extension of tumor can be eradicated, functional loss is decreased, and the need for anesthesia is avoided. Disadvantages are nerve and soft tissue damage and lack of cure of large tumors that are radiation resistant. Radiation doses in head and neck cancer range from 5,000 rad (50 Gy) for microscopic lesions to 7,500 rad (75 Gy) for advanced tumors (T3 and T4 lesions) given over 5 to 7½ weeks (Zagars & Norante, 1983).

Radiation causes mucositis of the treated area that begins during week 2 of treatment, continues until treatment is completed, and then gradually disappears. Most patients experience xerostomia, odynophagia, and ageusia during week 2 or 3 of treatment. These symptoms may be noted for several months to several years after treatment.

Xerostomia is usually permanent. The patient must be encouraged to experiment with food flavors, textures, and consistencies. Tart, acidic, salty, and spicy foods should be avoided to minimize pain during radiation treatment. Coarse foods or foods with rough edges may be irritating. Soft foods, such as cream soups, pudding, milk shakes, and mashed potatoes, are usually tolerated. Lukewarm or cold foods rather than hot foods are preferred by some patients. The use of nasogastric tubes for feeding should be considered during and after radiation if the patient is unable to meet nutrition needs.

Ulceration, pain, and esophageal stricture or spasm are delayed side effects of radiation treatment that may last from several months to several years (Coulston & Darbinian, 1986).

**Exhibit 7-3** Postgastrectomy Diet for Gastric Pull-Up

1. Begin oral intake with 5 to 6 meals. Limit to 4 to 6 oz of food per meal. Increase intake by 2 oz per meal every 3 to 5 days as tolerated.
2. Alternate liquids and solids (do not drink liquids with a solid meal).
3. Avoid simple carbohydrates.
4. Introduce high-fiber foods and milk products gradually. Add one new food at a time.

Liquid-only diets and pain medication may improve the ability to eat. Delayed swallowing reflex has also been reported as a side effect of radiation therapy. Osteonecrosis of the mandible is a major complication after delivery of more than 6,000 rad (60 Gy) of radiation when teeth have been extracted (Zagars & Norante, 1983). If dental extractions are indicated, the area should be healed completely before radiation therapy begins.

## Chemotherapy

Chemotherapy can improve local control, decrease tumor size, and eradicate metastatic foci. Chemotherapy agents being tested singly or in combination in head and neck cancer are methotrexate, cisplatin, 5-fluorouracil, bleomycin, hydroxyurea, cyclophosphamide, vincristine, and doxorubicin. The duration of response is relatively short, less than 3 months to 1 year (Zagars & Norante, 1983; Al-Sarraf, 1988). The most promising response rates occur with combination therapy regimens containing cisplatin (Zagars & Norante, 1983).

Chemotherapy-related problems (see Exhibit 7-2) in patients with head and neck cancer usually disappear after treatment is finished. Nausea and vomiting associated with some antineoplastic drugs, such as cisplatin, can be decreased or minimized with antiemetics. Antidiarrheals should be prescribed if diarrhea is a side effect of chemotherapy, such as with 5-fluorouracil. Aggressive nutrition intervention, by either tube feeding or total parenteral nutrition, should be considered (1) if a severely depleted nutrition status before treatment is noted, (2) when chemotherapy is repeated more frequently than every 3 to 4 weeks, (3) if the patient is unable to meet 60% of assessed calorie and protein needs for more than 7 days (Bell, Coffee, & Blackburn, 1986), or (4) if weight loss is severe (Kyle, 1988a).

Patients receiving chemotherapy can be nutritionally supported with nasogastric or nasointestinal tube feedings when anorexia results in inadequate food intake. Mild nausea controlled with antiemetics permits pump-assisted tube feeding. Severe nausea and vomiting are contraindications to tube feedings, however. Nasogastric tube feedings may be used to improve the nutrition status of the patient and to reverse ketosis and starvation associated with inadequate food intake. Anorexia may be the result of the disease, chemotherapy, or depression or be secondary to malnutrition.

## Immunotherapy

Immunotherapy is based on the principle that the host's immune system can recognize differences between normal and tumor cells and thereby can mount a protective response (Bakemeier & McCune, 1983). The benefits of immunotherapy for any cancer type, stage, or circumstance have not been demonstrated, however. Early trials of immunostimulation with Calmette-Guerin bacillus and *Corynebacterium parvum* in head and neck cancer have been abandoned (Zagars & Norante, 1983). Phase I trials with interleukin-2 in combination with cisplatin and 5-fluorouracil are under way.

Severe anorexia, possibly as a side effect of chills and fever or some biochemical reaction (Bell et al., 1986), has been noted after administration of immunotherapeutic agents such as interleukins or interferon. Calorie counts have revealed oral intakes of 400 to 700 kcal/day for some patients at the University of Texas M.D. Anderson Cancer Center who are receiving interleukins. Nasogastric tube feedings are used for nutrition support in some of these patients. Of estimated caloric needs, 80% to 100% can be met through the use of tube feedings without an increase in nausea, vomiting, or diarrhea. Pump-assisted feedings are usually better tolerated than bolus feedings and help ensure that caloric needs are met.

## SWALLOWING DISORDERS

Disease and treatment often cause swallowing abnormalities. Normal deglutition can be divided into four phases: (1) the oral preparatory phase, (2) the oral phase, (3) the pharyngeal phase, and (4) the esophageal phase (Logemann, 1983; Bowman, DuBrow, & Goepfert, 1988). During the oral phase, food is masticated, mixed with saliva, and held between the tongue and the hard palate. As the food moves posteriorly through the area of the tonsillar fossa, the swallowing reflex is activated. It triggers the following sequence of events, which prevents food from getting into the airway during the esophageal phase: (1) the soft palate moves upward and closes off the nasopharynx to prevent food from entering the nasal cavity; (2) the pharyngeal peristalsis (stripping waves) moves food through the pharynx to the esophagus; (3) the larynx moves upward and forward, and the epiglottic fold and false and true vocal cords close to prevent food from entering the airway; and (4) the cricopharyngeal sphincter opens to allow food to pass from the pharynx to the esophagus (Logemann, 1983).

Surgical and neurologic damage often causes compromised swallowing ability and airway protection and leads to increased risk of aspiration. Reduced tongue control and delayed or absent swallow reflex can cause aspiration before the swallow by allowing food to enter the unprotected airway (Logemann, 1983; Bowman et al., 1988). Treatment involves tongue exercises and stimulation of the swallowing reflex (Logemann, 1983). The oral diet should avoid thin liquids (water and juice), sticky or bulky foods, and foods that crumble and may cause airway obstruction (American Dietetic Association [ADA], 1988). Use of a thickening agent, such as "Thick it," may be beneficial in making food the desired consistency.

Open supraglottic fold and vocal cord sphincters can result in aspiration during the swallow. Treatment requires exercises to close the false and true vocal cords or injections of Teflon into the vocal cords to close the vocal cords (Logemann, 1983). Thin liquids and foods that crumble should be avoided.

Inadequate pharyngeal stripping waves and cricopharyngeal dysfunction may cause aspiration after the swallow by allowing food to pool in

the valleculae and to spill into the airway (Logemann, 1983). Liquids and pureed foods pass into the esophagus easily and are unlikely to spill over into the airway (ADA, 1988).

Patients can be taught to protect the airway, but pharyngeal stripping waves and soft palate closure of the nasopharynx cannot be initiated voluntarily. Supraglottic swallowing exercises are used to teach airway protection to patients with supraglottic laryngectomies or aspiration tendencies secondary to muscle or nerve damage. The patient is instructed to take a breath, hold it, swallow, cough hard with the breath held, and swallow again. The patient then checks his or her voice by saying "Ah." If the voice sounds gargly, coughing should be repeated to clear any food from the airway (Logemann, 1983). Caution must be exercised with liquids until the patient is proficient in clearing the airway. Many patients, however, are silent aspirators (Bowman et al., 1988).

Numerous other swallowing abnormalities occur after treatment for head and neck cancer. Before oral intake is permitted, all patients with subtotal laryngectomies or partial or total glossectomies should be evaluated with a modified barium swallow (videofluoroscopy) to determine whether there are swallowing abnormalities and what rehabilitation is necessary. A modified barium swallow can be videotaped to identify aspiration problems and to diagnose strictures (Bowman et al., 1988). Moreover, the video made during the swallow can be used as a teaching tool. Patients are able to see the passage of liquids when they swallow and how the throat can be cleared. The speech pathologist can direct swallowing as well as speech rehabilitation.

Patients with glossectomies should be evaluated for a palatal drop prosthesis. The prosthesis adds bulk to a denture to create a false palate and permits the tongue to make contact with it, which is necessary for eating and speech.

Delayed swallowing may be an indication for supplemental tube feeding. If the radiographic study indicates that each swallow takes more than 10 seconds, the patient may not be able to meet nutritional needs when eating by mouth only (Logemann, 1983).

## FISTULAS

Occasionally a chyle fistula is seen in patients with head and neck cancer as a result of damage to the thoracic ducts during surgery or tumor invasion of the thoracic duct (e.g., in lymphoma). Drainage of pale yellow chyle is reported after surgery. Chyle fistulas are treated with a low-fat diet or formula (<10 g of fat per day) (Teba, Dedhia, Bowen, & Alexander, 1985). Medium-chain triglyceride (MCT) oil or MCT-containing enteral formula may be used because MCT oil enters the systemic circulation without passing through the thoracic ducts and thereby decreases the lymphatic flow through the chyle leak. Total parenteral nutrition with the patient receiving nothing by mouth may be required if chyle drainage is not controlled with a low-fat diet (Ferguson, Little, & Skinner, 1985; Teba et al., 1985). The chyle fistula can be expected to heal in 2 to 6 weeks. Occasionally it may persist for several months.

Any fistula, including a chyle fistula, may be a major source of nutrient loss (Teba et al., 1985). The nutrition care plan must take such losses into consideration. At the University of Texas M.D. Anderson Cancer Center, providing up to three times the basal energy expenditure was necessary to achieve positive nitrogen balance and weight gain in patients with fistulas. If the patient is receiving total parenteral nutrition, the energy provided should not exceed twice the basal energy expenditure (Ota, Kleman, & Diamond, 1986).

## NUTRITION CARE

### Tube Feeding

The Department of Head and Neck Surgery at the University of Texas M.D. Anderson Cancer Center uses a postoperative nasogastric tube feeding protocol (Exhibit 7-4). Tube feedings are started 3 to 5 days after surgery. Intermittent gravity drip feedings of an isotonic, intact-protein, lactose-free formula are used. The advantages of a tube feeding protocol are (1) it allows timely initiation of a tube feeding, (2) it provides

**Exhibit 7-4** Tube Feeding Protocol

| | |
|---|---|
| Day 1 | Clear liquid, 240 mL three times per day |
| Day 2 | Isotonic, lactose-free formula (1 kcal/mL), 240 mL, and 240 mL of water three times per day; clear liquids (juice, broth, coffee) as desired |
| Day 3 | Isotonic formula, 480 mL three times per day; clear liquids as desired |
| Day 4 | Isotonic formula, 480 mL four times per day; clear liquids as desired |

If caloric requirements are greater than 2,200 kcal/day, the patient is changed to the following

| | |
|---|---|
| Day 5 | 1.5 kcal/mL formula, 240 mL, and 240 mL of isotonic formula (1 kcal/mL) four times per day; clear liquids as desired |
| Day 6 | 1.5 kcal/mL formula, 480 mL four times per day; clear liquids as desired |

*Source:* Courtesy of The Department of Head and Neck Surgery at the University of Texas M.D. Anderson Cancer Center.

for the timely adjustment of the volume or strength to meet the patient's estimated nutrition needs, and (3) it provides guidelines for physicians in training.

The dietitian determines which patients should not be placed on the tube feeding protocol when the physician orders the tube feeding to begin. Severely malnourished patients who have been able to eat little food are initially placed on pump-assisted formula delivery. Few patients can tolerate more than four feedings per day of two 8-oz cans given at 3- to 4-hour intervals. Patients requiring nutritional build-up can be given in excess of 3,000 cal/day by continuous pump infusion. Specialized tube feeding formulas are used as appropriate, such as high-fat, low-carbohydrate formulas for patients with chronic obstructive pulmonary disease; "blenderized" food formulas for diabetic patients; and decreased or modified fat or elemental formulas for patients with chyle fistulas. Fiber-containing formulas have recently been recommended for patients who experience diarrhea when receiving tube feedings. Clinicians were able to continue intermittent gravity drip tube feedings with fiber-containing formula in patients who experienced diarrhea of unknown etiology with isotonic formulas (Kyle, 1988b).

A percutaneous endoscopic gastrostomy (PEG) should be considered for patients who are likely to require tube feeding for several months or who are at risk for upper gastrointestinal obstruction secondary to tumor (e.g., inoperable tumors of the larynx or hypopharynx). Advantages of PEG are that swallowing is not impaired and throat irritation is decreased, and that it is more cosmetically acceptable than a nasogastric tube. The PEG can be placed under a local anesthetic, and the patient can begin feedings 24 hours later (Mamel, 1987). Subsequently, intermittent feeding throughout the day or 24-hour pump-assisted feedings can be administered. Possible side effects of PEG are similar to those of nasogastric tubes and include nausea and vomiting, bloating, cramping, abdominal pain, and diarrhea. Esophageal reflux is reported to be less common with gastrostomies (including PEG) than with nasogastric tubes (Torosian & Rombeau, 1980).

Jejunostomy feedings are indicated when gastric reflux causes aspiration, when the patient is unable to protect the airway from aspiration, when ulcerative or neoplastic disease or surgery involves the stomach, and when gastric emptying is impaired (Rombeau, Barot, Low, & Twomey, 1984). Tube feeding into the jejunum may be done through a nasojejunostomy, a PEG with the tube advanced into the jejunum, or a direct enteral jejunostomy placed during surgery.

A needle catheter jejunostomy, because of its small diameter, increases the risk of clogging; this can, however, be minimized with elemental formulas. These formulas are expensive and are not justified in the absence of maldigestion, malabsorption, or intolerance of polymeric formula secondary to malnutrition. Furthermore, Jones, Lees, Andrews, Frost, and Silk (1983) suggest that protein repletion occurs more effectively with polymeric than with elemental tube feeding formulas. Frequent flushing (every 4 to 6 hours) and minimal use of needle catheter jejunostomy tubes for medication administration decrease the chance for clogging of the tube by polymeric formulas. If the patient depends on the jejunostomy for administration of medication on discharge, an 8F feeding tube or larger should be chosen to minimize clogging.

Jejunostomy feedings generally require pump-assisted delivery of formula because bolus amounts or the hyperosmolarity of formulas contribute to diarrhea. Isotonic polymeric formulas are well tolerated if they are started at half strength at 25 to 50 mL/hour and increased by 25 mL/hour every 24 hours until the desired volume is reached; then the feeding is advanced to three-fourths and then to full strength (Ryan & Page, 1984). Initial small volumes (20 to 30 mL/hour) of full-strength isotonic formula are well tolerated by some patients. The feeding can be increased by 10 mL/hour every 12 hours to the desired volume. Others can tolerate concentrated (1.5 to 2.0 mL/hour) hyperosmolar formulas after intestinal adaptation. Before commercial formulas were developed, "blenderized" food was tolerated in jejunostomy feedings (Ryan & Page, 1984).

Formula-drug interaction resulting in delayed or reduced drug absorption is a contraindication for mixing a number of drugs with enteral formulas (Table 7-1) (Roe, 1979). In addition, physical incompatibilities with enteral formulas also contraindicate the addition of some drugs to enteral formulas (Exhibit 7-5) because of

**Table 7-1** Delayed or Reduced Drug Absorption with Food and Enteral Formulas

| Delayed | Reduced |
| --- | --- |
| Amoxicillin | Penicillin G |
| Cephalexin | Penicillin V (K) |
| Cephradine | Phenethicillin |
| Sulfanilamide | Ampicillin |
| Sulfadiazine | Amoxicillin |
| Sulfamethoxine | Tetracycline |
| Sulfamethoxypyridazine | Demethylchlortetracycline |
| Sulfisoxazole | Methacycline |
| Sulfasymazine | Oxytetracycline |
| Aspirin | Aspirin |
| Acetaminophen | Propantheline |
| Digoxin | Levodopa |
| Furosemide | Rifampin |
| Potassium ion | Doxycycline |
| | Isoniazid |
| | Phenobarbital |

*Source:* From "Interactions between Drugs and Nutrients" by D.A. Roe, 1979, *Medical Clinics of North America, 63*(5), p. 986. Copyright 1979 by W.B. Saunders Company. Reprinted by permission.

**Exhibit 7-5** Drug Additives That Change Physical Properties of Enteral Formulas

| | |
|---|---|
| Dimetapp elixir | Mandelamine suspension |
| Dimetane | Feosol elixir |
| Robitussin expectorant | Klorvess syrup |
| Sudafed syrup | KCl liquid |
| Cibalith-S syrup | |
| Thorazine | |
| Mellaril oral solution | |
| Neo-Calglucon | |

*Source:* From "Compatibilities of Enteral Products with Commonly Employed Drug Additives" by A.J. Cutie, E. Altman, and L. Lenkel, 1983, *Journal of Parenteral and Enteral Nutrition*, 7(2), pp. 186–191. Copyright 1983 by American Society for Parenteral and Enteral Nutrition. Adapted by permission.

increased incidence of tube clogging (Cutie, Altman, & Lenkel, 1983). No physical incompatibilities were reported when a number of drugs were mixed with elemental formulas (Burns, McCall, & Wirsching, 1988).

## Total and Peripheral Parenteral Nutrition

Total parenteral nutrition is necessary infrequently because patients with head and neck cancer usually have a functional gut below the tumor site. It may be used when complete upper gastrointestinal obstruction precludes access to the tract or if the patient has a history of paralytic ileus, chyle fistula that does not improve with fat-restricted diet or formula, or aspiration with tube feeding.

Peripheral parenteral nutrition should be considered in patients with head and neck cancer when short-term (1- to 2-week) complications, such as complete obstruction, paralytic ileus, severe nausea, or vomiting secondary to chemotherapy or anesthesia, prevent oral or enteral nutrition. Dextrose (3L, 10%) and amino acids (2.75%) provide 1,350 kcal and 82.5 g of protein. Daily lipids (500 mL, 20% for 1,000 kcal) can be given to increase caloric intake. Although peripheral parenteral nutrition cannot meet 100% of calorie needs, it can decrease nitrogen loss. Electrolyte, multivitamin, and mineral

preparations must be added to prevent deficiencies and to permit optimum use of nutrients.

## Hepatic Dysfunction due to Alcoholism

Long-term alcohol abuse can cause cirrhosis, ascites, and ultimately encephalopathy (Krause & Mahan, 1984). A high-calorie, high-protein diet should be prescribed for the cirrhotic patient who is not encephalopathic. Dietary sodium and fluids are restricted in the presence of ascites. Because the ascites displaces the stomach, early satiety is reported by many patients. Supplemental pump-assisted tube feedings are indicated if oral intake is inadequate. Vitamin supplementation (B complex) is indicated. Thiamin supplementation (50 to 100 mg/day) should be prescribed if beriberi, Korsakoff's psychosis, or polyneuritis is present. For patients with steatorrhea, fat-soluble vitamins—specifically A, D, and E—may have to be given in water-soluble form or intramuscularly (Krause & Mahan, 1984). Many chronic alcoholics require an alcohol drip after surgery to prevent alcohol withdrawal symptoms.

Cachexia is frequently noted in hepatic failure. The goal of therapy is to provide adequate calories and protein for liver regeneration. Energy needs of 1.5 to 1.75 times the basal energy expenditure may be required to achieve positive nitrogen balance. In the absence of encephalopathy, 1.5 g of protein per kilogram (dry weight) is recommended (Shronts, 1988). If no other cause of hepatic encephalopathy (e.g., infection, gastrointestinal bleeding, or electrolyte imbalance) is present, protein intake should be reduced to 0.5 g of high–biological value protein per kilogram per day during encephalopathy. Once mental status improves, the protein allowance is increased by 15 to 20 g/ day every 4 to 7 days until 60 to 80 g (1 g/kg/ day) of protein is being given per day (Krause & Mahan, 1984). The use of branched-chain amino acids in hepatic encephalopathy, although not demonstrated to be beneficial, is promising (Hiyama & Fischer, 1988). The diet must provide adequate calories to minimize endogenous protein catabolism, which may worsen the hepatic encephalopathy.

### Dumping Syndrome

A postgastrectomy diet (see Exhibit 7-3) with small (4- to 6-oz meals), frequent feedings appears to prevent nausea, vomiting, distention, and diarrhea associated with gastric pull-up. The patient is encouraged to increase oral intake gradually to help stretch the stomach. The elimination of simple carbohydrates is recommended to prevent osmotic diarrhea. The patient is encouraged to alternate solids and liquids as well. Daily calorie counts aid in determining the amount of food and total calories that the patient can tolerate. Most patients require supplemental jejunostomy tube feedings at discharge if estimated needs cannot be met by oral intake alone. The jejunostomy tube feeding is typically changed to supplemental nocturnal feedings once the patient starts eating. This stimulates oral intake during the day and allows the patient to be mobile.

## POTENTIAL COMPLICATIONS OF NUTRITION CARE

### Metabolic Abnormalities

Metabolic abnormalities seen in patients with head and neck cancer include glucose intolerance, hyperphosphatemia, and hypercalcemia. Glucose intolerance has been reported in cancer patients not previously diagnosed as diabetic because of insulin resistance (Heber, 1987), tumor load, sepsis, and stress. Short-term insulin administration may be necessary after surgery. The goal of therapy is to maintain blood glucose levels at less than 200 mg/dL.

Rapid refeeding of the malnourished patient can lead to low serum phosphate levels secondary to phosphate entering the cells (Sitrin & Wood, 1983). To prevent refeeding syndrome, serum phosphate levels must be monitored in all malnourished patients receiving tube feedings or total parenteral nutrition. Phosphate may be given as Neutra-Phos or Neutra-Phos-K. One tablet provides 250 mg of elemental phosphorus. The usual dosage is one or two tablets two or three times a day.

Hypercalcemia is associated with bone metastases in patients with head and neck cancer. Treatment includes rehydration and administration of mithramicin, calcitonin, or diphosphates (Arseneau & Rubin, 1983). Hypercalcemia cannot be controlled by restricting dietary calcium (ADA, 1981). Long-term therapy requires tumor removal.

### Electrolyte Imbalances

Electrolytes must be monitored by the dietitian during tube feeding. The low sodium content of some tube feeding formulas may result in hyponatremia. Low serum sodium levels can be corrected by adding table salt to the formula: 1 tsp of table salt provides 87.5 mEq of sodium ion and 85 mEq of chloride ion. The addition of 0.5 to 1 tsp of table salt per day is usually adequate to meet the patient's sodium needs.

### CONCLUSION

Nutrition care of the patient with head and neck cancer should be directed toward early intervention to provide adequate nutrition support as soon as is feasible. A multidisciplinary approach is essential for continued improvements in the diagnosis and treatment of head and neck cancer. There is increasing evidence that many cancers are preventable. The health care professional must help teach the public that tobacco, alcohol, and some dietary factors are preventable causes of cancer.

**REFERENCES**

Adams, F., Larson, D.L., & Goepfert, H. (1984). Does the diagnosis of depression in head and neck cancer mask organic brain disease? *Otolaryngology and Head and Neck Surgery, 92*(6), 618–624.

Al-Sarraf, M. (1988). Current treatment of head and neck cancer. *Mediguide to oncology* (Vol. 8, pp. 1–6). New York: Lederle.

American Dietetic Association. (1981). *Handbook of clinical dietetics*. New Haven, CT: Yale University Press.

American Dietetic Association. (1988). *Manual of clinical nutrition* (pp. 193–201). Chicago: Author.

Arseneau, J.C., & Rubin, P. (1983). Oncologic emergencies. In P. Rubin, (Ed.), *Clinical oncology* (6th ed., pp. 516–525). New York: American Cancer Society.

Bakemeier, R.F., & McCune, C.S. (1983). Basic principles of tumor immunology and immunotherapy. In P. Rubin (Ed.), *Clinical oncology* (6th ed., pp. 100–104). New York: American Cancer Society.

Bell, S.J., Coffee, L.M., & Blackburn, G.L. (1986). Use of total parenteral nutrition in cancer patients. *Topics in Clinical Nutrition, 1*, 37–49.

Bistrian, B.R. (1986). Some practical and theoretic concepts in the nutritional assessment of the cancer patient. *Cancer, 58*(8, Suppl.), 1863–1866.

Blackburn, G.L., Bistrian, B.R., Maini, B.S., Schlamm, H.T., & Smith, M.F. (1977). Nutritional and metabolic assessment of the hospitalized patient. *Journal of Parenteral and Enteral Nutrition, 1*, 11–22.

Bowman, J.B., DuBrow, R.A., & Goepfert, H. (1988). Modified barium swallow technique: A tool for diagnosing and evaluating swallowing disorders in cancer patients. *Cancer Bulletin, 40*(1), 59–62.

Brinson, R.R., & Kolts, B.E. (1987). Hypoalbuminemia as an indicator of diarrheal incidence in critically ill patients. *Critical Care Medicine, 15*(5), 506–509.

Burns, P.E., McCall, L., & Wirsching, R. (1988). Physical compatibilities of enteral formulas with various common medications. *Journal of the American Dietetic Association, 88*(9), 1094–1096.

Cann, C.I., Fried, M.P., & Rothman, K.J. (1985). Epidemiology of squamous cell cancer of the head and neck. *Otolaryngologic Clinics of North America, 18*(3), 367–388.

Coulston, A.M., & Darbinian, J.A. (1986). Nutritional management of patients with cancer. *Topics in Clinical Nutrition, 2*, 26–30.

Cutie, A.J., Altman, E., & Lenkel, L. (1983). Compatibilities of enteral products with commonly employed drug additives. *Journal of Parenteral and Enteral Nutrition, 7*(2), 186–191.

Eastern Cooperative Oncology Group. (1980). Prognostic effect of weight loss prior to chemotherapy in cancer patients. *American Journal of Medicine, 69*, 491–497.

Ferguson, M.K., Little, A.G., & Skinner, D.B. (1985). Current concepts in the management of postoperative chylothorax. *Annals of Thoracic Surgery, 40*(6), 542–545.

Grant, A., & DeHoog, S. (1985). *Nutritional assessment and support* (3rd ed.). Seattle: Authors.

Heber, D. (1987). Malnutrition in cancer. *UCLA Cancer Center Bulletin, 13*(3), 49–52.

Henrichs, M.H., & Schmale, A.H. (1983). Principles of psychosocial oncology. In P. Rubin (Ed.), *Clinical oncology* (6th ed., pp. 482–488). New York: American Cancer Society.

Hiyama, D.T., & Fischer, J.E. (1988). Nutritional support in hepatic failure. *Nutrition in Clinical Practice, 3*, 96–105.

Jones, B.J.M., Lees, R., Andrews, J., Frost P., & Silk, D.B.A. (1983). Comparison of an elemental and polymeric enteral formula in patients with normal gastrointestinal function. *Gut, 24*, 78–84.

Kelly, K. (1986). An overview of how to nourish the cancer patient by mouth. *Cancer, 58*(8, Suppl.), 1897–1901.

Krause, M.V., & Mahan, L.K. (1984). *Food, nutrition and diet therapy* (7th ed.). New York: Saunders.

Kyle, U.G. (1988a). Nutritional considerations in head and neck cancer. *Dietitians in Nutrition Support, 10*(5).

Kyle, U.G. (1988b). Unpublished data.

Logemann, J. (1983). *Evaluation and treatment of swallowing disorders*. San Diego: College-Hill.

Mamel, J.J. (1987). Percutaneous endoscopic gastrostomy. *Nutrition in Clinical Practice, 1*, 65–75.

Ota, D.M., Kleman, G., & Diamond, K. (1986). Practical considerations in the nutritional management of cancer patients. *Current Problems in Cancer, 10*(7), 348–398.

Rich, A.J. (1987). Nutritional status in cancer. *Anticancer Research, 7*, 271–280.

Roe, D.A. (1979). Interactions between drugs and nutrients. *Medical Clinics of North America, 63*(5), 985–1007.

Rombeau, J.L., Barot, L.R., Low, D.W., & Twomey, P.L. (1984). Feeding by tube enterostomy. In J.L. Rombeau (Ed.), *Clinical nutrition: Vol. 1. Enteral nutrition* (pp. 275–291). New York: Saunders.

Ryan, J.A., & Page, C.P. (1984). Intrajejunal feeding: Development and current status. *Journal of Parenteral and Enteral Nutrition, 8*(2), 187–198.

Shronts, E.P. (1988). Nutritional assessment of adults with end-stage hepatic failure. *Nutrition in Clinical Practice, 3*, 113–119.

Sitrin, M.D., & Wood, R.D. (1983). Clinical signs and management of hypophosphatemia. *Clinical Consultants in Nutrition Support, 3*(3), 1–6.

Teba, C., Dedhia, H.V., Bowen, R., & Alexander, J.C. (1985). Chylothorax review. *Critical Care Medicine, 13*(1), 49–52.

Torosian, M.H., & Rombeau, J.L. (1980). Feeding by enterostomy. *Surgery Gynecology and Obstetrics, 150*, 918–927.

Zagars, G., & Norante, J.D. (1983). Head and neck tumors. In P. Rubin (Ed.), *Clinical oncology* (6th ed., pp. 230–261). New York: American Cancer Society.

# Chapter 8

# Dysphagia and the Cancer Patient

*Kathryn Lee Bradford*

Dysphagia is described as the difficult passage of food from the mouth to the stomach. Dysphagia is secondary to the presence of neuromuscular disease, trauma, or pathologic or congenital conditions involving the head and neck. The diagnoses most frequently associated with dysphagia are stroke, cerebral palsy, multiple sclerosis, amyotrophic lateral sclerosis, and cancer of the head and neck. Dysphagia is life threatening because of its impact on nutrition status and safety during eating.

This chapter focuses on dysphagia as a symptom of or as a result of treatment for head and neck cancer. This type of dysphagia is particularly difficult to work with because in many cases the patient has had a surgical resection of the oral and esophageal structures that are essential for mastication and a successful swallow reflex.

The effects of cancer and its associated treatments on nutrition status have been well documented in the medical literature. Dysphagia further complicates the situation because the patient's ability to eat is compromised for an extended period of time and because the fear of choking adds to the patient's anxious state. This chapter is intended to educate the dietitian about the physiology of swallowing and in how to recognize dysphagic symptoms or their potential when associated with particular diagnoses.

Dysphagia has serious emotional and social consequences of which the medical team and patient's family must be aware. The inability to participate in eating, one of life's most social occasions, both safely and gracefully, generates a lot of frustration, anxiety, and depression (Pruyn, deJong, Bosman, & Van Poppel, 1986). An individual who cannot eat normally is likely to withdraw from social activities that involve eating. The patient's family must be counseled to be understanding and to find ways of making the patient feel comfortable sitting at the table and not eating or eating by means of whatever method is deemed safe. Every patient and family is different, and all members must give themselves time to adjust. In many cases, changes in feeding technique, body positioning, or food consistencies may be all that is required to solve the problem. Some patients, however, may require prosthetic devices or reconstructive surgery and an in-depth dysphagia training program. By taking the time to learn the diagnoses and treatments that are associated with dysphagia and by observing patients during mealtime, the dietitian can provide an invaluable service by identifying this frequently unrecognized nutrition problem.

## PHYSIOLOGY OF SWALLOWING

Swallowing is a complex process and requires approximately 10 seconds to complete. It is a reflexive act that is typically divided into three phases.

1. *Oral or voluntary phase.* The food is placed in the mouth on the tongue, the lips are closed, and the mandible is in a closed position. The food is manipulated by the tongue to the rear molars, where it is chewed by a rotary movement of the jaw. Once the food is chewed adequately, the tip of the tongue rises to the palate and propels the food to the back of the mouth, and through the coordination of the walls of the cheeks, tongue, and oropharynx the food is pushed into the oropharynx. Sensory receptors in the oropharynx react to the presence of food and initiate the second and third stages of swallowing. The oral phase is voluntary and requires approximately 1 to 2 seconds to complete.
2. *Pharyngeal phase.* The soft palate rises and the epiglottis descends, closing off the nasal pharynx and larynx, respectively. These protective movements prevent food from entering the nose (nasal regurgitation) or the larynx and trachea. There is a pause in the breathing cycle, and the food passes into the esophagus. This phase is involuntary and requires approximately 1 to 2 seconds to complete.
3. *Esophageal phase.* The soft palate and epiglottis return to their usual positions, and respiration continues. The bolus of food is now in the esophagus, where it passes into the stomach by peristalsis. The esophageal phase is involuntary and requires approximately 5 to 7 seconds to complete.

Radiographic studies may be required for those patients whose second and third phases of swallowing are prolonged.

The act of swallowing is under the control of the afferent and efferent functions of cranial nerves V, VII, IX, X, and XII. These nerves originate in the area of the medulla and pons of the brainstem. They provide sensory and motor innervation to the face, lips, tongue, oral cavity, and pharynx. Any disease, trauma, or treatment that affects these nerves can impair a person's ability to swallow.

### Trigeminal Nerve (Cranial Nerve V)

Cranial nerve V originates in the pons and innervates the temporal and masseter muscles of the jaw, which control chewing and jaw movement. The trigeminal nerve has three branches: ophthalmic, maxillary, and mandibular; these supply sensory innervation to the skin of the face, oral and nasal mucosa, and cornea of the eye. The sensations include touch, pain, heat, and cold. Cranial nerve V also provides proprioception to jaw muscles and the muscles of mastication. Damage to the trigeminal nerve may result in the inability to move the mandible and loss of the bite and jaw-jerk reflexes.

### Facial Nerve (Cranial Nerve VII)

Cranial nerve VII originates in the pons and innervates facial muscles and the taste receptors for the front two-thirds of the tongue. It does not, however, innervate the sensory receptors of the face or the muscles of the tongue. The facial nerve is responsible for facial expression and saliva and lacrimal secretions. Impairment of the facial nerve may result in loss of taste (sweet and sour), inability to change facial expression, decreased saliva production, mouth droop, and difficulty in manipulating food in the mouth.

### Glossopharyngeal Nerve (Cranial Nerve IX)

Cranial nerve IX originates in the medulla and innervates the pharyngeal muscles; it provides sensation to the esophagus and taste sensation for the posterior third of the tongue. The glossopharyngeal nerve works in concert with the vagus nerve. Impairment of the glossopharyngeal nerve can result in a decreased or absent gag reflex, difficulty in swallowing, and a loss of sensation in the throat, which may result in poor coughing and swallowing reflexes.

## Vagus Nerve (Cranial Nerve X)

Cranial nerve X originates in the medulla and innervates many of the same structures as the glossopharyngeal nerve. The vagus nerve is responsible for the motor functions of swallowing, vocal cord movement, and upward movement of the tongue, soft palate, and uvula. In addition, it is responsible for the sensory innervation of the posterior third of the tongue and the posterior wall of the pharynx. Impairment of the vagus nerve can also result in loss of the gag and cough reflexes, hoarseness, and nasal regurgitation of food.

## Hypoglossal Nerve (Cranial Nerve XII)

Cranial nerve XII originates in the medulla and supplies the extrinsic and intrinsic muscles of the tongue. Impairment of this nerve results in the inability to protrude the tongue or to move it laterally, mechanical dysphagia, and indistinct speech.

## ASSESSING THE PATIENT AND NUTRITION STATUS

The patient's nutrition status should be assessed as soon as possible by means of the standard parameters. It is imperative that the dietitian have an understanding of head and neck cancer diagnoses and their potential to cause dysphagia. For example, cancer of the larynx or the soft palate can result in nasal regurgitation, coughing, and choking events. The dietitian should ask such questions as the following: Has the patient's intake been affected by the presence of a tumor pressing on the cranial nerves or

impeding the passage of food along the esophagus? Has the patient complained of solid foods getting "clogged" in the throat or that it takes a long time for food to go down? Can the patient take solids and not liquids, or vice versa? Or can the dietitian expect the patient to develop dysphagia as a result of treatment?

Almost all patients with head and neck cancer are at high risk for dysphagia and consequent events of choking or aspiration because their reflexive abilities to protect themselves from these events are impaired or absent. The dietitian may be the first person to notice that a patient is having difficulty eating while observing the patient during meals. In addition, the dietitian should always ask patients during home or clinic visits whether they are having any difficulties chewing or swallowing. The dietitian must keep in mind that eating is a personal topic and that patients may be reluctant to discuss their problems. Symptoms of dysphagia include drooling, choking, coughing during or after meals, packing of food in the cheeks, inability to gag, aspiration of food or saliva, complaints of dry mouth or ulcerations of the oral mucosa, chronic upper respiratory infections, and weight loss. The medical or dysphagia team must determine whether the patient is mentally, emotionally, and physically able to begin dysphagia training. This assessment may include oral challenges with various food textures administered by the speech or occupational therapist or fluoroscopic examinations of the patient while swallowing radiographic foods or liquids given by the ENT physician or radiologist. Tube feedings or supplements are required for those patients who are unable to consume an adequate amount of food for any reason.

Any patient who is suspected of having a problem chewing or swallowing should be referred to a speech therapist for a complete examination. If a speech therapist is not available, the dietitian can assess the patient's lip and tongue control by asking the patient to perform the following:

- *tongue elevation*—ask the patient to articulate the sounds [*t*] or [*d*]

- *tongue retraction*—ask the patient to articulate the sounds [*ch*] or [*k*]
- *tongue protrusion*—ask the patient to thrust his or her tongue outward
- *tongue lateralization*—ask the patient to push his or her tongue into the sides of the right and left cheeks
- *lip closure*—ask the patient to articulate the sounds [*m*] or [*p*]

## DYSPHAGIA AS A RESULT OF TREATMENT

Surgical resection of the oral or esophageal structures interferes with the normal mechanisms of chewing and swallowing. In some cases, these deficits can be overcome with reconstructive surgery, the use of prosthetic devices, or dysphagia therapy. Some of the deficits that occur with head and neck surgery are as follows:

1. Surgical procedures involving the mandible interfere with mastication. These patients require either nasogastric or gastrostomy tube feedings until reconstructive surgery is completed.
2. Partial and total glossectomies impair the ability to manipulate food in the mouth. Food cannot be pushed posteriorly for the second phase of swallowing, nor can it be cleared from the cheeks. It is possible for glossectomy patients to learn to swallow, although with great difficulty. They can be taught to inject liquids or semisolids to the back of the mouth with a large bulb syringe or taught to swallow a feeding tube for intermittent feedings.
3. Surgery of the soft palate may result in nasal regurgitation.
4. Partial laryngectomies interfere with protecting the larynx and trachea and affect sensory innervation to this area. These patients can also learn to swallow, starting first with thick liquids and progressing to firmer textures. They must be taught to eat slowly and to avoid foods that contain pits or stringy, fibrous material.
5. Any surgical procedure to the oral cavity can cause significant scarring, which may further diminish structure and function by narrowing passageways and limiting movement.

The side effects of chemotherapy and radiation vary from patient to patient, as does each patient's ability to overcome the effects of these treatment modalities. Chemotherapeutic agents are known to alter taste acuity and to cause nausea and vomiting. A patient's ability to taste may also be altered or missing as a result of surgery or nerve damage.

Radiation to the oral cavity can decrease the production of saliva. A lack of saliva causes dry mouth, decreases taste acuity, impairs food bolus formation, impairs swallowing ability, increases the incidence of dental caries, and increases mucus viscosity. Xerostomia, mucositis, and stomatitis induced by radiation therapy or chemotherapy generally become evident 2 to 3 weeks after treatment is initiated. Any or all of these side effects may interfere with adequate nutrient intake.

## ORAL HYGIENE

Good oral hygiene is essential to the health and comfort of the dysphagic patient. It reduces the risk of oral infection and bacterial overgrowth and promotes the patient's comfort after surgery or therapy. The patient may complain of dry mouth and sore lips and gums and have difficulty chewing or wearing dentures. These side effects are best treated with nonirritating mouthwashes or swabs that can be recommended by the medical or dysphagia team.

Xerostomia, however, is a particularly difficult problem because saliva helps with bolus formation and lubricates the throat for easy passage of food. Saliva substitutes are available on the market and may be used before and during meals to aid in swallowing. Some patients find that sips of water or other liquids during the meal are just as helpful, however.

Dysphagic patients must be encouraged to rinse their mouths, brush their teeth, and examine the oral cavity for loose particles of food. This reduces the potential for dental caries or infection and minimizes the risk of the patient's aspirating a piece of food.

## POSITIONING FOR FEEDING

The medical team must decide on the proper body position for feeding the dysphagic patient. Good alignment of the alimentary canal and flexion assist in swallowing. If possible, the patient should be in a seated position with the feet flat on the floor. The head should be in the midline with the neck flexed. For bed-bound patients the head of the bed should be raised to approximately 75° and pillows used to help in securing a good head and body position. Some patients' ability to swallow can be improved through proper body alignment and by using gravity to aid in getting the food down.

Because of their condition, however, some patients cannot or should not sit up and must be fed in a reclining or semireclining position. In these cases precautions must be taken to minimize the potential of the patient's choking or aspirating (for example, rolling the patient onto one side). Suctioning equipment should be on hand and operational at all times.

## DYSPHAGIA DIET

Dysphagic patients are often afraid to eat. Many have been tube fed for so long that they are sure that they will choke even though there is no physiologic reason why such an event should occur. The dietitian should sit with such patients and coax them through each bite. A mirror should be set up on their table so that they can watch what they are doing. In addition, dysphagic patients are frequently embarrassed by their inability to complete such a natural function. Food should be served in a quiet atmosphere, and the patient should never be rushed. They should be reminded to concentrate on chewing or swallowing and not to be self-conscious.

Food should be appealing, mild tasting, and served at room temperature. This enhances the patient's desire to eat while decreasing the risk of burning the mouth on hot food because of a lack of oral sensation. Foods should be offered in small quantities so that the patient is not overwhelmed by the sight of a large portion. Foods of the appropriate consistency, texture, and temperature can help induce salivation and a swallow reflex and aid in strengthening the muscles of mastication. For example, small pieces of baked potato (without the skin) have some texture and require a minimal amount of chewing.

The consistency of the food offered depends on the patient's ability to control the food in the mouth and on any structural changes or obstructions in the oropharynx and esophagus. Clear liquids represent the most difficult food consistency to control during swallowing and are inappropriate for patients who lack good tongue control. Foods that stick together are easy to control and do not become lost in the patient's mouth. For example, macaroni and cheese usually forms a good bolus. As a member of the dysphagia team, the dietitian must be able to make food consistency recommendations on the basis of the foods that are available in the facility.

When writing menus for dysphagic patients, the dietitian must take into consideration patients' food preferences and any restrictions. Most dysphagic patients consume little food, however, so that many dietary restrictions are meaningless. The dietitian should consider the effort required of the patient to chew by trying the food beforehand or should mash the food offered before it is swallowed. For example, does a saltine cracker break up into pieces in the mouth or form a bolus? Does the chewed food require a lot of manipulation with the tongue to form a bolus? Cottage cheese breaks up into small pieces, but not if it is creamed in a blender. Does the institution's kitchen make a moist or dry meat loaf? Are the meat gravies thin or thick? The clinician should be familiar with the foods that the facility has to offer, but it must be remembered that once a patient goes home the food textures available will change as a result of the different preparation techniques used at home.

The menu items should be changed as often as possible to avoid boredom and possible reliance on particular foods. Each patient's tolerance and degree of ability is different and requires individual attention. The dietitian should always work closely with the speech or dysphagia therapist to determine appropriate food consistencies.

Eating is not enjoyable for the dysphagic patient. It is time consuming and requires a lot of effort. Combinations of food that will increase nutrient density while minimizing the quantity of food that the patient will have to consume should be sought. For example, carbohydrate or protein modules may be added to foods of the appropriate consistency, such as mashed potatoes, applesauce, or thick soup, to concentrate the calories and nutrients. The potential combinations are limitless.

Dysphagic patients are at risk for malnutrition and are candidates for nutrition support. Their ability to chew and swallow must be assessed before any nutrition therapy is implemented, however. Oral supplements may be appropriate for some patients who have control over their swallow and who are not at risk for aspiration. Tube feeding should be initiated with any patient who does not have an adequate oral intake. Patients with esophageal obstructions or pharyngeal sutures or who are at risk for aspiration may not be candidates for nasogastric feeding, however. They may require the placement of a gastrostomy or duodenal feeding tube. In some cases, feeding tubes should be routinely removed and reinserted to avoid pharyngeal irritation caused by an indwelling tube. Some patients may benefit from having the nasogastric tube reinserted because this process is a stimulus for the gag reflex and the muscles used for swallowing. A tube feeding should not be discontinued until a patient is able orally to sustain nutrition needs (caloric and fluid) as documented by a food intake record.

Tube feeding schedules should be arranged so as not to interfere with dysphagia therapy. Enteral feeding should be stopped at least one hour before dysphagia therapy because patients are more motivated when they are hungry. Supplemental liquids or puddings can also be incorporated into dysphagia training programs, if deemed appropriate.

Food consistency modifications for each patient should be determined by the dysphagia team. Initially, the patient receives small quantities of food (of the appropriate consistency) for dysphagia therapy sessions only. As therapy progresses foods may be sent at mealtime, and eating is supervised by the speech therapist, nurse, dietitian, or trained family member. As mentioned earlier, persons working with dysphagia patients should be trained to use suction equipment and should know proper procedures to deal with choking events, including the Heimlich maneuver.

Listed below are examples of food consistency modifications that have been successful (Lee-Bradford, 1981). Other versions are described in the literature (Bove & Kagel, 1983; Elizabethtown Hospital, 1984), but the individual foods included in each category of consistency modification are dependent on the philosophies of the particular dysphagia team, each patient's needs, and the ability of the institution's kitchen staff to prepare the modifications. Each category is defined by the degree of chewing or manipulation required by the patient or by dimensional size. The foods included in a category can vary from facility to facility and food to food depending on the preparation technique used. For example, meat loaf may be categorized as "chopped" in one hospital but as "chopped fine" in another. It is particularly important that the kitchen staff be trained and understand the differences among the categories so that they know what to prepare and send on a patient's tray when the word "chop" is written next to an item on the patient's menu.

1. *Pureed foods:* foods that are combined in a blender with a moderate amount of liquid to a creamy consistency, like that of thick soup, pureed foods require no chewing. Suggested foods: ice cream, ice milk, sherbet, thinned plain yogurt, mashed

potatoes, pureed soft cooked egg, cheese melted into other foods, "blenderized" cottage cheese, creamed wheat cereal, and pureed fruits and vegetables.
2. *Thick liquids:* nectar, sherbet, ice cream, custard, thickened soups, thinned plain yogurt, and eggnog.
3. *Ground foods:* foods put through a food grinder to break down the fiber and connective tissue content so that the food requires little or no chewing. Suggested foods: all ground meats, bite-sized vegetables, junior baby foods, soft canned fruits in bite-sized pieces, custards, moist cake, and soups without chunks of meat or vegetables. Avoid fibrous vegetables such as asparagus, celery, corn, peas, lettuce, and cabbage and fruits with pits, skins, or connective tissue such as oranges or grapefruit.
4. *Finely chopped foods:* foods chopped into pieces smaller than ¼ in, including meats, starches, and vegetables; some chewing is required. Finely chopped foods have the consistency of uncooked hamburger meat.
5. *Chopped foods:* foods chopped into ¼-in chunks, including meats, vegetables, and fruits, to decrease the content of fiber or connective tissue; chopped foods require a fair amount of chewing. They are good for patients who need texture in their diet to stimulate saliva production or sensation or who need to practice chewing. Suggested foods: all meats, flaked fish, bite-sized vegetables, soft canned fruits, some fresh fruits (cut in small pieces without the skin or membranes), tuna or egg salad, pasta or noodles, baked potato, scrambled or soft cooked egg, and hot cereals. Avoid fibrous, stringy vegetables, berries, cherries, and raisins.

6. *Cut foods:* foods that are cut into ½-in pieces for those patients who are unable to cut their food themselves.

It should be noted that making consistency modifications is a time-consuming task for the kitchen personnel, and they may become upset by the frequent and confusing requests for consistency changes. The dietitian should take the time to educate the kitchen staff about dysphagia and its treatment. The kitchen staff can also monitor a dysphagic patient's progress from the changes in the food consistencies being sent.

## CONCLUSION

Treatment of the dysphagic patient is a team effort. It requires the input of many health care professionals. The presence of a dysphagia team, either formal or informal, does not guarantee that the problem will be recognized. The dietitian is usually the first person to observe patients eating or trying to eat. As such, the dietitian should take the time to watch them. The dietitian should also know the patients' diagnoses and learn at least the basics of the physiology of chewing and swallowing. These are, after all, the prerequisites for all nutrition care.

**REFERENCES**

Bove, N., & Kagel, M. (1983). *Dysphagia diet.* Chester, PA: Crozer-Chester Medical Center.

Elizabethtown Hospital and Rehabilitation Center. (1984). *Dysphagia diet.* Elizabethtown, PA: Author.

Lee-Bradford, K. (1981). *Dysphagia and its dietary treatment—a review for dietitians.* New York: Author.

Pruyn, J.F., deJong, P.C., Bosman, L.J., & Van Poppel, J.W. (1986). Psychological aspects of head and neck cancer: A review of the literature. *Clinics in Otolaryngology, 11,* 469–474.

# Chapter 9

# Nutrition Implications in Esophageal and Gastric Cancer

*Abby S. Bloch*

Cancer of the esophagus and stomach profoundly affects the nutrition status of patients. Although the cure rate remains poor for both, the incidence of esophageal cancer is low in the United States (3.5 per 100,000 for white males) except among the Black population (13 per 100,000 for Black males). The incidence varies in different regions of the world, being high in Iran and certain provinces of China. No common cause has been linked with geographic occurrences. Factors that have been implicated include nitrosamines, alcohol, socioeconomic status, deficient diet, and exposure to opium tars and tobacco.

The incidence of gastric cancer has been decreasing in the United States since the 1930s, when it was the most frequent cause of cancer-related death (Lawrence, 1986). The mortality rates show a great deal of geographic variation. Although many studies have attempted to delineate the factors causing such variations, no etiologic factors have been clearly defined. The incidence of gastric cancer seems to increase as a function of distance from the equator. Poorer socioeconomic classes are more prone to develop gastric cancer than affluent ones. No rural-urban or occupational differences have been found to explain these findings, however (Haenszel & Correa, 1975).

## INCIDENCE AND CLINICAL FEATURES OF ESOPHAGEAL CANCER

Cancer of the esophagus accounts for 1% to 2% of all cancers, occurring three times as frequently in men as in women. Esophageal cancer occurs most often in those 70 to 80 years old. The tumors may not cause symptoms until the esophagus has been completely encompassed. Therefore, symptoms may be present for many months before diagnosis. As a result, 50% of patients already have metastases at the time of diagnosis. Squamous cell carcinoma accounts for 95% of cancers involving the body of the esophagus. When systemic spread occurs, the liver and lungs are commonly involved. Adenocarcinoma is common in the esophagogastric junction.

The average survival time of untreated patients is about 4 months. Dysphagia is the primary symptom and is usually the focus of palliation. Until early diagnosis is possible, long-term survival and cure will be difficult to achieve (Ellis, 1983).

Dysphagia becomes apparent first with ingestion of bulky foods and then progresses to soft foods and ultimately to liquids. Weight loss, regurgitation, and aspiration pneumonitis may also occur. Some patients experience hoarseness, coughing, fever, or choking. Other patients may have pain on swallowing. If a large mass is invading the lower esophageal sphincter, gastroesophageal reflux may occur.

The wide range of therapeutic regimens used in treating esophageal cancer reflects the overall poor results achieved with any form of therapy. All treatment modalities, including chemotherapy, radiation therapy, and surgery, are used alone or in combination together with palliative procedures for relief of dysphagia or pain.

## NUTRITION MANAGEMENT: ESOPHAGEAL CANCER PATIENTS

When evaluating a patient who presents with dysphagia or pain related to eating or swallowing, the clinician must determine the severity of the dysphagia. Is the patient's intake adequate to meet nutrition requirements? Would supplements of a nutritionally complete drink or snack augment an inadequate intake enough to meet the daily needs of the patient? To what degree is the patient able to eat solids? What kind of and how much fluid is being consumed? The patient may also be anorectic, a frequently concomitant occurrence.

The occurrence and degree of nausea or vomiting are also important for the clinician to discern. Does it occur before or only after ingestion of food? Does the patient experience symptoms after reclining or eating a large volume, or do they occur at specific times of the day?

On the basis of this initial screening and a weight history, other parameters of nutrition assessment, and the patient's medical history and physical examination, the clinician needs to evaluate the patient's degree of risk for malnutrition. Foods or drinks that are of high caloric density and of a texture tolerated by the patient may meet daily caloric and nutrient requirements. By being offered moist, soft, textured foods in small pieces that can be easily swallowed, the patient may be able to consume an adequate volume of food. Nevertheless, patients are usually afraid and reluctant to eat, so that strong encouragement and emphasis on the importance of eating must be given by the clinician and other members of the health care team.

Family members should be encouraged to be supportive without being overbearing. The patient is frequently depressed and overwhelmed by the disease and the accompanying debility. Family members who constantly harass the patient who has no appetite and finds eating a herculean task tend to create additional anxiety and tension for the dysphagic patient.

Another problem encountered by the esophageal cancer patient is reflux while eating or shortly after eating. Two mechanisms have been proposed to account for these symptoms: a weakening of the antireflux barrier by a direct reduction in pressure of the lower esophageal sphincter (LES), and a direct irritative effect of certain foods on the esophagus (Murphy & Castell, 1988). Tests to determine effects of various foods on LES pressure have shown that chocolates, fats, alcohol, coffee, and carminatives lower LES tone and thus cause the symptoms of heartburn, gas, and regurgitation (carminatives are defined as volatile oil extracts of plants used for flavoring foods such as oil of spearmint, peppermint, garlic, and onion [Murphy & Castell, 1988]).

Other foods reported to cause discomfort because of their high acid content (such as coffee, orange juice, and tomato juice) do not lower LES pressure and are not acidic in relation to gastric acid. The characteristics of these items that cause the irritation or problem appear to be related to their high osmolality, not their acidity. Proteins increase LES pressure, and carbohydrates cause no change in the pressure. Therefore, a high-protein, low-fat, high–complex carbohydrate diet and omission of those foods causing symptoms is advised.

When symptoms occur, the patient must be placed in a sitting or upright position while eating. Patients who are bedridden must be propped up enough to allow foods easy access to the stomach and gastrointestinal tract and to prevent reflux of foods and liquids into the esophagus. The patient must be advised to chew all foods thoroughly, to eat slowly, and to divide total daily food intake into small, frequent feedings rather than large meals (which usually discourage patients in their attempts to eat).

Like dysphagic patients, individuals with reflux should select foods that are high in caloric density if fat can be tolerated. Patients who have had vagotomies may be fat intolerant and must be evaluated for their ability to handle fats efficiently. If fat malabsorption is present, then care must be taken to prescribe a diet with a reasonable fat content that the patient can consume without developing steatorrhea. Loss of fat-soluble vitamins and minerals that bind with free fatty acids and form insoluble soaps may result (see Chapter 11 for a comprehensive review of malabsorption).

Another possible effect of vagotomies is gastric stasis. Patients experience early satiety and difficulty eating enough to meet daily nutrient needs. Distention and discomfort are usual symptoms when gastric stasis occurs. Diarrhea or frequent bowel activity may also be experienced by some patients. Queasiness or vomiting sometimes occurs. Small, frequent feedings and foods that do not cause additional distress should be selected. Some experimentation with food choices and response to foods is necessary to determine which foods are best tolerated by each individual. Foods that may create flatulence or distress should be eaten in small amounts until a confirmation of tolerance is made. Screening for foods that cause heartburn, abdominal pain, or aspiration should be included in the initial assessment. Taking a history for odynophagia (pain on swallowing), choking, or a feeling of food sticking in the throat may identify other limitations affecting the nutrition status of the patient.

Other medically related data include presence of fatigue, anemia, dehydration, esophageal varices, coughing on swallowing, and chronic obstructive pulmonary disease. Standard assessment procedures should be performed for these patients, and weight and laboratory values should be measured.

## SPECIFIC THERAPIES: ESOPHAGEAL CANCER PATIENTS

The reported results of radiation therapy vary widely, with 5-year survival rates ranging from 1% to 8%. Palliation of dysphagia is usually brief and occurs in 66% of treated patients or fewer (Ellis, 1983).

For patients undergoing radiation therapy, results of evaluation for esophagitis, stomatitis, xerostomia, early satiety, and reflux will influence the nutrition care plan. Patients should avoid possible irritants such as acidic foods, caffeine-containing items, and foods that are difficult to chew. Small, frequent feedings that have a high moisture content increase the total daily intake. Elevating the head and shoulders above the stomach decreases the risk of aspiration and reflux. Reflux esophagitis may cause vomiting and heartburn. A high-protein, moderate-fat diet eaten in small, frequent feedings is suggested. Any food that may be irritating to the esophagus should be avoided.

Chemotherapy can produce myelosuppression, cardiotoxicity, nephrotoxicity, and hepatotoxicity. Nausea, vomiting, xerostomia, constipation, and diarrhea are all possible depending on the type of chemotherapy and the protocol used. Adjustments in dietary recommendations should be consistent with the problem affecting the patient's nutrition status (see Chapter 16 for management options).

Surgery involving the esophagus may result in anemia, gastric atony or stasis, reflux esophagitis, diarrhea or steatorrhea, early satiety, or malabsorption syndrome. Vitamin $B_{12}$ and iron deficiencies may occur in this group. Therefore, patients with esophagectomies or esophagogastrectomies should be monitored for these nutrients. Laser surgery may also be used for palliation and dilatation. If oral intake is contraindicated for more than several days, enteral or parenteral nutrition should be instituted. Once oral intake resumes, the patient progresses from clear liquids to full liquids of 35 to 40 g of fat and low lactose content. The ultimate goal is five or six small, dry meals that are high in protein and contain 45 to 50 g of fat. As tolerance improves, meal size and fat content can be increased. Finally, fluids may be incorporated into the meal.

## DYSPHAGIA DIETS DESIGNED FOR ANTIASPIRATION

The goal of antiaspiration diets is to reduce the risk of aspiration and choking in patients with swallowing difficulties. This diet needs to provide foods that can be controlled and moved in the patient's mouth.

The diet progresses in stages according to consistency and texture of foods: liquids, thin and thick purees, soft foods, solid moist foods, and dry foods. Oral supplementation or enteral nutrition support may be needed to meet nutrition requirements because patients may be deficient in one or more nutrients as a result of the limited selection of items and volume consumed (see Chapter 8 on dysphagia). Exhibit 9-1 shows the diet levels and progressions that are used for managing dysphagic patients. The diet level used depends on the patient's ability to control the items offered. If appropriate, several stages may be collapsed into one for the maximum possible selection.

## INCIDENCE AND CLINICAL FEATURES OF GASTRIC CANCER

Since the 1930s, when gastric cancer was the most frequent cause of cancer-related death in the United States, the incidence of this disease has declined from 33 per 100,000 to 8 per 100,000 (Pocinki, 1988). Approximately 24,000 new cases are diagnosed each year. The disease is now the sixth most common cause of cancer-related death in the United States, but its mortality rate is declining. The drop in mortality is due to the decline in incidence, however, not to improvements in treatment. Each year about 14,000 people die of gastric cancer in the United States.

Gastric cancer remains relatively common in Japan, Chile, Colombia, Iceland, and Scandinavia; Nigeria, India, and the United States have the lowest rates. Stomach cancer is generally a disease of middle and later life, peaking in the age range from 50 to 60 years. Nonwhites develop the disease twice as often as whites (Pocinki, 1988). On the basis of studies of Japanese immigrants living in the United States, which show that the incidence of gastric cancer is as high as in the region in which the immigrants had spent their first 20 years of life, it is

suggested that dietary or other environmental factors are significant causes of gastric cancer.

Nitrate and nitrite consumption has been associated with increased incidences of stomach and esophageal cancer in Japan, Iran, China, the United States, England, Chile, and Colombia. Nitrosamines, which are carcinogenic, can be synthesized by bacteria in the stomach from ingested nitrates. These bacteria are usually killed by the acid present in normal stomachs; this may be why clinical conditions such as pernicious anemia, atrophic gastritis, hypochlorhydria, and achlorhydria have been associated with a high incidence of gastric cancer (Hitchcock, MacLean, & Sullivan, 1957).

Specific diets or dietary components in various populations appear to contain other carcinogenic agents. For example, salted meats and corn, which are eaten in large volumes in Colombia, may contain carcinogens. In Japan, talc-dusted rice containing asbestos has been linked to the high incidence of gastric cancer in that country. Consumption of smoked and singed foods (containing 3,4-benzopyrene), which is frequent among Icelanders, correlates with an increased incidence of gastric cancer.

The term stomach cancer usually refers to adenocarcinoma (arising in the glandular tissue). Adenocarcinomas account for 97% of all stomach cancers. The tumor can grow along the stomach wall into the esophagus or small intestine, or it may extend through the wall into the liver, pancreas, colon, peritoneum, or ovaries. Lymph nodes are frequently involved. If tumor cells enter the bloodstream, the liver, lungs, bone, and brain may become involved.

Most gastric cancers develop in the pylorus or lower portion of the stomach. The disease is less common in the body of the stomach and least common in the cardia. Recently, however, the number of cases occurring in the upper part of the stomach seems to be increasing.

Prognosis for gastric carcinoma remains poor because two-thirds of patients have either physical or operative findings at the time of diagnosis, which eliminates the possibility of surgical cure. Early gastric cancers are now increasingly diagnosed with the flexible fiberoptic gastroscope. Radiologic examination as well

**Exhibit 9-1** Dysphagia Diet Levels

Stage I—Dysphagia puree, no liquids
Stage II—Dysphagia puree plus thick liquids
Stage III—Dysphagia puree plus thin liquids
Stage IV—Dysphagia mechanical soft foods, no liquids
Stage V—Dysphagia mechanical soft foods plus thick liquids
Stage VI—Dysphagia mechanical soft foods plus thin liquids

**Stage I—Dysphagia Puree, No Liquids**

No liquids will be provided unless specified by physician's order. Includes smooth, moist, and pureed foods that require little or no chewing but form a moist, cohesive bolus.

| Food Group | Foods Allowed | Foods Avoided |
|---|---|---|
| Milk products | Pudding, custard, ice cream, plain or flavored yogurt (without fruit) | All others |
| Meat, poultry, and eggs | Pureed meat, chicken, fish; soufflés, soft cooked or poached eggs | All others |
| Vegetables and fruits | Pureed vegetables, fruits; applesauce | All others |
| Breads and cereals | Thick cooked cereals, mashed potato | All others |
| Fats | Butter, margarine, sour cream | All others |
| Miscellaneous | Salt, pepper, ketchup, mustard, jelly, gelatin dessert | None |

**Stage II—Dysphagia Puree Plus Thick Liquids**

Includes all foods allowed in stage I with the addition of the following *thick liquids*.

| Food Group | Liquids Allowed | Liquids Avoided |
|---|---|---|
| Milk products | Thickened eggnog, Carnation Instant Breakfast, milk shakes | All others |
| Soups | Thick creamed soups | Broth |
| Fruits | Thinned pureed fruits | All others |

**Stage III—Dysphagia Puree Plus Thin Liquids**

Includes all foods allowed in stage II with the addition of the following *thin liquids*.

| Food Group | Liquids Allowed | Liquids Avoided |
|---|---|---|
| Milk products | Eggnog, Carnation Instant Breakfast, milk | None |
| Soup | Thin creamed soups, broth | None |
| Beverages | Coffee, tea, soda, fruit juices | None |

*Note:* Once a patient has mastered stage III, the diet can be either progressed in consistency (i.e., to stage V) or changed to puree.

**Stage IV—Dysphagia Mechanical Soft Foods, No Liquids**

No liquids will be provided unless specified by physician's order. Includes minced and soft foods that require little or no chewing but form a soft, cohesive bolus.

| Food Group | Foods Allowed | Foods Avoided |
|---|---|---|
| Milk products | Pudding, custard, ice cream, cream pies; plain, flavored, fruited yogurt | All others |
| Cheeses | Small-curd cottage cheese, ricotta cheese, American cheese, grated cheese | All others |

*continues*

**Exhibit 9-1** continued

| Food Group | Foods Allowed | Foods Avoided |
|---|---|---|
| Eggs | Soft scrambled eggs, crustless quiche, soufflés, egg salad | All others |
| Meat, fish, and poultry | Ground meat or poultry with gravy; chicken or tuna salad (without celery); meat loaf; hamburger; baked or broiled fish; salmon loaf; pasta casseroles | |
| Vegetables | Cooked and diced carrots, beets, chopped or creamed spinach, butternut or acorn squash | Raw vegetables, other cooked vegetables |
| Potatoes, rice, and noodles | Mashed or baked (without skin) potatoes, macaroni and cheese, egg noodles, spaghetti with gravy or sauce | Rice, coarse grain (kasha, buckwheat, bran) |
| Fruit | Mashed banana, canned or cooked fruits cut into small pieces | Fruits with pits, raisins; all others |
| Breads and cereals | Bread, soft rolls, muffins, soft French toast, pancakes, cooked cereal, dry cereals soaked in milk, cakes without nuts | Dry crackers, breads with seeds, raisins, nuts |
| Fats | Butter, margarine, sour cream, gravy, mayonnaise | Nuts, seeds |

**Stage V—Dysphagia Mechanical Soft Foods Plus Thick Liquids**

Includes all food from stage IV with the addition of *thick liquids* as outlined in stage II.

**Stage VI—Dysphagia Mechanical Soft Foods Plus Thin Liquids**

Includes all food from stage IV with the addition of *thin liquids* as outlined in stage III.

*Note:* Once a patient has mastered stage VI, the diet can either be progressed in consistency (i.e., to regular) or changed to mechanical soft foods.

Patients at stages I and IV will need to have fluid status monitored and fluid requirements met by alternate means.

Milk products may not be tolerated by individuals who are susceptible to increased mucus production probably secondary to casein, a milk protein. If this becomes a problem, substitutes should be found.

Suggestions for dietitians:

1. A member of the medical or nursing staff or dysphagia team should be present at the bedside when a patient initially receives a dysphagia diet or advances to a higher stage to evaluate the patient's tolerance of the stage.
2. The dietitian should work closely with medical and nursing staff for continued evaluation of the patient's diet tolerance and progression.
3. Calorie counts are indicated to evaluate adequacy of intake and to justify the need for supplementation or nutrition support.
4. The dietitian should work closely with the dysphagia team for physiologic evaluation of the patient's ability to chew and swallow to select the correct diet stage.
5. The dietitian should encourage small, frequent meals, particularly in the first stages of the diet.
6. As a guide, the following list gives a progression of food consistencies in order of increasing swallowing difficulty:
   - stiff jelled consistency
   - standard jelled consistency
   - thick purees
   - applesauce consistency
   - thick soup consistency
   - nectar consistency
   - standard thin liquids
   - chunk consistency (ground or diced)

**Exhibit 9-1** continued

Eating tips:
1. Food should be taken in small portions (½ tsp at a time).
2. The patient should sit upright with hips flexed at a 90° angle.
3. If possible, the neck should be at a 90° angle and flexed slightly forward.
4. The patient should sit up for 15 to 30 minutes both before and after meals.
5. Food should be placed on the unaffected side when possible.
6. Cold or hot foods may be better tolerated than foods at room temperature.

*Source:* From "Antiaspiration-Dysphagia Diet" in the Memorial Sloan-Kettering Cancer Center *Diet Manual*, 1989. Reprinted by permission.

as computerized tomography and ultrasonography provide information about the size, location, and extent of the tumor. The extent of gastric resection can then be more accurately planned (Shiu, 1989). If a total gastrectomy is performed the type of reconstruction affects food passage, reservoir function, and proper mixing of food with duodenal, bile, and pancreatic juices while preventing bile reflux. Esophagoduodenal or jejunal anastomosis may cause severe reflux esophagitis. A jejunal pouch or interposition between the esophagus and duodenum provides good reservoir function. This enables better nutrition absorption and fewer problems than other procedures (Shiu, 1989).

Currently, no more than one-third of patients who are considered candidates for curative resection live 5 years or longer after treatment. (Lawrence, 1986). Gastric cancers that develop in the pyloric portion of the stomach tend to have a better prognosis than lesions in the upper or middle parts of the stomach (Shiu et al., 1987). Lesions requiring total gastrectomy or proximal gastrectomy generally have a poorer outlook than those requiring distal gastric resection. Patients with extensive lesions involving the entire stomach have the poorest prognosis (Lawrence, McNeer, Pack, Paglia, & Ashley, 1967). The presence of lymphatic metastases is the most significant prognostic variable. Patients without lymphatic metastases who are candidates for curative radical gastrectomy are the only group with a reasonably good prognosis: about 50% have long-term survival.

Gastric cancer is difficult to diagnose at an early stage because no identifying signs or symptoms are specifically associated with early gastric cancer. Most patients present with nonspecific gastrointestinal complaints such as vague gastric discomfort or indigestion. Some may experience vomiting, heartburn, or distention or complain of fullness or excessive belching. Patients may try to relieve these symptoms with antacids or by changing their diet. Of all patients, 5% to 10% have complaints similar to those of peptic ulcer disease; others may have nonspecific symptoms such as anemia, fatigue, or weight loss. Occasionally patients present with acute problems such as upper gastrointestinal bleeding, obstruction, or perforation.

## FUNCTIONS OF THE STOMACH

The stomach prepares food mechanically and chemically to move into the small intestine for digestion and absorption. The size of the stomach continually changes. When empty it is about the size of a sausage; when full it expands to many times that size. Sphincters control the openings at each end of the stomach. The esophageal sphincter allows food to move into the stomach. The pyloric sphincter allows food to pass into the duodenum.

The stomach is divided into four sections: the cardia, which surrounds the esophageal sphincter; the fundus, in the upper left quadrant of the stomach; the body, in the central region of the stomach; and the pylorus, which opens into the pyloric sphincter. The short part of the stomach is known as the lesser curvature and the outer bend as the greater curvature. Glands found in the mucosa lining the stomach wall secrete gastric juices made of mixtures of enzymes and hydrochloric acid, which are needed to digest food. Mucus, also secreted by the mucosa, protects the lining from the damaging effect of these secretions.

Several minutes after food enters the stomach, gentle rippling or agitation begins mixing the food with gastric juices. Peristalsis reduces the food to a thick slurry. As digestion continues, more vigorous mixing occurs in the body of the stomach and intensifies in the pylorus. Each wave forces a small amount of food through the pyloric sphincter into the duodenum. The normal stomach empties its contents in 2 to 4 hours after food is consumed.

The primary chemical activity of the stomach is to begin protein digestion by the action of gastric juices. The gastric glands secrete pepsinogen, the inactive form of pepsin, which is activated when it comes into contact with hydrochloric acid. This prevents the pepsin from digesting the lining of the stomach when food is not present. The stomach also secretes an intrinsic factor needed for the absorption of vitamin $B_{12}$.

## NUTRITION MANAGEMENT: GASTRIC CANCER PATIENTS

Once a general nutrition history and screening have been completed to establish the patient's baseline nutrition status, the clinician needs to develop a care plan that is based on the patient's therapeutic plans. If the patient is preoperative, a diet containing adequate protein and kilocalorie needs should be provided. If the patient has been identified as being at risk for malnutrition, then protein and kilocalorie requirements should be increased to provide appropriate needs before surgery. Patients are considered at risk if they have lost more than 15% body weight within 6 months or 10% within 3 months. Patients should be considered at risk if their weight is 15% or more below their desirable weight.

After the patient undergoes surgery, the clinician should determine whether both sphincters are intact. If not, then the possibility of reflux and rapid transit of food needs to be considered. Rapid transit may produce cramps, distention,

dumpinglike symptoms, and diarrhea. In such cases, patients are encouraged to eat slowly in small, frequent feedings. Eating solids separately from liquids may delay emptying somewhat. Foods with a high osmotic load may also cause increased activity of the bolus as it leaves the stomach. Therefore, foods high in concentrated sweets should be tested in small amounts before the consumption of normal portions. Exhibit 9-2 provides some further recommendations for diets for gastric cancer patients.

If the upper stomach has been removed, then the patient may experience early satiety as a result of the decreased capacity of the stomach. Small, frequent feedings similar to those described in Exhibit 9-2 should be recommended to the patient. If the esophagus was involved and if any of the problems mentioned in Exhibit 9-2 is present, management must address these as well. For patients with a partial gastrectomy, a high–caloric density drink or feeding is beneficial as a between-meal feeding. This increases caloric intake while decreasing symptoms of fullness, crampiness, and distention when too much food is consumed at one time. Providing adequate caloric intake and nutrient requirements must be carefully considered when patients' intake is diminished.

As with esophageal reflux, gastric reflux may occur as a result of the loss of the esophageal sphincter with a partial or total gastrectomy. Again, the patient should be counseled that chewing thoroughly, eating slowly, and positioning himself or herself upright while eating all decrease the possibility of reflux.

Fat intolerance may be seen in patients who have gastrectomies, especially if the vagus nerves were severed during surgery. A low-fat intake is advised until the patient begins to tolerate increased volumes of foods high in fat. Because of the high caloric potential of fat, decreased fat in the diet may significantly decrease caloric intake. Therefore, the patient will need to make a concerted effort to consume enough calories without the use of fat. Eating foods that contain complex carbohydrates such as flours, grains, and starches should be emphasized. Fat is inherent in most protein, so that increasing the protein content of the diet will

**Exhibit 9-2** Recommended Dietary Progressions for Patients with Gastric Cancer

Progress from clear liquids to regular liquids with between-meal feedings *after a proximal subtotal gastrectomy.* There is little potential for dumping because the pylorus is intact. Between-meal feedings are important to help offset inadequate caloric intake due to the reduced capacity of the stomach. Monitor for diarrhea and steatorrhea secondary to vagotomy.

*Postgastrectomy diet progression:* after a total gastrectomy, radical subtotal gastrectomy, or hemigastrectomy (pylorus removed), follow these recommendations:

1. Low–simple carbohydrate, clear-liquid diet.
   *Example:*   Coffee or tea (limit to 3 oz)
   Sugar substitute
   Apple juice (6 oz)
   Low-fat broth (3 oz)
   Sugar-free gelatin
   Sugar-free ginger ale
2. Advance to a low-lactose, low–simple carbohydrate, low-fat, full-liquid diet (five feedings).
   *Example:*   Apple juice (6 oz)
   Low-fat broth (3 oz)
   Eggs: soft, medium, or scrambled
   Cereal: farina, Cream of Wheat, Cream of Rice
   Mashed potatoes
   Low-lactose milk
   Tea or coffee with sugar substitute (limit to 3 oz)
   Sugar-free ginger ale
   Between-meal nourishments (unsweetened gelatin or custard)
3. Advance to a low-lactose, low–simple carbohydrate, high-protein, moderate-fat diet with liquids between meals (five feedings).
4. Gradually increase the fat content of the diet in 10-g increments.
5. Gradually test lactose tolerance with 5 to 6 g of lactose (equivalent to ½ c of milk).
6. Gradually increase vegetable and fruit content of the diet so that the patient is on a regular diet without concentrated sweets (five feedings) as tolerated.
7. Negative lymph nodes: recommend vitamin $B_{12}$ with iron supplementation to physician.
8. Positive lymph nodes: be less aggressive regarding vitamin and mineral supplementation.

Assess for signs of dumping:

1. Early (10 to 40 minutes after meals): bloating, pain, vomiting, diarrhea
2. Late (1 to 3 hours after meals): weakness, tiredness, faintness, dizziness, sweating, headaches, nausea, warmth, palpitations, dyspnea

It is common for postgastrectomy patients to complain of lack of appetite and early satiety. If the patient is unable to achieve adequate intake, ongoing dietary counseling will be necessary.

*Source:* From ''Process Criteria for Patients with Gastric Cancer'' in the Memorial Sloan-Kettering Cancer Center *Diet Manual,* 1989. Reprinted by permission.

tend to increase the fat content as well. If the patient will eat egg whites or fat-free dairy products, a wide selection of foods will be available.

Milk intolerance is also prevalent in many patients who have gastrectomies. The degree of intolerance is important to address in the nutrition advice given to the patient. If a mild intolerance appears to be present, then somewhat liberal use of products can be considered. A small amount of low-fat milk in coffee or cereal may be tolerated. Cheese may also cause little or no distress. Yogurt usually causes no problems for otherwise lactose-sensitive patients. Most patients can take some milk and milk-containing products. The clinician must determine how much is acceptable and to what degree the intolerance will become symptomatic.

When partial gastrectomies are in the lower remnant of the stomach, dumping syndrome is possible as a result of rapid transit of foods and liquids through the stomach and the dilutional response of the small remnant to high-osmotic bolus feedings. Again, small, frequent feedings must be recommended to these patients. Foods of low osmotic concentration should be encouraged. Generally, concentrated sweets such as sugar, jams, icings, frostings, and other sugar-containing foods are discouraged. These include honey, molasses, fructose, soft drinks, ices, and ice creams.

Separating liquids from solids frequently helps slow down the bolus leaving the stomach and prevents a rapid movement of the bolus through the gastrointestinal tract. In slowing down the bolus, the patient is spared the symptoms that accompany rapid transit such as cramping, distention, and diarrhea. If dumping syndrome is present, flushing, decreased blood pressure with tachycardia, and sweating may be experienced by the patient toward the end of the meal or immediately after eating. If dilution of the bolus increases transit through the gastrointestinal tract, then symptoms occur 1 to 1½ hours after the meal.

Because of the discomfort and embarrassment experienced by many patients after eating, they often elect not to eat rather than to suffer or be embarrassed. Nutrition is compromised for these reasons as well as inadequate intake and utilization. The clinician must monitor the patient for the possibility of nutrition deficit and institute nutrition management before the patient becomes malnourished and develops concomitant medical complications.

As was found in a recent study (Nishi et al., 1988), esophagectomy and esophagogastrectomy are associated with a high rate of complications, mainly pulmonary complications and anastomotic leakage. A preoperative nutrition assessment for these patients is mandatory. As the investigators in this study state, in recent years aggressive nutrition support and proper nutrition assessment during the perioperative period have become essential to achieving a satisfactory recovery because the operations for esophageal and gastric cancer have become more radical and more extensive. These investigators conclude that it is imperative to clarify the relationship between anastomotic leaks and the nutrition status in cancer patients (Nishi et al., 1988).

Experience has shown that many patients with esophageal or gastric cancer require enteral nutrition management to meet their nutrition needs. After all the above means have been exhausted, if the patient is still at nutrition risk enteral feeding should be instituted. Although nasoenteric feedings are the easiest and least invasive of enteric feeding methods, the use of percutaneous endoscopically placed gastrostomy (PEG) or jejunostomy (PEJ) tubes has been successful in this population (Shike, Schroy, Morse, & Richie, 1987). For long-term feeding, such tubes offer the patient a simple, unobtrusive means of nourishing himself or herself when oral intake is inadequate. (Shike et al., 1989). At Memorial Sloan-Kettering Cancer Center, PEG or PEJ feedings have been found to be a viable alternative to other modalities of nutrition support in this patient population. More than 200 home patients have used this method of management successfully; of these 25% were esophageal or gastric cancer patients. The complication rate in cancer patients with PEGs compares favorably with that for surgically placed gastrostomies and PEGs in patients with nonmalignant diseases, indicating that cancer patients are not at increased risk for developing complications from this procedure (Shike & Brennan, 1989).

## CONCLUSION

Both esophageal and gastric cancer create nutrition problems in the short and long term. Dietitians and nutritionists are faced with a challenge of providing solutions to physical and emotional roadblocks to adequate intake. Attention must be given at regular intervals to mechanical limitations, biochemical changes, nutrient deficiencies or depletion, and poor intake. Patients are at high risk for malnutrition from the time of diagnosis. Nutrition support should be an integral part of any medical management given. Patients and families need guidance and direction in daily selections and food choices. Having a responsive health professional who can give practical suggestions and hints about what to prepare and serve provides a much needed boost to these individuals during a stressful and difficult time.

## REFERENCES

Ellis, F.H. (1983). Carcinoma of the esophagus. *CA—A Cancer Journal for Clinicians, 33,* 4–21.

Haenszel, W., & Correa, P. (1975). Developments in the epidemiology of stomach cancer over the past decade. *Cancer Research, 35,* 3452–3459.

Hitchcock, C.R., MacLean, L.D., & Sullivan, A. (1957). The secretory and clinical aspects of achlorhydria and gastric atrophy as precursors of gastric cancer. *Journal of the National Cancer Institute, 18,* 795–811.

Lawrence, W.J. (1986). Gastric Cancer. *CA—A Cancer Journal for Clinicians, 36,* 5–25.

Lawrence, W.J., McNeer, G., Pack, G.T., Paglia, M.A., & Ashley, M.P. (1967). End results and prognosis. In G. McNeer & G.T. Pack (Eds.), *Neoplasms of the stomach* (pp. 447–491). Philadelphia: Lippincott.

Murphy, D.W., & Castell, D.O. (1988). Nutrition and gastrointestinal disease. In K. Jeejeebhoy (Ed.), *Current therapy in nutrition* (pp. 89–94). Toronto: Decker.

Nishi, M., Hiramatsu, Y., Koshiro, H., Kojima, Y., Samada, T., Yamanaka, H., & Yamamoto, M. (1988). Risk factors in relation to postoperative complications in patients undergoing esophagectomy or gastrectomy for cancer. *Annals of Surgery, 207,* 148–154.

Pocinki, K.M. (1988). *Cancer of the stomach* (Research Report #88-2978, pp. 1–18). Bethesda, MD: National Cancer Institute.

Shike, M., Berner, Y., Gerdes, H., Gerrold, F., Bloch, A., Sessions, R., & Strong, E. (1989). Percutaneous endoscopic gastrostomy and jejunostomy for long-term enteral feeding in patients with cancer of the head and neck. *Otolaryngology and Head and Neck Surgery, 103,* 549–554.

Shike, M., & Brennan, M.F. (1989). Supportive care of the cancer patient—Nutrition support. In V.T. DeVita, S. Hellman, and S.A. Rosenberg (Eds.), *Cancer: Principles and practice of oncology* (3rd ed., pp. 2029–2044). Philadelphia: Lippincott.

Shike, M., Schroy, P., Morse, R., & Richie, M.A. (1987). Percutaneous endoscopic jejunostomy in cancer patients with previous gastric resection. *Gastrointestinal Endoscopy, 33,* 372–374.

Shiu, M.H. (1989). Gastric tumors. In J.L. Cameron (Ed.), *Current surgical therapy—3* (pp. 44–51). Toronto: Decker.

Shiu, M.H., Moore, E., Sanders, M., Huvos, A., Freedman, B., Goodbold, J., Chaiyaphruk, S., Wesdorp, R., & Brennan, M. (1987). Influence of the extent of resection on survival after curative treatment of gastric carcinoma. *Archives of Surgery, 122,* 1347–1351.

# Chapter 10

# Nutrition Problems Caused by Pancreatic, Liver, or Renal Cancer

*Diana Fullen Bowers*

The pancreas, liver, and kidneys perform vital functions that are necessary to maintain the nutrition health of the body. Primary or metastatic carcinomas in these organs have the potential to disrupt their ability to regulate nutrition homeostasis. Little can be done to alter the systemic effects of cancer on nutrition status. The clinician can, however, provide a better quality of life for the patient through nutrition management of the various problems created by carcinomas arising from or metastasizing to these organs.

This chapter discusses the incidence and etiology of carcinoma of the pancreas, liver, and kidneys; nutrition problems created by cancer in these organs; and methods of management of identified nutrition problems.

## NUTRITION CONCERNS IN CANCER OF THE PANCREAS

### Anatomy and Function of the Pancreas

The pancreas is a lobular, elongated gland located in the retroperitoneum (Fig. 10-1). It ranges from 15 to 20 cm in length and can weigh 80 to 90 g (Tersigni & Toledo-Pereyra, 1985; Mackie & Moossa, 1980). The pancreas is subdivided into five anatomic portions: the head, neck, body, tail, and ulcinate process. The ulcinate process is a part of the head that hooks around behind the pancreatic blood vessels (Tersigni & Toledo-Pereyra, 1985). Several ducts are embedded in the gland that join to supply the gastrointestinal tract with pancreatic digestive juices (Tersigni & Toledo-Pereyra, 1985; Cooper & Moossa, 1980). The main pancreatic duct, called the duct of Wirsung, begins close to the tail of the gland and crosses the body and head, eventually emptying into the gastrointestinal tract. This is the chief excretory duct of the pancreas. Other ducts, including the duct of Santorini and secondary pancreatic ducts, also help drain the pancreas and provide pancreatic juices to the gastrointestinal tract. The common bile duct extends on or through the pancreatic head from the gallbladder to the duodenal wall (Tersigni & Toledo-Pereyra, 1985). Bile salts necessary for the digestion of dietary fats are delivered to the intestine through this duct.

### The Exocrine Pancreas

The pancreas has both exocrine and endocrine functions. The major exocrine function of the pancreas is the secretion of enzymes and bicarbonate into the duodenum to facilitate the digestion of nutrients. This secretion is stimulated

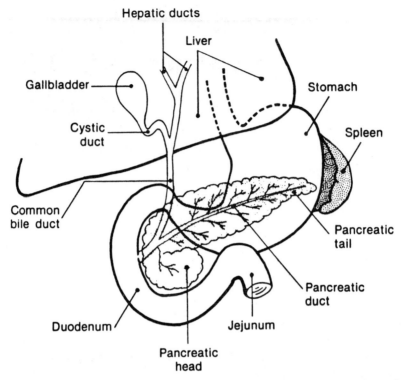

**Figure 10-1** Anatomical Location of the Pancreas. *Source:* From *Applied Biochemistry of Clinical Disorders* (p. 199) by A.G. Gornall (Ed.), 1986, Philadelphia: J.B. Lippincott Company. Copyright 1986 by J.B. Lippincott Company. Reprinted by permission.

primarily by the gut hormones secretin and cholecystokinin-pancreozymin (CCK-PZ) (Cooper & Moossa, 1980; Onstad & Bubrick, 1985). The pancreas has such a large reserve capacity in terms of its exocrine secretion that pancreatic function must be decreased by approximately 90% before the digestion of protein and fat is clearly impaired (Onstad & Bubrick, 1985; Greenberger & Toskes, 1987).

The exocrine cells of the pancreas produce two types of secretions. The first type contains fluid with a high concentration of bicarbonate. The bicarbonate acts to lower the acid content of the chyme coming into the duodenum from the stomach so that the pancreatic enzymes can work. This fluid also contains sodium, potassium, and, to a lesser extent, calcium, zinc, and magnesium. From 1.5 to 4 L of this fluid is produced per day from cells that are found along the ducts of the pancreas (Onstad & Bubrick, 1985).

The second type of secretion from the exocrine pancreas contains a high concentration of pancreatic enzymes. These enzymes are synthesized and stored in the acinar cells of the pancreas and are required for normal digestion of carbohydrate, protein, and fat (Onstad & Bubrick, 1985). The enzyme α-amylase aids in the digestion of complex carbohydrates. Several other enzymes are present that break down proteins to amino acids. Triglyceride (fat) molecules are broken down by several enzymes, including lipase, phospholipase A, and cholesterol esterase. Altogether, 19 different enzymes have been identified in pancreatic exocrine secretions (Onstad & Bubrick, 1985).

A mixture of both secretions is produced in response to oral feeding. The sight and smell of food can produce a prompt increase in secretion. This is known as the cephalic phase and is stimulated by a neural response (Cooper & Moossa, 1980). Maximal secretion of pancreatic juice occurs when food enters the duodenum from the stomach. This is a hormonal response caused by the gastrointestinal hormones secretin and CCK-

PZ. As products of digestion reach the ileum and colon, pancreatic secretion is inhibited, signaling the end of the digestive process (Onstad & Bubrick, 1985).

## Bile Secretion

Bile is made by the liver and stored in the gallbladder. Bile is delivered from the gallbladder to the intestine intermittently in response to a meal through the common bile duct. The secretion of bile provides the bile salts necessary for dietary fat digestion and absorption. The bile duct is also the secretory pathway for many organic compounds, including bilirubin, the breakdown product of hemoglobin.

Pancreatic cancer can cause obstruction of the common bile duct, thus preventing the secretion of bile into the small intestine. When this happens, patients become jaundiced as a result of the build-up of bilirubin and develop fat malabsorption as a result of the absence of bile salts.

## The Endocrine Pancreas

The endocrine cells of the pancreas are grouped into cells known as the islets of Langerhans. These cells are diffusely distributed among the exocrine cells throughout the pancreas and are concentrated in the tail of the gland (Dhorajiwala, Reckard, & Moossa, 1980). Five types of endocrine cells have been identified, each of which secretes a different hormone (Friesen, 1985; Jaspan, Polonsky, Foster, & Rubenstein, 1980; Wynick, Williams, & Bloom, 1988; Foster & Rubenstein, 1987; Greenberger, Toskes, & Isselbacher, 1987). The two major hormones secreted are insulin, from the β cells, and glucagon, from the α cells. Insulin and glucagon play important roles in the regulation of carbohydrate, protein, and fat metabolism. When the endocrine cells become neoplastic or malignant, excessive amounts of their respective hormones can be secreted. Because of the important functions that pancreatic endocrine secretions play in nutrient metabolism, pancreatic endocrine tumors have great significance in nutrition (Table 10-1). The treatment of choice for pancreatic endocrine tumors is surgical resection of the affected area of the pancreas.

## Pancreatic Cancer: Incidence and Clinical Features

Cancer of the pancreas is the fourth most common cancer in the United States today, surpassed in frequency only by cancers of the lung,

**Table 10-1** Entopic Pancreatic Endocrine Tumors

| Cell Type | Hormone | Tumor Type | Symptoms |
|---|---|---|---|
| α | Glucagon | Glucagonoma | Mild diabetes, dermatitis, angular cheilosis, stomatitis, glossitis, weight loss, anemia, decreased plasma amino acids, venous embolisms |
| β | Insulin | Insulinoma | Severe, recurrent hypoglycemia |
| Δ | Somastatin | Somastatinoma | Mild diabetes mellitus, diarrhea, cholelithiasis, steatorrhea, hypochlorhydria, weight loss, dyspepsia, anemia |
| F | Pancreatic polypeptide | Pancreatic polypeptideoma | Asymptomatic |
| Enterochromaffin | Serotonin | Carcinoid syndrome | Hypotension, diarrhea, flushing, wheezing, tachycardia, alcohol intolerance, hepatomegaly, peripheral edema |

colon, and breast. Pancreatic cancer is the second most common malignancy of the gastrointestinal tract. The incidence of pancreatic cancer has increased 300% over the last three decades to approximately 11 cases per 100,000 population (Greenberger et al., 1987; Leichman, 1985).

The most common cancer of the pancreas is adenocarcinoma of ductal origin, which represents about 90% of all pancreatic cancers and mainly affects the exocrine pancreas (Leichman, 1985; Moossa, Lewis, & Bowie, 1980). The disease occurs 50% more frequently in males than in females, and peak incidence is in the age group of 60 to 70 years (Greenberger et al., 1987; Moossa et al., 1980). Risk factors for the development of pancreatic cancer include cigarette smoking, diabetes mellitus, industrial exposure to chemical irritants, alcoholism, dietary factors, exposure to radiation, and ethnic and racial factors (Leichman, 1985; Buncher, 1980). Gold et al. (1985), in a study of dietary risk factors for pancreatic cancer, found significantly decreased risks associated with the consumption of raw fruits and vegetables and diet soda. Significantly increased risk was associated with the consumption of white bread. Risk ratios for coffee consumption were not significantly different (i.e., number of cups per day up to more than five cups per day did not correlate with increased incidence), but there appeared to be a dose-response relationship in women. Many dietary factors have been proposed to play an important role in the initiation or promotion of cancer, but definite cause-and-effect relationships remain to be shown conclusively.

Most pancreatic carcinomas (65%) occur in the head of the pancreas, 30% involve the body and tail, and only 5% are localized in the tail only. The disease is nearly impossible to detect before symptomatic presentation, and at the time of diagnosis approximately 60% of patients have demonstrated distinct metastases. The prognosis for pancreatic cancer is extremely poor, with the median survival time being 6 months from the time of diagnosis. Various diagnostic tests are being evaluated in an attempt to identify at-risk populations and to facilitate early diagnosis in the asymptomatic patient (Leichman, 1985; Malt, 1983).

Classic symptoms of pancreatic cancer include significant weight loss (greater than 10% of normal body weight), abdominal pain, anorexia, jaundice, and constipation or diarrhea (Greenberger et al., 1987; Moossa et al., 1980; Beazley, 1985). Symptoms are usually caused by tumor compression or obstruction of the common bile duct or duodenum. The weight loss associated with pancreatic cancer is approximately 25 pounds (Beazley, 1985) and cannot be explained solely on the basis of malabsorption and anorexia. Abdominal pain is usually mild initially and is confined to the epigastrium or right upper quadrant, occasionally radiating through to the back (Greenberger et al., 1987). As the tumor grows, pain becomes more intense and steady (Janowitz & Banks, 1976).

Anorexia, which further exacerbates weight loss, is associated with reluctance to eat because of postprandial discomfort, pain, or the metabolic effects of the carcinoma. Some patients experience intermittent nausea and vomiting accentuated by food intake. Others may experience a sense of fullness in the upper abdomen or nausea and dyspepsia, which is occasionally relieved by dietary management including small feedings or a bland diet and antacids. Nausea and vomiting often result from invasion of the tumor into the stomach or common bile duct or by blockage of the pancreatic duct, which impairs digestion by inhibiting the secretion of bile and pancreatic juices into the small intestine (Janowitz & Banks, 1976).

Constipation is associated with a decrease in food and fluid intake. The use of narcotic agents for control of pain can also cause constipation (Janowitz & Banks, 1976). Diarrhea can result from fat malabsorption caused by a decrease in pancreatic enzyme secretion or obstruction of the common bile duct. Fat malabsorption is known as steatorrhea. Invasion of the tumor into the stomach, duodenum, or transverse colon can cause gastrointestinal bleeding.

Jaundice occurs in 90% of patients with carcinoma of the head of the pancreas. Patients become jaundiced because of invasion and blockage of the common bile duct, which causes a build-up of bilirubin. Jaundice is a late manifestation in cancers involving the body and tail of the pancreas and indicates that the tumor has spread to the head of the pancreas and is obstructing the common bile duct.

Psychologic or emotional disturbances have been described in patients with pancreatic cancer and may include depression, anxiety, insomnia, restlessness, rage, and a sense of impending doom. These symptoms appear to be associated to a greater extent with pancreatic cancer than with any other malignant or nonmalignant disease. In most patients, these symptoms appear after organic symptoms (Greenberger et al., 1987; Beazley, 1985).

## Nutrition Therapy in the Treatment of Pancreatic Cancer

Surgery is the treatment of choice in pancreatic cancer and can involve either partial or total resection of the pancreas and surrounding organs. In some cases, the disease may be so widespread that pancreatic resection is of no benefit. In these cases, biliary diversion for palliative measures is usually performed. In addition to surgery, some patients may receive chemotherapy or radiation therapy (or both).

Many of the nutrition obstacles encountered in persons with pancreatic cancer are related to the systemic effects of malignancy and chemotherapy or radiation therapy. These may include nausea, vomiting, early satiety, anorexia, depression, and inflammation with destruction of the gastrointestinal mucosa.

Surgical resection as a treatment modality for pancreatic cancer creates several nutrition challenges: malabsorption caused by inadequate or absent exocrine pancreatic secretions or obstruction of the common bile duct (or both), diabetes mellitus resulting from resection of the endocrine pancreatic cells, and protein-calorie malnutrition, which develops secondary to malabsorption.

## Presurgical Considerations

Before surgery, patients may experience diarrhea (due to fat malabsorption), constipation (due to decreased intake and drug therapy), nausea, vomiting, early satiety, or anorexia. By this point, most patients have already sustained significant weight loss. Every effort should be made to optimize their nutrition status before surgery. For patients who are able to tolerate an oral diet, small, frequent feedings with supplements should be offered. Depending on the extent of the disease, some patients require a pancreatic enzyme replacement or a low-fat diet (or both). A multivitamin and mineral supplement may be of benefit, especially if symptoms of malabsorption are present. In patients with obstructive jaundice, supplemental vitamin K may be necessary, because of the lack of bile salts, to facilitate the gastrointestinal absorption of the vitamin.

Patients who cannot tolerate oral feedings may be candidates for enteral nutrition support. Various monomeric enteral formulas are available for use through small-bore nasoenteric feeding tubes (Table 10-2). The tip of the feeding tube should be placed into the small bowel to avoid stimulation of pancreatic enzyme secretion induced by intragastric nutrients. If enteral nutrition support cannot be achieved, total parenteral nutrition may be of benefit to optimize the patient's nutrition status before surgery (Grant, James, Grabowski, & Trexler, 1984).

## Partial Pancreaticoduodenectomy: The Whipple Procedure

The Whipple procedure involves the removal of the head of the pancreas, the distal portion of the common bile duct (from the pancreas to the duodenum), the distal portion of the stomach, and the entire duodenum (Fig. 10-2). A segment of the jejunum is brought up and sewn to the remaining portion of the stomach, common bile duct, and pancreas to maintain the integrity of the gastrointestinal tract (Tersigni & Toledo-Pereyra, 1985).

As mentioned, up to 90% of the pancreas must be resected before clinical symptoms of malabsorption result. Therefore, patients undergoing the Whipple procedure may or may not require a pancreatic enzyme replacement to aid in diges-

**Table 10-2** Enteral Formulas for Potential Use in Pancreatic Disease

| Nutrient Provided | Criticare HN (Mead Johnson) | Isotein HN (Sandoz Nutrition) | Osmolite HN (Ross) | Vivonex T.E.N. (Norwich-Eaton) | Vital HN (Ross) |
|---|---|---|---|---|---|
| Calories (kcal/mL) | 1.06 | 1.2 | 1.06 | 1.0 | 1.0 |
| Protein (%) | 14 | 23 | 16.7 | 15.3 | 16.7 |
| Fat (%) | 4.5 | 25 | 30 | 2.5 | 9.4 |
| Carbohydrate (%) | 81.5 | 52 | 53.3 | 82.2 | 73.9 |
| Protein (g/L) | 38 | 67.8 | 44.4 | 38.2 | 41.7 |
| Ratio of nonprotein calories to nitrogen | 149 | 86 | 125 | 149 | 125 |
| Fat (g/L) | 5 | 33.9 | 36.8 | 2.8 | 10.8 |
| Carbohydrate (g/L) | 220 | 156 | 141 | 206 | 185 |
| Sodium (mEq/L) | 28 | 27 | 40.5 | 20 | 20.3 |
| Potassium (mEq/L) | 34 | 27.4 | 40.3 | 20 | 34.2 |
| Osmolality (mOsm/kg) | 650 | 300 | 300 | 630 | 500 |
| Protein source | Hydrolyzed casein, free amino acids | Delactosed lactalbumin, sodium caseinate | Sodium and calcium caseinates, soy protein isolate | Free amino acids | Partially hydrolyzed meat, whey, soy protein; free amino acids |
| Fat source | Safflower oil | Soybean oil, medium-chain triglyceride (MCT), monoglycerides and diglycerides | MCT, corn oil, soy oil | Safflower oil | Safflower oil, MCT, monoglycerides and diglycerides |
| Carbohydrate source | Maltodextrin, corn starch | Fructose, maltodextrin | Glucose polymers | Maltodextrin | Sucrose |

*Note:* These formulas may be somewhat preferable for use in patients with acute pancreatitis because crystalline amino acids may stimulate pancreatic secretion less than polypeptides.

*Source:* From *Nutritional and Metabolic Support of Hospitalized Patients* (p. 210) by M.A. Bernard, D.O. Jacobs, and J.L. Rombeau, 1986, Philadelphia: W.B. Saunders Company. Copyright 1986 by W.B. Saunders Company. Adapted by permission.

tion and to help prevent malabsorption. Pancreatic enzyme replacements are available as either pancrelipase or pancreatin (Digestive enzymes, 1987; Enteral nutritional therapy, 1985). Both help digest and absorb fats, proteins, and carbohydrates. Pancrelipase has greater lipase activity than pancreatin and can therefore help control steatorrhea at low doses. Several products are available from different manufacturers that are either pancrelipases or pancreatins (Table 10-3).

Because the common bile duct is reconnected to the jejunum, bile salts can reach the gastrointestinal tract so that fat malabsorption often is not a problem postoperatively. Jaundice is usually resolved as well. If steatorrhea persists, it may be resolved or controlled with the administration of a pancreatic enzyme replacement along with a low-fat diet (Table 10-4). The use of cimetidine may be necessary to control severe steatorrhea (Bernard, Jacobs, & Rombeau, 1986; Levin & Kinzie, 1980).

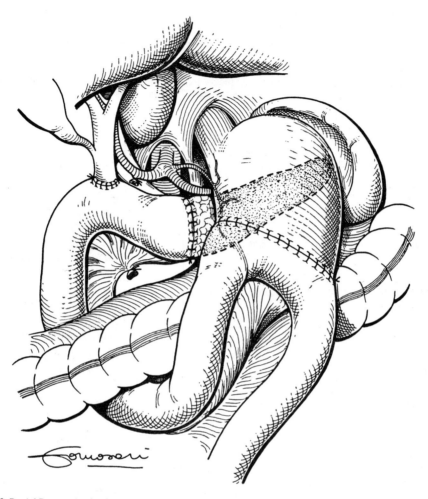

**Figure 10-2** Partial Pancreaticoduodenectomy (Whipple Procedure). *Source:* From *The Pancreas: Principles of Medical and Surgical Practice* (p. 45) by L. Toledo-Pereyra (Ed.), 1985, New York: Churchill Livingstone Inc. Copyright 1985 by Churchill Livingstone Inc. Reprinted by permission.

Calories can be added to the diet in the form of medium-chain triglyceride (MCT) oil. MCTs are more rapidly digested than conventional food fat and require less bile acids from the gallbladder for their digestion. In addition, they are absorbed directly into the circulation and do not require the more complicated steps for absorption that other fats do. MCT oil can be mixed with fruit juices, used on salads and vegetables, incorporated into sauces, or used in baking or cooking (Exhibit 10-1). Because it is heat sensitive, however, MCT oil is not appropriate for use in cooking at high temperatures (such as frying). MCT oil can also be added to enteral formulas for patients who are being fed through small-bore feeding tubes.

**Exhibit 10-1** Ways of Using MCT Oil as an Ingredient in Foods

Cooked vegetable seasoning (add spices and herbs)

Salad dressings

Barbecue sauces

Cream sauces

Marinades

Pie crust

Cakes and cookies

Fruit juices

*Source:* U.S. Department of Health and Human Services Publication No. (NIH) 76-111. National Heart and Lung Institute, Bethesda, MD. Revised 1973.

**Table 10-3** Pancreatic Enzyme Replacements

**PANCRELIPASE**

**Administration and Dosage:**

*Capsules and tablets:* Take 1 to 3 before or with meals and snacks. In severe deficiencies, the dose may be increased to 8 if no nausea, cramps or diarrhea results.

*Powder:* 0.7 g with meals.

Content given per capsule, tablet or 0.7 g powder.

| Product and Distributor | Lipase (units) | Protease (units) | Amylase (units) | Other Content | How Supplied | C.I.* |
|---|---|---|---|---|---|---|
| *Rx* **Pancrease Capsules** (McNeil Pharm.) | 4,000 | 25,000 | 20,000 | | Dye free. Enteric coated microspheres. (#McNeil Pancrease). White. In 100s and 250s. | 345 |
| *Rx* **Cotazym-S Capsules** (Organon) | 5,000 | 20,000 | 20,000 | | Enteric coated spheres. (#Organon 388). Clear. In 100s and 500s. | 286 |
| *otc* **Festal II Tablets** (Hoechst-Roussel) | 6,000 | 20,000 | 30,000 | | Enteric coated. (#Hoechst 72). White. In 100s and 500s. | 241 |
| *Rx* **Ku-Zyme HP Capsules** (Kremers-Urban) | 8,000 | 30,000 | 30,000 | | (#Kremers-Urban 525). White. In 100s. | 309 |
| *Rx* **Viokase Tablets** (Robins) | | | | | (#Viokase AHR/9111). Tan. In 100s and 500s. | 172 |
| *Rx* **Creon Capsules** (Reid-Rowell) | 8,000 | 13,000 | 30,000 | | Enteric coated microspheres. (#Reid Rowell Creon). Brown and yellow. In 100s and 250s. | 339 |
| *Rx* **Ilozyme Tablets** (Adria) | 11,000 | 30,000 | 30,000 | | (#Adria 200). Buff. In 250s. | 271 |
| *Rx* **Viokase Powder** (Robins) | 16,800 | 70,000 | 70,000 | | In 120 and 240 g. | 334 |
| *Rx* **Cotazym Capsules** (Organon) | 8,000 | 30,000 | 30,000 | 25 mg calcium carbonate | Regular. (#Organon 381). Green. In 100s & 500s. Cherry flavor (#Organon 386). White/red. In 100s. | 209 209 |

The recommended dosage of MCT oil is 15 mL (1 tbsp) three to four times per day. Each tablespoon of MCT oil provides approximately 100 kcal. MCT oil is manufactured by Mead Johnson and is available in 1-qt bottles. It can be ordered for stock by most pharmacies. MCT oil should not be used by patients with advanced cirrhosis and encephalopathy because of adverse effects of its altered metabolism in these disease states (Enteral nutritional therapy, 1985; Bernard et al., 1986).

Some patients undergoing the Whipple procedure develop diabetes mellitus because of the loss of endocrine pancreatic function (Beazley, 1985). Diabetes mellitus does not usually develop until more than 70% of the pancreas is removed. Insulin is required to maintain blood glucose levels within normal ranges. A low–simple sugar diet should be provided to aid in blood sugar control along with small, frequent feedings (Exhibit 10-2).

Small, frequent feedings are needed by patients undergoing the Whipple procedure to achieve optimal caloric intake. Partial resection of the stomach and total resection of the duodenum result in a decreased volume capacity and

**Table 10-3** continued

PANCREATIN
    **Administration and Dosage:**
      *Tablets:* Take 1 to 3 after meals.

Content given per tablet.

| | Product and Distributor | Pancreatin (mg) | Lipase (units) | Protease (units) | Amylase (units) | How Supplied | C.I.* |
|---|---|---|---|---|---|---|---|
| otc sf | **Hi-Vegi-Lip Tablets** (Freeda) | 2,400 | 12,000 | 60,000 | 60,000 | In 100s and 250s. | 199 |
| otc | **Pancreatin Enseals (Tablets)** (Lilly) | 1,000 | 2,000 | 25,000 | 25,000 | Enteric coated. In 100s and 500s. | 224 |
| otc | **Pancreatin Tablets** (Lilly) | 325 | 650 | 8,125 | 8,125 | In 100s and 1000s. | 136 |
| otc | **Dizymes Tablets** (Recsei Labs) | 250 | 6,750 | 41,250 | 43,750 | Enteric coated. In 100s, 500s and 1000s. | 105 |

*Cost Index based on cost per capsule, tablet or gram of powder.
#Product identification code.
sf—Sugar free.

*Source:* Used with permission from Drug Facts and Comparisons. 1989 ed. St. Louis: Facts and Comparisons, a Division of the J.B. Lippincott Company.

absorptive area of the gastrointestinal tract. Fluids may be limited initially to ½-c servings taken 1 to 2 hours after the dry portion of the meal. In addition, simple sugars are limited to help control osmotically induced diarrhea (dumping syndrome) caused by a decrease in the absorptive area and volume capacity of the gastrointestinal tract (Exhibit 10-3).

### Total Pancreatectomy

In some cases, the entire pancreas and duodenum may be resected in an effort to remove all malignant cells (Beazley, 1985). In this procedure, a segment of the jejunum is sewn to the remaining common bile duct and stomach (Fig. 10-3). All patients undergoing total pancreatectomy require insulin to regulate blood glucose and a pancreatic enzyme replacement to avoid maldigestion and malabsorption.

Nutrition therapy should consist of a low–simple sugar diet (see Exhibit 10-2) with small,

frequent feedings to achieve maximal caloric intake and to prevent large fluctuations in blood glucose level. Fat malabsorption should not be a problem once the optimal dose of pancreatic enzyme replacement is achieved. If steatorrhea persists, however, a low-fat diet (see Table 10-4) or cimetidine (or both) may be in order. MCT oil may be added to the diet as a caloric supplement.

### Palliative Management

Most pancreatic carcinomas are unresectable. Patients with unresectable pancreatic cancer are often jaundiced as a result of tumor obstruction of the common bile duct and require biliary diversion for palliation of symptoms. This can be achieved by means of various surgical bypass procedures, including the Roux-en-Y surgical procedure, or by percutaneous transhepatic perduodenal drainage with a catheter or prosthesis placed under radiologic control (Malt, 1983;

**Table 10-4** Guidelines for a Low-Fat Diet

| Type of Food | Food Included | Food Excluded |
|---|---|---|
| Beverages (nondairy) | Coffee, tea, carbonated beverages, fruit and vegetable juice. | None. |
| Breads | Whole wheat, white, rye, or pumpernickel breads; also oatmeal bread, raisin bread, Italian bread, French bread, English muffins, matzo, saltines, graham crackers, and pretzels. Baked goods and other products containing no whole milk or egg yolk or fat. | Egg or cheese bread. Biscuits, muffins, sweet rolls, cornbread, pancakes, and waffles. French toast. High-fat rolls. Corn chips, potato chips, cheese crackers, and other flavored crackers. |
| Cereals | All cereals; also grain products such as rice, noodles, macaroni, spaghetti, and flour. | None. |
| Dairy products | Skim (nonfat) milk, skim milk powder, and evaporated skim milk; buttermilk, cottage cheese, yogurt, and specially prepared cheese containing up to 1% fat. Sherbet (1% to 2% fat). Sapsago cheese. | Whole milk and whole milk products, including chocolate milk, evaporated and condensed milk, cream (sweet or sour), ice cream, and ice milk. Nondairy substitutes for cream, sour cream, and whipped topping. Cream cheese and all other cheese made from cream or whole milk. Regular creamed cottage cheese unless substituted for meat (¼ cup = 1 oz of meat). |
| Desserts | Fruit ices (water ices), sherbet (1% to 2% fat), gelatin dessert, fruit whips, meringues, and angel food cake (including the mix). Cakes, pies, cookies, pudding, and frostings made with allowed ingredients such as skim milk and egg whites. Junket made with skim milk. | Commercial cakes, pies, cookies, and mixes. Ice cream, ice milk. Desserts that contain whole milk, fat, and egg yolks. |
| Fats | None (MCT is a special fat that can be used, but only on physician's recommendation). | All fats and oils; gravies and cream sauces containing fat; salad dressings and mayonnaise; whipped toppings. |
| Fruits | Any fresh (except avocado), canned, frozen, or dried fruit or juice. | Avocado. |
| Meat, poultry, fish, and eggs | Limit to 5 oz/day: Lean, well-trimmed meat such as beef, pork, lamb, liver, veal, chicken, turkey; fish and water-packed salmon or tuna; shellfish. Egg white, dried or chipped beef, and dry (no-fat) cottage cheese may be used as desired. One egg yolk may be substituted for 1 oz of meat. Limit egg yolks to 3 per week. | Fried meats; fried fish; fatty meats such as bacon, cold cuts, sausage, luncheon meats, hot dogs, corned beef; goose, duck, poultry skin; fish canned in oil; pork and beans; spareribs; regular ground beef or hamburger; meats canned or frozen in sauces or gravy; frozen or packaged dinners and prepared products (convenience foods) containing fat. |
| Soups | Bouillon, clear broth, fat-free vegetable soup, cream soup made with skim milk, and packaged dehydrated soups (broth base). | All others. |
| Sweets | Pure sugar candy such as gum drops, jelly beans, hard candy, marshmallows, and mints (not chocolate). Also jam, jelly, honey, and syrup (containing no fat). | All other candy. |

**Table 10-4** continued

| Type of Food | Food Included | Food Excluded |
|---|---|---|
| Vegetables | Any fresh, frozen, or canned without fat. Vegetarian baked beans. | Buttered, creamed, or fried vegetables. Pork and beans. |
| Miscellaneous | Pickles, salt, spices, herbs, cocoa (limit to 1 tbsp dry cocoa per day). | Nuts, olives, peanut butter, coconut, chocolate. |

*Source:* U.S. Department of Health and Human Services Publication No. (NIH) 76-111. National Heart and Lung Institute, Bethesda, MD. Revised 1973.

Beazley, 1985). Either procedure will allow bile salts to reach the intestine, thus relieving jaundice and limiting fat malabsorption.

Patients undergoing palliative biliary diversion may require pancreatic enzyme replacement if a large portion of the pancreas has tumor involvement. A low-fat diet with small, frequent feedings may also be of benefit.

### Chemotherapy

Four classes of antineoplastic agents have demonstrated effects against disseminated pancreatic adenocarcinoma. They include 5-fluorouracil, mitomycin-C, adriamycin, and chloroethyl nitrosoureas. These drugs appear to be most efficacious in patients demonstrating a good performance status, that is, those who are asymptomatic or symptomatic and either fully ambulatory or in bed less than 50% of the day (Leichman, 1985; Klaassen, MacIntyre, Catton, Engstrom, & Moertel, 1985). Even so, the response rate is only 20% to 40%, and the median survival rate is rarely greater than 6 months (Leichman, 1985).

### Radiation Therapy

Radiation therapy has been successful for both reduction in tumor size and palliation of pain (Leichman, 1985). Some investigators have demonstrated long-term survival in patients receiving radiation therapy for unresectable pancreatic cancer (Leichman, 1985). Survival seems to be improved when radiation is used in combination with chemotherapy.

## NUTRITION CONCERNS IN CANCER OF THE LIVER

### Anatomy and Function of the Liver

The liver is located in the right upper quadrant of the abdomen with its lower edge behind the right costal (rib) margin (Goldberg & Gornall, 1980). It has a large right lobe and a smaller left lobe and represents approximately 3% of the body mass (Goodman, 1974).

The liver is unique among organs in that it has a dual blood supply, consisting of the hepatic arterial system and the hepatic portal vein. The hepatic artery supplies approximately 25% of the hepatic circulation with oxygen-rich blood. Of the hepatic circulation, 75% originates from the hepatic portal vein. Blood from the hepatic portal vein has an oxygen saturation of approximately 70%, which is 25% less than that originating from the hepatic artery. The blood supply of the hepatic portal vein contains the entire venous drainage of the gastrointestinal tract and pancreas (Goodman, 1974). Because of its location and vascular supply, the liver is the first organ to receive dietary nutrients from the gastrointestinal tract. Accordingly, it is the primary organ responsible for the assimilation and storage of carbohydrate, protein, and fat and is the primary regulator of their metabolism.

The liver maintains a constant level of blood glucose despite a fluctuating supply of dietary carbohydrate. Glucose homeostasis is achieved through liver uptake of excessive blood glucose and conversion of this glucose into its storage form, glycogen. Conversely, when blood glucose is low the liver breaks down glycogen and

**Exhibit 10-2** Guidelines for a Low–Simple Sugar Diet

The purpose of this diet is to help you control your blood sugar. To do this you need to:

- avoid sugar and foods that are high in sugar. Examples are table sugar, honey, jelly, syrups, ice cream, gelatin, pie, cake, cookies, candy, and soda pop.
- limit fruits and milk to the amounts recommended.
- include starches, but limit them to one to two servings per meal. Examples are breads, cereals, potatoes, rice, corn, and noodles.
- eat three balanced meals. Try to eat at the same time each day, and **do not** skip meals.

Select various foods from the following groups:

1. *Meat and meat substitutes:* meat, poultry, fish, eggs, cheese, cottage cheese, peanut butter, lunch meat, weiners. Recommended: one serving at each meal.
2. *Breads and starches:* bread, cereals (not sugar coated), crackers, rice, noodles, macaroni, spaghetti, soup, popcorn, starchy vegetables (potatoes, peas, lima beans, corn, mixed vegetables, dried beans). Recommended: one to two servings at each meal.
3. *Vegetables:* any cooked or raw vegetable may be used as desired except starchy vegetables. Recommended: one to two servings per day.
4. *Fruits:* unsweetened juices, fresh fruit, canned fruit packed in natural juice, canned fruit packed in light syrup *if rinsed and drained*, unsweetened frozen fruit. Recommended: two to three servings per day. One serving is ½ c or one small fruit.
5. *Milk:* milk, buttermilk, plain yogurt. Recommended: one to two servings per day.
6. *Fats:* butter, margarine, salad dressing, mayonnaise, bacon, lard, shortening, nuts, oil, olives, sour cream, creamer, cream cheese. Recommended: Allowed as desired, but use *sparingly* if you are trying to control weight.

Foods allowed as desired:

- Bouillon
- Catsup
- Coffee, tea
- Diet gelatin
- Dill pickles
- Herbs and spices
- Mustard
- Raw vegetables, cooked nonstarchy vegetables
- Sugar-free gums and mints
- Sugar-free soda pops
- Sugar substitutes
- Tomato juice, vegetable juice
- Vinegar

Foods to avoid:

- Alcoholic beverages (unless permitted by physician), sweet liqueurs, sweetened cocktail mixes
- Candy
- Chocolate milk, instant breakfast mixes, instant cocoa mixes
- Frosting
- Gelatin
- Granola, granola products, sugar-coated cereal
- Honey, molasses, syrup

**Exhibit 10-2** continued

- Ice cream, ice milk, sherbet, frozen yogurt, ices
- Jams, jellies, preserves
- Marshmallows
- Milk shakes, malts
- Pie, cake, cookies, doughnuts, pastries, pudding
- Soda pop, fruit drinks made with sugar
- Sugar, brown sugar, fructose
- Yogurt (fruit flavored)

*Source:* From *Manual of Clinical Dietetics* by The Clinical Section of the Columbus Dietetic Administrative Council, 1985, Columbus, OH: Vision Printing. Copyright by Columbus Dietetic Administrative Council. Reprinted by permission.

releases glucose into the bloodstream. If glycogen stores are depleted, the liver is capable of making glucose from amino acids, which are the building blocks of protein.

Protein synthesis is an important function of the liver. The liver is a major source of proteins called enzymes, which help regulate the metabolism of carbohydrate, protein, and fat. The liver also synthesizes most of the proteins found in blood plasma, including albumin, lipoproteins, and transferrin.

Degradation of proteins, including those of skeletal muscle, also occurs in the liver when energy and glucose are needed for the body. During periods of starvation the use of glucose by the peripheral tissues decreases, and less glucose is made from amino acids in the liver. These changes in metabolism promote the conservation of body protein. In cancer patients, however, the rate of glucose synthesized from amino acids increases, as does the degradation of muscle protein. The reasons for this increased glucose use and production from amino acids are unknown. The tumor itself, however, appears to use glucose at a rapid rate, resulting in depletion of body protein and fat (Bernard et al., 1986).

Fat metabolism is intimately controlled by the liver. During fed states, excess dietary carbohydrate is converted into fat for storage. This fat, along with other dietary fat, is sent from the liver through the bloodstream to adipose tissue for storage. During periods of starvation, adipose tissue releases the stored fat as fatty acids, which are sent back to the liver and converted into energy.

**Exhibit 10-3** Postgastrectomy Diet

*Purpose:* To alleviate the symptoms of postgastrectomy surgery, including dumping syndrome, diarrhea, and reactive hypoglycemia.

*Characteristics:* Small, frequent meals low in simple sugars. Fluid volume is often restricted to ½-c servings at meals to prevent rapid transit of the food bolus. Fluids are encouraged between meals to maintain adequate hydration and can be gradually increased as patient tolerance allows. Raw fruits and vegetables and other foods high in fiber may need to be avoided during the initial postoperative period. Caffeine and chocolate should be avoided because of their gastric secretory potential.

*Sample menu:*

Breakfast: 1 egg with margarine or MCT oil
1 slice of toast
½ c of milk
Midmorning snack: ½ c of milk
¾ c of unsweetened cereal
Lunch: ½ toasted cheese sandwich
¼ c of unsweetened canned fruit
½ c of milk
Midafternoon snack: ½ c of diet baked custard
six crackers with margarine
Dinner: 1 to 2 oz of tender meat
½ c of mashed potatoes with margarine or MCT oil
¼ c of unsweetened canned fruit
½ c of milk
Bedtime snack: 1 oz of low-fat cheese
six crackers

*Source:* From *Manual of Clinical Dietetics* by The Clinical Section of the Columbus Dietetic Administrative Council, 1985, Columbus, OH: Vision Printing. Copyright by Columbus Dietetic Administrative Council. Reprinted by permission.

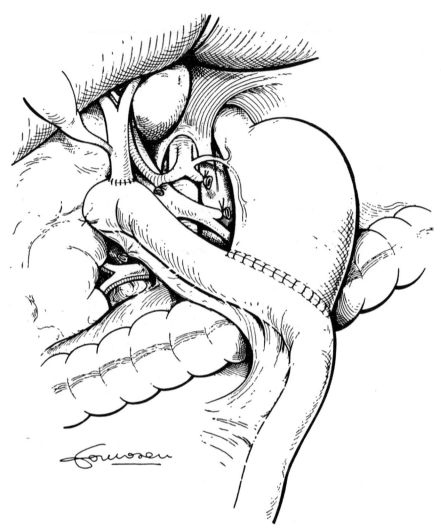

**Figure 10-3** Total Pancreatectomy. *Source: The Pancreas: Principles of Medical and Surgical Practice* (p. 46), L. Toledo-Pereyra (Ed.), 1985, New York: Churchill Livingstone Inc. Copyright 1985 by Churchill Livingstone Inc. Reprinted by permission.

The liver is also the primary site of cholesterol synthesis and degradation. The rate of cholesterol synthesis by the liver varies according to the amount of dietary cholesterol. Dietary cholesterol intake is generally not of concern in cancer patients.

The liver is the primary site of storage and metabolism of vitamins A, B complex (especially $B_6$ and $B_{12}$), D, and K (Goldberg & Gornall, 1980). The metal ions iron and copper are also tightly regulated by the liver. Other important functions of the liver include the synthesis, secretion, and excretion of bile, detoxification of potentially injurious substances, and synthesis of compounds needed for blood coagulation (Goldberg & Gornall, 1980).

### Primary Liver Cancer: Incidence and Etiology

Primary carcinomas of the liver may arise from liver cells (hepatocellular carcinoma) or from bile duct cells (cholangiocellular carcinoma). Primary liver cancers represent 1% to 2% of all malignancies in the United States. Hepatocellular carcinoma accounts for 80% to 90% of primary liver carcinomas. It is two to four times more prevalent in men than in women, and its peak incidence occurs between 50 and 70 years of age (Alpert, 1976; Alpert & Isselbacher, 1987).

The etiology of hepatocellular cancer remains unknown, although several factors have been associated with the disease. Approximately two-thirds of patients in this population have had some type of underlying chronic liver disease, whether metabolic, alcoholic, viral, or idiopathic. Alcoholic and postnecrotic cirrhosis are the most common forms of underlying liver disease in patients with liver cancer in the United States (Alpert & Isselbacher, 1987). Viral hepatitis, mycotoxins, hormonal factors, and iatrogenic factors are also associated with the development of liver cancer (Linsell, 1987).

## Symptoms and Clinical Features

Hepatic cancers often escape clinical recognition because in most patients the signs and symptoms are associated with progression of the underlying liver disease. Hepatomegaly with abdominal pain in the right upper quadrant is the most common complaint (Alpert, 1976; Alpert & Isselbacher, 1987). Other nonspecific symptoms include anorexia, weight loss, muscle wasting, weakness, and fatigue. Approximately 25% of patients complain of a sense of fullness or heaviness. Severe jaundice is present in patients with cholangiocarcinoma, but jaundice is relatively uncommon in hepatocellular carcinoma. If the portal vein is obstructed, ascites and gastrointestinal bleeding from esophageal varices may result (Alpert, 1976).

Anemia and an elevated alkaline phosphatase level are commonly found laboratory abnormalities (Alpert, 1976; Alpert & Isselbacher, 1987). Almost all patients with hepatocellular cancer have high levels of α-fetoprotein, a protein that is undetectable in normal adults (Alpert, 1976; Alpert & Isselbacher, 1987). The prognosis for patients with primary liver cancer is grim. Most patients die within 4 to 6 months of diagnosis as a result of gastrointestinal hemorrhage from ruptured esophageal varices, progressive cachexia, or hepatic failure.

## Treatment

Tumors of primary hepatic carcinomas are generally large and encompass both lobes of the liver by the time a diagnosis is made (Alpert, 1976). The tumor may respond to brief periods of systemic or intra-arterial hepatic perfusion chemotherapy, but the overall results are poor (Alpert, 1976; Alpert & Isselbacher, 1987). Surgical resection may be of benefit if the tumor is small and localized. Liver transplantation may be considered a therapeutic option, but recurrence of tumor and appearance of metastases after transplantation have limited the usefulness of this procedure (Alpert & Isselbacher, 1987).

## Secondary Tumors of the Liver

The liver is the second most common site of primary tumor metastases. The incidence of metastatic carcinoma of the liver is at least 20 times greater than that of primary carcinomas, encompassing one-third to one-half of all patients with known primary carcinomas. Primary carcinomas of the pancreas, colon, and stomach (all of which are drained by the portal system) along with carcinomas of the lung and breast and melanomas are the most frequent sources of metastatic liver carcinoma (Alpert, 1976; Alpert & Isselbacher, 1987; Wanebo, 1987). Nearly all types of neoplasms, with the exception of primary brain carcinomas, can metastasize to the liver.

Anorexia, nausea, weight loss, and weakness are the most frequent symptoms of liver metastases, with hepatomegaly being the most frequent physical sign (Alpert, 1976). Approximately 50% of patients are jaundiced. Mild abnormalities in liver function tests are common, with hypoalbuminemia and anemia occurring in more widespread disease.

Most metastatic carcinomas are diffuse and invade both lobes of the liver, rendering them inoperable. They respond poorly to all forms of medical therapy, although systemic chemotherapy may slow tumor growth and reduce symptoms. Surgical resection may be beneficial for localized metastases. Hepatic dearterialization is used as a method of palliative treatment for both primary and secondary hepatic cancers (Cady, 1982). This method of treatment reduces the tumor load by inducing ischemic necrosis of the tumor.

## Nutrition Management of Liver Cancer

### Changes in Carbohydrate Metabolism

Primary or secondary cancer of the liver can potentially alter the liver's capacity to regulate carbohydrate metabolism. The most serious side effect of the altered carbohydrate metabolism is hypoglycemia, or low blood sugar. Patients experiencing recurrent hypoglycemia have symptoms of weakness, dizziness, clamminess, headache, shakiness, confusion, and, in extreme cases, loss of consciousness. A low–simple sugar diet with small, frequent feedings will help prevent hypoglycemia. The diet is similar to the postgastrectomy diet (see Exhibit 10-3) except that fluids need not be limited and can be taken with meals. Foods high in sugar are avoided so that excessive insulin secretion from the pancreas is not stimulated.

### Fat Malabsorption

Steatorrhea is a common manifestation of malabsorption in patients with liver cancer and underlying cirrhosis. It may be the result of the direct effects of ethanol, an altered pancreatic response to a fatty challenge, or bile salt abnormalities (or all three). In patients without cirrhosis the hepatic tumor may obstruct the biliary drainage system, preventing the secretion of bile salts into the gastrointestinal tract. Dietary management includes a low-fat diet (see Table 10-4) with discretionary use of MCT oil as a caloric supplement. Patients with advanced cirrhosis or encephalopathy should not receive MCT oil as a caloric supplement because of its altered metabolism in severe liver disease (Enteral nutritional therapy, 1985; Bernard et al., 1986).

### Vitamin and Mineral Deficiencies

The efficacy of vitamin and mineral supplementation in cancer therapy is unknown. Vitamin deficiencies may result from inadequate intake, intestinal malabsorption, or reduced hepatic storage capacity. The presence of steatorrhea can induce deficiencies of fat-soluble vitamins. In severe cases of liver injury hypervitaminosis can occur, but these cases are extremely rare. Patients with inadequate oral intakes or malabsorption syndromes may benefit from therapeutic multivitamin and mineral supplements. Megadoses of vitamins and minerals are not recommended.

### Ascites

Malignant ascites is the second most common cause of ascites (Conn, 1976). It can develop as a result of extensive intrahepatic metastases, compression of the hepatic veins or vena cava, or obstruction of the portal vein. Dietary management of ascites may consist of a sodium restriction of up to 2 g (87 mEq) of sodium per day (Table 10-5) and/or a fluid restriction of 1 to 1.5 liters per day (Exhibits 10-4 and 10-5). The need for a dietary sodium restriction should be evaluated not only in terms of medical management but also in terms of actual oral intake. Often, cancer patients do not eat enough food to amount to 2 g of sodium per day, thus negating the need for salt-free foods. In some cases, small amounts of table salt can be added to the diet to increase palatability.

### Hepatic Encephalopathy

The two basic hypotheses regarding the pathogenesis of hepatic encephalopathy in liver disease are that it results from the accumulation of specific neurotoxins and that physiologic changes resulting from liver failure alter the brain's normal neurotransmitter function and thus change mental status (Bernard et al., 1986). Protein intake must be adjusted individually in patients with hepatic encephalopathy. Too severe a restriction may actually exacerbate the encephalopathy, and too liberal of an intake may worsen it as well. Generally, patients with hepatic encephalopathy and mental status changes are not fed orally because of their increased risk of aspiration. Enteral or parenteral nutrition support may or may not be indicated, depending on the patient's overall prognosis.

**Table 10-5** Daily Meal Plans for Sodium-Restricted Diets

| Food Group | Amount of Sodium | | | | | |
|---|---|---|---|---|---|---|
| | 250 mg (11 mEq) | 500 mg (22 mEq) | 1,000 mg (43 mEq) | 2,000 mg (87 mEq) | 4,000 mg (173 mEq) | 6,000 mg (261 mEq) |
| Milk, regular | None | 1 c | 2 c | 2 c* | 2 to 4 c* | As desired |
| Milk, low sodium | 2 c | As desired | As desired | As desired | As desired | As desired |
| Fruit† | As desired | As desired | As desired | As desired | As desired | As desired |
| Vegetables, canned | None | None | None | None | As desired‡ | As desired |
| Vegetables, salt free | 2§ | 2§ | As desired | As desired | As desired | As desired |
| Wheat, salt free | 4 oz | 5 oz | 6 oz | 8 oz | 8 oz | As desired |
| Eggs | As meat substitute | One | One | One | One | As desired |
| Fat, regular | None | None | None | 6 tsp | As desired | As desired |
| Fat, salt free | As desired | As desired | As desired | As desired | As desired | As desired |
| Bread, regular | None | None | Three slices | Five slices | As desired | As desired |
| Bread, salt free | Three slices | Five slices | As desired | As desired | As desired | As desired |
| Salt-free gravy and broth | One serving | One serving | As desired | As desired | As desired | As desired |
| Desserts, sodium free‖ | One serving | Two servings | As desired | As desired | As desired | As desired |
| Desserts, regular | None | None | One serving | Two servings | As desired | As desired |
| Salt | None | None | None | None | ½ tsp for cooking | Use freely in cooking; none at table |

*Buttermilk may be calculated into the diet plan.
†Maraschino cherries and dried fruits containing sodium compounds may be restricted.
‡Vegetables processed with salt (e.g., pickles, olives, sauerkraut) should be avoided.
§The following vegetables have a sodium content higher than most other vegetables: beets, celery, carrots, greens (beet, dandelion, kale, spinach). These should be taken into consideration when calculating diets of 500 mg or less.
‖A sodium-free dessert has less than 12 mg (0.5 mEq) sodium per average serving.

*Source:* From *Manual of Clinical Dietetics* by the Clinical Section of the Columbus Dietetic Administrative Council, 1985, Columbus, OH: Vision Printing. Copyright by Columbus Dietetic Administrative Council. Reprinted by permission.

---

## NUTRITION CONSIDERATIONS IN RENAL CANCER

### Renal Function

The kidneys perform many physiologic functions that are needed to maintain homeostasis in the body. The process of urine formation allows regulation of the composition of body fluids and removal of metabolic waste. Thus the kidneys can regulate blood osmolality, fluid volume, sodium and potassium balance, hydrogen ion concentration, and calcium and phosphorus balance through the formation of urine. The kidneys filter approximately 170 to 180 L of body fluid per day to create an average of 1.5 L of urine.

The formation of urine is the means whereby the kidney excretes waste products of metabolism, especially those of nitrogen metabolism. These waste products include creatinine, urea, and uric acid. The elimination of various drugs and toxins also occurs through the action of the kidney.

Several endocrine secretions that have a broad impact on the regulation of body systems originate in the kidney. The final conversion of vitamin D to its most active metabolite, 1,25-dihydroxycholecalciferol, occurs in the kidney. This metabolite affects the processes of calcium absorption from the gastrointestinal tract and bone reabsorption. Renin, which functions to control blood pressure, is synthesized in the

**Exhibit 10-4** Restriction of Dietary Fluid

1. A measured amount of fluid is allowed per 24 hours.
2. Foods are classified as fluid if they are liquid at room temperature and include:
   - alcoholic beverages
   - carbonated beverages
   - coffee
   - cream
   - ice (melts to $\frac{9}{10}$ of its initial volume)
   - ice cream or ice milk (melts to $\frac{1}{2}$ of its initial volume)
   - gelatin
   - juices
   - milk
   - flavored ices
   - sherbet (melts to $\frac{2}{3}$ of its initial volume)
   - soups
   - tea
   - water
3. Items that melt to a volume less than the initial volume (e.g., ice, sherbet) should be counted as the smaller volume.
4. Gravies, sauces, and salad dressing should be used sparingly because of their fluid content, and amounts may be calculated into the fluid restriction.
5. The water content of foods that are solid at room temperature accounts for approximately 500 to 800 mL/day. This amount approximates insensible water loss and is not counted toward the daily fluid limit.

*Source:* From *Manual of Clinical Dietetics* by The Clinical Section of the Columbus Dietetic Administrative Council, 1985, Columbus, OH: Vision Printing. Copyright by Columbus Dietetic Administrative Council. Reprinted by permission.

**Exhibit 10-5** Helpful Hints for Fluid Control

1. Avoid salty foods: you will be less thirsty.
2. Get the most nutrition from your allowed liquids: instead of coffee, tea, soft drinks, and alcoholic beverages, use milk, soups, or juices.
3. Try sliced lemon wedges to stimulate saliva and to moisten a dry mouth.
4. Use sour hard candies and chewing gum to moisten your mouth.
5. Rinse your mouth with water, but don't swallow the water.
6. Use small cups and glasses for beverages and other liquids.
7. When thirsty, try eating something such as bread and margarine with jelly before taking liquids. Food may moisten a dry mouth as well as a liquid.
8. To measure the amount of fluid in ice:
   - One ice cube = 2 tbsp (1 oz) of water.
   - One c of crushed ice = $\frac{1}{2}$ c (4 oz) of water.
9. Take medications with mealtime liquids.
10. Try putting lemon juice in ice cubes: you will use fewer ice cubes that way. Use about half a lemon per tray of water.

*Source:* From *Manual of Clinical Dietetics* by The Clinical Section of the Columbus Dietetic Administrative Council, 1985, Columbus, OH: Vision Printing. Copyright by Columbus Dietetic Administrative Council. Reprinted by permission.

kidney. The kidney is also intimately involved in the maintenance of normal red blood cell production through its synthesis of erythropoietin. Erythropoietin stimulates the maturation of red blood cells and the synthesis of hemoglobin.

The kidneys, like the pancreas and liver, have a large reserve capacity. Up to 55% of renal function must be lost before a patient begins to be symptomatic. As renal function deteriorates, symptoms of azotemia (excessive amounts of nitrogen components in the blood), loss of ability to concentrate urine, anemia, and impaired ability to maintain electrolyte and acid-base balance become manifest. Tumors of the kidney have the potential to affect all the physiologic processes that the organ performs. Thus symptoms of acute or chronic renal failure or symptoms of excessive or deficient renal endocrine secretions may be present in patients with tumors of the kidney.

## Renal Cancer

Four different types of cancer affect the kidney, and each involves different types of cells: renal cell carcinoma (discussed below), Wilms' tumor, various types of sarcoma, and epithelial tumors of the renal pelvis (Javadpour, 1984b). Renal cell carcinoma accounts for 85% of all primary renal neoplasms and is the third most common urologic cancer (Javadpour, 1984a; Garnick & Brenner, 1987). The disease occurs two to three times as frequently in men as in women, and peak incidence is in the fifth and sixth decades of life. The progression of renal cell cancer is slow as a result of a slow tumor-doubling time. Suspected risk factors for the development of renal cell carcinoma include aromatic hydrocarbons, aromatic amines, aflatoxins, hormones, lead compounds, radiation, certain viruses, and cigar smoking (Javadpour, 1984a). Renal cell carcinoma originates from renal tubular epithelial cells and spreads by direct extension or through the venous and lymphatic channels (Javadpour, 1984c). Common sites of metastasis include lung, mediastinum, bone, skin, liver, central nervous system, thyroid, and liver (Garnick & Brenner, 1987; Khoury & Saul, 1986).

## Symptoms of Renal Cell Carcinoma

Hematuria is the most common symptom of renal cell carcinoma, occurring in approximately 60% of all cases. Other symptoms, including flank pain and a palpable abdominal mass, are usually late manifestations of the disease. Fatigability, weight loss, and cachexia are found in approximately 50% of patients (Garnick & Brenner, 1987). Renal cell carcinomas may produce hormones or hormonelike substances that stimulate hypercalcemia, hypertension, or glucose intolerance.

## Treatment of Renal Cell Carcinoma

The treatment for renal cell carcinoma is radical nephrectomy (Garnick & Brenner, 1987; Javadpour, 1984c). Partial nephrectomy can be performed in cases in which the tumor involves both kidneys. Chemotherapy and radiation therapy have not been shown to be effective against renal cell carcinoma (Garnick & Brenner, 1987; Javadpour, 1984c). Patients with tumors that are confined in the kidney (stage I) have the best 5-year survival rates (60% to 75%). Approximately 30% of patients with renal cell carcinomas have distant metastases (stage IV) at the time of diagnosis. The survival time for patients with stage IV disease is 6 to 9 months (Khoury & Saul, 1986).

## Nutrition Management

### Hypertension

Hypertension is present in up to 40% of patients with renal adenocarcinoma (Sufrin, Golio, & Murphy, 1986) and may result from various mechanisms, including hyperreninemia, renal arteriovenous fistulae, polycythemia, hypercalcemia, ureteral obstruction, or elevated intracranial pressure secondary to cerebral metastases. Hypertension is usually associated with early-stage, low-grade clear cell carcinoma. Reductions in plasma renin levels or elimination of arteriovenous fistulae by means of radical nephrectomy is associated with reduced levels of hypertension (Sufrin et al., 1986). Dietary sodium and fluid management is of modest, if any, benefit in controlling hypertension before surgical removal of the tumor and elimination of the underlying etiologic factors. Sodium and fluid management may be of benefit in the perioperative period until homeostasis of fluid volume is achieved (see Table 10-5 and Exhibits 10-4 and 10-5).

### Hypercalcemia

Hypercalcemia is associated with malignancies in general and is present in 3% to 13% of patients with renal cell carcinoma. The etiology of the hypercalcemia is varied and may involve multiple factors, including osteoclast activating factor, 1,25-dihydroxycholecalciferol, prostaglandins, direct erosion of bone by tumor cells, or excess parathyroid hormone (Sufrin et al., 1986). Symptoms of hypercalcemia can be nonspecific and may include weakness, anorexia, and mental status changes.

Medical management of hypercalcemia associated with renal cell carcinoma may include saline infusion, furosemide-induced diuresis, and administration of corticosteroids or mithramycin (Mundy et al., 1984; Buescu, Dimich, & Myers, 1975). Dietary calcium restriction is of little therapeutic benefit in the management of malignancy-induced hypercalcemia. Adequate fluid intake is necessary to avoid dehydration in patients receiving diuretics to induce renal calcium excretion.

## Acute Renal Failure

Acute renal failure may be defined as an abrupt decrease in renal function that is sufficient to result in azotemia and an increase in serum creatinine levels. The etiology of acute renal failure may be related to prerenal, intrinsic, or postrenal function and anatomy. The prerenal type occurs in response to hypoperfusion of functionally intact nephrons resulting from hypovolemia, peripheral vasodilation, impaired cardiac function, extrarenal vascular occlusion, or disorders of intrarenal circulation. This form of acute renal failure is frequently encountered in cancer patients who tend to have depleted extracellular fluid as a result of inadequate dietary intake, gastrointestinal losses, the diuretic effect of hypercalcemia, hypoalbuminemia, or third-spacing from malignant effusions.

Intrinsic acute renal failure results from abnormalities of the renal glomeruli, tubules, interstitium, or blood vessels. Renal failure secondary to cancer chemotherapy or radiation therapy is classified as intrinsic and is related to glomerular and tubular injury. Intrinsic acute renal failure that cannot be related to primary anatomic lesions of the glomeruli, blood vessels, or renal interstitium is referred to as acute tubular necrosis. Acute tubular necrosis can result from renal toxicity of some anticancer agents.

The postrenal form of acute renal failure is the result of mechanical obstruction of the ureters, bladder, or urethra.

Patients with acute renal failure may not excrete any urine or may have a urine output of greater than 3 L/day. Anuria is defined as the excretion of less than 100 mL of urine per 24-hour period, or less than 4 mL/hour. Anuria is commonly associated with postrenal obstruction or bilateral renal arterial or venous occlusion. Oliguria describes the excretion of 100 to 400 mL of urine per 24-hour period, or less than 20 mL/hour. This condition may reflect a state of dehydration or occur as a pathologic consequence of urinary obstruction or intrinsic renal disease.

A urine output greater than 3 L/day is described as polyuria. Polyuria may occur despite rising serum levels of blood urea nitrogen and creatinine and results from a simultaneous reduction in glomerular filtration rate and salt and water reabsorption (Jenkins & Rieselbach, 1982). This condition is associated with non-oliguric acute tubular necrosis, the postrenal form of acute renal failure due to prostatic obstruction, or solute diuresis in the presence of extracellular fluid volume depletion, including glycosuric states.

## Nutrition Management of Acute Renal Failure

Nutrition support of patients with acute renal failure may involve sodium, potassium, protein, or fluid restrictions. The diet must be individualized for each patient and varies according to the etiology of the disease and the amount of urine excreted.

### Sodium

Sodium restriction is necessary in acute renal failure to aid in controlling extracellular fluid volume. Expansion of the extracellular fluid volume due to excessive sodium intake may lead to hypertension, peripheral edema, cardiomegaly, pulmonary congestion, or pulmonary edema (Jenkins & Rieselbach, 1982). A daily intake of 2 g (87 mEq) of sodium is usually sufficient to avoid any expansion of extracellular fluid volume. Many medications are hidden sources of sodium that must be considered part of the overall sodium intake (Tables 10-6 and 10-7). The efficacy of a therapeutic sodium intake is monitored by taking daily weights and intake and output values as well as by measuring central venous pressure, pulmonary artery diastolic pressures, or capillary wedge pressures, if available.

Hyponatremia is described as a serum sodium level of less than 130 mEq/L. This condition may develop secondary to a positive fluid balance or when the quantity of water in the extracellular fluid increases without a proportionate increase in extracellular fluid sodium content. Hyponatremia becomes symptomatic when the serum sodium level falls to less than 120 mEq/L. Symptoms of hyponatremia include confusion,

**Table 10-6** Sodium Content of Selected Oral Medications

| Medication | Sodium Content |
|---|---|
| Alka-Seltzer, antacid | 567 mg per tablet |
| Alka-Seltzer, effervescent antacid | 311 mg per tablet |
| Alka-Seltzer, pain reliever | 506 mg per tablet |
| Alka-Seltzer Plus | 506 mg per tablet |
| Fleet Phospho-Soda | 554 mg per 5 mL |
| K-Phos Neutral | 298 mg per tablet |
| K-Phos Original | Sodium free |
| Phenergan | 57 mg per 5 mL |
| Rolaids | 53 mg per tablet |

*Source:* From *Food Medication Interactions*, 6th ed., by A. Allen and D. Powers, 1988, Phoenix, AZ: FMI Publishing. Copyright 1988 by FMI Publishing. Reprinted by permission.

**Table 10-7** Sodium Content of Selected Parenteral Medications

| Drug | Sodium Content |
|---|---|
| Ampicillin sodium | 2.8 to 3.4 mEq/g |
| Carbenicillin disodium | 5.2 to 6.5 mEq/g |
| Cefamandole nafate | 3.3 mEq/g |
| Cefoxitin sodium | 2.3 mEq/g |
| Metronidazole (500 mg per 100 mL) | 14 mEq per 100 mL |
| Methylprednisolone sodium succinate | 2.01 mEq/g |
| Mezlocillin sodium | 1.85 mEq/g |
| Nafcillin sodium | 2.9 mEq/g |
| Penicillin G sodium | 2 mEq per $10^6$ U |
| Piperacillin sodium | 1.98 mEq/g |
| Ticarcillin disodium | 5.2 to 6.5 mEq/g |
| Saline solutions | |
| 0.9% Sodium chloride | 154 mEq/L |
| 5% Dextrose, 0.2% sodium chloride | 34 mEq/L |
| 5% Dextrose, 0.45% sodium chloride | 77 mEq/L |
| 5% Dextrose, 0.9% sodium chloride | 154 mEq/L |
| Ringer's solution | 147 mEq/L |
| Lactated Ringer's solution | 130 mEq/L |
| Sodium bicarbonate solutions | |
| Sodium bicarbonate (4%) | 2.38 mEq per 5 mL |
| Sodium bicarbonate (5%) | 297.5 mEq per 500 mL |
| Sodium bicarbonate (7.5%) | 44.6 mEq per 50 mL |
| Sodium bicarbonate (8.4%) | 50 mEq per 50 mL |

*Source:* "Sodium Content of Commonly Administered Intravenous Drugs" by G. Raymond, P. Day, and M. Rabb, 1982, *Hospital Pharmacy, 17,* pp. 560–561. Copyright 1982 by J.B. Lippincott Company. Reprinted by permission.

lethargy, stupor, coma, and seizures. Strict fluid restriction is the first-line management for the treatment of hyponatremia (see Exhibits 10-4 and 10-5). In severe cases, however, the administration of hypertonic saline solutions or dialysis (or both) may be necessary. Sodium administration as a treatment modality for hyponatremia is reserved for the most severe cases.

*Fluid*

Oliguric or anuric patients need fluid restrictions to prevent a positive water balance. Insensible water loss is approximately 800 mL/day. This amount increases in the presence of fever, hyperventilation, or gastrointestinal losses due to nausea, vomiting, or diarrhea. A fluid intake of 800 mL plus the amount of urine volume per day is generally sufficient to prevent a positive water balance. Exhibits 10-4 and 10-5 list suggestions to aid with the management of dietary fluid restrictions.

*Potassium*

The usual dietary potassium intake approximates 1 mEq per kilogram of body weight, or roughly 50 to 100 mEq/day. Of this potassium intake, 90% to 95% is excreted in the urine and 5% to 10% is excreted in the stool.

The kidney has a tremendous capacity to secrete potassium into the urine by the distal nephron segments. Almost all the potassium in urine is secreted by the kidneys. In addition, the fecal excretion of potassium in patients with renal failure can range from 20% to 50% of the ingested load. Therefore, dietary potassium restriction is usually not necessary until urine volume is less than 1,000 mL/day or when the glomerular filtration rate is less than 10 mL/minute. When needed, dietary potassium restrictions should equal 1 mEq of potassium per kilogram of ideal body weight. For patients who are less than their ideal body weight, the amount of potassium should be based on actual body weight. Potassium intake generally should not exceed 65 mEq/day in patients who require a potassium restriction. Table 10-8 provides the potassium and caloric content of selected foods.

**Table 10-8** Potassium Content of Selected Foods

| Food Group | Amount | Potassium Content (mEq) | Calories |
|---|---|---|---|
| Dairy products | | | |
| Skim milk | 1 c | 9 | 88 |
| Whole milk | 1 c | 9 | 159 |
| Plain yogurt | 1 c | 9 | 113 |
| Meats | | | |
| Beef | 3 oz | 7 | 222 |
| Lamb | 3 oz | 6 | 237 |
| Pork | 3 oz | 6 | 308 |
| Poultry | 3 oz | 9 | 167 |
| Fish | 3 oz | 10 | 190 |
| Tuna (water pack) | 3 oz | 7 | 126 |
| Salmon | 3 oz | 7 | 145 |
| Starches | | | |
| White bread | One slice | 0.5 | 68 |
| Whole wheat bread | One slice | 2 | 61 |
| Pasta | ½ c | 1 | 77 |
| Brown rice | ½ c | 2 | 116 |
| Oatmeal | ½ c | 2 | 66 |
| Fruits | | | |
| Fresh apricots | Two medium | 5 | 36 |
| Canned apricots (heavy syrup) | Four halves | 7 | 97 |
| Dried apricots (uncooked) | Four large halves | 5 | 50 |
| Avocado, raw | 1 c, cubed | 23 | 250 |
| Banana | Half small (7 in) | 5 | 40 |
| Cantaloupe | 1 c, cubed | 10 | 48 |
| Honeydew melon | 1 c, cubed | 11 | 56 |
| Grapefruit juice (unsweetened) | ½ c | 6 | 53 |
| Fresh nectarine | One medium | 10 | 88 |
| Fresh orange | One medium | 8 | 71 |
| Orange juice (unsweetened frozen concentrate, diluted) | ½ c | 6.5 | 44 |
| Pineapple juice (canned, unsweetened) | ½ c | 4 | 69 |
| Prunes (uncooked) | Two medium | 3 | 43 |
| Prune juice | ½ c | 7 | 98 |
| Raisins | 2 tbsp | 4 | 52 |
| Dates (pitted) | Two medium | 3 | 44 |
| Vegetables | | | |
| Carrots (raw) | One large | 6 | 30 |
| Mushrooms (raw, diced) | 1 c | 7 | 20 |
| Tomato (raw) | One medium | 8 | 27 |
| Spinach (frozen leaf, cooked) | ½ c | 7 | 46 |
| Kale (frozen leaf, cooked) | ½ c | 3 | 45 |
| Mustard greens | ½ c | 3 | 47 |
| Collards | ½ c | 5 | 45 |
| Winter squash (cooked) | ½ c | 6 | 44 |
| Potatoes | | | |
| Irish (baked in skin) | One medium | 20 | 145 |
| Sweet potato (baked in skin) | One medium | 9 | 161 |
| French fried (2 to 3½ in long) | 10 | 11 | 137 |
| Potato chips | 1 oz | 8 | 161 |
| Lentils (dried, split) | ½ c | 6 | 106 |
| Split peas | ½ c | 8 | 115 |

**Table 10-8** continued

| Food Group | Amount | Potassium Content (mEq) | Calories |
|---|---|---|---|
| Navy beans | ½ c | 10 | 112 |
| Lima beans | ½ c | 9 | 94 |
| Pinto beans | ½ c | 8 | 110 |
| Miscellaneous | | | |
| Nuts | | | |
| Almonds | 10 whole nuts | 3 | 89 |
| Brazil nuts | Four medium | 3 | 92 |
| Peanuts | 20 whole nuts | 2 | 53 |
| Pecans | Two whole | 1 | 25 |
| Molasses, blackstrap | 1 tbsp | 15 | 43 |
| Wheat bran | 1 tbsp | 1 | 9 |
| Wheat germ | 1 tbsp | 1.5 | 23 |
| Salt substitute | 1 tsp | 50 | 0 |

*Source:* From *Manual of Clinical Dietetics* by The Clinical Section of the Columbus Dietetic Administrative Council, 1985, Columbus, OH: Vision Printing. Copyright by Columbus Dietetic Administrative Council. Reprinted by permission.

*Protein*

Protein intake should be limited to 0.5 to 0.8 g per kilogram of ideal body weight in persons with acute renal failure to avoid exacerbation of the accumulation of nitrogenous waste products. For persons who are less than their ideal body weight, the amount of protein should be based on actual body weight. Protein of high biological value should make up most of the dietary protein provided. Provision of adequate nonprotein kilocalories is essential to achieve optimal utilization of the nitrogen provided. Caloric requirements may approach 50 kcal/kg/day, and a nitrogen:kilocalorie ratio of 1:300 to 1:450 is recommended (Blackburn, Etter, & MacKenzie, 1978). Exhibit 10-6 lists foods low in sodium, potassium, and protein that can be added to the diet to increase caloric intake.

**Chronic Renal Failure**

Chronic renal failure may result from neoplastic disease or its treatment. Cancer may lead to chronic renal failure by (1) membranous nephropathy associated with solid tumors; (2) amyloidosis associated with multiple myeloma; (3) cancer chemotherapy; (4) radiation-induced interstitial nephropathy; (5) nephropathy due to hypercalcemia associated with bone

**Exhibit 10-6** Good Caloric Sources for Sodium-, Potassium-, and Protein-Restricted Diets

Butter
Candy canes
Candy corn
Corn starch
Cotton candy
Divinity candy (no nuts)
Fondant
French creams, buttercreams (not chocolate)
Gumdrops
Hard candy (unfilled)
Honey
Jam
Jelly
Jellybeans
Lemon drops
Lifesavers
Lollipops
Marshmallows
Mints (not chocolate)
Pancake syrup
Sugar (granulated or powdered)
Taffy (made without salt)
Wheat starch
Whipping cream
Whipped topping

*Source:* From *Manual of Clinical Dietetics* by The Clinical Section of the Columbus Dietetic Administrative Council, 1985, Columbus, OH: Vision Printing. Copyright by Columbus Dietetic Administrative Council. Reprinted by permission.

metastasis, production of parathyroid hormone–like polypeptides, increased prostaglandins, or release of osteoclast-activating factor in multiple myeloma; or (6) urinary tract obstruction from various tumors (Schwartz & Klahr, 1982).

Many of the dietary restrictions needed to manage acute renal failure may be less stringent or not necessary in patients with chronic renal failure who undergo routine dialysis. Although a controlled sodium intake is still needed, a diet containing 4 to 6 g of sodium (see Table 10-5) may provide adequate control of extracellular fluid volume. Fluid and potassium restrictions are necessary in oliguric or anuric patients, as described for the management of acute renal failure. Protein intake can be liberalized to 1 g per kilogram of ideal body weight (or actual body weight if less than ideal). The provision of adequate nonprotein kilocalories remains necessary to achieve optimal nitrogen utilization.

## CONCLUSION

The pathogenesis of cancer of the pancreas, liver, or kidney can result in many metabolic aberrations, most of which have significant effects on nutrition. Although many of the nutrition problems created by these malignancies can be treated by specific nutrition regimens, the efficacy of diet therapy should be evaluated not only from a medical viewpoint but from an emotional and psychologic viewpoint as well. Because the prognosis for patients with pancreatic, liver, or renal carcinoma is grim, diet therapy should parallel the goals of the medical team and family wishes. When palliation of symptoms through surgery or drug therapy becomes the primary goal, diet therapy should then be directed toward patient comfort rather than control of metabolic aberrations.

### REFERENCES

Alpert, E. (1976). Tumors of the liver. In J.P. Sanford & J.M. Dietschy (Eds.), *The science and practice of clinical medicine: Disorders of the gastrointestinal tract, disorders of the liver, nutritional disorders* (Vol. 1, pp. 328–333). New York: Grune & Stratton.

Alpert, E., & Isselbacher, K.J. (1987). Tumors of the liver. In E. Braunwald, K.J. Isselbacher, R.G. Petersdorf, J.D. Wilson, J.B. Martin, & A.S. Fauci (Eds.), *Harrison's principles of internal medicine* (pp. 1351–1353). New York: McGraw-Hill.

Beazley, R.M. (1985). Pancreatic cancer: Surgical aspects. In L.H. Toledo-Pereyra (Ed.), *The pancreas: Principles of medical and surgical practice* (pp. 307–337). New York: Wiley.

Bernard, M.A., Jacobs, D.O., & Rombeau, J.L. (1986). *Nutritional and metabolic support of hospitalized patients*. Philadelphia: Saunders.

Blackburn, G.L., Etter, G., & MacKenzie, J. (1978). Criteria for choosing amino acid therapy in acute renal failure. *American Journal of Clinical Nutrition, 31*, 1841.

Buescu, A., Dimich, A.B., & Myers, W.P.L. (1975). Cancer hypercalcemia—A pragmatic approach. *Clinical Bulletin (Memorial Sloan-Kettering Cancer Center), 5*, 91.

Buncher, C.R. (1980). Epidemiology of pancreatic cancer. In A.R. Moossa (Ed.), *Tumors of the pancreas* (pp. 415–427). Baltimore: Williams & Wilkins.

Cady, B. (1982). Selection of treatment for liver metastases. In L. Weiss & H.A. Gilbert (Eds.), *Liver metastasis* (pp. 275–293). Boston: Hall.

Conn, H.O. (1976). Differential diagnosis of ascites. In J.P. Sanford & J.M. Dietschy (Eds.), *The science and practice of clinical medicine: Disorders of the gastrointestinal tract, disorders of the liver, nutritional disorders* (Vol. 1, pp. 261–263). New York: Grune & Stratton.

Cooper, M.J., & Moossa, A.R. (1980). Cellular composition and physiology of the exocrine pancreas. In A.R. Moossa (Ed.), *Tumors of the pancreas* (pp. 21–28). Baltimore: Williams & Wilkins.

Dhorajiwala, J.M., Reckard, C.R., & Moossa, A.R. (1980). Cellular composition and physiology of the islets of Langerhans. In A.R. Moossa (Ed.), *Tumors of the pancreas* (pp. 29–35). Baltimore: Williams & Wilkins.

Digestive enzymes. (1987). *Facts and Comparisons, 6*, 309–310.

Enteral nutritional therapy: Modular supplements. (1985). *Facts and Comparisons, 4*, 56.

Foster, D.W., & Rubenstein, A.H. (1987). Hypoglycemia, insulinoma, and other hormone-secreting tumors of the pancreas. In E. Braunwald, K.J. Isselbacher, R.G. Petersdorf, J.D. Wilson, J.B. Martin, & A.S. Fauci (Eds.), *Harrison's principles of internal medicine* (pp. 1800–1807). New York: McGraw-Hill.

Friesen, S.R. (1985). Endocrine tumors. In L.H. Toledo-Pereyra (Ed.), *The pancreas: Principles of medical and surgical practice* (pp. 339–357). New York: Wiley.

Garnick, M.B., & Brenner, B.M. (1987). Tumors of the urinary tract. In E. Braunwald, K.J. Isselbacher, R.G. Petersdorf, J.D. Wilson, J.B. Martin, & A.S. Fauci (Eds.), *Harrison's principles of internal medicine* (pp. 1218–1221). New York: McGraw-Hill.

Gold, E.B., Gordis, L., Diener, M.D., Seltser, R., Boitnott, J.K., Bynum, T.E., & Hutcheon, D.F. (1985). Diet and other risk factors for cancer of the pancreas. *Cancer, 55*, 460–467.

Goldberg, D.M., & Gornall, A.G. (1980). Hepatobiliary disorders. In A.G. Gornall (Ed.), *Applied biochemistry of clinical disorders* (pp. 164–192). Hagerstown, MD: Harper & Row.

Goodman, H.M. (1974). The pancreas and regulation of metabolism. In V.B. Mountcastle (Ed.), *Medical physiology* (Vol. 2, pp. 1776–1807). St. Louis: Mosby.

Grant, J.P., James, S., Grabowski, V., & Trexler, K.M. (1984). Total parenteral nutrition in pancreatic disease. *Annals of Surgery, 200*, 627–631.

Greenberger, N.J., & Toskes, P.P. (1987). Approach to the patient with pancreatic disease. In E. Braunwald, K.J. Isselbacher, R.G. Petersdorf, J.D. Wilson, J.B. Martin, & A.S. Fauci (Eds.), *Harrison's principles of internal medicine* (pp. 1368–1372). New York: McGraw-Hill.

Greenberger, N.J., Toskes, P.P., & Isselbacher, K.J. (1987). Diseases of the pancreas. In E. Braunwald, K.J. Isselbacher, R.G. Petersdorf, J.D. Wilson, J.B. Martin, & A.S. Fauci (Eds.), *Harrison's principles of internal medicine* (pp. 1372–1384). New York: McGraw-Hill.

Janowitz, H.D., & Banks, P.A. (1976). Tumors of the pancreas. In J.P. Sanford & J.M. Dietschy (Eds.), *The science and practice of clinical medicine: Disorders of the gastrointestinal tract, disorders of the liver, nutritional disorders* (Vol. 1, pp. 211–216). New York: Grune & Stratton.

Jaspan, J.B., Polonsky, K.S., Foster, D.W., & Rubenstein, A.H. (1980). Clinical features and diagnosis of islet cell tumors. In A.R. Moossa (Ed.), *Tumors of the pancreas* (pp. 469–504). Baltimore: Williams & Wilkins.

Javadpour, N. (1984a). Natural history, diagnosis, and staging of renal cancer. In N. Javadpour (Ed.), *Cancer of the kidney* (pp. 5–13). New York: Thieme-Stratton.

Javadpour, N. (1984b). Overview of renal cancer. In N. Javadpour (Ed.), *Cancer of the kidney* (pp. 1–3). New York: Thieme-Stratton.

Javadpour, N. (1984c). Surgical management of renal cancer. In N. Javadpour (Ed.), *Cancer of the kidney* (pp. 69–80). New York: Thieme-Stratton.

Jenkins, P.G., & Rieselbach, R.E. (1982). Acute renal failure: Diagnosis, clinical spectrum, and management. In R.E. Rieselbach & M.B. Garnick (Eds.), *Cancer and the kidney* (pp. 103–179). Philadelphia: Lea & Febiger.

Khoury, S., & Saul, A. (1986). Metastatic renal adenocarcinoma. In J.B. deKernion & M. Pavone-Macaluso (Eds.), *Tumors of the kidney* (pp. 194–204). Baltimore: Williams & Wilkins.

Klaassen, D.J., MacIntyre, J.M., Catton, G.E., Engstrom, P.F., & Moertel, C.G. (1985). Treatment of locally unresectable cancer of the stomach and pancreas: A randomized comparison of 5-fluorouracil alone with radiation plus concurrent and maintenance 5-fluorouracil—An Eastern Cooperative Oncology Group study. *Journal of Clinical Oncology, 3*, 373–378.

Leichman, L.P. (1985). Pancreatic cancer: Medical aspects. In L.H. Toledo-Pereyra (Ed.), *The pancreas: Principles of medical and surgical practice* (pp. 285–305). New York: Wiley.

Levin, B., & Kinzie, J.J. (1980). Adjuvant therapy of pancreatic tumors. In A.R. Moossa (Ed.), *Tumors of the pancreas* (pp. 521–531). Baltimore: Williams & Wilkins.

Linsell, A. (1987). Primary liver cancer: Epidemiology and etiology. In H.J. Wanebo (Ed.), *Hepatic and biliary cancer* (pp. 3–15). New York: Marcel Dekker.

Mackie, C.R., & Moossa, A.R. (1980). Surgical anatomy of the pancreas. In A.R. Moossa (Ed.), *Tumors of the pancreas* (pp. 1–19). Baltimore: Williams & Wilkins.

Malt, R.A. (1983). Treatment of pancreatic cancer. *Journal of the American Medical Association, 250*, 1433–1437.

Moossa, A.R., Lewis, M.H., & Bowie, J.D. (1980). Clinical features and diagnosis of pancreatic cancer. In A.R. Moossa (Ed.), *Tumors of the pancreas* (pp. 429–442). Baltimore: Williams & Wilkins.

Mundy, G.R., Ibbotson, K.J., D'Souza, S.M., Simpson, E.L., Jacobs, J.W., & Martin, T.J. (1984). The hypercalcemia of cancer. *New England Journal of Medicine, 310*, 1718.

Onstad, G.R., & Bubrick, M.P. (1985). Physiology. In L.H. Toledo-Pereyra (Ed.), *The pancreas: Principles of medical and surgical practice* (pp. 51–66). New York: Wiley.

Schwartz, J.C., & Klahr, S. (1982). Chronic renal failure: Pathophysiology, complications, and medical management. In R.E. Rieselbach & M.B. Garnick (Eds.), *Cancer and the kidney* (pp. 180–213). Philadelphia: Lea & Febiger.

Sufrin, G., Golio, A., & Murphy, G.P. (1986). Serologic markers, paraneoplastic syndromes, and ectopic hormone production in renal adenocarcinoma. In J.B. deKernion & M. Pavone-Macaluso (Eds.), *Tumors of the kidney* (pp. 51–71). Baltimore: Williams & Wilkins.

Tersigni, R., & Toledo-Pereyra, L.H. (1985). Surgical anatomy of the pancreas. In L.H. Toledo-Pereyra (Ed.), *The pancreas: Principles of medical and surgical practice* (pp. 31–50). New York: Wiley.

Wanebo, H.J. (1987). Surgical management of liver metastases. In H.J. Wanebo (Ed.), *Hepatic and biliary cancer* (pp. 461–476). New York: Marcel Dekker.

Wynick, D., Williams, S.J., & Bloom, S.R. (1988). Symptomatic secondary hormone syndromes in patients with established malignant pancreatic endocrine tumors. *New England Journal of Medicine, 319*, 605–607.

# Chapter 11

# The Gastrointestinal Tract: Small Bowel and Colon

*Mindy Hermann-Zaidins*

The impact of cancer on the small and large intestine is more reflective of treatment, specifically surgery and radiation, than of the tumor itself. Small bowel tumors are relatively uncommon as a primary disease, and newly diagnosed colon cancer rarely affects directly a patient's ability to absorb nutrients. Nevertheless, the acute and chronic nutrition-related effects of bowel resection and lower abdominal radiation therapy present a constant challenge for the dietitian.

## DIGESTIVE, ABSORPTIVE, AND METABOLIC CONSEQUENCES

### Duodenum and Jejunum

Duodenal and jejunal resections or partial bypass are rare as isolated events; instead, they often accompany excision of other gastrointestinal (GI) tract organs. Total or partial gastric resections may circumvent the duodenum. Pancreatic surgery often includes removal of both the duodenum and portions of the jejunum.

*Note:* Portions of this chapter were adapted from "Malabsorption" by M.G. Hermann-Zaidins in *Dietitian's Handbook of Enteral and Parenteral Nutrition* (pp. 417–433) by A. Skipper (Ed.), 1990, Rockville, MD: Aspen Publishers, Inc. Copyright 1990 by Aspen Publishers, Inc.

Exhibit 11-1 lists a few of the surgical procedures that involve the upper small bowel. All these procedures may cause hypergastrinemia and gastric hypersecretion and thereby may result in inactivation or dilution of pancreatic enzymes, impairment of micelle formation, and rapid transit of food boluses (Tilson, 1980; Weser, 1983).

Radiation damage, adhesions, or fistulae may severely impair portions of the duodenum or jejunum, potentially necessitating surgical removal. The radiation-induced acute and chronic changes listed in Exhibit 11-2 often lead to functional aberrations in mucosal water and electrolyte transport, enzyme production, motility, and, ultimately, macronutrient absorption. Adhesions that partially or totally obstruct the bowel can lead to anorexia, nausea, vomit-

**Exhibit 11-1** Surgical Procedures That Include Duodenal Excision or Bypass

| |
|---|
| Partial gastrectomy with gastrojejunostomy |
| Total gastrectomy |
| Billroth II |
| Total gastrectomy with Roux-en-Y esophagojejunostomy |
| Pancreatoduodenectomy (Whipple procedure) |
| Regional pancreatectomy |

Exhibit 11-2 Radiation-Induced Bowel Changes

Short term
  Shortening of villi
  Mucosal thickening
  Mucosal ulcerations
  Reduced absorptive surface

Long term
  Ischemic stenosis
  Bowel obstruction
  Fistula formation

ing, diarrhea, and the blind loop syndrome. Diarrhea, steatorrhea, and weight loss may be associated with gastrocolic, enteroentero, or enterocutaneous fistulae.

The effects of bowel surgery on nutrient digestion and absorption depend on the extent and site of the resection, integrity of the ileum, and function of the remainder of the GI tract.

## Ileum

Ileal resections often are necessitated by metastatic disease, fistulae, or radiation damage. They have the greatest adverse effect, compared to duodenal or other resections, on nutrition status because of the ileum's slow transit, ability to reabsorb bile salts, and ability to absorb vitamin $B_{12}$ (Weser, 1983); these functions cannot be assumed by other parts of the small bowel. Additionally, the ileocecal valve prolongs transit time by regulating flow and minimizes bacterial migration from the colon (Tilson, 1980; Weser, 1983). Absorption is least affected by ileal resections of less than 100 cm; a common consequence is watery diarrhea containing small amounts of fat (Weser, 1983; Hofmann & Poley, 1972). Excision of more than 100 cm causes bile salt losses that exceed the liver's capacity for resynthesis.

Ileal hypertrophy is greatest after duodenal or jejunal resections (Ostrov & Balint, 1980; Williamson, 1978). Factors stimulating growth include the physical presence of nutrients (Tilson, 1980; Weser, 1979, 1983; Weser, Fletcher, & Urban, 1979), the effect of enteric

hormones (Tilson, 1980; Weser et al., 1979; Weser, Bell, & Tawil, 1981; Young, Cioletti, Winborn, Traylor, & Weser, 1980; Schwartz & Storozuk, 1985), and pancreatobiliary secretions (Weser, 1983; Weser et al., 1979). For these reasons, use of the enteral feeding route is recommended wherever possible.

## Colon

Partial or total colectomies may induce profound losses of fluid and electrolytes, the severity of which is related to the length and site of resection (Mitchell et al., 1980). Potassium depletion appears to be related to the length of colon lost, in contrast to sodium, which is dependent on the ileum (Mitchell et al., 1980).

## General Effects

Intestinal lymphomas thicken and ulcerate the small bowel mucosa, reducing its absorptive ability and often creating a protein-losing enteropathy. The distal ileum, with its rich aggregation of lymphatic tissue, commonly is involved.

Prior GI surgery or active disease processes may further affect absorption. Systemic or localized infectious agents often cause watery diarrhea or malabsorption (or both). Bacterial overgrowth from anatomic abnormalities or blind loops leads to malabsorption of vitamin $B_{12}$ and deconjugation of bile salts. Carbohydrate absorption likewise may be affected.

The panmalabsorption observed after radiation therapy (Reeves, Sanders, Isley, Sharpe, & Baylin, 1959; Duncan & Leonard, 1965; Donaldson, 1984) passes through acute and chronic phases. Whereas acute radiation enteritis abates within a short period of time, chronic mucosal changes may develop long after radiation therapy has been completed and may not reverse themselves. Chemotherapeutic agents that induce malabsorption by causing villous shortening, crypt hypertrophy, and mucosal convolutions include methotrexate (Williamson, 1978) and neomycin (Green & Tall, 1979).

## Ostomies

The behavior of an ostomy relates directly to the factors discussed above. Ileostomies and jejunostomies cause great increases in GI fluid loss because they bypass the colon, which is the major site of fluid absorption. If macronutrient malabsorption also is present, output may become excessive. Colostomies may have little effect on bowel movements, especially if a significant amount of large bowel is functional.

## EVALUATING THE SEVERITY OF MALABSORPTION

### Clinical Signs and Symptoms

The clinical signs and symptoms of malabsorption reflect the patient's inability to utilize nutrients in the diet. Because many patients receive little or no nutrition guidance before the development of absorption problems, their self-selected diets often are completely inappropriate for their condition.

Weight loss usually occurs in spite of marked changes in appetite. Although anorexia is common among cancer patients, hypergeusia of more than 10,000 cal/day is not unheard of. Physical manifestations of vitamin and mineral deficiencies include tetany, severe dry skin, and positive Chvostek's and Trousseau's signs (Table 11-1).

Stool changes may reflect the etiology of malabsorption. Table 11-2 summarizes common aberrations, most of which relate to fat loss. Although dietitians may find questioning patients, caretakers, and nurses about patients' bowel movement characteristics to be unpleas-

**Table 11-2** Stool Color and Consistency Changes in Small Bowel and Colon Disease

| Characteristics | Absorptive Defect |
| --- | --- |
| Watery, brown | Carbohydrates, lactose, electrolytes, water |
| Yellow, normal form | Fat |
| Yellow, foamy, oily | Fat and other nutrients |
| Foul smelling | Fat |
| Silver, gray | Fat, secondary to biliary obstruction |

ant, they will learn a tremendous amount about patients' absorptive problems by doing so. This knowledge in turn facilitates the planning of nutrition intervention. Dietitians may find it helpful to develop a chart of sample colors so that the patient can readily identify his or her characteristic stool color.

### Laboratory Tests

Abnormal laboratory test results are similar to those observed in chronic malnutrition. The most serious aberrations are in serum cholesterol, folate, $B_{12}$, iron, calcium, magnesium, and fat-soluble vitamins. Abnormal values reflect the impaired absorption and loss of these nutrients in the stool.

### The Malabsorption Work-Up

Quantitative and qualitative tests of absorption aid the practitioner in formulating a diagnosis, assessing the severity of the absorptive defect, and developing appropriate medical and nutrition care plans. Several clinicians have prioritized testing through the use of decision trees (Krejs & Fordtran, 1983; Dobbins, 1980; Olsen, 1979). These guides suggest a logical progression of tests to avoid excessive costs and unnecessary procedures.

The importance of a thorough assessment of the patient's medical history and clinical presentation should not be underestimated. This assessment is based on discussions with the patient, interdisciplinary meetings, and a comprehensive review of the patient's medical chart. Often the

**Table 11-1** Vitamin and Mineral Deficiencies Common in Small Bowel and Colon Disease

| Sign or Symptom | Vitamin or Mineral |
| --- | --- |
| Tetany | Calcium |
| Chvostek's sign | Calcium |
| Trousseau's sign | Magnesium |
| Paresthesia | Magnesium |
| Dry skin | Essential fatty acids |

dietitian picks up valuable information during patient evaluation and monitoring that is instrumental in identifying the patient's absorptive defects. A small number of select tests then can be performed to confirm the clinical observations.

*Fat Absorption*

The normal small bowel absorbs approximately 95% of a typical 60- to 100-g fat intake (Gray, 1983). Tests of fat malabsorption, namely Sudan stain, fecal fat test, and labeled carbon breath test, identify abnormal losses, but they cannot identify the etiology of the absorptive defect (e.g., pancreatic insufficiency rather than short bowel syndrome).

1. *Sudan stain.* Sudan stain calls for preparation and staining of a small sample of stool and examination of it for a specified number and size of fat globules (Drummey, Benson, & Jones, 1961). This test can qualitatively identify moderate malabsorption (Gray, 1983) but cannot predict the amount of fat lost in the stool. Sudan stain often is falsely negative in patients with nonsevere malabsorption.
2. *Labeled carbon breath test.* The labeled carbon breath test qualitatively evaluates fat absorption as it relates to carbon dioxide exhalation. A designated amount of isotopically labeled fat, usually [$^{14}$C]triolein, is mixed with an unlabeled carrier and administered to the patient, after an overnight fast, in a beverage carrier of known fat composition. Breath samples are collected over 5 to 6 hours and analyzed for $^{14}CO_2$. The lower the $^{14}CO_2$ content, the greater the fat malabsorption. Delayed gastric emptying, chronic pulmonary disease, diabetes mellitus, hyperlipidemia, obesity, liver disease, and other lung or metabolic disorders can affect the accuracy of the test (Newcomer, Hofmann, DiMagno, Thomas, & Carlson, 1979).
3. *Fecal fat test.* The fecal fat test usually is performed on an inpatient basis only and requires the provision of an 80- to 100-g fat diet for several days. Stools are collected for 48 or 72 hours and analyzed for fat content. This test also is considered qualitative. One investigator has observed that daily excretion of more than 40 g of fat may indicate defective lipolysis from pancreatic disease or massive ileal resection and that loss of 25 to 30 g of fat may signify mucosal damage (Ryan & Olsen, 1983).

Accurate test results are difficult to obtain because of incomplete or inaccurate calorie counts or stool collections and fluctuations in fat intake (Thorsgaard Pedersen & Halgreen, 1984). Staff resistance to this test reflects its poor aesthetic value and labor intensity. Fecal collections should be avoided in patients with acquired immunodeficiency syndrome or other diseases potentially communicable through stool.

The results of fecal fat and labeled carbon tests correlate well with severe malabsorption (West, Levin, Griffin, & Maxwell, 1981; Benini et al., 1984). The fecal fat test is more sensitive to mild steatorrhea than the breath test, although the latter may become more popular because it can be performed on outpatients.

*Small Bowel Function*

Evaluation of small bowel function is done by means of tests specific for the duodenum and jejunum rather than the ileum. The duodenum and jejunum are targeted with the D-xylose test. The Schilling test, best known for examining vitamin B$_{12}$ absorption, also is used to evaluate ileal viability.

*D-Xylose test.* Xylose, a pentose, does not require digestion before absorption. Therefore, normal results in a patient with steatorrhea usually signify that malabsorption is from impaired digestion (pancreatic insufficiency, depleted bile salt pool, and the like) rather than from an absorptive defect. Abnormal serum, urine, and stool levels point toward malabsorption; the normal stool should contain almost no xylose. Renal disease, bacterial overgrowth, age, and fluid retention affect the reliability of test results.

*Schilling test.* The Schilling test calls for concurrent administration of an unlabeled vitamin $B_{12}$ dose intramuscularly and a labeled $B_{12}$ dose orally (Adams & Cartwright, 1963). A 24-hour urine collection is started, and specimens are later analyzed for radioactivity. Several malabsorption-related syndromes affect the results of the Schilling test. Bacterial overgrowth, pancreatic insufficiency, or absence of intrinsic factor must be compensated for before this test is used to evaluate malabsorption (Gray, 1983).

### Disaccharidase Activity and Stool Carbohydrate

Lactose intolerance commonly is observed in the patient with malabsorption. Any impairment of small bowel integrity may compromise villous lactase production, thereby causing watery diarrhea after ingestion of lactose. A peak rise in breath hydrogen during the lactose tolerance test may indicate insufficient lactase activity (Ravich & Bayless, 1983).

Tests of disaccharidase activity and other measures of stool carbohydrate, such as stool *p*H, are not extremely sensitive (Ryan & Olsen, 1983; Anderson, Levine, & Levitt, 1981; Perman, Modler, Barr, & Rosenthal, 1984; Stephen, Haddad, & Phillips, 1983; Welsh & Griffiths, 1980). Fecal carbohydrate usually is not measurable directly.

### Bacterial Overgrowth

The $^{14}C$-labeled bile acid and the labeled D-xylose breath tests detect bacterial overgrowth in the small bowel, which is ordinarily a site of minimal contamination. The bile acid test identifies abnormal bacterial deconjugation of bile acids in the ileum, which results in the appearance of $^{14}CO_2$ in the breath. Under normal conditions the labeled bile acid would be absorbed, not deconjugated, before absorption. This test is not sensitive, especially in the presence of ileal damage and rapid transit (Isaacs & Kim, 1979; King, Toskes, Guilarte, Lorenz, & Welkos, 1980). The labeled D-xylose test appears to be more sensitive (King et al., 1980).

### Mucosal Integrity

Abdominal x-ray examinations, computerized axial tomography scans, barium studies, and intestinal biopsy assess the viability of the small bowel mucosa. One study categorizes roentgenographic abnormalities as follows (Munyer & Moss, 1980). Small bowel dilation with normal folds is consistent with sprue and collagen diseases. Thickened folds are observed in radiation enteritis, parasitic diseases, lymphoma, and Crohn's disease. Disaccharidase deficiency, biliary disease, and pancreatic disease usually do not affect small bowel x-ray results because they represent defects in digestion but not absorption.

## NUTRITION INTERVENTIONS

A thorough assessment of malabsorption, including clinical evaluation and the absorption work-up, establishes initial guidelines for nutrition management. Feeding the cancer patient with malabsorption is a dynamic process that can be both challenging and frustrating. Many patients, particularly those with resections limited to the duodenum or jejunum, improve in their ability to handle nutrients as the remaining small bowel expands its absorptive capacity. Others, especially those with chronic radiation damage, may experience a worsening of malabsorptive symptoms over time, especially if their symptoms are accompanied by progressive malnutrition. This necessitates major dietary modifications, including the use of enteral or parenteral feeding.

Philosophies of dietary manipulation vary in the type of nutrient restriction, degree of macronutrient hydrolysis, and use of alternate feeding modalities (Weser et al., 1979; Jeejeebhoy, 1983; Woolf, Miller, Kurian, & Jeejeebhoy, 1983; Young, 1983; Greenberger, 1978; Shils, 1984). Table 11-3 summarizes dietary recommendations for complications associated with cancer treatment.

Most patients, except those with severe malabsorption, can be managed successfully on oral feeding. Furthermore, it is important to provide

**Table 11-3** Nutrition Management Options

| Nutrient Modification | Diagnoses |
|---|---|
| Moderate fat plus medium-chain triglyceride (MCT) oil | Bile salt diarrhea, ileal resection (<100 cm) |
| Low fat plus MCT oil | Rapid transit, ileal resection (>100 cm), ileal damage, mucosal alterations |
| Low lactose | Lactose intolerance, rapid transit, mucosal alterations |
| Low osmolality | Rapid transit, ileal damage, ileal resection (>100 cm) |
| Low oxalate | Ileal damage, colon intact; ileal resection (>100 cm), colon intact |
| Hydrolyzed enteral | Acute malabsorption, mucosal alterations, ileal resection (>100 cm), massive resection |

*Source:* Adapted from *Clinical Management of Gastrointestinal Cancer* (pp. 303–326) by J.J. DeCosse and P. Sherlock (Eds.), 1984, Boston: Martinus Nijhoff. Copyright 1984 by Martinus Nijhoff.

the patient with oral or enteral nutrients early in the course of management to stimulate intestinal hypertrophy (Feldman, Dowling, McNaughton, & Peters, 1976), hyperplasia (Feldman et al., 1976), and brush border enzyme activity (Levine, Deren, Steiger, & Zinno, 1974).

Nutrition regimens rarely can be standardized and instead must be tailored to the individual patient. The coexistence of conditions or complications (e.g., short bowel with radiation enteritis or bacterial overgrowth with bile salt diarrhea) complicates management. It is crucial for nutrition and medical personnel to collaborate in developing a comprehensive care plan for the patient.

The relationship between the etiology of malabsorption and the patient's ability to handle specific nutrients must be fully understood to formulate a successful nutrition care plan. The initial diet prescription should be conservative because it is far easier to begin with a skeletal base diet and add or increase nutrients as tolerated by the patient.

## General Macronutrient Manipulations

### Carbohydrate

Carbohydrate intake may require modification, especially if the patient has developed a watery, osmotic-type diarrhea of normal color. Common recommendations include elimination of lactose (Shils, 1984), restriction of simple sugars to control osmotic load (Greenberger, 1978), and limitation of insoluble dietary fiber (Donaldson, 1984; Dutta & Hlasko, 1985) such as that found in whole wheat products, fruits, vegetables, and legumes. The type and amount of dietary carbohydrate permitted depend on the patient's tolerance of feeding and on the specific absorptive deficit. Recent findings suggest that carbohydrate malabsorption may be more problematic than fat malabsorption because of its impact on fluid and electrolyte balance (Woolf et al., 1983; Ameen, Powell, & Jones, 1987).

Dietary disaccharides, specifically lactose, often must be restricted (Shils, 1984), particularly in patients with radiation enteritis or bowel resections. Some patients can use lactose-reduced products, in which approximately 60% of the lactose has been converted to glucose and galactose, to enable nearly normal consumption of dairy products. Other more compromised individuals may be required to eliminate all sources of lactose, including yogurt and certain cheeses. Lactase enzyme preparations can be utilized to ensure 100% breakdown of the lactose in regular or modified lactose milks. As the villi regenerate and regain some ability to synthesize lactase, lactose tolerance may improve somewhat but probably never will return to normal.

Restriction of simple carbohydrates has been recommended to decrease the dietary osmotic load in short gut–induced rapid transit (Greenberger, 1978) and to reduce malabsorption of nutrients. Artificial sweeteners may be added to increase palatability, and oligosaccharide modules may be used to enhance caloric intake.

High-fiber diets usually are discouraged because they have been shown to aggravate malabsorption (Donaldson, 1984; Dutta & Hlasko, 1985). Some patients may benefit from pectin-containing foods, however, such as oatmeal and applesauce, or psyllium supplements, which help solidify the stool by adsorbing water.

*Protein*

Protein absorption usually is not affected in mild to moderate malabsorption if the activities of proteolytic enzymes and amino acid–absorptive systems have not been affected by the disease process. The more impaired patient may require hydrolyzed protein to maximize absorption, however. Hydrolyzed formulas have been recommended for patients with radiation enteritis (Heymsfield, Horowitz, & Lawson, 1980; Beer, Farr, & Halsted, 1985), massive small bowel resection (Heymsfield et al., 1980; Iles, 1984), or high-output intestinal fistulae (Rocchio, Cha, Haas, & Randall, 1974). Patients on these formulas should be fed enterally because hydrolyzed protein is extremely unpalatable; as such, poor compliance with an oral prescription can be expected.

The overuse of formulas with hydrolyzed protein has been criticized by practitioners who hold that their relative benefits have not been sufficiently demonstrated (Koretz & Meyer, 1980). This formula class is expensive and may not be well tolerated because of its hypertonicity. An additional drawback is that these formulas usually are started at low concentrations and slow infusion rates, a practice that increases the time necessary for the patient to reach calorie and nutrient goals. One group examining hydrolyzed and polymeric products observed more rapid bowel adaptation after feeding with an intact protein formula (Fairfull-Smith, Abunassar, Freeman, & Maroun, 1980).

*Fat*

*Long-chain fat.* The digestion and absorption of long-chain fat commonly are impaired to a greater degree than those of other nutrients. Any significant interruption in dietary fat incorporation, including enzymatic lipolysis, micelle formation, absorption, or reabsorption of bile salts, causes mild to severe fat losses in the stool. These losses also tend to induce depletion of fat-soluble vitamins and certain minerals. As such, dietary fat modification is a crucial step in managing the patient with bowel impairment.

Fat restriction has been prescribed to reduce losses of fluids and electrolytes (Greenberger, 1978; Andersson, Isaksson, & Sjogren, 1974; Bochenek, Rodgers, & Balint, 1970), divalent cations (calcium, zinc, magnesium, and copper) (Ovesen, Chu, & Howard, 1983), and bile acid. Deconjugation by colonic bacteria of malabsorbed bile acids causes colonic secretion of water and sodium (Hofmann & Poley, 1972). A long-chain fat restriction of 30 to 40 g daily, or approximately 15% to 20% of the total calories, is widely recommended (Tilson, 1980; Ostrov & Balint, 1980; Weser et al., 1979; Greenberger, 1978; Shils, 1984; Andersson et al., 1974; Ovesen et al., 1983; Cello, 1983; Griffin, Fagan, Hodgson, & Chadwick, 1982), especially to reduce the steatorrhea, diarrhea (Winawer, Broitman, Woolchow, Osborne, & Zamcheck, 1966), and bile salt losses (Winawer et al., 1966) caused by small bowel resection or radiation enteritis.

A recent controversy has developed regarding the use of low-fat diets in patients with fat malabsorption. Several investigators found no significant changes in stool volume (Ovesen et al., 1983; Simko, McCarroll, Goodman, Weesner, & Kelley, 1980), electrolyte and mineral losses (Weser, 1979; Ovesen et al., 1983), and percentage fat absorption (Weser, 1979) when patients were switched from low-fat to high-fat diets. Their thinking was that if the percentage of fat absorbed remains stable, regardless of total dietary content, then the patient will benefit from the high-fat regimen because the total calories absorbed would be greater. Additionally, the high-carbohydrate, high-osmolality diet created when fat is restricted actually may aggravate diarrhea. Palatability also becomes an issue in extremely low-fat diets.

Where fat restriction is indicated, one should begin with only enough long-chain fat to prevent essential fatty acid deficiency. Dietary fat can be increased gradually as tolerated by the patient. The patient's ability to handle dietary fat may improve as the remaining bowel hypertrophies (Woolf, Miller, Kurian, & Jeejeebhoy, 1987). The patient whose absorption improves significantly eventually can return to a nearly normal diet. Patients who are unable to tolerate long-chain fat must be observed for signs of mineral and fat-soluble vitamin deficiencies that can develop over time.

*Medium-chain triglycerides.* Medium-chain triglyceride (MCT) oil often is recommended (Ostrov & Balint, 1980; Greenberger, 1978; Shils, 1984; Williams & Dickson, 1972) solely as an additional calorie source; for cooking; for adding to foods in place of oil, butter, or margarine; or frozen for use as a spread. It must be added gradually, beginning at no more than 20 to 30 g daily, to minimize abdominal discomfort and diarrhea (Shils, 1984). Many patients on enteral feeding do not tolerate MCTs. For such patients, the dietitian may prefer to utilize low-fat formulas to which MCT oil or an MCT-containing module can be added as tolerated. MCT oil does not contain essential fatty acids.

## Micronutrients

### Electrolytes

Patients with significant losses of small bowel or colon function may lose large amounts of sodium and potassium in the stool. Malabsorbed bile salts, free fatty acids, and carbohydrate residues impair further the colon's ability to handle electrolytes (Woolf et al., 1987). Additional sodium may be added to the patient's diet or formula as needed. Potassium is less palatable but may be taken as an elixir, in tablet form, or mixed into an enteral formula.

### Minerals

Magnesium, calcium, and zinc commonly are malabsorbed. Additional magnesium can be pro-

vided as Epsom salts (magnesium sulfate) or magnesium chloride; small doses should be spread throughout the day to minimize the cathartic effect of this mineral. Calcium supplementation becomes even more important for the patient on limited dairy product consumption. The carbonate form of calcium is often used because of its high concentration of elemental calcium. Table 11-4 lists several generic calcium compounds that may be utilized.

### Vitamins

Malabsorption of fat-soluble vitamins is common among patients with steatorrhea. Vitamin $B_{12}$ deficiency develops over time in those with gastric resections, ileal impairment, or bacterial overgrowth, which necessitates intravenous or intramuscular supplementation. Multiple B-vitamin deficiencies often arise from general malnutrition. Folate levels may drop as a result of villous atrophy.

Vitamin and mineral supplementation must be individually adjusted on the basis of serum levels, stool losses, and clinical deficiency symptoms. The literature provides sample regimens (Gray, 1983; Greenberger, 1978) that include the B vitamins and vitamins A and D in aqueous or fat-soluble form, sodium, potassium, calcium, magnesium, zinc, and iron (Table 11-5).

## Fluid

Increased fluid needs arise in those with significant colon resections. These needs are even greater if ileal viability or the ileocecal valve has been lost. Some patients benefit from the prescription of psyllium fiber supplements such as Metamucil, which adsorb water, solidify the

**Table 11-4** Calcium Supplements

| Supplement | Calcium Content (mg per 1 g) |
| --- | --- |
| Calcium carbonate | 401 |
| Calcium lactate | 130 |
| Calcium phosphate | 158 |
| Glubionate calcium (Neo-Calglucon) | 23 (per 1 mL) |

**Table 11-5** Sample Vitamin and Mineral Regimen for Patients with Malabsorption

| Nutrient | Recommended Daily Dosage | Route of Administration |
|---|---|---|
| Vitamin A, fat soluble | 25,000 to 50,000 U | Oral |
| Vitamin D, fat soluble | 15,000 to 30,000 U | Oral |
| Vitamin $B_{12}$ | 100 μg (monthly) | Intramuscular |
| Calcium | 300 to 1500 mg | Oral |
| Magnesium | 8 to 48 mEq | Oral or intravenous |
| Other nutrients as needed (B vitamins, potassium, zinc, iron) | | |

*Source:* From *Gastrointestinal Disease: Pathophysiology, Diagnosis, Management*, 3rd ed. (pp. 228–256) by M.H. Sleisinger and J.S. Fordtran (Eds.), 1983, Philadelphia: W.B. Saunders Company. Copyright 1983 by W.B. Saunders Company; "State of the Art: The Management of the Patient with Small Bowel Syndrome" by N.J. Greenberger, 1978, *American Journal of Gastroenterology, 70*, pp. 528–540. Copyright 1978 by Williams & Wilkins Company.

stool, and possibly enhance fluid resorption. It may be necessary to supplement the patient with intravenous infusions if absorptive capacity for oral fluids is inadequate.

## Special Dietary Regimens

### Diet for Rapid Transit

The overall objective for controlling rapid transit of food boluses is to minimize intake of dietary components that tend to stimulate bowel movement. Dietary fiber and fat often are restricted. Many patients, especially those in the acute phase of malabsorption, benefit from the separation of dietary liquids and solids, with intake of liquids being limited to at least 1 hour before or after the meal (Woolf et al., 1987).

Small, frequent feedings also may be effective in controlling rapid transit. The patient should be instructed to divide up a typical day's volume of food into five to six equally sized meals of similar composition. Many patients have trouble adapting to this type of diet regimen and may lose weight initially from either underestimating nutrient needs or skipping feedings. Small, frequent feedings, although often recommended to anorectic cancer patients, may not be entirely successful if the patient's appetite wanes during the day regardless of meal size.

Restrictions on salt and concentrated sweets help control transit by reducing the osmolality of the postprandial luminal contents. This intervention should be combined with the avoidance of fluids with meals to reduce the dissolved solute load presented to the intestine.

### Low Fiber

Fiber-restricted diets are indicated for a number of conditions, including radiation enteritis, rapid transit, and partial bowel obstruction. The fiber restriction should be strictly enforced in the early stages of management to stabilize the patient. It may be possible to liberalize the diet over time after monitoring changes in bowel movements and diet tolerance.

Foods high in insoluble fiber tend to stimulate bowel movement or to increase stool bulk and often are restricted for the long term. Patients with partial bowel obstruction require intensive diet instruction because they are at risk of total obstruction from extremely fibrous foods. Other patients may find that soluble fiber, such as that found in apples, oats, and potatoes, either helps solidify the stool or has no positive or negative effect.

### Low Fat, Low Fiber, and Low Lactose

Patients with mild to moderate radiation enteritis have been managed successfully on diets restricted in fat, fiber, and lactose. Dietary fat content is limited to less than 40 g/day. Fruits and vegetables containing more than 2 g of fiber per serving are eliminated, as are breads, grains, and cereals containing more than 1.5 g of fiber. Only lactose-free or lactase-treated low-fat dairy products are permitted. Tolerance of yogurt varies from patient to patient; patients are encouraged to try a small amount and to monitor themselves for changes in symptoms.

Some patients will be able to liberalize the diet without adverse effects. Additional foods should be tried one at a time to enable identification of specific intolerances.

## Other Factors in Management

### Oxalate

Patients with ileal resections or other causes of marked steatorrhea but with an intact colon are at high risk of developing hyperoxaluria and renal oxalate stones from the colonic absorption of free oxalate (Shils, 1984). The stones are caused by fat malabsorption and the formation of calcium soaps, allowing oxalate, a compound ordinarily bound with calcium, to be absorbed by the colon (Hofmann, Laker, Dharmasathaphorn, Sherr, & Lorenzo, 1983). The free oxalate circulates to the kidney, where it recomplexes with the calcium filtering through the renal tubules.

Shils (1984) has outlined a dietary and supplement regimen to reduce the incidence of oxalate stone formation. Modifications include restricting long-chain fat and oxalate-containing foods and increasing intake of calcium, magnesium, and citrate. Magnesium and citrate solubilize calcium and inhibit the formation of calcium oxalate.

### Adjunct Medical Therapies

Adjunct medical therapies may be necessary for optimal control of the patient's symptoms and to maximize the effects of nutrition support.

*Pancreatic enzymes.* Pancreatic enzymes often are administered to patients whose pancreatic function has been partially or totally compromised by cancer or its treatments. These products, in combination with a low-fat diet,

may reduce diarrhea by increasing fat absorption and decreasing fecal bile salt losses (Dutta, Anand, & Gadacz, 1986). Meal size and fat content together with medication type (capsule or tablet) and effect on the patient's symptoms dictate the dosage necessary to achieve maximal response with minimal side effects of abdominal cramping and discomfort (Perry & Gallagher, 1985). Shils (1984) recommends administering small enzyme doses at the beginning, middle, and end of a meal to improve absorption through the relatively continual mixing of enzymes and food.

Antacids, sodium bicarbonate, or cimetidine (Cortot, Fleming, & Malagelada, 1979) administered concurrently with the pancreatic enzyme preparation may neutralize gastric acid and prevent the denaturation of non–enterically coated products (Durie, Bell, & Linton, 1980).

*Cholestyramine.* Cholestyramine with (Tilson, 1980; Cello, 1983; Williams & Dickson, 1972; Chary & Thomson, 1984) or without (Hofmann & Poley, 1969, 1972; Shils, 1984) dietary fat restriction may be effective in controlling diarrhea from bile acid losses or radiation enteritis. It is less effective in patients with extensive resections and after depletion of the bile acid pool has occurred.

*Antidiarrheal agents.* Antidiarrheal agents, including kaolin-pectin, codeine, tincture of opium, and anticholinergics, are widely prescribed in conjunction with dietary modification. Kaolin-pectin compounds help solidify a liquid stool; the other preparations slow bowel peristalsis.

## PARENTERAL AND ENTERAL FEEDINGS

### Parenteral Feeding

Short-term total parenteral nutrition (TPN) may be utilized to support patients postoperatively, during acute phases of malabsorption, and while the malabsorption work-up is in progress. TPN may be provided after GI resection or when bowel rest is prescribed until bowel sounds return and the patient is stabilized on an oral diet. The feasibility of weaning a patient off TPN depends on the degree of gut adaptation, which may take weeks to months (Weser et al., 1979; Sheldon, 1979) and requires the presence of nutrients in the gut (Williamson, 1978; Guedon et al., 1986).

Long-term TPN benefits a subset of patients. Those with severe diarrhea or steatorrhea from radiation or chronic malnutrition often cannot be managed orally or enterally, especially in the early stages of their nutrition rehabilitation. Other patients who require TPN include those with high-output GI fistulae (Randall, 1984), small remnants of small bowel (Heymsfield et al., 1980), or frequent, voluminous diarrhea (Tilson, 1980), in which fluid and nutrient losses far exceed absorptive capacity.

## Enteral Feeding

Patients with moderate to severe malabsorption may be best supported by enteral feeding. Shils (1984) uses the results of the D-xylose test as a screening tool, attempting feeding if urinary xylose excretion exceeds 1.2 to 1.6 g and monitoring the patient carefully. As a rule, slow-drip, pump-controlled feedings are preferable to maximize absorption and to minimize side effects.

Enteral products for patients with malabsorption can be classified into three groups: hydrolyzed, intact nutrient, and modular.

Hydrolyzed formulas, which are enzymatically predigested and generally low in fat, have been well tolerated by patients with radiation enteritis (Heymsfield et al., 1980; Beer et al., 1985), massive resections (Beer et al., 1985; Iles, 1984), and high-output fistulae (Rocchio et al., 1974). These products can be utilized when the patient's tolerance of feeding is being assessed because they are absorbed easily and do not challenge the gut with large amounts of fat. Dilution of the formula to half strength for the first day reduces the osmotic load and may diminish side effects.

Some patients, especially those with mild malabsorption, are able to tolerate a moderate-fat, intact-nutrient product. Patients are started slowly, at approximately 50 mL/hour, and are monitored closely while the feeding rate is increased by 10 to 20 mL/hour. Any significant changes in stool frequency, volume, odor, or color may signify an aggravation of the patient's malabsorption.

Modules may be added to a complete formula or combined to create a customized feeding. Fat sources include emulsified MCT and long-chain products and nonemulsified cooking oils. They can be used to increase or modify a formula's fat content. Carbohydrates, such as liquid or powdered oligosaccharides, increase caloric density without significantly adding to a product's osmotic load.

## MODIFICATIONS AND PATIENT MONITORING

All intakes and outputs must be monitored extremely closely during the early stages of refeeding, usually while the patient is hospitalized. Monitoring will identify nutrient imbalances and assess whether infused fluids are being absorbed. Members of the medical staff, the patient, and significant others should be instructed to notify the dietitian of any output changes during this period. Diet and formula modifications can be recommended on the basis of tolerance and evaluated while the patient is easily accessible. Laboratory tests, including measures of electrolyte and mineral status, should be evaluated at least twice weekly throughout the refeeding period.

If well tolerated, feedings can be advanced slowly by gradually increasing food variety and meal size or by raising the enteral formula infusion rate by 10 to 20 mL/hour. The key to successful feeding is to progress slowly, monitor carefully, and never discontinue one feeding modality until the patient can handle enough calories of the target regimen. It may be necessary to use two feeding modalities over a prolonged period of time to meet the patient's nutrient and fluid needs. Overnight enteral or parenteral infusions can compensate for mild malabsorption of oral nutrients and fluids taken during the day and will allow the patient to return to normal daytime activities.

Management of malabsorption requires continual patient evaluation and monitoring. Abdominal discomfort, flatulence, diarrhea, or steatorrhea may signify intolerance of the selected regimen. Modifications of dietary fat content and type, osmolality, meal size, formula category, or infusion rate probably will be necessary to alleviate the patient's symptoms.

Communication among the patient, significant others, the dietitian, and additional members of the medical team is essential to successful patient management. All diet modifications, expected outcomes, and potential symptoms of intolerance should be explained to the patient. The patient and significant others must be encouraged to bring all problems and questions to the attention of the medical team. Periodic serum chemistry evaluations should be performed regularly in house or on an outpatient follow-up basis to monitor for signs of fluid, electrolyte, and nutrient imbalances. Mineral, vitamin, and electrolyte preparations can be added to the nutrition regimen as indicated; again, tolerance should be monitored closely.

Regularly scheduled clinic visits or follow-up telephone calls enable the clinician to follow closely the progress of patients at home. Exhibit 11-3 lists suggested components of an outpatient assessment.

The malabsorption work-up can be repeated, partially or in its entirety, after 2 to 3 months (Ostrov & Balint, 1980) to assess progress and to guide further nutrition modifications. Absorption should improve over time, except in cases in which ileal function has been significantly lost (Kovisto & Miettinen, 1986).

## CONCLUSION

Feeding the cancer patient with malabsorption is a long-term challenge to the dietitian and members of the health care team. It requires

**Exhibit 11-3** Outpatient Assessment

Current weight
Weight changes
Bowel movements (color, odor, frequency, consistency)
Calorie count (diet diary or 24-hour recall)
Changes in diet or feeding regimen
Medications (types and dosages)
Symptoms, side effects, or problems
Activity level

thorough understanding of the absorptive process and of the impact of cancer and its treatments on the incorporation of nutrients. The most satisfying aspect of patient management is observing the dramatic improvements in nutrient tolerance, and thus in the quality of life, that result from formulation of the correct regimen.

## REFERENCES

Adams, J.F., & Cartwright, E.J. (1963). The reliability and reproducibility of the Schilling test in primary malabsorptive disease and after partial gastrectomy. *Gut, 4*, 32–36.

Ameen, V.Z., Powell, G.K., & Jones, L.A. (1987). Quantification of fecal carbohydrate excretion in patients with short bowel syndrome. *Gastroenterology, 92*, 493–500.

Anderson, I.H., Levine, A.S., & Levitt, M.D. (1981). Incomplete absorption of the carbohydrate in all-purpose wheat flour. *New England Journal of Medicine, 304*, 891–892.

Andersson, H., Isaksson, B., & Sjogren, B. (1974). Fat-reduced diet in the symptomatic treatment of small bowel disease. *Gut, 15*, 351–359.

Beer, W.H., Farr, A., & Halsted, C.H. (1985). Clinical and nutritional implications of radiation enteritis. *American Journal of Clinical Nutrition, 41*, 85–91.

Benini, L., Scuro, L.A., Menini, E., Manfrini, C., Vantini, I., Vaona, B., Brocco, G., Talamini, G., & Cavallini, G. (1984). Is the [14]C-triolein breath test useful in the assessment of malabsorption in clinical practice? *Digestion, 29*, 91–97.

Bochenek, W., Rodgers, J.B., & Balint, J.A. (1970). Effects of changes in dietary lipids on intestinal fluid loss in short-bowel syndrome. *Annals of Internal Medicine, 72*, 205–213.

Cello, J.P. (1983). Inflammatory and malignant diseases of the small bowel causing malabsorption. *Clinics in Gastroenterology, 12*, 511–532.

Chary, S., & Thomson, D.H. (1984). A clinical trial evaluating cholestyramine to prevent diarrhea in patients maintained on low-fat diets during pelvic radiation therapy. *International Journal of Radiation Oncology Biology and Physics, 10*, 1885–1890.

Cortot, A., Fleming, C.R., & Malagelada, J.-R. (1979). Improved nutrient absorption after cimetidine in small bowel syndrome with gastric hypersecretion. *New England Journal of Medicine, 300*, 79–81.

Dobbins, W.O. (1980). When and how to evaluate the patient with malabsorption. *Practical Gastroenterology, 4*, 4–11.

Donaldson, S.M. (1984). Nutritional support as an adjunct to radiation therapy. *Journal of Parenteral and Enteral Nutrition, 8*, 302–310.

Drummey, G.D., Benson, J.A., & Jones, C.M. (1961). Microscopic examination of the stool for steatorrhea. *New England Journal of Medicine, 264*, 85–87.

Duncan, W., & Leonard, J.C. (1965). The malabsorption syndrome following radiotherapy. *Quarterly Journal of Medicine, 34*, 319–329.

Durie, P.R., Bell, L., & Linton, W. (1980). Effect of cimetidine and sodium bicarbonate on pancreatic replacement therapy in cystic fibrosis. *Gut, 21*, 778–786.

Dutta, S.K., Anand, K., & Gadacz, T.R. (1986). Bile salt malabsorption in pancreatic insufficiency secondary to alcoholic pancreatitis. *Gastroenterology, 91*, 1243–1249.

Dutta, S.K., & Hlasko, J. (1985). Dietary fiber in pancreatic disease: Effect of high fiber diet on fat malabsorption in pancreatic insufficiency and in vitro study of the interaction of dietary fiber with pancreatic enzymes. *American Journal of Clinical Nutrition, 41*, 517–525.

Fairfull-Smith, R., Abunassar, R., Freeman, J.B., & Maroun, J.A. (1980). Rational use of elemental and nonelemental diets in hospitalized patients. *Annals of Surgery, 192*, 600–603.

Feldman, E.J., Dowling, R.H., McNaughton, J., & Peters, T.J. (1976). Effects of oral versus intravenous nutrition on intestinal adaptation after small bowel resection in the dog. *Gastroenterology, 70*, 712–719.

Gray, G.M. (1983). Maldigestion and malabsorption: Clinical manifestations and specific diagnosis. In M.H. Sleisinger & J.S. Fordtran (Eds.), *Gastrointestinal disease—Pathophysiology, diagnosis, management* (3rd ed., pp. 228–256). Philadelphia: Saunders.

Green, P.H.R., & Tall, A.R. (1979). Drugs, alcohol and malabsorption. *American Journal of Medicine, 67*, 1066–1076.

Greenberger, N.J. (1978). State of the art: The management of the patient with small bowel syndrome. *American Journal of Gastroenterology, 70*, 528–540.

Griffin, G.E., Fagan, E.F., Hodgson, H.J., & Chadwick, V.S. (1982). Enteral therapy in the management of massive gut resection complicated by chronic fluid and electrolyte depletion. *Digestive Diseases and Sciences, 27*, 902–908.

Guedon, C., Schmitz, J., Lerebours, E., Metayer, J., Avdran, E., Hemet, J., & Colin, R. (1986). Decreased brush border hydrolase activities without gross morphologic changes in human intestinal mucosa after prolonged total parenteral nutrition of adults. *Gastroenterology, 90*, 373–378.

Heymsfield, S.B., Horowitz, J., & Lawson, D.H. (1980). Enteral hyperalimentation. In J.E. Berk (Ed.), *Developments in digestive diseases* (pp. 59–83). Philadelphia: Lea & Febiger.

Hofmann, A.F., Laker, M.F., Dharmasathaphorn, K., Sherr, H.P., & Lorenzo, D. (1983). Complex pathogenesis of hyperoxaluria after jejunoilial bypass surgery. *Gastroenterology, 84*, 293–300.

Hofmann, A.F., & Poley, J.R. (1969). Cholestyramine treatment of diarrhea associated with ileal resection. *New England Journal of Medicine, 281*, 397–402.

Hofmann, A.F., & Poley, J.R. (1972). Role of bile acid malabsorption in pathogenesis of diarrhea and steatorrhea in patients with ileal resection. *Gastroenterology, 62*, 918–934.

Iles, M. (1984). Effective use of total parenteral nutrition in an ileostomy patient. *Journal of the American Dietetic Association, 84*, 1324–1328.

Isaacs, P.E.T., & Kim, Y.S. (1979). The contaminated small bowel syndrome. *American Journal of Medicine, 67*, 1049–1057.

Jeejeebhoy, K.N. (1983). Therapy of the short-gut syndrome. *Lancet, 1*, 1427–1430.

King, C.E., Toskes, P.P., Guilarte, T.R., Lorenz, E., & Welkos, S.L. (1980). Comparison of the one-gram D-[$^{14}$C]xylose breath test to the [$^{14}$C]bile acid breath test in patients with small intestine bacterial overgrowth. *Digestive Diseases and Sciences, 25*, 53–58.

Koretz, R.L., & Meyer, J.H. (1980). Elemental diets—Facts and fantasies. *Gastroenterology, 78*, 393–410.

Kovisto, P., & Miettinen, T.A. (1986). Adaptation of cholesterol and bile acid metabolism and vitamin B$_{12}$ absorption in the long-term follow-up after partial ileal bypass. *Gastroenterology, 90*, 984–990.

Krejs, G.J., & Fordtran, J.S. (1983). Diarrhea. In M.H. Sleisinger & J.S. Fordtran (Eds.), *Gastrointestinal disease—Pathophysiology, diagnosis, management* (3rd ed., pp. 257–279). Philadelphia: Saunders.

Levine, G.M., Deren, J.J., Steiger, E., & Zinno, R. (1974). Role of oral intake in maintenance of gut mass and disaccharidase activity. *Gastroenterology, 67*, 975–982.

Mitchell, J.E., Breuer, R.I., Zuckerman, L., Berlin, J., Schilli, R., & Dunn, J.K. (1980). The colon influences ileal resection diarrhea. *Digestive Diseases and Sciences, 25*, 33–41.

Munyer, T.P., & Moss, A.A. (1980). Radiologic evaluation of the malabsorption syndrome. *Practical Gastroenterology, 4*, 12–17.

Newcomer, A.D., Hofmann, A.F., DiMagno, E.P., Thomas, P.J., & Carlson, G.L. (1979). Triolein breath test. *Gastroenterology, 76*, 6–13.

Olsen, W.A. (1979). A pathophysiological approach to diagnosis of malabsorption. *American Journal of Medicine, 67*, 1007–1013.

Ostrov, A.H., & Balint, J.A. (1980). Management of the short-bowel syndrome. *Practical Gastroenterology, 4*, 36–42.

Ovesen, L., Chu, R., & Howard, L. (1983). The influence of dietary fat on jejunostomy output in patients with severe bowel syndrome. *American Journal of Clinical Nutrition, 38*, 270–277.

Perman, J.A., Modler, S., Barr, R.G., & Rosenthal, P. (1984). Fasting breath hydrogen concentration: Normal values and clinical application. *Gastroenterology, 87*, 1358–1363.

Perry, R.S., & Gallagher, J. (1985). Management of maldigestion associated with pancreatic insufficiency. *Clinical Pharmacology, 4*, 161–169.

Randall, H.T. (1984). Enteral nutrition: Tube feeding in acute and chronic illness. *Journal of Parenteral and Enteral Nutrition, 8*, 113–136.

Ravich, W.J., & Bayless, T.M. (1983). Carbohydrate absorption and malabsorption. *Clinics in Gastroenterology, 12*, 335–356.

Reeves, R.J., Sanders, S.P., Isley, J.K., Sharpe, K.W., & Baylin, G.J. (1959). Gastrointestinal tract in patients undergoing radiation therapy. *Radiology, 73*, 398–401.

Rocchio, M.A., Cha, C.-J.M., Haas, K.F., & Randall, H.T. (1974). Use of chemically defined diets in the management of patients with high output gastrointestinal cutaneous fistulas. *American Journal of Surgery, 127*, 148.

Ryan, M.E., & Olsen, W.A. (1983). A diagnostic approach to malabsorption syndromes: A pathophysiological approach. *Clinics in Gastroenterology, 12*, 533–550.

Schwartz, M.S., & Storozuk, R.B. (1985). Enhancement of small intestine function by gastrin. *Journal of Surgical Research, 38*, 613–617.

Sheldon, G.F. (1979). Role of parenteral nutrition in patients with short bowel syndrome. *American Journal of Medicine, 67*, 1021–1029.

Shils, M.E. (1984). Nutritional repletion after major gut excision. In J.J. DeCosse & P. Sherlock (Eds.), *Clinical management of gastrointestinal cancer* (pp. 303–326). Boston: Martinus Nijhoff.

Simko, V., McCarroll, A.M., Goodman, S., Weesner, R.E., & Kelley, R.E. (1980). High-fat diet in a short bowel syndrome. *Digestive Diseases and Sciences, 25*, 333–339.

Stephen, A.M., Haddad, A.C., & Phillips, S.F. (1983). Passage of carbohydrate into the colon. *Gastroenterology, 85*, 589–595.

Thorsgaard Pedersen, N., & Halgreen, H. (1984). Faecal fat and faecal weight: Reproducibility and diagnostic efficiency of various regimens. *Scandinavian Journal of Gastroenterology, 19*, 350–354.

Tilson, M.D. (1980). Pathophysiology and treatment of short bowel syndrome. *Surgical Clinics of North America, 60*, 1273–1284.

Welsh, J.D., & Griffiths, W.J. (1980). Breath hydrogen test after oral lactose in postgastrectomy patients. *American Journal of Clinical Nutrition, 33*, 2324–2327.

Weser, E. (1979). Nutritional aspects of malabsorption. *American Journal of Medicine, 67*, 1014–1020.

Weser, E. (1983). Nutritional aspects of malabsorption: Short gut adaptation. *Clinics in Gastroenterology, 12*, 443–461.

Weser, E., Bell, D., & Tawil, T. (1981). Effects of octapeptide-cholecystokinin, secretin, and glucagon on intestinal mucosal growth in parenterally nourished rats. *Digestive Diseases and Sciences, 26*, 409–416.

Weser, E., Fletcher, J.T., & Urban, E. (1979). Short bowel syndrome. *Gastroenterology, 77*, 572–579.

West, P.S., Levin, G.E., Griffin, G.E., & Maxwell, J.D. (1981). Comparison of simple screening tests for fat malabsorption. *British Medical Journal, 282*, 1501–1504.

Williams, C.N., & Dickson, R.C. (1972). Cholestyramine and medium-chain triglycerides in prolonged management of patients subjected to ileal resection or bypass. *Canadian Medical Association Journal, 107*, 626–631.

Williamson, R.C.N. (1978). Intestinal adaptation (part I): Structural, functional and cytokinetic changes. *New England Journal of Medicine, 298*, 1393–1402.

Winawer, S.J., Broitman, S.A., Woolchow, D.A., Osborne, M.P., & Zamcheck, N. (1966). Successful management of massive small-bowel resection based on assessment of absorption defects and nutritional needs. *New England Journal of Medicine, 274*, 72–78.

Woolf, G.M., Miller, C., Kurian, R., & Jeejeebhoy, K.N. (1983). Diet for patients with a small bowel: High fat or high carbohydrate? *Gastroenterology, 84*, 823–828.

Woolf, G.M., Miller, C., Kurian, R., & Jeejeebhoy, K.N. (1987). Nutritional absorption in short bowel syndrome. *Digestive Diseases and Sciences, 32*, 8–15.

Young, E.A. (1983). Short bowel syndrome: High-fat versus high-carbohydrate diet. *Gastroenterology, 84*, 872–874.

Young, E.A., Cioletti, L.A., Winborn, W.B., Traylor, J.B., & Weser, E. (1980). Comparative study of nutritional adaptation to defined formula diets in rats. *American Journal of Clinical Nutrition, 33*, 2106–2118.

# Chapter 12

# Low-Microbial Diets for Patients with Granulocytopenia

*Gaile L. Moe*

Immunocompromised patients are individuals at increased risk of infection, often of a life-threatening nature. Immunocompromised patients include those with cancer, acquired immunodeficiency syndrome, myeloproliferative disorders, burns, diabetes, or severe trauma and those receiving immunosuppressive therapy. Exhibit 12-1 describes the defects in host defense that cause the patient to become a compromised host.

Much of the medical care of the immunocompromised patient is aimed toward the prevention or treatment of infection. This chapter briefly discusses infection in granulocytopenic patients, the role that the microorganisms in food may play in the etiology of these infections, and the indications for and production of a diet with a reduced microbial content.

## GRANULOCYTOPENIA

Granulocytopenia is commonly seen in the cancer patient as a result of underlying disease, chemotherapy, or radiation therapy (Newman & Schimpff, 1987; Pizzo, 1984). Granulocytes (basophils, eosinophils, and polymorphonuclear leukocytes or neutrophils) are phagocytic cells that are the first line of systemic defense against bacterial invasion. Neutrophils represent 70% of a normal total white blood cell count of 4,500 to 10,000 per microliter. Although the factors listed in Exhibit 12-1 are important risk factors for infection, the incidence of serious infection is most closely associated with the degree and duration of granulocytopenia. The frequency of infection increases as the granulocyte count drops to less than $1,000/\mu L$ and increases further as the count approaches zero. Severe infections are likely to occur when the count is less than $100/\mu L$ and when the duration of granulocytopenia exceeds 7 days.

---

**Exhibit 12-1** Defects in Host Immune Defense Leading to Immunocompromise

Granulocytopenia
Cellular immune dysfunction
Humoral immune dysfunction
Damage to alimentary canal and respiratory tract
  mucosa
Disruption of normal microbial flora
Obstruction to natural body passages
Breach of body barriers

*Source:* From *Clinical Approach to Infection in the Compromised Host,* 2nd ed. (pp. 5–40) by R.H. Rubin and L.S. Young (Eds.), 1988, New York: Plenum Medical Book Company. Copyright 1988 by Plenum Medical Book Company.

Patients with acute leukemia undergoing remission induction or bone marrow transplantation lack circulating granulocytes for 14 days or longer (Newman & Schimpff, 1987; Meyers & Thomas, 1988). Infectious organisms are primarily the aerobic Gram-negative rods *Pseudomas aeruginosa, Escherichia coli*, and *Klebsiella pneumoniae* and to a lesser degree the Gram-positive organisms *Staphylococcus epidermidis* and *S. aureus*. After a prolonged period of immunosuppression, infections from yeast (*Candida albicans, C. tropicalis*, and *Torulopsis glabrata*) and filamentous fungi (*Aspergillus* spp.) are more prominent (Newman & Schimpff, 1987).

Microbial colonization often precedes infection during granulocytopenia (Cohen et al., 1983). Microbial colonization is promoted by mucosal damage along the alimentary tract and reduction of the normal anaerobic flora of the lower gastrointestinal tract. This flora protects against colonization by the elaboration of antibioticlike substances, the production of short-chain fatty acids (which are inhibitory to microbial growth), and the creation of an environment with an unfavorable oxidation-reduction potential (Panosian & Gorbach, 1985). Normal peristaltic action protects against bacterial overgrowth by enabling gastric fluids to dislodge loosely attached bacteria from the mucosa and into the colon (Abraham & Beachey, 1985). The use of narcotics and antidiarrheal agents can contribute to decreased intestinal peristalsis. An obstruction to a natural body passage, such as an intestinal obstruction, can result in infection from the stasis of body fluids and consequent overgrowth of organisms (Wade & Schimpff, 1988). An increase in gastric $pH$ and a decrease in function of the local lymphoid tissue resulting in diminished mucosal immunoglobulin production can also promote bacterial colonization (Wade & Schimpff, 1988).

Mucosa damaged by chemotherapy, radiation therapy, or gastrointestinal infections is susceptible to colonization by Gram-negative bacilli (Newman & Schimpff, 1987). The damaged mucosa may further serve as a portal of systemic entry for these organisms with resultant secondary bacteremias. In the marrow transplant patient gastrointestinal graft-versus-host disease, a result of cytotoxicity against host tissue by immunologically competent donor marrow T lymphocytes, can also result in severe mucosal damage (McDonald, Shulman, Sullivan, & Spencer, 1986). Dietch, Winterton, Li, and Berg (1987), by use of the mouse model, have demonstrated that under certain conditions the indigenous bacteria colonizing the gastrointestinal tract are able to pass through the epithelial mucosa to infect the mesenteric lymph nodes and systemic organs, a process termed bacterial translocation. Factors promoting bacterial translocation include bacterial overgrowth, impaired host immunity, physical disruption of the gut mucosal barrier, trauma, and endotoxemia. In the burned mouse model, 30% total body surface burn plus endotoxin injection resulted in lethal systemic infection from the uncontrolled spread of bacteria translocating from the gut (Dietch & Berg, 1987).

The administration of broad-spectrum intravenous antibiotics, which is a routine practice in granulocytopenic febrile patients, can lead to the suppression of the normal enteric flora and allow for overgrowth of yeasts and colonization of the gut by antibiotic-resistant microorganisms. Van der Waaij (1979) demonstrated that the oropharynx of patients on ampicillin rapidly becomes colonized by Gram-negative bacilli.

## INFECTION PREVENTION STRATEGIES

Pizzo (1984) and Wade and Schimpff (1988) reviewed techniques commonly employed to reduce infection in immunosuppressed patients. Nearly half the infections in severely granulocytopenic patients with cancer are caused by hospital-acquired organisms; the other infections result from organisms already colonizing the body, especially along the alimentary canal. Thus infection prevention strategies focus on the prevention of acquisition of new organisms and on the suppression of endogenous pathogenic enteric organisms.

The most intensive strategy employed to prevent infection in patients with prolonged granulocytopenia is total reverse isolation in a laminar air flow (LAF) room. LAF isolation typically includes the use of topical antibiotic preparations and the routine ingestion of oral, liquid, nonabsorbable antibiotics (often gentamicin, vancomycin, and nystatin). This strategy attempts both to suppress the existing microbial flora of the patient with the antibiotic regimens and to limit the acquisition of new organisms with the high-efficiency LAF particulate air filters. These filters eliminate all bacteria and fungi and some of the large viruses. All medical and personal items, food, and water that enter the room must be sterile or have low counts of microorganisms. A sizeable reduction in infection has been shown with the use of this strategy (Petersen et al., 1988). Care for patients in LAF rooms is costly (close to $1,500 per patient per day). High costs coupled with failure to decrease overall mortality limit the widespread use of LAF rooms.

Standard reverse isolation (single room isolation with staff and visitors required to wear masks, gowns, and booties) prevents transfer of organisms from staff to patient but has no impact on the acquisition of organisms from water, food (unless a low-microbial diet is employed), air, or supplies (Nausef & Maki, 1981).

## ROLE OF FOOD IN INFECTION

Foodborne illness in the general population is recognized as being widespread, with between 24 and 81 million cases of foodborne diarrheal disease reported in the United States each year (Institute of Food Technologists' Expert Panel, 1988). The occurrence of foodborne enteric pathogens such as *Salmonella*, *Shigella*, and *Vibrio* organisms, *Campylobacter fetus jejuni*, *Yersinia enterocolitica*, enteropathogenic *E. coli*, *Staphylococcus aureus*, and *Clostridium perfringens* and *C. botulinum* is for public health reasons a well-studied subject. On the other hand, although studies have implicated food as a source of new exogenous organisms in the granulocytopenic patient, quantitative studies are sparse. Little is known about how organisms from food colonize and infect individual patients. Even less is known regarding the role of intervention (i.e., providing low-microbial diets) in reducing infection.

## NORMAL FLORA IN FOODS

Microorganisms are naturally present in the soil, water, and air; thus the exterior surfaces of plants and animals are contaminated with various microorganisms. Food is an ideal medium for supporting the growth of microorganisms. Each processing step subjects raw foods to additional opportunities for contamination.

*Pseudomonas, Enterobacter, Klebsiella, Citrobacter*, and *Serratia* organisms are among the Gram-negative rods often found on vegetables, including tomatoes, radishes, celery, carrots, and lettuce (Remington & Schimpff, 1981). Shooter, Faiers, Cooke, Breaden, and O'Farrell (1971) isolated *E. coli, Klebsiella* organisms, and *Pseudomonas aeruginosa* from food in hospitals, canteens, and schools. Salads had a high frequency of contamination by these three types of organisms. Kominos, Copeland, Grosiak, and Postic (1972) examined vegetables from the kitchen of a general hospital in Pittsburgh. *Pseudomonas aeruginosa* was isolated from 82% of whole tomato samples and 27% of tomato salads. *Pseudomonas aeruginosa* was found on all types of vegetables, with tomatoes having the largest degree of contamination. Subsequent investigations revealed *Klebsiella* organisms in 46%, *Enterobacter agglomerans* in 85%, and *Enterobacter cloacae* in 48% of salad samples (Wright, Kominos, & Yee, 1976). The investigators concluded that these microorganisms were natural flora of vegetables. Cooked foods have also been implicated as a source of *P. aeruginosa*. Subramaniam and Shriniwas (1987) evaluated cooked Indian foods for the presence of *P. aeruginosa* and found that 12 of 68 foods samples yielded the organism. Of the 12 positive samples, 6 produced enterotoxin. The role of enterotoxigenic strains in gastrointestinal infection has not been completely established, however.

The gastrointestinal tract of animals contains large numbers of organisms that can contaminate interior muscle tissue if improper slaughtering and dressing procedures are used. A heterogenous flora exists on raw red meats, poultry, and fish as a result of contamination from the animal or processing environment. Raw poultry is frequently contaminated with *Salmonella* and

*Campylobacter* organisms. The pseudomonads and the closely related aerobic, psychrophilic Gram-negative bacteria are responsible for spoilage in these foods. Conventional cooking of meats to an internal temperature of 85°C (185°F) results in thermal destruction of these pathogens (Crespo & Ockerman, 1977). Enterococci in concentrations as high as $10^6$/g may be found in certain cheeses and sausages (Subcommittee on Microbiological Criteria, 1985).

Pinegar and Cooke (1985) examined 4,246 samples of retail processed foods for the presence of *E. coli*. Twenty-eight percent of the cake and confectionery products and 9% of the meats and meat-based products were found to be contaminated. Of the contaminated foods, 27% contained more than $10^3$ *E. coli* per gram. St. Louis et al. (1988) found raw shell eggs to be contaminated with *Salmonella enteritidis*.

The pasteurization of milk should result in the destruction of all non–spore-forming pathogens. Fleming et al. (1985) reported, however, that pasteurized whole and 2% milk was the vehicle of infection in an outbreak of listeriosis in 49 patients. Seven of the cases were fetuses or infants; the other 42 were immunosuppressed adults. When the Public Health Service–Food and Drug Administration's chemical, bacteriologic, and temperature standards for grade A milk and milk products are followed, the bacterial limits for these products (except cultured products) are less than 20,000/mL with coliforms not exceeding 10/mL. Grade A aseptically processed milk and milk products should have no growth of bacteria and are shelf stable without refrigeration until opened (Subcommittee on Microbiological Criteria, 1985).

Thermophilic spore-forming bacteria are found in severely heat-processed, low-acid canned foods. Dry spices contain large numbers of aerobic spore-forming bacteria. Molds and yeasts predominate in dried fruits.

The indigenous microflora of bottled drinking water usually consists of Gram-negative bacteria belonging to genera such as *Pseudomonas, Cytophaga, Flavobacterium*, and *Alcaligenes*. Distilled water is often used to store cultures of *P. aeruginosa* because they will remain viable in it for many months. Good-quality drinking water usually contains less than 100 bacteria per milliliter at the time of bottling (Subcommittee on Microbiological Criteria, 1985).

Cross-contamination with organisms in food preparation areas may occur. Casewell and Phillips (1978) demonstrated that equipment, utensils, and working surfaces in a hospital kitchen contaminated with *Klebsiella* organisms led to the contamination of salads prepared in the kitchen. *Campylobacter fetus jejuni* from raw chicken parts contaminated work surfaces and floors but could be removed by sanitization with hot water, detergent, and drying, thus preventing cross-contamination (Dawkins, Bolton, & Hutchinson, 1984).

## MICROBIAL EVALUATION OF FOODS FOR PATIENTS WITH GRANULOCYTOPENIA

Pizzo, Purvis, and Waters (1982) evaluated the microbiologic profiles of 236 food items for patients undergoing gastrointestinal decontamination who were being maintained in protective isolation. The criteria for acceptance into the diet (<500/mL of *Bacillus* spp.) were empirically derived. The acceptability of food items varied among different food categories. Almost all the beverages and breads were acceptable, whereas 70% or fewer canned food products, cereals, frozen, and snack items were acceptable. Only 20% of processed meats and 30% of fresh fruits and vegetables were acceptable. The microbiologic profiles frequently varied by manufacturer, and some of the foods were autoclaved before culturing whereas others were not.

At the Fred Hutchinson Cancer Research Center and Swedish Hospital Medical Center, 198 foods prepared by means of conventional preparation methods only were evaluated for acceptability on a low-microbial diet served to marrow transplant patients undergoing gastrointestinal decontamination in LAF rooms (Moe, Johnson, & Tari, 1988). Foods were cultured a minimum of three times each from three different manufacturing lots. The acceptance criteria, defined as the absence of organisms or a total of not more than $10^4$ colony-forming units of *Bacillus* organisms, diphtheroids, or micrococci per milliliter and not more than $10^3$ colony-forming units of coagulase-negative staphylococci or *Streptococcus viridans* per milliliter, were more liberal than those employed by Pizzo (1984). More than 80% of beverages, starches, breads and cereals, cooked fresh meats, and mixed cooked entrees and frozen vegetables were acceptable. Only 36% of pasteurized dairy products and 42% of dessert and snack items met these acceptance criteria, however. Of particular concern was the presence of 17 different species of Gram-negative rods in concentrations as high as $10^6$/mL in pasteurized, nonfermented dairy products including milk, pudding, and ice cream. Bottled, distilled water also contained more than $10^3$ *Pseudomonas* organisms per milliliter. The diet derived from this microbiologic evaluation of foods is presented in Table 12-1.

In another study, Ayers, Hancock, Buesching, and Tutschka (1986) performed 309 quantitative cultures on 60 potentially nonsterile commercial and routine hospital kitchen–prepared food products. Cultures of all products showed 37% with no growth, 13% with *Bacillus* organisms only, 15% with consistent contamination, and 35% with variable contamination. Microbe-free foods or foods containing *Bacillus* organisms only were put on the diet and served to marrow transplant patients who were in protected environments and on antibiotic prophylaxis during the high-risk period for infection. Of these patients, 41% became transiently colonized with *Bacillus* organisms; no infections with *Bacillus* organisms or other food-borne pathogens occurred.

## STERILE DIETS

A sterile diet consists of food that has no bacterial or fungal growth on culture. If a food is not commercially canned, then sterility is achieved by steam autoclaving or oven baking (Aker & Cheney, 1983; Frankmann, Beck, & Schomburg, 1984). It is well known that $\gamma$ irradiation at a dose of 10 to 50 kGy (1 to 5 Mrad) can also sterilize foods, but this sterilization method has not been approved by the Food and Drug Administration (Aker, 1984; Schweigert, 1987).

The microwave cooking (500 W for 10 minutes) of uncooked, individually packaged and frozen meals in Japan resulted in complete sterilization of the meals even when 100-g portions of the meals were inoculated with $10^6$ *E. coli* and *B. subtilis* before microwaving (Fujita & Kohzuki, 1983). Microwave cooking as a method of food sterilization has not been reported in the United States. The effects of microwaves on microorganisms in foods have been reported as being more food dependent than the effects of conventional heating, and high levels of microorganisms may not be destroyed within manufacturers' recommended cooking times (Fung & Cunningham, 1980). Lindsay, Krissinger, and Fields (1986) compared the bacterial content of chicken cooked to an internal temperature of 85°C (185°F) to 91°C (195°F) in microwave and conventional ovens. Sixty-six percent of the fresh chickens yielded positive cultures for *Salmonella* organisms; no cultures were positive after cooking in the conventional oven, but five of the nine (56%) microwave-cooked samples were positive for *Salmonella* organisms. Microwave cooking as a means to reduce significantly the bacterial content of foods cannot now be recommended, but further investigations would be useful.

Systematic bacteriologic monitoring of foods on the sterile diet in each individual institution is usually done. If the food is cultured, a representative sample of that food must be free of all bacterial and fungal growth after 7 days of microbiologic testing. An indirect and relatively inexpensive method of monitoring uses spore strips impregnated with heat- and cold-resistant spores. The spore strips are inserted into the densest part of the food before oven baking or autoclaving. The spore strip is removed from the food after processing, inoculated into liquid growth medium, and incubated for 48 hours. No growth indicates that the food is sterile.

Food preparation and tray assembly are done aseptically, preferably in a protected environment such as an LAF hood, to prevent bacterial fallout from the air. All tray service items, utensils, cookware, and paper goods must be sterilized. Trays should be wrapped in sterile packaging for delivery to the patient to prevent contamination en route.

**Table 12-1** Low-Microbial Diet

| Food Group | Foods Allowed | Foods Omitted |
|---|---|---|
| Beverages | Coffee, instant coffee; tea, instant tea; fruit-flavored powdered drink mixes; carbonated beverages; canned fruit-ades; pasteurized beer; bottled seltzer waters; sterile water and ice | Nonpasteurized beer; wine; bottled, distilled water |
| Milk and dairy products | Ultra–heat-treated milk; instant hot cocoa mix; commercial sterile milk shake products; canned milk; half-and-half creamer; American cheese; creamed cheese in individual packets; processed, pasteurized cheese spread and cheese food spread; canned puddings | Whipped cream, nondairy whipped topping, pasteurized milk, yogurt, cheese (except American), buttermilk, ice cream (all varieties), sherbet, cottage cheese, sour cream, powdered instant breakfast drinks, homemade and commercially prepared refrigerated puddings |
| Fruits and fruit juices | Canned fruit, canned and bottled fruit juices, baked apples | Fresh fruits and juices; raisins, all other dried fruits |
| Vegetables and vegetable juices | All canned vegetables and vegetable juices, canned bean salad, frozen vegetables (well cooked), baked fresh squash | Fresh vegetables, onion rings |
| Potato and potato substitutes | Cooked white or sweet potatoes, yams, french fries, hash brown potatoes; instant mashed potatoes; rice, pasta, noodles cooked in sterile water; chow mein noodles | Raw potato; au gratin potatoes; rice, pasta, potatoes cooked in nonsterile water; potato salad; macaroni salad |
| Breads and cereals | All breads, English muffins, bagels (except onion), hamburger and hot dog buns, dinner rolls; tortillas; hot and cold cereals (except as noted); pancakes; waffles; French toast; blueberry and plain muffins; crackers | All raisin- and nut-containing cereals and breads, cinnamon rolls, sweet rolls, doughnuts, onion bagels |
| Meat, meat substitutes, and mixed entrees | All hot, well-cooked beef, pork, poultry, fish; canned meats, fish, shellfish; hot dogs (well cooked); spaghetti sauce; frozen commercial mixed entrees, heated thoroughly (chicken and beef pot pies, macaroni and cheese, beef stroganoff, spaghetti with meat suace); peanut butter (smooth); canned beans, legumes, refried beans; baby food in jars | Deli meats; processed luncheon meats; raw eggs; dried meats (beef jerky); rare and medium-cooked meats, seafood; lasagna; pizza |
| Soups | All hot canned and dehydrated packaged soups, broths, bouillons | Homemade soups, commercial refrigerated and frozen soups, cold soups |
| Fats and oils | Margarine; vegetable oil; fat for deep fat frying; shortening; mayonnaise, tartar sauce from individual packets; canned gravy, sauces | Butter; homemade gravy; hollandaise sauce; mayonnaise, tartar sauce from multiserving containers |
| Condiments and spices | Individually packaged mustard, ketchup, taco sauce, lemon juice, salad dressings, jam, jelly, cranberry sauce, honey, syrup; sugars; salt; canned chocolate syrup; dill pickles; canned black olives; seasonings, spices, pepper added before cooking | Condiments from multiserving containers; green olives; sweet pickle relish; seasonings, spices, pepper added after cooking |
| Desserts and snacks | Pound and angel food cakes, commercial cookies (ginger snaps, frosting-filled sandwich cookies, shortbread, vanilla wafers), corn and tortilla chips, crackers, popcorn, canned dips, individually packaged cupcakes, individually | All other cakes, all other cookies, candy-coated popcorn, pies, nuts (all varieties), potato chips, pretzels, ice cream bars, candy made with nuts or dried fruits, candy bars |

**Table 12-1** continued

| Food Group | Foods Allowed | Foods Omitted |
|---|---|---|
| | packaged fruit pies, flavored ices off the stick, gelatin, custard (homemade), candy (hard candies, jelly beans, gum drops, orange slices, gummi bears, lemon drops, marshmallows, peanut butter cups, plain chocolate disc candies), chewing gum | |
| Nutrition supplements | Glucose polymers, powdered supplements reconstituted with sterile water, all canned supplements | |

Many factors deter institutions from implementing sterile food services, including the lack of data demonstrating therapeutic benefit (i.e., a reduction in infection) compared to less stringent diets. Other deterrents include increased training requirements of food service personnel, the need for a separate kitchen, high patient meal costs, a lack of standardized guidelines, and a lack of foods and supplies necessary to produce the diet (Dezenhall, Curry-Bartley, Blackburn, De Lamerens, & Khan, 1987).

## LOW-MICROBIAL DIETS

The objectives of the low-microbial diet are to prevent acquisition of new pathogenic organisms from foods and to provide a palatable and nutritionally adequate diet without significantly increasing patient meal costs. Consultation with infectious disease personnel about the degree of microbial restriction desired for individual patient populations is recommended. Those patients maintained in LAF environments or undergoing gastrointestinal decontamination are often managed with a stringent regimen that may include the use of a diet with a defined and known microbial content and certain aseptic food preparation techniques used in the production of a sterile diet. Such procedures may include (1) the use of LAF hoods and or a separate kitchen for food preparation, (2) sterilization of the outside of leak-proof food containers by soaking them in an iodine-based germicidal solution for 5 minutes with subsequent rinsing with sterile water, and (3) the use of steam- or ethylene oxide–sterilized dishes, utensils, and cookware. These procedures increase meal costs; research demonstrating their effectiveness is lacking.

Diets with a reduced bacterial content can vary widely in content. The simplest low-microbial diet in use is a house diet with fresh, raw vegetables and most fresh fruits excluded. Freshly peeled, thick-skinned fruits such as oranges, grapefruit, bananas, and melons may be allowed. This type of diet is not a true low-microbial diet; it probably contains large numbers of pathogens because fresh dairy products, spices, nuts, and other pathogen-containing foods are not limited.

The low-microbial diet in Table 12-1 contains foods that are sterile or have low numbers of organisms not usually considered pathogenic. Brand names are not included on this diet, but it is likely that not all brand preparations of the same food product have the same microbiologic profile. This type of diet can be produced in a hospital main kitchen. Guidelines for food preparation, serving, and storage of a low-microbial diet are presented in Exhibit 12-2.

### Nutrition Adequacy

Low-microbial and sterile diets can provide adequate energy, protein, and minerals if they are carefully planned by the dietitian and appropriately selected by the patient. It is recommended that the patient be monitored for actual food and nutrient intake. A multivitamin supplement should be provided because heat-labile vitamins in the food may be destroyed by heat processing.

**Exhibit 12-2** Guidelines for Food Preparation, Serving, and Storage for Low-Microbial Diets

1. Personnel preparing food wash their hands with a bactericidal soap before food preparation and observe other food service hygiene measures (e.g., wearing hair restraints).
2. Foods are handled with clean or sterile utensils (tongs held in alcohol) or sterile, gloved hands.
3. Raw foods such as meats, poultry, and entrees should be cooked well done (i.e., to an internal temperature of 85°C [185°F]).
4. Cooked foods are not served if left at room temperature for more than 1 hour.
5. Cooked foods may be frozen for reheating at a later time.
6. For patients in ultraisolation environments, exterior wrappers (e.g., cereal box or candy wrapper) should be removed before serving.
7. Canned beverages such as canned fruit juices should be poured from the original container into a clean glass because the exterior of the container may be contaminated.
8. Sterile water is used to reconstitute powdered drinks and soups. Sterile water is used for drinking and ice making. Ice can be made by pouring 60 mL of sterile water into a sterile specimen cup and freezing. The specimen cups can be resterilized.
9. Cooked foods prepared outside the hospital are not allowed because the cooking time and temperatures and the holding times cannot be ascertained. Eating out is not allowed until the low-microbial diet is discontinued.
10. Meals are served on sterile or very clean tableware. Dishes washed at high temperatures (71°C [160°F]) with an 82°C (180°F) rinse should be acceptable after washing, eliminating the need for steam sterilization. Flatware, cups, glasses, trays, straws, baby bottles, and paper goods are either sterile or very clean. Individual disposable tray service is not required. Trays should be covered during delivery to the patient.

## Efficacy and Use of Low-Microbial Diets

Aker and Cheney (1983) reviewed studies of immunosuppressed cancer patients that compared the rates of infection, morbidity, mortality, and response to therapy in LAF, protective isolation, and standard hospital care with sterile, low-microbial, or regular diets. They concluded that the protective benefit of a sterile or low-microbial diet compared to the general diet has not been established because of a lack of

controlled trials designed to answer this question. The data suggest, however, that sterile food is not required for gut sterilization when oral, nonabsorbable antibiotics are administered and that the provision of low-microbial diets as a means to reduce the acquisition of new exogenous organisms to the granulocytopenic patient, regardless of environment, is a reasonable measure that should neither substantially increase costs nor compromise the patient's nutrition status. The need for a low-microbial diet with patients with immune deficiencies other than granulocytopenia is unknown.

Few data exist on the actual usage of low-microbial or sterile diets for immunosuppressed patients. Dezenhall et al. (1987) surveyed food service practices of 20 U.S. hospitals performing marrow transplants. All the institutions served some form of low-microbial diet regardless of the type of isolation employed. Only one of the hospitals served exclusively sterile foods. Four of the hospitals did bacteriologic monitoring of foods. The data suggested a decrease in the use of strictly sterile diets; four centers reported changing from a sterile food service to a more liberal, modified bacteria diet or a house diet without fresh fruits and vegetables.

## Acceptance of Low-Microbial Diets

Acceptance of the low-microbial diet may be minimal, but this issue has not been fully investigated. Cheney, Aker, and Lenssen (1988) examined the effect of ultraisolation environments and low-microbial or sterile diets on oral intake in 469 patients undergoing allogeneic marrow transplantation. Of these, 259 patients were maintained in simple protective isolation and received a regular diet, and 210 patients were maintained in LAF rooms and underwent gastrointestinal decontamination with oral, nonabsorbable antibiotics and received either a low-microbial or a sterile diet. Because the transplant regimen adversely affects oral intake, all patients received total parenteral nutrition but were encouraged to eat as tolerated. There was no difference in oral intake between the two groups, but patients in the LAF environment attained an oral intake containing 10 g of protein per day slightly sooner overall. These data suggest that sterile and low-microbial diets do not inhibit food intake or delay the refeeding process after reliance on parenteral nutrition.

## REFERENCES

Abraham, S.N., & Beachey, E.H. (1985). Host defenses against adhesion of bacteria to mucosal surfaces. In J.I. Gallin & A.S. Fauci (Eds.), *Advances in host defense mechanisms: Vol. 4* (pp. 63–88). New York: Raven.

Aker, S.N. (1984). On the cutting edge of dietetic science. *Nutrition Today, 19*(4), 24–27.

Aker, S.N., & Cheney, C.L. (1983). The use of sterile and low microbial diets in ultraisolation environments. *Journal of Parenteral and Enteral Nutrition, 7*, 390–397.

Ayers, L.W., Hancock, D., Buesching, W., & Tutschka, P. (1986). Development and evaluation of diets using nonsterile but controlled microbial content foods for control of nosocomial infections in bone marrow transplant patients. *Abstracts of the annual meeting, American Society for Microbiology* (p. 414). Washington, DC: American Society for Microbiology.

Casewell, M., & Phillips, I. (1978). Food as a source of *Klebsiella* species for colonisation and infection of intensive care patients. *Journal of Clinical Pathology, 31*, 845–849.

Cheney, C.L., Aker, S.N., & Lenssen, P. (1988). The effect of ultraisolation environment on oral intake after marrow transplantation [Abstract]. *Journal of the American College of Nutrition, 7*, 415.

Cohen, M.L., Murphy, M.T., Counts, G.W., Buckner, C.D., Clift, R.A., & Meyers, J.D. (1983). Prediction by surveillance cultures of bacteremia among neutropenic patients treated in a protective environment. *Journal of Infectious Diseases, 147*, 789–793.

Crespo, L.F., & Ockerman, H.W. (1977). Thermal destruction of microorganisms in meat by microwave and conventional cooking. *Journal of Food Protection, 40*, 442–444.

Dawkins, H.C., Bolton, F.J., & Hutchinson, D.N. (1984). A study of the spread of *Campylobacter jejuni* in four large kitchens. *Journal of Hygiene, Cambridge, 92*, 357–364.

Dezenhall, A., Curry-Bartley, K., Blackburn, S.A., De Lamerens, S., & Khan, A.R. (1987). Food and nutrition services in bone marrow transplant centers. *Journal of the American Dietetic Association, 87*, 1351–1353.

Dietch, E.A., & Berg, R.D. (1987). Endotoxin but not malnutrition promotes bacterial translocation of the gut flora in burned mice. *Journal of Trauma, 27*, 161–166.

Dietch, E.A., Winterton, J., Li, M., & Berg, R. (1987). The gut as a portal of entry for bacteremia: Role of protein malnutrition. *Annals of Surgery, 205*, 681–691.

Fleming, D.W., Cochi, S.L., MacDonald, K.L., Brondum, J., Hayes, P.S., Plikaytis, B.D., Holmes, M.B.,

Audurier, A., Broome, C.V., & Reingold, A.L. (1985). Pasteurized milk as a vehicle of infection in an outbreak of listeriosis. *New England Journal of Medicine, 312*, 404–407.

Frankmann, C., Beck, J., & Schomburg, R. (1984). Feeding in protected environments. In J.C. Rose (Ed.), *Handbook for health care food service management* (pp. 241–250). Rockville, MD: Aspen.

Fujita, S., & Kohzuki, E. (1983). Microwave food processing for bioclean room patients. *Japanese Journal of Clinical Oncology, 13*(Suppl. 1), 127–132.

Fung, D.Y.C., & Cunningham, F.E. (1980). Effect of microwaves on microorganisms in foods. *Journal of Food Protection, 43*, 641–650.

Institute of Food Technologists' Expert Panel on Food Safety & Nutrition. (1988). Bacteria associated with foodborne diseases. *Food Technology, 42*(4), 1–19.

Kominos, S.D., Copeland, C.E., Grosiak, B., & Postic, B. (1972). Introduction of *Pseudomonas aeruginosa* into a hospital via vegetables. *Applied Microbiology, 24*, 567–570.

Lindsay, R.E., Krissinger, W.A., & Fields, B.F. (1986). Microwave vs. conventional oven cooking of chicken: Relationship of internal temperature to surface contamination by *Salmonella typhimurium*. *Journal of the American Dietetic Association, 86*, 373–374.

McDonald, G.B., Shulman, H.M., Sullivan, K.M., & Spencer, G.D. (1986). Intestinal and hepatic complications of human bone marrow transplantation: Part I. *Gastroenterology, 90*, 460–477.

Moe, G., Johnson, M., & Tari, S. (1988). Unpublished data.

Meyers, J.D., & Thomas, E.D. (1988). Infection complicating bone marrow transplantation. In R.H. Rubin & L.S. Young (Eds.), *Clinical approach to infection in the compromised host* (pp. 525–556). New York: Plenum Medical.

Nausef, W.M., & Maki, D.G. (1981). A study of the value of simple protective isolation in patients with granulocytopenia. *New England Journal of Medicine, 304*, 448–453.

Newman, K.A., & Schimpff, S.C. (1987). Hospital hotel services as risk factors for infection among immunocompromised patients. *Reviews of Infectious Diseases, 9*, 206–213.

Panosian, C.B., & Gorbach, S.L. (1985). Infectious diseases of the gastrointestinal tract. In J.I. Gallin & A.S. Fauci (Eds.), *Advances in host defense mechanisms: Vol. 4* (pp. 165–187). New York: Raven.

Petersen, F., Thornquist, M., Buckner, C., Counts, G., Nelson, N., Meyers, J., Clift, R., & Thomas, E. (1988). The effects of infection prevention regimens on early infectious complications in marrow transplant patients: A four-arm randomized study. *Infection, 16*, 199–208.

Pinegar, J.A., & Cooke, E.M. (1985). *Escherichia coli* in retail processed food. *Journal of Hygiene, Cambridge, 95*, 39–46.

Pizzo, P.A. (1984). Granulocytopenia and cancer therapy: Past problems, current solutions, future challenges. *Cancer, 54*, 2649–2661.

Pizzo, P.A., Purvis, D.S., & Waters, C. (1982). Microbiological evaluation of food items. *Journal of the American Dietetic Association, 81*, 272–279.

Remington, J.S., & Schimpff, S.C. (1981). Please don't eat the salads. *New England Journal of Medicine, 304*, 433–435.

Schweigert, B.S. (1987). Food irradiation: What is it? Where is it now? Where is it going? *Nutrition Today, 22*(6), 13–19.

Shooter, R.A., Faiers, M.C., Cooke, E.M., Breaden, A.L., & O'Farrell, S.M. (1971). Isolation of *Escherichia coli, Pseudomonas aeruginosa*, and *Klebsiella* from food in hospitals, canteens, and schools. *Lancet, 2*, 390–392.

St. Louis, M.E., Morse, D.L., Potter, M.E., Demelfi, T.M., Guzewich, J.J., Tauxe, R.V., & Blake, P.A. (1988). The emergence of grade A eggs as a major source of *Salmonella enteritidis* infections: New implications for the control of salmonellosis. *Journal of the American Medical Association, 259*, 2103–2107.

Subcommittee on Microbiological Criteria, Committee on Food Protection, Food and Nutrition Board, National Research Council. (1985). *An evaluation of the role of microbiological criteria for foods and food ingredients.* Washington, DC: National Academy Press.

Subramaniam, L., & Shriniwas, S.N.V. (1987). Food as a likely source of *Pseudomonas aeruginosa. Indian Journal of Medical Research, 85*, 617–619.

Van der Waaij, D. (1979). The colonization resistance of the digestive tract in man and animals. In T.M. Fliedner, H. Heit, D. Neithammer, & H. Pflieger (Eds.), *Clinical and experimental gnotobiotics: Proceedings of the VIth international symposium on gnotobiology* (pp. 155–161). Ulm, Germany: Association for Gnotobiotics.

Wade, J.C., & Schimpff, S.C. (1988). Epidemiology and prevention of infection in the compromised host. In R.H. Rubin & L.S. Young (Eds.), *Clinical approach to infection in the compromised host* (2nd ed., pp. 5–40). New York: Plenum Medical.

Wright, C., Kominos, S.D., & Yee, R.B. (1976). Enterobacteriaceae and *Pseudomonas aeruginosa* recovered from vegetable salads. *Applied Environmental Microbiology, 31*, 453–454.

# Chapter 13

# Pediatric Oncology Nutrition Support

*Nancy Costlow*

Although rare, cancer is the second most common cause of death in children (second only to accidental death). The types of malignancies in children are vastly different from those in adults. In general the prognosis is much better for children than for adults. The overall cure rate approaches 60% to 65%, and for some types it is as high as 90% to 95%. In the past decade, significant advances have been made in the diagnosis, treatment, and prognosis of pediatric cancer patients. New chemotherapeutic agents, imaging techniques, and treatment protocols and better supportive care including nutrition support have contributed to these advancements.

Most cancer in children is of relatively acute onset, which affects nutrition status at diagnosis. Carter et al. (1983) studied 277 children at diagnosis and concluded that initial nutrient intake as well as weight for height of children with cancer at diagnosis are similar to those of the general population. Although weight loss may be a presenting symptom in adults with cancer, this study found a low incidence of malnutrition in children with newly diagnosed tumors, and if malnutrition was detected it was of caloric or energy etiology, not inadequate protein status. Thus malnutrition in pediatric oncology patients is primarily due to treatment or tumor progression (Carter et al., 1983).

Effective therapy for pediatric cancer requires multimodal treatment protocols necessitating referral to specialized diagnostic and treatment centers. Because the incidence of each tumor type is low, several large study groups have been formed. The Pediatric Oncology Group and the Children's Cancer Study Group are two large, multi-institutional groups involved in the study of various pediatric tumors. The National Wilms' Tumor Study and the Intergroup Rhabdomyosarcoma Study are two national study groups for specific solid tumor types.

The philosophy of treatment in pediatric oncology is to use an aggressive, multimodal approach. The key for providing appropriate nutrition support is to prevent nutrition depletion by early intervention rather than to institute nutrition support when the patient is already malnourished. This requires knowledge of treatment plans, including all aspects of treatment that will be involved (surgery, chemotherapy, or radiation therapy), and knowledge of expected side effects, length of therapy, and intervals between treatments. Much of this information can be obtained by reading the protocols written for each specific treatment, which include a background of the disease, treatment plans, and specific drugs and doses that are given. It is important to understand different tumor types, especially in terms of which tumors result in a high risk for depleted nutrition status either from the tumor itself or from the intensive treatment planned. In general, patients with advanced disease or those who have relapsed or not responded to treatment are most likely to be at nutrition risk. Also, certain treatments such as abdominal radiation, surgery, and intense, frequent cycles of chemotherapy or the presence of severe infections or pain predispose the patient to increased nutrition risk. Side effects of each chemotherapy drug or area to be irradiated are numerous. The specific nutrition effects of these treatments should be anticipated to predict interference with eating and to plan appropriate means of nutrition support.

A discussion of the most common pediatric tumor types and their treatment follows. This will be helpful in determining the effect on nutrition status of different tumor types and the anticipated need for nutrition intervention.

## LEUKEMIA

Leukemia is the most common type of cancer in children, with an incidence of approximately 2,000 new cases diagnosed per year. Acute lymphocytic leukemia (ALL) is the most prevalent subtype in children. Recent treatment protocols have had good results: overall there is a cure rate of approximately 60% to 65%. Treatment usually consists of chemotherapy with an intensive induction phase and a fairly long-term, less intensive maintenance phase lasting approximately 2 to 3 years. Methotrexate, a mainstay of leukemia treatment, can cause severe mucositis, which may impair oral intake. In general, however, the nutrition risk for patients with ALL undergoing initial treatment is minimal.

In contrast, acute nonlymphocytic leukemia, infant leukemia, and T-cell leukemia (which is a subtype of ALL) have a much poorer prognosis than ALL. These require aggressive treatment that results in extended periods of neutropenia. Infection is a major life-threatening complication of treatment, which affects nutrition status. Early nutrition assessment and intervention are recommended.

## SOLID TUMORS

Brain tumors are the most prevalent solid tumor in children. Although some types are cured with surgery alone, many brain tumors are incurable, causing progressive neurologic deterioration and leading to death. Recent advances have led to increased disease-free survival and improved quality of life. A combination of surgery, radiation therapy, and chemotherapy is often used to treat brain tumors. Steroid use is common and causes a host of nutrition complications, such as severe obesity with depleted protein reserves, metabolic abnormalities, and the like. Neurologic problems such as inability to suck or swallow may complicate eating, possibly requiring enteral alimentation by means of feeding tubes.

Neuroblastoma is a malignancy of neural crest origin. The primary site is the adrenal gland. Early dissemination often occurs with metastasis to bone marrow, lymph nodes, bone, liver, or skin. A good prognosis can be expected in localized or completely excised tumors and in children younger than 1 year of age. Patients with disseminated disease have a poor prognosis, so that aggressive treatment is given in an attempt to improve the outcome. Intensive chemotherapy is used and includes extremely emetogenic drugs such as cyclophosphamide and cisplatin. An initial abdominal mass effect, as well as possible surgical procedures, often compromise oral intake. Abdominal radiation or bone marrow transplant are other treatment options with deleterious effects on nutrition status. Thus advanced neuroblastoma requires intensive treatment, during which nutrition assessment and support are important adjuncts.

Wilms' tumor is a pediatric kidney cancer that is treated according to protocols from the National Wilms' Tumor Study. This disease has a relatively good prognosis and a prolonged disease-free survival of more than 80%. Prompt surgery and postoperative radiation therapy and chemotherapy have contributed to these good results. Nausea and vomiting are common side effects of drugs used to treat Wilms' tumor, and absorption difficulties may result from abdominal radiation. Because the prognosis for Wilms' tumor is good, maintenance of adequate nutrition status to allow complete medical treatment is essential.

Other common tumors of childhood include lymphoma, rhabdomyosarcoma (a tumor arising from striated muscle), Ewing's sarcoma (a malignant tumor of bone), and osteosarcoma (another malignant tumor of bone with a different histology). These tumors require intensive multimodal treatment with surgery, chemotherapy, and radiation therapy that often interferes with nutrition status. Hodgkin's disease, retinoblastoma, and early stage nonmetastatic tumors often are treated with less intensive treatment regimens that pose less of a nutrition risk.

Bone marrow transplants are used for leukemia and some solid tumors to allow maximal chemotherapy. This involves long-term hospitalization and possible severe complications such as graft-versus-host disease, infections, venocclusive disease of the liver, pneumonia, and mucositis. Nutrition support with on-going assessment and monitoring should be a routine part of the care of each bone marrow transplant patient.

## NUTRITION ASSESSMENT

Nutrition assessment of the pediatric oncology patient is similar to that of the adult oncology patient in many respects; several frequently used nutrition assessment parameters are not appropriate, however. Total lymphocyte count or any other hematologic indicator such as hematocrit, hemoglobin, and serum iron are altered by transfusions and the effect of treatment on bone marrow function rather than nutrition status. Therefore, these values should not be used in assessment of nutrition status in pediatric oncology patients.

Criteria with which to assess patients include weight and height, both of which can be followed over time. Weight measurements should be interpreted as percentage weight changes because a 2-kg weight change in a 70-kg adult is insignificant but in a 15-kg child is significant. Hydration status and use of steroid therapy must be accounted for in analyzing this parameter. Also, assessment of weight for height should be plotted on standard growth charts and monitored throughout treatment. Several types of growth charts are available; the ones most commonly used were compiled from the National Center for Health Statistics of the Public Health Service. Several charts are available and incorporate age

(birth to 36 months and 2 to 18 years) and sex differences. Sequential monitoring is useful in following a child's overall growth pattern. When weight or height deviates from that child's previous pattern, an assessment of nutrition status is indicated.

Other anthropometric measurements such as triceps skin fold, midarm muscle circumference, or subscapular skin fold thickness may be utilized for detailed assessment of body fat and muscle reserves. Biochemical measurement of serum albumin and transferrin levels is used to assess visceral protein status. Serial values can help predict trends in individual nutrition status, but these values may be influenced by hydration status, infection, and liver disease.

Each nutrition assessment parameter by itself can be affected by various external components, as mentioned above. Therefore, it is necessary for a skilled nutritionist to combine all data that are available with the patient's current clinical picture to formulate an accurate assessment of nutrition status.

## LEARNED FOOD AVERSIONS

Bernstein (1978), in a classic study, demonstrated that children undergoing abdominal radiation or chemotherapy (causing gastrointestinal toxicity) acquired food aversions to an unusual flavor of ice cream that they consumed before treatment. In this randomized study, pediatric oncology patients were offered a novel flavor of ice cream before receiving chemotherapy. This group of children had a significantly lower likelihood of accepting that specific ice cream flavor again compared to children who previously received treatment without sampling the ice cream or children who sampled the ice cream without subsequent toxic therapy. Learned food aversions may contribute to the anorexia and weight loss that are often encountered in oncology patients. Avoiding favorite or nutrient-dense foods before treatments that cause gastrointestinal toxicity should be considered in an attempt to prevent acquired aversions to these foods. Fasting or eating a light meal before chemotherapy is often recommended to reduce vomiting as well.

## ANTICIPATORY NAUSEA AND VOMITING

Another problem that often affects older children and adolescents undergoing cancer treatment is anticipatory nausea and vomiting. This may take the form of mild or severe symptoms of nausea or actual vomiting before administration of intravenous chemotherapy and is paired with anxiety-producing stimuli. For example, some patients experience nausea or vomiting upon walking into the clinic or even driving toward the hospital. This is most likely to occur in the teenaged population, especially among patients who have had many previous cycles of emetogenic chemotherapy. Symptoms are most severe in patients who have had an extended and severe period of postchemotherapy emesis. The overall incidence of anticipatory symptoms was 33% in a study conducted at an adult ambulatory oncology clinic (Stefanek, Sheidler, & Fetting, 1988).

Teenagers receiving treatment for osteosarcoma or Hodgkin's disease or intensive chemotherapy for leukemia are candidates for developing anticipatory symptoms. Treatment includes the use of relaxation techniques when anticipatory symptoms begin. An antiemetic or antianxiety drug given before the onset of symptoms may prevent or lessen the severity of symptoms.

## NUTRITION PRIORITIES

During periods of treatment, food and eating habits often become a much emphasized area of conflict, and sometimes a battle ground, between the child and his or her parents. Nausea, vomiting, mucositis, pain, food aversion, taste changes, and anticipatory symptoms of nausea and vomiting are just a few of the obstacles that prevent a child from eating normally. Parents often feel helpless at this time because they have no control over their child's disease or treatment. Because they have maintained control of their child's diet before the illness, they often put too much emphasis on eating habits after the onset of

illness, which leads to conflict and a struggle for control between parents and child.

During treatment children often become picky eaters. They may undergo short periods of eating only a few different items (often nonnutritious or "junk" foods). Health care professionals must counsel parents that these are common behaviors experienced by pediatric oncology patients and that they should avoid conflict with the child over this issue. Parents should understand that short periods of time without a proper diet will not adversely affect their child's overall nutrition status and that "bad days" can be compensated for on better days. Furthermore, parents should be reminded that food fetishes are common in many children without a diagnosis of cancer. Thus to keep eating from becoming a battle ground the child should be allowed to maintain control, and parents should be assured that, although balanced nutrition is important, all attempts should be made to avoid conflict while providing the maximal intake possible.

Nutrition priorities must change during cancer treatment. Parents should concentrate on providing high-calorie, high-protein foods that are nutrient dense rather than the usually prescribed well-balanced diet from all four food groups. It often takes much counseling to help parents understand that they may encourage their child to eat cholesterol-rich, high-fat foods such as butter or margarine, ice creams, cheeses, and rich sauces as concentrated calorie sources rather than avoid these items because of their much publicized cardiovascular risks. After treatment is completed, a switch back to previous priorities is indicated. Also, parents may feel less pressured to improve their child's intake if they are aware that nutrition support is available as a back-up if adequate oral intake is not possible.

## NUTRITION SUPPORT

Several options exist for providing nutrition support to pediatric oncology patients. Oral feeding is preferable if tolerated. Individual counseling with emphasis on anticipated nutrition problems according to the specific treatment plan is optimal. High-protein, high-calorie, nutrient-dense foods should be encouraged during treatment-free periods, with less emphasis on oral intake during periods of chemotherapy. Vitamin supplements must be approved by the child's physician because they can interfere with the mechanism of certain chemotherapeutic drugs and possibly with radiation therapy.

Working with each patient in choosing appropriate menu items and offering high-calorie "super shakes" and other supplements such as puddings, ice cream, and snack foods can significantly improve caloric intake. Also, allowing parents to bring food from home to hospitalized children provides the child with familiar, less institutionalized meals, which may promote better oral consumption. Further, motivation to eat is improved by explaining the importance of eating to the child in terms that he or she understands while at the same time giving "permission" not to eat during times of vomiting, mucositis, and so forth. Graphing calorie counts in an attractive chart form to display on a child's wall provides a visual display of intake and provides positive reinforcement for improvement (for example, stickers may be put on the chart to indicate intake that exceeds a certain goal calorie level).

Tube feeding can provide nutrition support in patients with adequate gastrointestinal function but suboptimal oral intake. Nasogastric or nasoduodenal tubes are most frequently used, but gastrostomy or jejunostomy feedings are optimal for long-term feedings or when the nasopharynx must be bypassed. Small-bore, flexible feeding tubes and various feeding formulas that are easy to tolerate and can be given slowly through feeding pumps are available. There are numerous formulas available for tube feedings, each with specific indications (e.g., lactose free, high fiber, elemental, or modular feedings). The formula should be chosen after thorough assessment of the patient's medical and nutrition status. This enables tube feeding to be administered without complications of vomiting, diarrhea, or nasopharyngeal irritation. Home care companies enable families to administer enteral nutrition support at home by educating them about administration of the feedings, providing formulas and equipment, and monitoring blood work and physical assessments as directed. Nightly tube feeding with self-placement and self-removal of the tube is an option that allows adequate nutrition support without the stigma of a tube protruding from the nose.

Total parenteral nutrition (TPN) is an intravenous infusion of a concentrated solution of dextrose, amino acids, lipid, vitamins, minerals, and trace elements given through central venous catheters. TPN is indicated when the patient's nutrition status cannot be maintained by the enteral route. This may occur with tumors producing gastrointestinal tract obstruction, severe mucositis, or protracted nausea and vomiting. Central venous access must be obtained and used solely for nutrient infusion to reduce the incidence of infection. The TPN should be advanced slowly over several days. Precise monitoring is essential and must include daily evaluations of weight, intake and output, temperature, and urine parameters to assess tolerance to the infusions. Frequent evaluation of blood counts and blood chemistries is necessary to monitor for metabolic complications and hepatic dysfunction. Serial assessments of nutrition status are indicated to document nutrition repletion or maintenance. Home care companies are useful in enabling a stable patient to receive parenteral alimentation in the comfort of his or her own home. Cycling the infusions at night is often well tolerated and encourages the patient to be mobile and functional during the day, which promotes much needed normalization in the life of a child with cancer.

## REFERENCES

Bernstein, I.L. (1978). Learned taste aversions in children. *Science, 200,* 1302–1303.

Carter, P., Carr, D., van Eys, J., Ramirez, I., Coody, D., & Taylor, G. (1983). Energy and nutrient intake of children with cancer. *Journal of the American Dietetic Association, 82,* 610–615.

Stefanek, M.E., Sheidler, V.R., & Fetting, J.H. (1988). Anticipatory nausea and vomiting: Does it remain a significant clinical problem? *Cancer, 62,* 2654–2657.

# Chapter 14

# Nutrition in Children with Cancer: A Case Study Approach

*Juliene B. Burgess and Amy Austin Brewer*

Although childhood cancer is rare, it is recognized as the chief cause of death from disease in children past infancy (American Cancer Society, 1988). Approximately 6,600 children were newly diagnosed with cancer in the United States in 1988. Eighteen hundred deaths were attributed to childhood cancer in that year; half those deaths were from leukemia. Nevertheless, the prognosis for many of the typical childhood cancers has been steadily improving over the past 25 years. Survival of children with acute lymphocytic leukemia (ALL) rose from 4% in 1960 to 56% in 1985; that of children with bone cancer, from 20% to 45%; with brain and central nervous system cancers, from 35% to 53%; with neuroblastoma, from 25% to 53%; with Hodgkin's disease, from 52% to 88%; and with Wilms' tumor, from 57% to 82% (National Institutes of Health, 1985).

The role of nutrition support in the medical management of children with cancer has kept pace with the advances in antineoplastic therapy. No longer does a child need to experience malnutrition because of severe mucositis and gastritis. Gone too is the attitude that malnutrition is an obligatory consequence of a diagnosis of cancer. Although malnutrition does not occur any more frequently at diagnosis in children with cancer than in those with benign disease (Carter, Carr, van Eys, & Coody, 1983), it has been shown to have a negative effect on prognosis and outcome (Donaldson et al., 1981). Therefore, the prevention or reversal of malnutrition has become an accepted part of the medical management of children with malignancies.

A child's physiologic demands for nutrition are unequalled by those at any other stage in life. So much cell growth and tissue formation occurs that any interference with substrate availability can have long-term effects. Therefore, issues of growth and development must be considered alongside issues of disease and acute stress in the child with cancer.

The American Academy of Pediatrics' (AAP) Committee on Nutrition appointed a special task force to report on the special nutrition needs of children with malignancies. Their report, which was published by the academy in 1987, deals comprehensively with the why, when, and how of nutrition support of children with cancer. The American Dietetic Association (ADA) published *Quality Assurance Criteria for Pediatric Nutrition Conditions: A Model* in 1988 as guidelines for dietitians. These publications as well as other reports in the medical literature provide a superb foundation for those seeking documentation of practice standards in the area of nutrition and childhood cancer.

There are four major requisites for the success of nutrition support in the pediatric population. First is an appreciation of the importance of the social and psychologic parameters of a child's life, in addition to his or her medical history, at the time of diagnosis. Second is familiarity with treatment protocols—surgical procedures, radiation therapies, and chemotherapies—and the expected toxicities of each. Third is the use of definitive clinical guidelines, such as those published by the AAP or the ADA, to establish nutrition intervention strategies. Fourth is an understanding of the necessity of early and consistent interaction of the nutrition staff with the child and family.

The social and psychologic factors that may confound treatment issues cannot be underestimated. Although these issues are not absent in adult populations, they are particularly pronounced in the pediatric setting. As in adults, the diagnosis of cancer makes a sudden and abrupt intrusion into a child's life. There are changes in family routine, new and traumatic medical procedures, hospitalizations, and so on. These all have an impact on family relationships as well as on a child's interaction with his or her peers. In the traditional nuclear family these are complex issues. In single-parent homes or homes with combined families these issues take on even more complexity. It is not uncommon for siblings to have a difficult time adjusting to this new change as well. Behavior and emotional problems often arise. Young children may experience behavior regression. Adolescents, with their natural preoccupation with body image, may refuse to comply with their nutrition care plan for fear of weight gain or because they view their loss of appetite as the perfect opportunity to diet. Behavior problems relating to food can have significant effects on a child's nutrition status, and an awareness and sensitivity on the part of the nutrition staff is invaluable to the achievement of nutrition goals.

Complex issues of control can and do arise around the area of nutrition. Sometimes it is the patient and sometimes it is the family who "acts out" the frustration and the need to exert control over the frightening turn of events in their lives. Power struggles between parents or spouses can be as common as power struggles between parent and child. Therefore, compliance with nutrition therapy by either the patient or the family can never be assumed.

Antineoplastic therapy may well induce learned food aversions that lead to inadequate intake or anticipatory vomiting. These aversions can develop at any time and in children of any age. They most often occur when a food is eaten around the time of a particularly toxic treatment. These psychologic associations of food with nausea and vomiting are best dealt with by preventive measures because reason does little to stem the involuntary reaction. Changes in taste perception as well as changes in food preferences are also common. This can be particularly baffling to care givers who are struggling to find ways to nurture and nourish a child through difficult times.

The success of nutrition support is dependent on the clinician's commitment to act to prevent, as opposed to reacting to, crisis. To this end, it is imperative that the nutrition staff be familiar with antineoplastic treatment protocols: the drugs, the side effects, the timing, and so forth. Because many cancer therapies have side effects with predictable onsets and durations, preventive action can be taken on the basis of these parameters.

Children experience great substrate demands at times of rapid growth. Antineoplastic therapy can alter substrate utilization, thus negatively affecting the child's nutrition status and overall growth. Norton and Peter (1989) present a schematic that illustrates the multifactoral nature of malnutrition in young cancer patients (Fig. 14-1). Altered metabolism, antineoplastic therapy, tumor substrate consumption, growth demands, and hypophagia all contribute to cachexia and its attendant morbidity in this population.

The AAP's task force report lists five criteria for nutrition intervention in children with malignancies:

1. an interval or total weight loss of more than 5% of the preillness body weight
2. a relative weight for height of 90% or less, or when the weight for height percentile determined from the National Center for Health Statistics growth charts is in the 10th percentile channel or lower
3. serum albumin level of 3.2 mg/dL or less

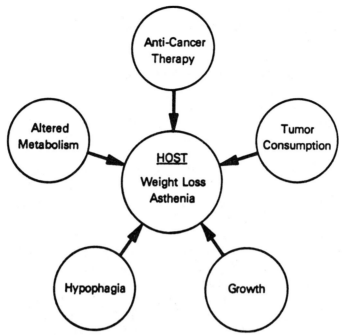

**Figure 14-1** Schematic Representation of the Origin of Cachexia in a Pediatric Oncology Patient. *Source:* From *Principles and Practice of Pediatric Oncology* (p. 871) by P.A. Pizzo and D.G. Poplack (Eds.), 1989, Philadelphia: J.B. Lippincott Company. Copyright 1989 by J.B. Lippincott Company. Reprinted by permission.

4. energy reserves (as estimated by arm fat area or subscapular skin folds) of the 5th percentile or less for age and sex
5. a current percentile for weight or height that is 2 percentile channels lower than the preillness percentile

These guidelines can help clinicians identify which of their patients are at risk nutritionally and thus help them prioritize their efforts.

All children diagnosed with cancer are at some nutrition risk by virtue of the fact that they will be undergoing therapy that will disrupt their normal lifestyle. Some diagnoses, however, such as Ewing's sarcoma, are typically accompanied by weight loss, so that the need for nutrition intervention is obvious from the start. Other diagnoses, such as acute myelocytic leukemia, are treated with such aggressive chemotherapy regimens that patients are unable to maintain adequate nutrition status by oral intake. Generally, children with the poorest prognoses are treated with the most aggressive therapies and therefore are at greatest risk of developing mal-

nutrition (Lingard et al., 1986). Guidelines for intervention also provide an objective view of risk for patients with less apparent need for nutrition support.

The journey from the list of criteria for nutrition intervention to the bedside, where nutrition therapy will be implemented, is never as simple as it appears to be on the printed page. The methods of intervention are the same as those used in adults: enteral, including volitional oral feeding and feeding by tube; and parenteral, including peripheral and central venous alimentation. Nevertheless, a significant difference between treating adults and treating children is the wide range of ages and therefore abilities to understand, consent, and cooperate. Further, no matter what the age of the child, there is usually at least one set of parents to include in the treatment plan. Maintaining adequate nutrition status in the pediatric population requires an appreciation for human development and family dynamics. Accordingly, patience and persistence are the first two requirements of nutrition intervention strategies.

Goals established by the AAP for nutrition rehabilitation of pediatric patients include the following:

- current body weight greater than the ideal body weight
- arm fat area greater than or equal to the 10th percentile for age and sex
- serum albumin level of 3.2 mg/dL or greater

Realistic, individual objectives for nutrition support and rehabilitation based on a child's social, psychologic, and medical history and in concert with the antineoplastic therapy plan provide a means to measure success for both patient and staff. Erratic intervention produces little if any positive effects. Similarly, stamping the medical record with a nutrition plan that does not take into consideration the context of a child's treatment will be ineffective as well as damaging to the credibility of the nutrition staff as an integral part of the health care team.

Early and consistent contact of the patient by the nutrition staff is essential for the prevention of therapy-related nutrition problems. These can arise at any point in a child's treatment. If the family members have been apprised of the possible problems, they are usually much easier to handle. Early introduction of the role of nutrition in the child's therapy helps establish its importance in the minds of the patient and family. Not all newly diagnosed patients need immediate nutrition attention, but information provided in an initial interview can plant the idea that nutrition is important and bears observation as therapy progresses. Often nutrition issues are of primary importance to parents, and they are relieved to know that their child will be monitored. Studies in adult cancer patients (Padilla & Grant, 1985) have demonstrated that quality of appetite, ability to eat, and control of nausea and vomiting were more important to patients' perception of quality of life than ability to work, degree of strength, or pain control. Indeed, parents of pediatric cancer patients often consider appetite, eating behavior, and weight status indicative of their child's response to therapy (Lingard et al., 1986).

The four following case studies illustrate representative nutrition problems and approaches to support that incorporate these requisites for nutrition support.

## CASE 1

D.H. was a very thin 17-year-old white adolescent boy who presented to his local doctor with general malaise, back pain, abdominal pain, fever, night sweats, pruritus, and a 24-lb weight loss over a 3-month period. He was referred to a cancer research center, where his diagnostic work-up revealed stage IV B Hodgkin's disease, nodular sclerosis subtype. At the time of diagnosis he had hepatosplenomegaly, mediastinal lymph node involvement, and disease metastatic to the vertebrae at L-4, L-5, T-1, and T-7. He was treated according to the center's protocol for Hodgkin's disease IV B with thoracic and abdominal radiation to 35 Gy and with the chemotherapeutic agents cyclophosphamide, vincristine, and ABVD (adriamycin, bleomycin, vinblastine, dacarbazine).

D.'s most significant medical problem during therapy was weight loss. In addition to his extreme initial weight loss, he lost 8.5 lb over a 6-day period with his first course of ABVD. A coincidental viral infection was in part responsible for this additional weight loss. He was hospitalized in an attempt to arrest and reverse his weight loss.

D. was typical of many teenagers. Adolescence is an especially difficult time to be diagnosed with a life-threatening disease. Physically unable to join his peers in normal activity and distressed by the dramatic change in appearance that his weight loss caused, D. was depressed and withdrawn. The erythema and hyperpigmentation of his skin caused by radiation therapy and the hair loss induced by chemotherapy served to aggravate his emotional state.

D. was included in the formulation of his nutrition intervention strategies from the beginning of his treatment. Although his weight loss was serious enough to warrant immediate nasogastric tube feedings, D. was, at his request, allowed a period of several days to attempt oral renourishment. It was agreed that if he was able to consume 2,000 calories per day by the end of that time he would be discharged on oral therapy alone. Because he was motivated and cooperative, D. was able to reverse his weight loss by eating nutrient-dense foods and supplements while he was still undergoing chemotherapy. With intensive counseling and support from the dietitians, D. learned to count calories and to maximize his intake during the "good" times between cycles of therapy. By adding glucose polymers to beverages and by drinking fortified milk shakes between meals, he was able to consume up to 4,500 calories on his best days.

As is often the case with patients with Hodgkin's disease, as D.'s therapy controlled his disease he began to feel much better between his courses of therapy and actually achieved normal weight while he was still undergoing therapy.

For D., it was the support group for teens and the persistence of the health care team that made the difference. The support group provided him the assurance that he was not the only teen confronting cancer and loss of "normalcy" as well as a peer group for social activity around the hospital and clinic. The health care team determined to offer him the opportunity to take as much control over his circumstances as possible, and he responded well to the responsibility.

Successful rehabilitation of a malnourished patient with a volitional oral feeding program is extremely labor intensive. Nevertheless, by teaching D. how, in effect, to treat himself, his rehabilitation was swift, complete, and far more pleasant for all concerned than is typical of such cases. He learned to count calories in his favorite foods and to use supplements to boost his intake whenever he was able. He also learned to avoid food aversions by limiting his oral intake around the time of any therapy that was particularly toxic gastrointestinally (in his case, administration of ABVD). Further, he became an effective peer counselor for other teens with nutrition problems.

Eight years after diagnosis, D. is disease free, well nourished, and happily married.

## CASE 2

R.D. was a 5-year-old white boy who was referred with a diagnosis of embryonal rhabdomyosarcoma stage II C. By the staging system employed for rhabdomyosarcoma, this meant local or regional disease with involvement of contiguous organs or regional lymph nodes. R.'s disease involved his nasopharynx with extension to the pterygoid fossa, ethmoid sinus, base of the skull, maxillary sinus, and uvula. The extent of his disease required placement of a tracheostomy at the time of his diagnostic surgery.

Rhabdomyosarcoma is the most common soft tissue sarcoma in children and adolescents. Head and neck and genitourinary sites are the primary disease sites, and peak incidence is between ages 3 and 12 years.

Because R.'s therapy would include head and neck radiation therapy to 45 Gy, the decision was made to place a percutaneous gastrostomy during his surgery for central venous catheter placement before beginning therapy. The sequelae of head and neck radiation, which can be subject to recall by subsequent chemotherapy, can preclude adequate oral intake for months. Oral mucosal changes (ulcerations, mucositis, infections, gingivitis, and glossitis) are acute side effects of radiation therapy. Children of R.'s age are especially susceptible to the long-term problems that can significantly affect nutrition status. These include xerostomia, dental caries, delayed tooth eruption, exfoliation of teeth, cessation of root development, osteoradionecrosis, and facial skeletal hypoplasia. A percutaneously placed gastrostomy tube provided the optimal solution to the challenges presented by R.'s disease and therapy.

In addition to radiation therapy, R. was treated according to a protocol for rhabdomyosarcoma with alternating cycles of dacarbazine plus adriamycin and cyclophosphamide, vincristine, and dactinomycin. Throughout the expected sequelae of head and neck radiation, when he was able to take little to nothing by mouth, R. was maintained nutritionally with a complete liquid formula through his gastrostomy tube. Chemotherapeutic toxicities other than weight loss (primarily leukopenia) caused some delays in R.'s treatment schedule. Despite the use of therapy that was as aggressive as he could tolerate, his disease progressed.

Although R. died a year after his diagnosis from complications of disease metastatic to his liver, the quality of his life during his year of therapy was significantly enhanced by his feeding gastrostomy. Any patient receiving head and neck radiation should be reviewed as a potential candidate for a percutaneous gastrostomy. Frequently, the side effects of radiation, which are often more pronounced in children compared to adults, so interfere with adequate intake that nutrition support is obligatory. Especially for young children such as R., in whom the ability to cooperate with a treatment plan is minimal, a percutaneous gastrostomy can be invaluable for facilitating nutrition support.

## CASE 3

K.D. was 15 years old the summer that she was diagnosed with stage II large cell non-Hodgkin's lymphoma with mediastinal involvement. Of average height and weight (5 ft 3 in, 115 lb), she gave a 6-week history of decreased appetite with a report of an undetermined amount of recent weight loss. She complained of general fatigue, and a power struggle with her mother over the issue of eating was apparent from the first interview.

K. began induction therapy with radiation to the lungs (15 Gy fractionated over 10 days) with subsequent cycles of cyclophosphamide, adriamycin, vincristine, and prednisone. Once in remission, K. received cycles of maintenance chemotherapy for 15 months.

K.'s weight at admission was satisfactory, but dietary supplements were prescribed throughout radiation therapy for weight maintenance. She experienced decreased appetite and mild epigastric pain during radiation therapy but complied readily with supplementation in an effort to avoid weight loss. Despite her best efforts, however, at the completion of her radiation therapy, K. had lost 2 lb.

Induction chemotherapy included a cycle of prednisone, and K. was encouraged to take advantage of its appetite-stimulating properties to attempt to regain weight. She did well and gained 4 lb. Nevertheless, she experienced severe nausea with cyclophosphamide and adriamycin treatment and began losing weight again. Eating once again became a focus of conflict between her and her mother. After a loss of 7% from her prediagnosis weight, a decision

was made to supplement K.'s oral intake with nightly nasogastric tube feedings on an outpatient basis. A nasogastric tube was placed, and K. was taught to set up her feedings and to operate an enteral pump for 10 hours at night. One week later, she returned to the clinic with a further weight loss of 2 lb.

On questioning, K. admitted that she had been turning the pump off at night because of feelings of bloating and nausea and that she was eating little during the day because of discomfort and embarrassment at having the tube dangling around her face. She was admitted to the hospital and fed continuously by nasogastric tube until a 5-lb weight gain was achieved. During this admission, K. was instructed to place her own small-bore Silastic feeding tube so that after discharge she could place and remove the tube for supplemental feedings as needed. She was discharged after 3 weeks to resume chemotherapy and tube feedings as needed for weight maintenance.

K. repeatedly used nasogastric feedings through the remaining months of her maintenance chemotherapy and successfully avoided chronic progressive weight loss. Three years later, she remains in remission and at a healthy weight for her height with a normal lifestyle.

This case again illustrates the need for vigilance on the part of the nutrition staff. Making note of family dynamics that were producing aberrant behavior on K.'s part, steps were taken to prevent her negative behavior from seriously endangering her nutrition status. In fact, K. was admitted to a psychiatric hospital for behavior problems twice during the course of her maintenance chemotherapy. Allowing K. a certain amount of responsibility for, and control over, her nutrition therapy was successful in averting a nutrition crisis.

## CASE 4

H.P. was a well-nourished, normally developed, 7-year-old white girl when she was diagnosed as having acute nonlymphocytic leukemia (ANLL). She presented with central nervous system involvement and a white cell count of 100,000, factors indicating a poor prognosis.

Her history revealed that she had experienced depressed appetite, gastrointestinal distress, and bone pain for about 6 weeks before diagnosis. At admission her height was 48 in and her weight was 53 lb. Immediately after diagnosis H. was taken to surgery for placement of a central venous catheter. This would be used in the upcoming months not only for chemotherapy but also for parenteral nutrition support.

H. was started right away on several cycles of etoposide, cytarabine, daunomycin, 6-thio-guanine, and intrathecal methotrexate. After the second cycle, she began exhibiting the predicted gastrointestinal toxicities: severe mucositis, stomatitis, ulcerations, anorexia, nausea, vomiting, and diarrhea. Total parenteral nutrition was initiated immediately and she was given nothing by mouth until her blood counts recovered and her toxicities subsided.

As she recovered, H. became interested in eating more. Her parenteral support was gradually worked into a cycling schedule of 12 hours on and 12 hours off, allowing her to be "free" during the day. As her routine became more normalized her appetite increased, and she was weaned completely from parenteral support and discharged home with a net weight gain of 5 lb.

H. experienced a relapse of ANLL within several weeks and was placed on a second regimen of chemotherapy. This one consisted of cycles of teniposide, amsacrine, cytarabine, etoposide, and daunomycin. Again parenteral support was initiated after the second cycle to maintain adequate nutrition status. Because of the severe gastrointestinal toxicities that H. experienced with the reinduction chemotherapy, she remained on parenteral support for several months. Her medical course during this admission was complicated by a fungal infection treated with amphotericin B. Again she was discharged in remission, with a net weight gain and an adequate oral intake.

H.'s second remission lasted only 3 months. Conventional therapy for her disease having been exhausted, H. was placed on phase I antineoplastic agents while continuing to be supported on parenteral nutrition. A remission could not be reinduced. Her parents were instructed in the use of the parenteral pump, and H. was able to go home on supportive care between medical crises. H. died of her disease 2 years after her diagnosis.

Parenteral nutrition support was a vital ingredient in the treatment plan that prolonged H.'s life for those 2 years. Remission induction therapy for ANLL is extremely aggressive and usually carries severe side effects. Toxicity onset can be rapid, and H. often went from total oral intake to total parenteral support in a matter of days. Cycling the parenteral support to nighttime feeding allowed H. a degree of freedom and normalcy of schedule, which helped her psychologic outlook during her long hospitalizations. The ability to offer home parenteral support added greatly to the quality of her last days as well.

## CONCLUSION

These case studies are real life examples of the challenges to be met in the nutrition management of children with cancer. They illustrate that, although nutrition intervention may not change the course of disease, it is invaluable in the treatment process and in quality of life issues. An appreciation of a child's social and psychologic history, in addition to the medical history, is primary in this endeavor. Familiarity with the surgical procedures, radiation therapies, chemotherapies, and probable toxicities for individual patients is essential. A nutrition care plan, with definitive clinical guidelines by which to evaluate progress, is imperative. Finally, early intervention and consistent monitoring is crucial to the success of nutrition management of these children.

Efficacy of nutrition intervention in the pediatric cancer patient is extensively reviewed in the AAP Task Force report (1987). The literature bears out clinical observations that the efficacy of nutrition support in maintaining or restoring nutrition status varies widely with diagnosis, antineoplastic therapy, and nutrition intervention employed.

Although there is not much that distinguishes malnutrition in the cancer patient from the malnutrition seen in other children, it is clear that aggressive antineoplastic therapies lead frequently to complications that predispose a child to malnutrition. Because nutrition status has been shown to be prognostic for disease outcome of children with cancer, intervention is appropriate for any child undergoing antineoplastic therapy. Whether malnutrition is the cause of increased mortality or a symptom of aggressive disease is as yet an unresolved issue. Nevertheless, it is apparent that nutrition intervention alone does not change the outcome of disease. Malnutrition is no more acceptable in a child with cancer than in a child with benign disease and should be prevented or treated.

## REFERENCES

American Academy of Pediatrics, Committee on Nutrition. (1987). *Report of the Task Force on Special Nutritional Needs of Children with Malignancies*. Chicago: Author.

American Cancer Society. (1988). *Cancer facts and figures*. New York: Author.

American Dietetic Association. (1988). *Quality assurance criteria for pediatric nutrition conditions: A model*. Chicago: Author.

Carter, P., Carr, D., van Eys, J., & Coody, D. (1983). Nutritional parameters in children with cancer. *Journal of the American Dietetic Association, 82*, 616–622.

Donaldson, S.S., Wesley, M.N., DeWys, W.D., Suskind, R.M., Jaffe, N., & van Eys, J. (1981). A study of the nutritional status of pediatric cancer patients. *American Journal of the Diseases of Childhood, 135*, 1107–1112.

Lingard, C.D., Rickard, K.A., Jaeger, B.L., Weetman, R.M., Coates, T.D., & Baehner, R.L. (1986). Planning and implementing a nutrition program for children with cancer. *Topics in Clinical Nutrition, 1*(2), 71–86.

National Institutes of Health. (1985). *Cancer rates and risks* (NIH publication no. 85-691). Rockville, MD: Department of Health and Human Services.

Norton, J.A., & Peter J. (1989). Nutritional supportive care. In P.A. Pizzo & D.G. Poplack (Eds.), *Principles and practice of pediatric oncology* (chap. 40). Philadelphia: Lippincott.

Padilla, G.V., & Grant, M. (1985). Psychosocial aspects of artificial feeding. *Cancer, 65*(Suppl.), 301–304.

# Chapter 15

# Nutrition Management of the Patient with Breast Cancer

*Jacalyn See*

The nutrition management of the patient with breast cancer depends on the presence or absence of active disease, stage of disease, treatment, weight status, other medical problems, and overall prognosis. Like other cancer patients, breast cancer patients with advanced disease may experience anorexia and weight loss. The management of nutrition problems in the malnourished breast cancer patient is similar to that in other cancer patients.

Obesity and weight gain are commonly seen among patients with localized breast cancer as well as those with advanced disease; this is often identified as a greater problem than weight loss in most breast cancer patients. Because of the possible link between obesity and the development of breast cancer, obesity is a common finding in breast cancer. Weight gain in patients receiving adjuvant chemotherapy has also been widely observed in clinical practice and is identified as a problem for patients with early breast cancer. Whether or not weight reduction is appropriate for these patients is a question frequently faced by dietitians and physicians. This chapter focuses on the problems of weight gain and obesity in the patient with primary breast cancer.

## DIETARY RISK FACTORS FOR BREAST CANCER

### Obesity

Several studies have reported that obesity is a risk factor for the development of breast cancer (Hirayama, 1978; Committee on Diet, 1982; Butrum, Clifford, & Lanza, 1988; Albanes, 1987a; Kalish, 1984). Some have associated height as well as weight with breast cancer risk and have proposed that large body mass is implicated. The association with height suggests a role of nutrition effects mediated through childhood diet. It has been suggested that nutrition factors influencing height and weight may, in turn, affect age at menarche. Early menarche is strongly associated with an increased risk of developing breast cancer (Wynder & Rose, 1984).

Although the evidence is less strong for height as a risk factor, the bulk of evidence supports the importance of obesity and increased body mass as risk factors. This correlation of body weight to breast cancer incidence is mainly confined to postmenopausal women and is believed to be due to estrogen production in adipose tissue.

There is considerable evidence incriminating estrogens as potential tumor promotors (Wynder & Rose, 1984; James, Folkerd, Bonney, Beraneck, & Reed, 1982). Several animal studies, particularly in mice and rats, have also demonstrated that overnutrition significantly increases the frequency of spontaneous and chemically induced mammary tumors (Wynder & Rose, 1984; Albanes, 1987b).

In addition to its role in the development of breast cancer, obesity at diagnosis has been noted to be a risk factor for relapse of breast cancer (Donegan, Hartz, & Rimm, 1978; Boyd et al., 1981; Eberlein, Simon, Fisher, & Lippman, 1985; Zumoff et al., 1982), an effect that is also most marked in postmenopausal women. It is not known whether weight gained after diagnosis has a similar effect on early disease recurrence. Excessive weight gain has been identified as a possible prognostic factor, but reports are conflicting (Heasman, Sutherland, Campbell, Elkahim, & Boyd, 1985; Goodwin, Panzarella, & Boyd, 1988; Camoriano et al., in preparation). Likewise, it is not clear whether a patient who was obese at the time of diagnosis would have an improved prognosis if she lost weight after her diagnosis. There is some evidence that obese patients are more likely to have a greater incidence of positive axillary node involvement at diagnosis than those of normal weight, suggesting that subsequent weight loss may have no effect on survival (Donegan et al., 1978; Boyd et al., 1981; Eberlein et al., 1985; Zumoff et al., 1982).

### Dietary Fat

Some reviewers have attributed the association of obesity and breast cancer to a high-fat diet, which in itself is thought to be a risk factor for breast cancer. A number of sources show strong positive correlations between a high-fat diet and breast cancer risk. The evidence comes mainly from epidemiologic data and animal experimental studies (Hirayama, 1978; Committee on Diet, 1982; Butrum et al., 1988; Wynder & Rose, 1984; Albanes, 1987b; Miller et al., 1978; Lubin et al., 1981). As with obesity, animal studies support the hypothesis that dietary fat may be relevant to the development of breast cancer. Thus the incidence of mammary cancer in rats that are on a high-fat diet is greater than in rats fed a low-fat diet (Committee on Diet, 1982; Wynder & Rose, 1984; Albanes, 1987b; Miller et al., 1978).

Cancer incidence and mortality data from geographic correlation studies demonstrate a strong relationship between breast cancer incidence and per capita fat consumption. In general, these studies indicate that total fat intake, not the specific type of fat, is responsible for the observed effects. Studies of immigrants suggest that differences in cancer rates are due largely to environmental factors, including diet. The effects of acculturation, including dietary change, are observed in populations that migrate from a country with a low incidence to a country with a high incidence of breast cancer as they acquire the cancer rates of their host country (Wynder & Rose, 1984; Miller et al., 1978).

A definite positive relationship of fat intake to breast cancer remains to be demonstrated. Nevertheless, the evidence regarding the etiologic role of a high-fat intake is strong enough that the National Academy of Sciences has recommended interim dietary guidelines to reduce dietary fat intake from its present level of 40% of the calories in the typical American diet to 30% (Plamer & Bakshi, 1983; Executive summary, 1983). This reduction can be achieved without a major disturbance of dietary habits.

### PRIMARY BREAST CANCER: EFFECTS OF SYSTEMIC ADJUVANT CHEMOTHERAPY

Systemic adjuvant therapy involving the use of chemotherapy or hormonal therapy or both is now generally recommended for many women with primary breast cancer (Adjuvant chemotherapy, 1985; Kinne, Harris, Hellman, & Henderson, 1987). The acute toxicities from adjuvant chemotherapy include varying degrees of nausea and vomiting, fatigue, diarrhea, mucositis, alopecia, and myelosuppression. The side effects may be moderate to severe. Patients are often relatively asymptomatic compared to patients with advanced breast cancer or with many other cancers, however. Thus the side effects are usually well tolerated by most women and can be effectively managed without hospitalization.

Weight gain is another troublesome effect of chemotherapy reported by many women. Several studies have indicated that weight gain occurs in most women receiving such chemotherapy (Heasman et al., 1985; Goodwin et al., 1988; Camoriano et al., in preparation; Dixon, Moritz, & Baker, 1978; DeConti, 1982; Knobf, Mullen, Xistris, & Moritz, 1983; Bonadonna et al., 1985; Foltz, 1985; Huntington, 1985; Knobf, 1986). Indeed, weight loss among this patient population is rare. The median reported weight gain during adjuvant chemotherapy is $\pm 4$ kg, but several studies have reported a weight gain of more than 10 kg in approximately 25% of subjects during 1 year of adjuvant chemotherapy (Camoriano et al., in preparation; DeConti et al., 1982; Knobf et al., 1983).

The weight gain seems to occur regardless of the specific type of chemotherapy drugs used. Prednisone is notoriously associated with weight gain and has been blamed for the weight gain seen in some breast cancer patients. Various regimens both with and without steroids, however, have been associated with weight gain (Heasman et al., 1985; Goodwin et al., 1988; Camoriano et al., in preparation; Dixon et al., 1978; DeConti, 1982; Knobf et al., 1983; Bonadonna et al., 1985; Foltz, 1985; Huntington, 1985; Knobf, 1986). Age and pretreatment weight seem to have little influence on this weight gain. Many studies demonstrate a greater weight gain in premenopausal than in postmenopausal women, however (Heasman et al., 1985; Camoriano et al., in preparation; Bonadonna et al., 1985; Huntington, 1985). Bonadonna et al. (1985) observed an average weight gain of 4 kg in 706 women treated with CMF (cyclophosphamide, methotrexate, and 5-fluorouracil). A weight gain of 3 kg was noted in patients receiving CMF for 6 months, and a gain of 5 kg and 3 kg, respectively, was seen in menopausal and postmenopausal women on CMF for 12 months. Subjects on CMFP (CMF

plus prednisone) for 6 months gained an average of 4 kg.

DeConti (1982) reported a weight gain in excess of 10% of pretreatment weight in 45% of 53 patients treated with CMF (cytoxan, methotrexate, and 5-fluorouracil) with or without PT (prednisone plus tamoxifen). Weight gain exceeded 10 kg in 25% of the patients. The median weight gain was 4 kg with CMF compared to a median gain of 8.8 kg with CMFPT regimens. No correlation was found between weight gain and menopausal status.

Data from an unpublished North Central Cancer Treatment Group–Mayo Clinic study are consonant with other findings (Camoriano et al., in preparation). In 662 patients treated with CFP (cyclophosphamide, 5-fluorouracil, and prednisone) or CFPT, median weight gains of 5.5 kg in premenopausal and 3.2 kg in postmenopausal women occurred. Twenty percent of premenopausal and 6% of postmenopausal women gained more than 10 kg during 1 year of adjuvant chemotherapy.

Weight changes in patients with primary breast cancer who are not receiving adjuvant chemotherapy have not been well documented. Nevertheless, the limited reports available indicate an average weight gain of 1.5 to 2.0 kg in untreated patients after 1 year (Goodwin et al., 1988; Camoriano et al., in preparation). These data suggest that factors other than the influence of chemotherapy may play a role in the weight gain observed in primary breast cancer patients.

Weight gain may also be one of the most distressing side effects of chemotherapy. For many women, unwanted weight gain can significantly affect their self-esteem when it is superimposed on a change in body image due to the loss of a breast and the other toxicities associated with breast cancer therapy. Furthermore, the weight gained is not easily lost after completion of chemotherapy.

The underlying pathophysiologic basis for this weight gain is unclear. It is probably multifactoral. Proposed mechanisms include increased food intake, decreased energy expenditure, and hormonal changes. Psychologic factors such as anxiety and depression may be associated with changes in food intake and have been cited as being responsible for the observed weight gain (Foltz, 1985; Knobf, 1986). Eating in response to emotional distress has long been noted as an etiologic factor in weight gain, and emotional morbidity manifested by the presence of mild to moderate depression or anxiety is a common finding among breast cancer patients (Knobf, 1986; Meyerowitz, Sparks, & Spears, 1979; Sinsheimer & Holland, 1987). In a study by Knobf (1986), weight gain correlated with a less happy mood and a more worried outlook. These data suggest that emotional distress is common during adjuvant chemotherapy and may in some way contribute to weight gain.

Lifestyle changes due to illness and treatment may also affect food intake. A change in both social and employment activities because of fatigue or weakness may result in altered eating habits as well as a reduction in energy expenditure. With more unoccupied time available, a patient may find herself eating more frequently than she had when she was involved in activities outside the home. Smoking cessation after the diagnosis of breast cancer may also be a contributing factor because weight gain is a common sequela of smoking cessation (Stamford, Matter, Fell, & Papanek, 1986). Patients may also deliberately eat more. Patients and family members frequently associate chemotherapy or cancer with weight loss and weight loss with a poor outcome. Thus patients may eat more in an effort to improve their prognosis, often at the advice of well-meaning family members and health care professionals. Finally, nausea or alterations in taste induced by chemotherapy may be associated with an increased food intake. Eating frequently often helps alleviate a feeling of nausea or remove a bad taste in the mouth.

Increased intake is only one of the mechanisms that facilitate weight gain. As mentioned above, decreased energy expenditure in the form of a lowered basal energy expenditure or a decrease in physical activity may be a contributing factor. Alterations in metabolic rate in breast cancer patients have not been well substantiated in the literature. Decreased activity, however, is well documented (Foltz, 1985; Huntington, 1985; Meyerowitz et al., 1979) and may be the result of both psychologic and physiologic factors. Indeed, depression may not only be associated with an increased food intake but may well be accompanied by a decrease in activity, as noted earlier.

Fatigue is a common physical symptom and may contribute to weight gain because of its effects on activity and decreased mobility. Failure to return to preillness work-related or athletic activities as a result of an inability to perform these activities raises the possibility that weight gain is a function of a decrease in physical activity due to fatigue or weakness. Additionally some patients may have a tendency to eat more, thinking that it will give them a lift of energy.

Hormonal influences as etiologic factors in weight gain have been postulated, but data are not conclusive (Foltz, 1985). Adjuvant chemotherapy is known to decrease ovarian function (Rose & Davis, 1977). It has been speculated that the reduction in estradiol levels resulting from suppression of ovarian function accounts for the weight gain, but this relationship is not clear. Changes in estradiol levels may also explain the difference in weight gain in premenopausal compared to postmenopausal patients. Further research is needed to investigate this potential mechanism for weight gain during adjuvant chemotherapy.

## MANAGEMENT OF WEIGHT GAIN

Because of the high frequency of weight gain, its psychologic impact, and its associated health risks, efforts to control obesity and weight gain are beneficial to breast cancer patients. Weight control interventions should be directed at overweight patients and those who are gaining weight.

Exhibit 15-1 summarizes the management of weight problems in the breast cancer patient.

### Nutrition Assessment

A thorough nutrition assessment consisting of a weight history, diet history, and lifestyle and activity history should be included in the initial evaluation (Exhibit 15-1). The information obtained in the nutrition assessment can then be

**Exhibit 15-1** Weight Management Guidelines for the Patient with Breast Cancer

Nutrition assessment

- Weight history
  Date of onset of obesity
  History of dieting
- Diet history
  Eating patterns
  Nutrition composition of diet
  Attitudes, beliefs, meaning of food
  24-hour recall
- Lifestyle and activity history
  Changes in physical and social activities
  Smoking cessation

Nutrition counseling

- Diet
  Calories: to maintain or achieve desirable weight
  Fat: <30% of calories
  Carbohydrates: >50% of calories
  Protein: 15% to 20% of calories
  Discuss rationale for low-fat, high-carbohydrate diet
  Discuss food selection and preparation to reduce fat, increase carbohydrate intake
  Discourage quick–weight loss diets
  Discuss relationship of diet and weight to other health risks
  Modify diet as needed for diabetes, hypertension, hyperlipidemia, other health problems
  Use exchange diet, if appropriate
- Exercise and activity
  Discuss benefits
  Identify appropriate amounts and types of aerobic exercise
  Encourage previous social and physical activities or suitable alternatives
- Behavior modification
  Identify eating patterns and behaviors
  Explore emotional and environmental reasons for overeating or snacking
  Plan interventions to break or weaken undesirable eating patterns

Managing acute side effects

- Give suggestions for low-calorie foods to help counteract nausea and reduce a bad taste in the mouth

Follow-up

- Every 4 to 6 weeks

used to identify factors such as inactivity, improper eating habits, and inappropriate attitudes or beliefs that may be contributing to the weight problem. The weight history should include the date of obesity onset and a history of previous efforts at weight control. The patient with a history of weight problems may be at a greater risk of weight gain, especially during times of stress, than the patient who has not experienced these problems.

The diet history should include a review of the patient's eating habits, frequency of eating, and the meaning of food to the individual (e.g., use of food as reward, comfort, anxiety, defense against cancer, and so forth). A 24-hour recall can be used to identify usual food intake. Changes in the patient's activity, including housework, employment, and involvement in social, community, and sports activities, should also be noted.

After the initial assessment, the dietitian can provide the necessary interventions to help the patient with weight control. Often, simply increasing the patient's awareness of factors that may contribute to weight gain may have a prophylactic effect. The role of obesity and weight gain in disease recurrence is not yet known. Therefore, caution must be used to avoid provoking feelings of guilt or anxiety when counseling patients. As for any patient attempting weight loss or control, it is important to plan a program that will result in a permanent change in eating and exercise habits and long-term weight control.

## Eating Habits

A healthy diet de-emphasizing fat should be encouraged (Exhibit 15-1). Although there is no evidence that dietary fat intake has an influence on prognosis of established breast cancer, it has been associated with the development of breast cancer. Thus reducing fat to approximately 30% of the total calories as recommended by the National Academy of Sciences seems to be appropriate (Plamer & Bakshi, 1983; Executive summary, 1983). A reduction of fat intake can be accomplished by encouraging intake of more complex carbohydrates (bread, pasta, rice, potatoes, cereals, and other grain products), vegetables, and fruits. This type of diet is also less calorically dense and thus promotes weight control. The rationale for replacing high-fat foods with those high in starch and fiber for its effects on weight control, breast cancer risk, and general good health should be explained to the patient. The dietitian should also discuss food selection, food preparation, and meal planning to achieve these goals if improvements in these areas are needed. Most patients appreciate helpful suggestions about shopping for low-fat foods, modifying cooking techniques, and planning meals. They may also need to learn how to identify hidden sources of fat such as bakery goods, snack foods, nuts, and the like.

The use of low-calorie, low-carbohydrate diets and other quick–weight loss diets should be discouraged. The negative consequences of such dieting in terms of reduced rate of energy metabolism, increased likelihood of binge eating, and increased rate of recidivism as well as the nutrition deficits associated with these diets should be explained to the patient. Patients with breast cancer should be assured that they are not likely to become malnourished, as do some cancer patients, and that there is no need to eat more protein, calories, or other nutrients because of the presence of cancer or its treatment. Some patients need to learn how to cope with ''sabotage.'' Well-meaning family members and friends may use food as a sign of affection or reward or encourage patients to eat for stamina to overcome disease or treatment effects.

If the patient is motivated to lose weight, a modest calorie reduction resulting in a weight loss of approximately 0.5 to 0.75 lb/week can be prescribed. If the patient is hesitant about attempting weight loss at the time or is depressed, however, weight loss efforts should be deferred until after the completion of treatment, when the chances for successful weight loss may be much greater. If the patient has complications from obesity or weight gain such as diabetes, hypertension, hyperlipidemia, or degenerative joint disease, the relationship of excessive weight to these other health problems should be discussed and the weight control diet planned with modifications to meet these special needs.

If the patient is eating more because of a complaint of increase in appetite, suggestions for behavior modification techniques such as eating more slowly, filling dinner plates in the kitchen instead of serving family style, and the like may help with appetite and portion control. Again, high-fiber, high–complex carbohydrate foods should be encouraged because they tend to be more filling and less calorically dense. Food cravings may occur as a side effect of treatment or may stem from an emotional need. The dietitian can help the patient by defining limitations on these foods or by identifying low-calorie alternatives, such as frozen low-fat yogurt or fruit instead of ice cream and sugar-free hot cocoa instead of chocolate desserts or candies. If the patient is snacking more because of having more time (i.e., out of boredom), activities such as crafts, hobbies, or physical exercise should be suggested and involvement in preillness social activities and other activities outside the home encouraged. Having the patient keep records or food diaries to become aware of her eating patterns and to identify times associated with eating may help her learn to differentiate between appetite and hunger. The patient may need to be told when and how much snacking is appropriate and given suggestions for healthy snacks (e.g., raw vegetables, fresh fruit, and air-popped popcorn). A program of behavior modification (Brownell, 1988) can be a valuable guide for nutritionists in helping patients identify and change eating behaviors.

If the patient has recently stopped smoking, she may need counseling about how to prevent excessive weight gain as a result of this. Measures to minimize snacking and oral cravings that often replace the urge to smoke are helpful and may include the behavior modification techniques for appetite and portion control mentioned above, planning alternate activities when one has a tendency to snack or smoke, and use of low-calorie snacks. An increase in exercise, as tolerated, can also help by counteracting the decrease in metabolism that may occur as a result of smoking cessation (Stamford et al., 1986).

People often misinterpret an emotion or some other sensation as hunger and may eat for comfort or as a reaction to anxiety over upcoming cancer treatment. If the patient is eating for comfort, solace, or reward, the dietitian should try to increase her awareness of the problem by exploring emotional reasons for overeating or snacking. Sometimes simply making the patient aware of the problem can help her control or manage it. It may be helpful to discuss the ill consequences and futility of eating to counteract emotional distress. Again, having the patient keep records or food diaries may help her increase her awareness of emotions and situations associated with eating. The dietitian should discuss other practices or material objects that may be gratifying, such as buying new clothes or jewelry or taking a vacation. If the patient is eating more because of anxiety or depression, other methods of coping such as relaxation techniques, hobbies, or physical exercise should be explored. Her physician may refer her for psychologic counseling if the anxiety or depression is persistent or severe.

## Activity and Exercise

Barring severe fatigue or physical immobility, previous social and physical activities or suitable alternatives should be encouraged (Exhibit 15-1). Not only will this help control weight gain by increasing the patient's calorie expenditure, it may also keep her occupied and help reduce anxiety and depression. The benefits of aerobic exercise should be discussed, and the most appropriate type of exercise for the individual should be recommended. The patient's physician should be consulted regarding any exercise limitations or restrictions. For example, some forms of exercise such as tennis, swimming, or other activities that make vigorous use of the arm muscles may not be suitable for a patient with lymphedema. These patients may benefit from counseling from a physical therapist. Care should be taken not to provoke guilt or anxiety in patients if they are not able to exercise because of fatigue. Walking and biking are practical forms of exercise for most patients, however, and should be encouraged for a minimum of 15 to 20 minutes three or four times a week.

## Managing Acute Side Effects

Patients may need advice about how to prevent excessive calorie intake while trying to control side effects such as nausea or a bad taste in the mouth (Exhibit 15-1). High-carbohydrate, low-fat foods such as plain pasta, rice, potatoes, bread, and cereals tend to be tolerated better than rich, high-fat foods. Patients who are eating more frequently to counteract nausea also appreciate suggestions for low-calorie snacks. A few soda crackers, some sugar-free gelatin dessert, sugar-free carbonated beverages, sugar-free hard candies, dry popcorn, a piece of dry toast, or a handful of dry cereal are often just as effective in controlling nausea as their high-calorie counterparts. Sugar-free gum or candies or frequent sips of sugar-free lemonade or other soft drinks are helpful in reducing a bad taste in the mouth.

## Follow-Up

Because many of these patients are likely to have a long history of obesity, frequent follow-up visits are encouraged to monitor their progress in weight control and to provide reinforcement. Most patients are on a 4- to 6-week treatment cycle, which provides a good time frame for dietary counseling as well (Exhibit 15-1).

## The Underweight Patient

The dietitian may occasionally encounter an underweight patient on adjuvant chemotherapy. Weight gain for these individuals is appropriate. They may also need counseling about how to maintain an adequate intake in spite of nausea, mucositis, and other side effects of chemotherapy.

## Radiation Therapy

Radiation therapy for breast cancer is usually well tolerated from a nutrition standpoint.

Weight gain is normally not seen in patients undergoing radiation for breast cancer, as it is in patients on adjuvant chemotherapy. Patients undergoing radiation treatments should receive adequate protein, calories, and other nutrients to promote maintenance and repair of body tissue. For obese patients, weight loss should be discouraged until after the completion of treatment. Again, underweight individuals or those with weight loss need to be counseled about measures to ensure nutrition adequacy.

### After Treatment

The guidelines for assessment and counseling given in Exhibit 15-1 for patients undergoing adjuvant chemotherapy can be used for weight loss and control after treatment as well. For patients who have successfully completed treatment and who are disease free, weight reduction to achieve ideal body weight is recommended to reduce the risk of developing other health problems related to obesity and, possibly, to improve prognosis.

## PATIENTS WITH ADVANCED CANCER

Breast cancer can recur both locally and at distant metastatic sites. The most common sites of distant metastatic relapse are bone, lung, and liver. Although metastatic breast cancer is not considered a curable disease, systemic therapy can result in significant palliation (Smith, 1987). Patients with advanced breast cancer experience toxicities from treatment similar to those seen in treatment for primary breast cancer, but the toxicities may be less well tolerated because the patients are often symptomatic. Pain occurs in approximately 65% of patients with bone metastasis and may contribute to weight loss through its effect on appetite (Smith, 1987).

Because hormonal therapy is less toxic than chemotherapy, it is often favored as the first treatment modality in patients with metastatic disease (Canellos, Petrek, McCormick, & Henderson, 1987; Ingle, 1987; Carter, 1987). Tam-

oxifen, with its minimal toxicity, is probably the most widely used hormonal agent. Megestrol acetate is another frequently used and well-tolerated hormonal agent whose only notable side effect is weight gain. Although the degree of weight gain may be comparable to that seen in patients on adjuvant chemotherapy, it may be less of a potential clinical problem because of the stage of the disease. Other common second-line hormonal agents are also reasonably well tolerated.

Chemotherapy is utilized in patients in whom hormonal therapy has failed or in patients who are not candidates for hormonal therapy because of the site, extent, or growth of disease (e.g., with rapid progression of metastatic tumor in the liver or lung) (Canellos et al., 1987). As in early breast cancer, combinations of drugs are often used because they produce better response rates than single-agent therapy (Canellos et al., 1987; Carter, 1987). Thus side effects can be quite severe. After acute treatment-related toxicities resolve, however, an increase in appetite may accompany an improvement in quality of life as a result of symptom relief.

Radiation therapy is often used for palliation in patients with advanced disease, especially those with osseous metastasis. Thus, if the patient is anorectic because of severe pain, radiation therapy may enhance the patient's appetite and ability to eat by helping alleviate this pain. Depending on the site of administration, however, radiation may produce anorexia while it is being given.

Bone is the most common site of metastasis in patients with breast cancer (Ingle, Sim, Schray, Wold, & Beaubout, 1988). The spread of breast cancer to bone can result in considerable morbidity in terms of pain and decreased mobility. Patients with breast cancer whose disease is limited to the bone, however, generally have a favorable response to treatment and may live for a considerable period of time. In metastatic disease of the breast, pathologic fractures of the femur and hips as well as spinal compression fractures can occur. Prevention of weight gain in this subset of patients may help reduce the risk of further fractures. It may also help the patients maintain mobility with minimal functional disability during their remaining time of survival.

## REFERENCES

Adjuvant chemotherapy for breast cancer. (1985). *National Institutes of Health consensus development conference statement*. Bethesda, MD: National Cancer Institute.

Albanes, D. (1987a). Caloric intake, body weight, and cancer: A review. *Nutrition and Cancer, 9*, 199–217.

Albanes, D. (1987b). Total calories, body weight, and tumor incidence in mice. *Cancer Research, 47*, 1987–1992.

Bonadonna, G., Valagussa, P., Rossi, A., Tancini, G., Brambilla, C., Zambetti, M., & Veronesi, U. (1985). Ten-year experience with CMF-based adjuvant chemotherapy in resectable breast cancer. *Breast Cancer Research and Treatment, 5*, 95–115.

Boyd, N.F., Campbell, J.E., Germanson, T., Thomson, D.B., Sutherland, D.J., & Malkin, J.W. (1981). Weight and prognosis in breast cancer. *Journal of the National Cancer Institute, 67*, 785–789.

Brownell, K. (1988). *The LEARN program for weight control*. Philadelphia: University of Pennsylvania School of Medicine.

Butrum, R.P., Clifford, C.K., & Lanza, E. (1988). NCI dietary guidelines: Rationale. *American Journal of Clinical Nutrition, 48*, 888–895.

Camoriano, J.K., Loprinzi, C.L., Ingle, J.N., Therneau, T.M., Everson, L.K., & Krook, J.E. (In preparation). Weight change in women treated with adjuvant therapy or observed following mastectomy for node-positive breast cancer.

Canellos, G.P., Petrek, J.A., McCormick, B., and Henderson, I.C. (1987). Treatment of metastases. In J.R. Harris, S. Hellman, I.C. Henderson, & D.W. Kinne (Eds.), *Breast Diseases* (pp. 385–479). Philadelphia: Lippincott.

Carter, S.K. (1987). Hormone and chemotherapy: Fundamental clinical concepts. In I.M. Ariel & J.B. Cleary (Eds.), *Breast cancer: Diagnosis and treatment* (pp. 358–378). New York: McGraw-Hill.

Committee on Diet, Nutrition, and Cancer, Assembly of Life Sciences, National Research Council. (1982). *Diet, nutrition, and cancer*. Washington, DC: National Academy Press.

DeConti, R.D. (1982). Weight gain in the adjuvant chemotherapy of breast cancer. *Proceedings of the American Society of Clinical Oncology, 1*, 73.

Dixon, J., Moritz, D.A., & Baker, F.L. (1978). Breast cancer and weight gain: An unexpected finding. *Oncology Nursing Forum, 5*, 5–7.

Donegan, W.L., Hartz, A.J., & Rimm, A.J. (1978). The association of body weight and recurrent cancer of the breast. *Cancer, 41*, 1590–1594.

Eberlein, T., Simon, R., Fisher, S., & Lippman, M.E. (1985). Height, weight and risk of breast cancer relapse. *Breast Cancer Research and Treatment, 5*, 81–86.

Executive summary of the Committee on Diet, Nutrition, and Cancer: Diet, nutrition and cancer. (1983). *Cancer Research, 43*, 3018–3023.

Foltz, A.T. (1985). Weight gain among stage II breast cancer patients: A study of five factors. *Oncology Nursing Forum, 12*, 21–26.

Goodwin, P.J., Panzarella, T., & Boyd, N.F. (1988). Weight gain in women with localized breast cancer—A descriptive study. *Breast Cancer Research and Treatment, 11*, 59–66.

Heasman, K.Z., Sutherland, H.J., Campbell, J.A., Elkahim, T., & Boyd, N.F. (1985). Weight gain during adjuvant chemotherapy for breast cancer. *Breast Cancer Research and Treatment, 5*, 195–200.

Hirayama, T. (1978). Epidemiology of breast cancer with special reference to role of diet. *Preventive Medicine, 7*, 173–195.

Huntington, M.O. (1985). Weight gain in patients receiving adjuvant chemotherapy for carcinoma of the breast. *Cancer, 56*, 472–474.

Ingle, J.N. (1987). Hormone and chemotherapy selection of specific options. In I.M. Ariel & J.B. Cleary (Eds.), *Breast cancer: Diagnosis and treatment* (pp. 379–392). New York: McGraw-Hill.

Ingle, J.N., Sim, F.H., Schray, M.F., Wold, L.E., & Beaubout, J.W. (1988). Breast cancer. In F.H. Sim (Ed.), *Diagnosis and management of metastatic bone disease—A multidisciplinary approach* (pp. 251–263). New York: Raven.

James, V.H.T., Folkerd, E.J., Bonney, R.D., Beranek, P.A., & Reed, M.J. (1982). Factors influencing estrogen production and metabolism in postmenopausal women with endocrine cancer. *Journal of Endocrinological Investigation, 5*, 335–345.

Kalish, L.A. (1984). Relationships of body size with breast cancer. *Journal of Clinical Oncology, 2*, 287–293.

Kinne, D.W., Harris, J.R., Hellman, S., & Henderson, I.C. (1987). Primary treatment of breast cancer. In J.R. Harris, S. Hellman, I.C. Henderson, & D.W. Kinne (Eds.), *Breast diseases* (pp. 259–358). Philadelphia: Lippincott.

Knobf, M.K. (1986). Physical and psychological distress associated with adjuvant chemotherapy in women with breast cancer. *Journal of Clinical Oncology, 4*, 678–684.

Knobf, M.K., Mullen, J.C., Xistris, D., & Moritz, D.A. (1983). Weight gain in women with breast cancer receiving adjuvant chemotherapy. *Oncology Nursing Forum, 10*, 28–33.

Lubin, J.H., Burns, P.E., Blot, W.J., Ziegler, R.G., Lees, A.W., & Fraumeni, J.F. (1981). Dietary factors and breast cancer risk. *International Journal of Cancer, 28*, 685–689.

Meyerowitz, B.E., Sparks, F.C., & Spears, I.K. (1979). Adjuvant chemotherapy for breast carcinoma, psychosocial implications. *Cancer, 43*, 1613–1618.

Miller, A.B., Kelly, A., Choi, N.W., Matthews, V., Morgan, R.W., Munan, L., Burch, J.D., Feather, J., Howe, G.R., & Jain, M. (1978). A study of diet and breast cancer. *American Journal of Epidemiology, 107*, 499–509.

Plamer, S., & Bakshi, K. (1983). Diet, nutrition, and cancer: Interim dietary guidelines. *Journal of the National Cancer Institute, 70*, 1151–1170.

Rose, D.P., & Davis, T.E. (1977). Ovarian function in patients receiving adjuvant chemotherapy for breast cancer. *Lancet, 1*, 1174–1176.

Sinsheimer, L.M., & Holland, J.C. (1987). Psychological issues in breast cancer. *Seminars in Oncology, 14*, 75–82.

Smith, I.E. (1987). Recurrent disease. In J.R. Harris, S. Hellman, I.C. Henderson, & D.W. Kinne (Eds.), *Breast diseases* (pp. 369–384). Philadelphia: Lippincott.

Stamford, B.A., Matter, S., Fell, R.D., & Papanek, P. (1986). Effects of smoking cessation on weight gain, metabolic rate, caloric consumption, and blood lipids. *American Journal of Clinical Nutrition, 43*, 486–494.

Wynder, E.L., & Rose, D.P. (1984). Diet and breast cancer. *Hospital Practice, 14*, 73–88.

Zumoff, B., Gorzynski, G., Katz, J.L., Weiner, H., Levin, J., Holland, J., & Fukushima, D.K. (1982). Nonobesity at the time of mastectomy is highly predictive of 10-year disease-free survival in women with breast cancer. *Anticancer Research, 2*, 59–62.

# Part III

# Treatment Modalities

# Chapter 16

# Impact of Chemotherapy on the Nutrition Status of the Cancer Patient

*Jeanne A. Darbinian and*
*Ann M. Coulston*

Chemotherapeutic drugs constitute one of three major oncologic treatment modalities. These agents exert their antineoplastic effects by inhibiting or disrupting cellular DNA, RNA, or protein synthesis. Although certain drugs act at a specific phase in the cell cycle, others may be cytotoxic at different stages of cellular synthesis or replication (Carter, 1987). Treatment regimens frequently employ multiple agents or combination chemotherapy to increase tumoricidal efficacy.

Antineoplastic agents have a narrow therapeutic index, meaning that they act against and are thus toxic to both malignant tissues and normal host cells that have a high replication rate. These include cells in the bone marrow; hair follicles; oral, esophageal, and gastrointestinal mucosa; and reproductive system (specifically, ovaries and testes) (Mitchell & Schein, 1982). Damage to the epithelial cells lining the alimentary tract may have significant nutrition consequences if mucosal insult precludes adequate intake or absorption of energy and nutrients (Mitchell & Schein, 1982; Laszlo, Stevenson, & Lucas, 1986).

In addition to this direct effect on host nutrition status, chemotherapeutic drugs may indirectly alter food intake or utilization by inducing nausea, vomiting, anorexia, and learned food aversions (Laszlo et al., 1986; Stoudemire, Cotanch, & Laszlo, 1984; Bernstein, 1978; Bernstein & Bernstein, 1981; Bernstein, Webster, & Bernstein, 1982). Finally, the effects that these agents may have on host cellular protein turnover, energy metabolism, and, ultimately, lean body mass remain to be elucidated (Herrmann, Garnick, Moore, & Wilmore, 1981; Drott, Unsgaard, Schersten, & Lundholm, 1988; Lerebours et al., 1988). This chapter identifies the nutrition sequelae associated with chemotherapy-induced toxicities and discusses practical approaches to the nutrition management of patients who incur these complications.

## NAUSEA AND VOMITING

The two most common acute effects associated with antineoplastic therapy are nausea and vomiting. As is well recognized, untoward gastrointestinal symptoms resulting from chemotherapy are dependent on drug dosage, duration of treatment, and individual response. Nevertheless, there are specific agents that are highly emetogenic and (can potentially) induce vomiting in virtually all patients (Laszlo et al., 1986). These are classified in Table 16-1 as severe and include dactinomycin, daunorubicin, cisplatin, mechlorethamine (nitrogen mustard), nitrosoureas (lomustine, carmustine, and streptozocin), and dacarbazine. Onset of symptoms can be immediate or delayed; duration can range from several hours to days.

**Table 16-1** Nutrition-Related Toxicities of Antineoplastic Drugs

| Drug | Nausea and Vomiting | Mucositis or Stomatitis | Altered Taste or Smell | Diarrhea (D) or Constipation (C) | Other |
|---|---|---|---|---|---|
| Alkylating agents | | | | | |
|   Alkyl sulfonates | Mild | | | | |
|   Cisplatin | Severe | | | | |
| Nitrogen mustards | | | | | |
|   Chlorambucil | Mild | Mild | | | |
|   Cyclophosphamide | Moderate* | Mild to moderate* | † | Mild (D)* | |
|   Mechlorethamine | Severe | | | Mild (D) | |
|   Phenylalanine mustard | Mild | | | Mild (D) | |
| Nitrosoureas | | | | | |
|   Lomustine | Moderate to severe | | | | |
|   Carmustine | Moderate to severe | | | | |
|   Streptozocin | Severe | | | Mild (D) | Hepatitis |
| Antibiotics | | | | | |
|   Bleomycin | Mild | Mild | † | | |
|   Dactinomycin | Moderate to severe | Moderate to severe | | Moderate (D) | |
|   Daunorubicin | Severe | Severe | | Moderate (D) | |
|   Doxorubicin | Moderate | Severe | | Moderate (D) | |
|   Mitomycin | Moderate | Mild | | Mild (D) | |
|   Plicamycin | Severe | Moderate | | Mild (D) | Hepatitis |
| Antimetabolites | | | | | |
|   Cytosine arabinoside | Moderate* | Moderate* | | Severe (D)* | |
|   5-Fluorouracil | Mild to moderate* | Moderate to severe* | † | Severe (D) | |
|   Hydroxyurea | Mild* | Mild* | | Mild (D and C)* | |
|   6-Mercaptopurine | Mild* | Moderate* | † | Moderate (D) | Cholestasis |
|   Methotrexate | Mild to severe* | Mild to severe* | † | Moderate (D)* | Hepatitis* |
|   6-Thioguanine | Mild* | Moderate* | | Moderate (D)* | |
| Plant products | | | | | |
|   Vinblastine | Mild | Moderate to severe | † | Severe (C) | |
|   Vincristine | Mild | Moderate | | Severe (C) | Neuropathy |
|   Etoposide | Mild to moderate | | | | |
| Hormones | | | | | |
|   Tamoxifen | Mild | | | | |
| Miscellaneous | | | | | |
|   Asparaginase | Moderate | | † | | Pancreatitis |
|   Procarbazine | Moderate | Moderate | † | Mild (D) | |
|   Dacarbazine | Moderate to severe* | | | | |

*Dose dependent.
† Drug with associated side effect but extent unknown.

*Source:* Adapted from "Nutrition Management of Patients with Cancer" by A.M. Coulston and J.D. Darbinian, 1986, *Topics in Clinical Nutrition, 1*(2), p. 31. Copyright 1986 by Aspen Publishers, Inc.

Chemotherapy-induced vomiting is ultimately mediated by the emetic center, which is located in the lateral reticular formation in the medulla oblongata (Seigel & Longo, 1981; Penta, Poster, & Bruno, 1983; Borison & McCarthy, 1983). Situated nearby, in the floor of the fourth ventricle of the brain, is the chemoreceptor trigger zone (CTZ), which is believed to be the major source of afferent fibers to the emetic center. The exact mechanism whereby the emetic effect of blood-borne drugs and toxins is mediated through the CTZ remains unknown.

In addition to the CTZ two other sites with input to the emetic center are the periphery (principally the pharynx and gastrointestinal tract), with afferent impulses transmitted primarily by the vagus nerve, and the cortex. The latter may play a role in such phenomena as anticipatory vomiting, which appears to involve higher brain loci. Although the CTZ is believed to be a primary mediator, trigger sites of most antineoplastic agents are unknown. Elucidation of how specific chemotherapeutic drugs cause vomiting would serve to optimize antiemetic therapy by permitting effective combinations of agents that act at different but relevant loci in the emetic pathway (Penta et al., 1983).

Nausea and vomiting, if not controlled, can result in electrolyte imbalance, dehydration, weight loss, and weakness (Laszlo et al., 1986; Stoudemire et al., 1984; Dennis, 1983). Combination antiemetic therapy, which is often employed prophylactically, can be effective in minimizing these toxic side effects (Laszlo et al., 1986; Stoudemire et al., 1984; Penta et al., 1983). Nevertheless, some patients experience severe symptoms that may be temporarily refractory to pharmacologic intervention. When this occurs, the patient should not be given food or fluids enterally. Intravenous hydration should be instituted or increased to cover gastrointestinal losses. Serum electrolyte levels should be carefully monitored and deficits corrected by means of intravenous replacement (Dennis, 1983; Grant, 1986). If symptoms subside or resolve within 24 to 48 hours, parenteral nutritional intervention is probably unnecessary; if symptoms are protracted, however, this intervention is usually indicated. Patients who present for therapy in a severely malnourished or depleted state and children, whose growth and development are contingent on adequate nutrient intake, are of particular concern in this regard.

Tube feeding may be tolerated if a flexible feeding tube can be passed nasoenterically (i.e., distal to the Treitz ligament) and its tip location confirmed radiographically. The tube may move proximally into the stomach, however, thus placing the patient at risk for aspiration should a particularly severe and prolonged emesis bout occur after or during infusion of formula (Grant, 1986). Moreover, such patients are usually sedated to alleviate symptoms, which also potentiates the risk of aspiration. Peripheral or central venous parenteral nutrition may be the appropriate modality to employ initially. Tolerance to substrates and serum electrolytes should be carefully monitored as caloric and protein support is progressively increased. Even with eventual resolution of symptoms, appetite may be slow to return and oral intake inadequate to provide sufficient energy and nutrients to maintain or rehabilitate the malnourished patient. Thus supplemental parenteral nutrition or tube feedings may be warranted as an interim measure during this transitional period (Grant, 1986).

For the chemotherapy patient who experiences nausea and vomiting but not to the extreme that oral intake is precluded or severely compromised, there are still many obstacles to surmount. Learned food aversions may develop as a consequence of exposure to foods (novel or familiar) before receiving chemotherapeutic drugs that resulted in nausea and vomiting (Bernstein & Bernstein, 1981; Herrmann et al., 1981; Bernstein et al., 1982). This untoward effect may exacerbate preexisting therapy-associated anorexia because many patients abstain from or limit intake to avoid further gastrointestinal distress. Dysgeusia or hypogeusia may ensue from the effect of blood- or saliva-borne chemotherapeutic agents on taste buds (e.g., methotrexate and cyclophosphamide) (McAnena & Daly, 1986; Steele et al., 1979; Juma, Rogers, & Trounce, 1979). Moreover, some drugs (e.g., procarbazine) may adversely affect salivary flow with resultant xerostomia (McDonald & Tirumali, 1984). These unpleasant symptoms can aggravate the underlying nausea and propensity for emesis, thereby limiting oral intake to an even greater extent.

Nausea and vomiting can be alleviated, perhaps minimized, if a common-sense and gentle approach to eating is taken. In view of the impressive experimental and empiric evidence that learned food aversions are real, it is recommended that food be withheld, if feasible, during the period when acute toxicities typically manifest themselves (i.e., just before, during, and after chemotherapy administration). Similarly, introduction of new items that may subsequently be potential allies (e.g., palatable liquid nutrition supplements) should be deferred until after the nausea and vomiting have substantially subsided. A careful and accurate diet history of each patient should be obtained before institution of chemotherapy to avoid untimely exposure of the patient to his or her food preferences or aversions.

Effort should be made to identify and remove any offending odors that may precipitate nausea or vomiting. If possible, the patient should not be in the same room where food is prepared. Common examples of foods with odors that are particularly nauseating to patients include cooked cruciferous vegetables (e.g., broccoli, cauliflower, Brussels sprouts), fish, casserole dishes with strong cheeses, and fried foods. Another variable affecting the intensity of food odors is the length of time between preparation and serving. This is especially relevant in the hospital setting because institutional food services utilize dome-shaped plate covers in which odors may become trapped. The problem only worsens the longer the food is allowed to stand at room temperature. Thus it is important to deliver or serve food that is ready for consumption as soon as feasible.

Dysgeusia should also be ruled out as a contributory factor to nausea and vomiting. Not uncommonly, patients receiving chemotherapy complain of a lingering bitter or metallic aftertaste (Trant, Serin, & Douglass, 1982). Moreover, taste threshold abnormalities of the four taste qualities (sweet, sour, salty, and bitter) may develop (Trant, 1986). Foods identified as exacerbating these symptoms (e.g., meats and chocolate) should be excluded, appropriately modified, or substituted. It is best to offer patients small, frequent meals and alternate dry foods (e.g., crackers or toast) with liquid items. Cool, essentially nonodorous foods such as clear, nonacidic liquids (e.g., ginger ale), flavored ices, boiled or baked potatoes, plain rice, cool broth from which all visible fat has been removed, dry cereal, and crackers are often well tolerated.

Gastrointestinal motility may be transiently altered after periods of acute nausea and vomiting. For this reason, high-fat items, although of great caloric density, should be provisionally limited or excluded so as not to delay gastric emptying and thus contribute to a feeling of fullness or exacerbate underlying early satiety. Food should be consumed slowly, and meals should be served in a relaxed, nonthreatening atmosphere, which is often a difficult feat in the hospital milieu. Most important, portion sizes should be carefully controlled to avoid overwhelming the patient and provoking a sense of defeat.

It should again be emphasized that responses to chemotherapy-associated nausea and vomiting are highly individual. Many patients are quite resilient, demonstrating satisfactory tolerance to food shortly after the acutely toxic phase has passed. Others, however, experience considerable difficulty that is compounded by perhaps psychologic as well as physiologic determinants. It has been estimated that anticipatory nausea and vomiting occurs in approximately 25% of treated patients (Morrow, 1982; Morrow, Arseneau, Asbury, Bennett, & Boros, 1982). For these individuals, relaxation techniques or other behavor therapies may be useful and may even facilitate their nutrition management and care (Morrow & Morrell, 1982; Cotanch, 1983).

Exhibit 16-1 summarizes care of the cancer patient who is experiencing chemotherapy-related nausea and vomiting.

## ORAL AND ESOPHAGEAL MUCOSITIS

The rapidly proliferating cells lining the alimentary tract are prime targets of several antineoplastic agents (Table 16-1). Drug-induced mucosal sloughing can produce stomatitis, cheilosis, glossitis, pharyngitis, and esophagitis. The severity and extent of injury or ulceration are related to drug dosage and schedule and may be significantly augmented by prior or concurrent irradiation (Mitchell & Schein, 1982; McDonald & Tirumali, 1984). Radiation injury to the skin and squamous epithelia of the oral cavity, pharynx, and esophagus may be potentiated by dactinomycin and doxorubicin, whereas an additive toxic effect has been observed with vinblastine, hydroxyurea, procarbazine, methotrexate, 5-fluorouracil, bleomycin, and 6-mercaptopurine. The synergistic effect of dactinomycin and esophageal

**Exhibit 16-1** Nutrition Care Summary for Nausea and Vomiting

1. Do not offer foods when the patient is nauseated or vomiting. This practice may cause the patient to become discouraged or depressed, induce learned food aversions, and increase the risk of aspiration.
2. Obtain a thorough diet history that clearly identifies food preferences and aversions. Avoid items that exacerbate symptoms.
3. Encourage small, frequent meals when symptoms of nausea and vomiting subside sufficiently. Alternate dry with liquid items; avoid serving hot and cold foods simultaneously. Choose foods that are easily digested, cool or at room temperature, and have little or no odor. Examples include clear, nonacidic liquids (e.g., ginger ale); flavored ices; canned fruit; boiled or baked potatoes; rice; cold, skimmed broth; and dry bread products (e.g., crackers, cereal, and bread sticks).
4. Avoid highly fatty or fried foods, excessively sweet items, and rich desserts.
5. Identify offending odors or abnormal taste sensations, and remove or appropriately modify corresponding foods.
6. Avoid food preparation in the same room where the patient is present. Whenever possible, serve food soon after it is ready for consumption.
7. Keep portion sizes small, and present meals in a relaxed, nonthreatening, unhurried atmosphere.
8. Consider administrating intravenous fluids if vomiting persists beyond 36 hours and if losses cannot be replaced enterally. Parenteral nutrition may be indicated for patients who are malnourished and have prolonged and refractory emesis.
9. Do not permit the patient to lie down for at least 1 hour after eating.

irradiation can result in strictures, which may necessitate placement of a feeding gastrostomy tube to permit adequate fluid and nutrient intake.

The toxic effects of chemotherapeutic drugs on oral and esophageal epithelia are usually transient, with recovery taking place in 2 to 3 weeks (McDonald & Tirumali, 1984). Mucosal regeneration may be delayed if there are supervening viral (e.g., herpes simplex virus) or fungal (e.g., candidiasis) infections. The latter may be colonized throughout the alimentary tract, resulting in patchy exudates with fissures in the oropharynx and diffuse erosions and ulcerations in the esophagus and stomach (Mitchell & Schein, 1982). Prophylactic antiviral and topical antifungal therapies may prevent or minimize such infections in particularly susceptible individuals (i.e., those receiving multimodal antineoplastic therapy including corticosteroids and antimicrobial antibiotics). When these infections occur, they can range from mild discomfort to severe oral pain, dysphagia, odynophagia, upper gastrointestinal bleeding, and retrosternal pain. Frequently, there is concomitant nausea and vomiting. Oral intake may be severely limited if not precluded by both physical injury and anorexia.

Fastidious mouth care, performed at regular intervals throughout the day, is an important first line of defense against infection or tissue necrosis. Specially formulated solutions are available with which to bathe oral tissues, conferring antiseptic protection without provoking further irritation or pain. Topical antifungal agents available as troches or liquid suspensions are frequently employed as prophylaxis or treatment against oropharyngeal candidiasis. Proper use requires that the medication ultimately be swallowed to permit coating of the esophagus (and stomach). Although this procedure may be well tolerated by some patients, for others it creates another source of nausea and vomiting. Add to this regimen oral (nonabsorbable) antibiotics, which are a frequent therapeutic component for immunosuppressed patients undergoing high-dose chemotherapy and irradiation, and yet another potentially untoward factor is introduced.

Typically, patients may be too uncomfortable to consume adequate nutrients and fluids orally. Nutrition intervention by means of tube feeding may be indicated if the patient can tolerate the presence of a feeding tube in the nasopharynx or oropharynx, has sufficient intestinal absorptive surface area, and has minimal nausea and vomiting. Before the advent of the presently available soft, flexible, and fine-bore feeding tubes, use of this modality in the thrombocytopenic, immunocompromised chemotherapy patient was contraindicated. Now, however, tube feeding has been successfully performed and sustained in such individuals with minimal complaints or irritation. The new tubes can remain in place for up to 2 weeks without stiffening and thus increasing the risk of intestinal perforation (if placed nasoenterically).

If it is determined that the patient has a functioning gastrointestinal tract, tube feeding should be considered. This may be instituted with an iso-osmotic, low-residue formula instilled at a slow rate with a feeding pump to permit a slow, continuous infusion. Bolus administration is contraindicated in nasoenteric regimens. Patients who are still capable of oral intake may require nocturnal supplementation to minimize interference with eating efforts during the day. Careful documentation of oral caloric, protein, and fluid intake permits proper adjustments in the tube feeding regimen to be made.

Some patients incur such severe and protracted mucositis in conjunction with nausea and vomiting that enteral intake is precluded. For these individuals, total parenteral nutrition is indicated to prevent weight loss and dehydration. Each regimen must be tailored to the individual under consideration, with special attention being paid to the patient's nutrition history and current nutrition status.

For patients with less severe cases of oropharyngeal mucositis, it is possible that nutrient and fluid requirements may be met with oral intake if appropriate modifications or adjustments in food selections and meal patterns are made. Such individuals may benefit from foods of soft consistency and texture that are not excessively acidic, salty, or spicy and are served at the correct temperature for the patient's tolerance. Examples of well-tolerated foods include mildly spiced casseroles; blended cold or strained (cream) soups; custard; pudding; soft cooked eggs; mashed potatoes; milk shakes; mildly flavored, smooth yogurts ( e.g., vanilla); plain ice cream or sherbet; cooked cereal; and pureed or "blenderized" meats and vegetables with a high moisture content (i.e., with sufficient added water, gravy, or sauce). A confounding factor may be concomitant hypogeusia, which could exacerbate underlying anorexia if the patient is being given a bland diet. Similarly, altered taste sensation may render liquid nutrition supplements unpalatable even if they do not aggravate oral or esophageal discomfort.

Nutrition management often entails a creative combination of texture, temperature, and flavor that is both acceptable and beneficial to such patients. Variety, even within the constraints of some patients' narrow tolerance, is essential to avoid or minimize taste fatigue. Nonacidic, fruit-flavored milk shakes made by combining sherbet, sorbet, ice cream, or yogurt with milk and canned or fresh fruit are often well accepted by patients.

Chemotherapeutic cycles usually occur at 3- to 4-week intervals to allow the patient sufficient recovery time from myelosuppressive effects. During these therapy-free periods, efforts to optimize intake should be escalated to offset interludes of food deprivation when treatment is resumed. Generous use of fat in acceptable and disguised forms is one important means of adding calories without markedly affecting volume. Gravies, cream sauces, butter, margarine, oil, mayonnaise, softened cream cheese, and sour cream should be included as tolerated. Consumption of fluids with few or no calories should be discouraged, and protein- and calorie-laden beverages (e.g., milk shakes and liquid nutrition supplements) should be emphasized over juices or soft drinks. Addition of glucose polymers to beverages and soups may also be helpful. Protein intake can be enhanced by cooking cereal in milk rather than water; adding dry milk solids to soups, milk, or shakes; adding dried or chopped meat, poultry, or fish to soups and casseroles; adding grated or melted cheese to vegetables, casseroles, and starches; and adding (coddled) eggs to hot cereal and milk shakes. If meats are distasteful to the patient, poultry or mild fish can be offered. Moreover, *tofu* (soybean curd) or bean dishes (in small quantities initially to minimize flatulence) may be well tolerated and accepted. Peanut butter spread on small pieces of soft fruit (e.g., banana coins or apple slices) or added to a milk shake can augment both calories and protein. Addition of powdered protein modules to soups, beverages, and pureed or "blenderized" foods should be considered, especially if the aforementioned foods are poorly tolerated or rejected by the patient.

It is important to emphasize that patients' food choices should not be restricted because the foods selected or preferred are not compatible with currently accepted dietary guidelines. Instead, although every effort should be made to maximize the diet's caloric and nutrient density, a fair amount of latitude should be afforded so that eating is a pleasant and positive experience.

Exhibit 16-2 presents guidelines for nutrition care of patients with oral and esophageal mucositis.

## INTESTINAL MUCOSITIS

DNA synthesis of rapidly dividing crypt cells of the intestinal mucosa is also inhibited by antineoplastic agents, with resultant alteration in cell structure and function. Clinical manifestations range from minimal symptoms to bloody diarrhea, abdominal pain, and protein-losing enteropathy (Table 16-1). The most severe cases have been observed with sequential administration of high-dose 5-fluorouracil and cytosine arabinoside. Gastrointestinal toxicity constitutes a major factor that limits dosages of these agents. In the absence of supervening infections, complete mucosal regeneration may occur 2 weeks after therapy is completed or discontinued (McDonald & Tirumali, 1984).

The effect of chemotherapeutic drugs on small bowel absorptive capacity is unclear because of patient variability and a relative paucity of clinical studies addressing this problem. Hyams, Batrus, Grand, and Sallan (1982) demonstrated the onset of secondary lactose malabsorption in children receiving chemotherapy for treatment of various malignancies. In another study of pediatric cancer patients treated with various antineoplastic drug regimens, Pledger, Pearson, Craft, Laker, and Eastham (1988) found a significant reduction in intestinal mannitol absorption (a measure of small bowel permeability and hence of mucosal integrity) relative to normal age-matched controls. Moreover, the decreased mannitol absorption correlated significantly with (poor) nutrition status. It is unclear whether the enteropathy was caused by malnutrition brought on by the disease and treatment or whether the chemotherapeutic drugs produced an enteropathy that resulted in secondary malnutrition. This unanswered question points to the complex interrelationships among antineoplastic drugs, gastrointestinal function, and nutrition status. Pretreatment nutrition status may be marginal as a result of underlying malignant disease. In this setting, intestinal absorption may already be tenuous while functional abnormalities remain subclinical. Subsequent addition of cytotoxic therapeutic drugs may well compound the problem, creating a vicious cycle: malnutrition-induced malabsorption and malnutrition exacerbated by malabsorption. Effective nutrition intervention is required to break this cycle because malnutrition correlates inversely with survival of cancer patients (Nixon et al., 1980; Eastern Cooperative Oncology Group, 1980).

Diarrhea necessitates close monitoring of fluid and electrolyte status to enable adequate replacement of losses and correction of derangements. It is difficult to stipulate what dietary restrictions should be imposed because there is considerable individual variation. Empiric restriction of lactose is usually indicated if diarrhea is significant. If small amounts of lactose-

---

**Exhibit 16-2** Nutrition Care Summary for Oral and Esophageal Mucositis

1. Encourage daily mouth care at appropriate intervals.
2. Offer nonacidic, bland foods with a high moisture content such as custard; puddings; cream soups; texturally smooth, mildly seasoned casseroles; soft cooked or scrambled eggs; ice cream; and milk shakes.
3. Vary the diet as much as possible to minimize taste fatigue. Experiment with new flavors that are nonirritating (e.g., avoid extra salt, pepper, cinnamon; consider using mild herbs).
4. Take advantage of therapy-free intervals to optimize or improve caloric and protein intake. Allow the patient sufficient dietary latitude so that efforts directed at and interest in eating are not stultified.
5. Consider tube feeding if oral intake is severely compromised but if the patient can tolerate the presence of a nasogastric feeding tube and has intact gastrointestinal function.
6. Consider total parenteral nutrition if enteral intake is precluded.

containing foods are permitted, careful observation of patient response should be made. There are various lactose-free, palatable liquid nutrition supplements and frozen products that may serve as acceptable substitutes and provide adequate calories and protein. Highly fatty or greasy foods may not be tolerated; their impact on diarrhea is variable but may exacerbate the problem. Normally, low-residue, easily digested, and easily absorbed foods should be emphasized and offered as small, frequent meals. Examples include cooked root vegetables, baked or boiled potatoes, bananas, applesauce, cooked cereal, rice, and refined bread products. Although consumption of fluids should be encouraged and lossed replaced, it is recommended that liquids be consumed between meals. Foods with a high caffeine content and those that produce gas and cause bloating (e.g., legumes and cruciferous vegetables) should be avoided.

Use of liquid elemental diets comprising partially hydrolyzed or chemically defined nutrients may be indicated for some patients who have sustained significant drug-induced mucosal injury and can tolerate enterally administered nutrition support. Some clinical investigators believe that these formulas may maintain intestinal mucosal integrity during chemotherapy and facilitate tissue repair once it is completed (Bouvous, 1987). A primary concern is whether the gastrointestinal tract is too fragile to tolerate feeding of any sort. If this is the case and if recovery is expected to be delayed, total parenteral nutrition should be instituted to preserve nutrition status and to promote healing. On the other hand, if enteral support is deemed an appropriate modality, a continuous drip may be initiated with an elemental (or semielemental) formula diluted to approximately an iso-osmolar concentration. Unless the fluid is required (e.g., in cases in which intravenous access is limited), it is recommended that the strength of the formula be advanced before the volume to maximize delivery of calories and nutrients.

Routes of delivery may be by nasogastric tube, nasoenteric tube, gastrostomy, or jejunostomy. Bolus administration should never by employed with nasoenteric or jejunostomy tube feedings. Some patients may be able to consume some or all of the formula orally, although the palatability of these formulas is generally poor. Furthermore, some formulas that may be best tolerated by the patient are not recommended for oral use. Tube feeding formulas that are lactose free and iso-osmolar and that comprise intact protein may also be well tolerated by patients with less severe cases of chemotherapy-induced diarrhea. Again, the volume and rate should be advanced carefully with consistent documentation of patient tolerance.

Exhibit 16-3 outlines nutrition care for cancer patients with intestinal mucositis.

## CONSTIPATION

Chemotherapy can directly or indirectly result in constipation. Frequent complications associated with use of the vinca alkaloids, particularly vincristine, are adynamic ileus, severe constipation, colicky abdominal pain, and distention, all of which are clinical manifestations of drug-induced neurotoxicity. Symptoms may appear within 3 days of drug administration and may not resolve for 2 to 3 weeks. Elderly patients and those receiving high doses of this agent are most susceptible to these toxicities. Other chemotherapy-associated causes of constipation include diminished oral intake and use of opiates (for pain) and anticholinergic medications (for treatment of diarrhea or emesis) (McDonald & Tirumali, 1984).

Nutrition implications can be significant, especially if abdominal pain and distention preclude oral or enteral intake. Parenteral nutrition should be considered as interim support if small bowel obstruction is suspected and if gut rest is imposed. Once obstruction and risk of perforation have been safely ruled out oral or enteral feeding can usually be resumed, but this must be done slowly and in conjunction with close monitoring of symptoms and tolerance. Stool lubricants or softeners such as mineral oil may be useful in preventing impaction and relieving symptoms of abdominal fullness. Adequate fluid intake should be encouraged and fiber gradually increased as patient tolerance allows. If the patient is receiving tube feedings, changing to a fiber-enriched formula (or mixing enteral formulas 1:1 with a low-residue preparation) may promote ease of elimination (Exhibit 16-4).

**Exhibit 16-3** Nutrition Care Plan for Intestinal Mucositis

1. Monitor fluid balance (intake and output) closely, and replace losses with warm or room-temperature, mild liquids (e.g., weak or herbal tea, broth, [diluted] fruit nectars) between meals.
2. Encourage small, frequent meals, and emphasize soft, bland, low-residue foods. Examples include cooked root vegetables; potatoes; rice; refined breads, crackers, grains, and cereals; lean, plain meats; bananas; and applesauce.
3. Minimize or avoid highly spiced or greasy foods, raw fruits and vegetables, foods that may produce flatulence (e.g., legumes, cruciferous vegetables), whole grains, and nuts. In general, avoid foods that are high in fiber unless it is of the soluble type such as that found in applesauce and bananas.
4. Limit or restrict lactose (milk and many dairy products), especially if consumption of these foods is associated with worsening of symptoms. Substitute lactose-free nondairy products or reduced-lactose milk (when treated with commercially available lactase, milk may be rendered 90% lactose free). Cheeses aged more than 90 days and yogurt with active bacterial cultures may be tolerated; introduce these gradually and individually.
5. Avoid foods and beverages with a high caffeine content.
6. Consider tube feeding with an elemental or chemically defined enteral formula if the patient's gastrointestinal tract is functional.
7. Impose bowel rest and institute total parenteral nutrition if mucosal injury is deemed extensive and if recovery is protracted.

**Exhibit 16-4** Nutrition Care Summary for Constipation

1. Administer adequate fluids (minimum of 64 oz/day for adults).
2. Encourage increased physical activity as tolerated.
3. Increase the fiber content of the patient's diet (gingerly at first) by including whole grain breads and cereals (e.g., wheat bran), fruits and vegetables, nuts and legumes.

## OTHER COMPLICATIONS

Several chemotherapeutic agents have been associated with hepatotoxicity (Table 16-1), although abnormalities are usually mild and transient. Occasionally, however, significant injury results and may adversely affect appetite (secondary to characteristic anorexia) or absorption (e.g., cholestasis). If cholestasis is prolonged, absorption of fat and fat-soluble vitamins, especially K and E, should be assessed and appropriate supplementation (with water-miscible preparations) started (Sokol, Balistreri, Hoofnagle, & Jones, 1983; Sokol, Heubi, Iannaccone, Bove, & Balistreri, 1984).

L-Asparaginase therapy can precipitate pancreatitis. This complication may necessitate provisional bowel rest until acute symptoms resolve. Vinca alkaloid administration may lead to peripheral neuritis with parasthesias, ataxia, and generalized muscle weakness and malaise. Patients may encounter difficulty with feeding themselves, masticating, or consuming food and fluids in general. Modifications in diet consistency or conversion to a predominantly liquid diet may be a necessary provisional measure.

## EFFECT OF CHEMOTHERAPY ON ENERGY AND NITROGEN BALANCE

As delineated in the foregoing discussion, the toxic effects of chemotherapeutic agents can interfere profoundly with normal host ingestion and absorption of nutrients. What is less well understood is the direct impact of these drugs on host cell metabolism. The clinically relevant concern is how these agents alter—if at all—energy and protein requirements to maintain lean body mass or, in the case of children, to promote growth. More important is the question of whether these effects, once identified, can be successfully overridden by provision of adequate nutrition support. Several studies have attempted to answer these important questions (Herrmann et al., 1981; Drott et al., 1988; Lerebours et al., 1988). Herrmann et al. (1981) demonstrated that patients with testicular cancer receiving nutrition support as total parenteral nutrition were able to maintain nitrogen equilibrium before administration of chemotherapy; negative nitrogen balance ensued once the drugs were given, however. Alterations in protein kinetics were also observed, suggesting drug-induced disruption in lean body mass.

It appears that ideal nutrition management of the cancer patient undergoing chemotherapy entails a multistage process, with the first step being to determine the level of energy and nitrogen intake required to offset the deleterious effects of the drugs. Energy and protein requirements are generally estimated to be 40% to 80% more than the patient's calculated basal energy expenditure (derived from the equation of Harris and Benedict [1919]) and 1.2 to 1.5 g of protein per kilogram of (ideal) body weight, respectively. Predicted (basal) energy expenditure, however, may be inaccurate as a result of the aberrations in energy metabolism and considerable individual variation observed in cancer patients (Knox et al., 1983). For this reason, resting energy expenditure measured by bedside indirect calorimetry may afford accurate baseline data from which targeted levels of caloric intake may be extrapolated. Whenever feasible, this method should be employed in an effort to optimize nutrition support and to avoid complications associated with overfeeding. After determining the targeted caloric and protein requirements, the second step is to achieve these goals by some combination of tolerated nutrition support. Finally, patient response to nutrition support must be carefully and consistently assessed by serial monitoring of changes in nutrition assessment and body composition parameters.

Choosing the appropriate modalities can at times present a dilemma. The adage "If the gut works, use it" still substantially applies. Gastrointestinal function may be too limiting and the nutrition status too depleted, however, to permit delivery of adequate fluid and nutrients as a result of cytotoxic insult. In these instances, supplemental or total parenteral nutrition support should be considered. The problem of central venous access may be obviated by the fact that many chemotherapy patients already have an indwelling catheter that can be used for such purposes as nutrition support.

Overall patient outcome is ultimately contingent on many factors, and the effect of nutrition status on this endpoint remains unclear. Nevertheless, prognosis may be favorably influenced by provision of adequate nutrients to preserve lean body mass and adipose tissue stores in the face of malignant disease and the cytotoxic agents used to treat it.

## REFERENCES

Bernstein, I.L. (1978). Learned taste aversions in children receiving chemotherapy. *Science, 200,* 1302–1303.

Bernstein, I.L., & Bernstein, I.D. (1981). Learned food aversions and cancer anorexia. *Cancer Treatment Reports, 65*(Suppl. 5), 43–47.

Bernstein, I.L., Webster, M.M., & Bernstein, I.D. (1982). Food aversions in children receiving chemotherapy for cancer. *Cancer, 50,* 2961–2963.

Borison, H.L., & McCarthy, L.E. (1983). Neuropharmacologic mechanisms of emesis. In J. Laszlo (Ed.), *Antiemetics and cancer chemotherapy* (pp. 6–20). Baltimore: Williams & Wilkins.

Bouvous, G. (1987). Elemental diets during cancer chemotherapy: A commentary. *Anticancer Research, 7,* 1225–1228.

Carter, B.L. (1987). Commonly used chemotherapeutic agents. *Primary Care, 14,* 293–315.

Cotanch, P.H. (1983). Relaxation techniques as antiemetic therapy. In J. Laszlo (Ed.), *Antiemetics and cancer chemotherapy* (pp. 164–176). Baltimore: Williams & Wilkins.

Dennis, V.W. (1983). Fluid and electrolyte changes after vomiting. In J. Laszlo (Ed.), *Antiemetics and cancer chemotherapy* (pp. 34–42). Baltimore: Williams & Wilkins.

Drott, C., Unsgaard, B., Schersten, T., & Lundholm, K. (1988). Total parenteral nutrition as an adjuvant to patients undergoing chemotherapy for testicular carcinoma: Protection of body composition—A randomized, prospective study. *Surgery, 103,* 499–506.

Eastern Cooperative Oncology Group. (1980). Prognostic effect of weight loss prior to chemotherapy in cancer patients. *American Journal of Medicine, 69,* 491–497.

Grant, J.P. (1986). Preventing complications of surgery: Emphasis on nutritional factors. In J. Laszlo (Ed.), *Physician's guide to cancer care complications: Prevention and management* (pp. 37–59). New York: Marcel Dekker.

Harris, J.A., & Benedict, F.G. (1919). *A biometric study of basal metabolism in man* (Publication No. 279 of the Carnegie Institution of Washington). Washington, DC: Carnegie Institution of Washington.

Herrmann, V.M., Garnick, M.B., Moore, F.D., & Wilmore, D.W. (1981). Effect of cytotoxic agents on protein kinetics in patients with metastatic cancer. *Surgery, 90,* 381–387.

Hyams, J.S., Batrus, C.L., Grand, R.J., & Sallan, S.E. (1982). Cancer chemotherapy-induced lactose malabsorption in children. *Cancer, 49,* 646–650.

Juma, F.D., Rogers, H.J., & Trounce, J.R. (1979). The kinetics of salivary elimination of cyclophosphamide in man. *British Journal of Clinical Pharmacology, 8,* 455–458.

Knox, L.S., Crosby, L.V., Feurer, I.D., Buzby, G.P., Miller, C.L., & Mullen, J.L. (1983). Energy expenditure in malnourished cancer patients. *Annals of Surgery, 197,* 152–162.

Laszlo, J., Stevenson D., & Lucas, V.S. (1986). Chemotherapy. In J. Laszlo (Ed.), *Physician's guide to cancer care complications: Prevention and management* (pp. 61–145). New York: Marcel Dekker.

Lerebours, E., Tilly, H., Rimbert, A., Delarus, J., Pignet, H., & Colin, R. (1988). Change in energy and protein status in patients with acute leukemia. *Cancer, 61,* 2412–2417.

McAnena, O.J., & Daly, J.M. (1986). Impact of antitumor therapy on nutrition. *Surgical Clinics of North America, 66,* 1213–1228.

McDonald, G.B., & Tirumali, N. (1984). Intestinal and liver toxicity of antineoplastic drugs. *Western Journal of Medicine, 140,* 250–259.

Mitchell, E.P., & Schein, P.S. (1982). Gastrointestinal toxicity of chemotherapeutic agents. *Seminars in Oncology, 9,* 52–64.

Morrow, G.R. (1982). Prevalence and correlates of anticipatory nausea and vomiting in chemotherapy patients. *Journal of the National Cancer Institute, 68,* 585–588.

Morrow, G.R., Arseneau, J.C., Asbury, R.F., Bennett, J.M., & Boros, L. (1982). Anticipatory nausea and vomiting with chemotherapy. *New England Journal of Medicine, 306,* 431–432.

Morrow, G.R., & Morrel, C. (1982). Behavioral treatment for the anticipatory nausea and vomiting induced by cancer chemotherapy. *New England Journal of Medicine, 307,* 1476–1480.

Nixon, D.W., Heymsfield, S.B., Cohen, A.E., Kutner, M.H., Ansley, J., Lawson, D.H., & Rudman, D. (1980).

Protein-calorie undernutrition in hospitalized cancer patients. *American Journal of Medicine, 68,* 683–690.

Penta, J., Poster, D., & Bruno, S. (1983). The pharmacologic treatment of nausea and vomiting caused by cancer chemotherapy: A review. In J. Laszlo (Ed.), *Antiemetics and cancer chemotherapy* (pp. 53–92). Baltimore: Williams & Wilkins.

Pledger, J.V., Pearson, A.D.J., Craft, A.W., Laker, M.F., & Eastham, E.J. (1988). Intestinal permeability during chemotherapy for childhood tumours. *European Journal of Pediatrics, 147,* 123–127.

Seigel, L.J., & Longo, D.L. (1981). The control of chemotherapy-induced emesis. *Annals of Internal Medicine, 95,* 352–359.

Sokol, R.J., Balistreri, W.F., Hoofnagle, J.H., & Jones, E.A. (1983). Vitamin E deficiency in adults with chronic liver disease. *American Journal of Clinical Nutrition, 41,* 66–72.

Sokol, R.J., Heubi, J.E., Iannaccone, S.T., Bove, K.E., & Balistreri, W.F. (1984). Vitamin E deficiency with normal serum vitamin E concentrations in children with chronic cholestasis. *New England Journal of Medicine, 310,* 1209–1212.

Steele, W.H., Stuart, J.F.B., Whiting, B., Lawrence, J.R., Calman, K.C., McVie, J.G., & Baird, G.M. (1979). Serum, tear, and salivary concentrations of methotrexate in man. *British Journal of Clinical Pharmacology, 7,* 207–211.

Stoudemire, A., Cotanch, P., & Laszlo, J. (1984). Recent advances in the pharmacologic and behavioral management of chemotherapy-induced emesis. *Archives of Internal Medicine, 144,* 1029–1033.

Trant, A.S. (1986). Taste and anorexia in cancer patients: A review. *Topics in Clinical Nutrition, 1,* 17–25.

Trant, A.S., Serin, J., & Douglass, H.O. (1982). Is taste related to anorexia in cancer patients? *American Journal of Clinical Nutrition, 36,* 45–58.

# Chapter 17

# The Impact of Radiation Therapy on the Nutrition Status of the Cancer Patient: An Overview

*Bonnie Terrill Ross*

## THERAPEUTIC RADIATION

Radiation has been used in a medical setting since the early 1900s. It has been referred to as x-ray therapy, teletherapy, radiation therapy, and cobalt therapy. Radiation therapy treatment machines, regardless of their name, produce external radiation of high energies that is used in treating various malignancies. Radiation is a form of electromagnetic energy that can effect change in human tissue. Radiation therapy techniques are quite sophisticated, and the technology has been rapidly advancing over the last several decades.

Radiation may be utilized as a definitive or adjuvant form of cancer treatment. The goal of radiation therapy treatments may be cure of the disease or palliation of symptomatic disease. More than 50% of all patients diagnosed with cancer receive radiation therapy treatments sometime throughout the course of their illness. Approximately 30% of those patients who receive radiation therapy treatments require another course of radiation in the future, usually for metastatic disease.

The radiation dose and the number of treatments are prescribed by the radiation oncologist. Treatment courses may be only one single treatment or may last as long as 7 weeks. The average course of treatment, however, ranges between 4 and 5 weeks. Usually the treatments

are given daily, 5 days per week. Actual treatment times are short, usually less than a few minutes.

Many patients already have nutrition problems before they begin radiation therapy treatments. These problems are often the result of the disease process itself combined with the psychologic distress that accompanies a cancer diagnosis. Those patients who are recovering from surgery or have received chemotherapy often have profound nutrition difficulties. Nutrition risk is compounded in patients receiving concurrent radiation therapy and chemotherapy treatments.

## NUTRITION OVERVIEW

Historically, cancer patients have not received the nutrition attention that they deserve despite the high percentage of oncology patients with devastating nutrition problems that make up the hospital inpatient and outpatient population. This may be due to a lack of insight on the part of clinicians into the unique nutrition needs of the cancer patient and failure to provide adequate dietitian coverage on the oncology units and in cancer treatment departments. It may also be due to a shortage of available dietitians who have training and experience in oncology nutrition care and who feel comfortable with and are dedicated to working with cancer patients. In this era of hospital cost containment, recommendations for new or expanded dietitian positions in cancer departments often meet with resistance. In the adult cancer patient population, aggressive nutrition support may not greatly affect long-term patient survival rates.

Nevertheless, many far-reaching benefits of proper nutrition care exist. These include a reduction in morbidity of patients who achieve and maintain adequate nutrition and a decrease in the incidence and severity of treatment-related side effects. Adequate nutrition may also help preserve immunologic function in the radiation-treated patient. Patients who achieve or maintain a satisfactory nutrition state during their radiation therapy have a shorter recovery period after treatments compared to undernourished patients. Likewise, patients who preserve their nutrition status during radiation treatments are certainly more physiologically equipped to tolerate any additional type of cancer therapy that they may need in the future.

Concerns and questions about proper nutrition are universal among cancer patients confronting cancer treatment. Without nutrition counseling, patients are left with a void in their cancer care. Poor nutrition may result in interruptions and delays in a patient's course of radiation therapy, chemotherapy, and recovery from major surgery. Prolonged hospital stays, delayed rehabilitation, and increased morbidity can often be traced to inadequate nutrition care.

Frustrated patients and family members may seek assistance outside the institution for nutrition counseling. All too often patients and their families turn to unorthodox cancer therapies, which almost always involve scientifically unsound and unsafe practices but offer the patient the nutrition regimen that may be lacking in institutionalized cancer care protocols.

## SIDE EFFECTS OF RADIATION THERAPY

The extent of nutrition problems in cancer patients receiving radiation therapy varies widely. Some patients may experience serious eating difficulties while others have few or no side effects. Unlike chemotherapy, which is systemic, radiation therapy is directed at a designated body site. Most radiation therapy patients experience side effects in relation to their site of treatment and the dose of radiation received.

Along with killing cancer cells, radiation can damage normal tissue in the field of treatment. Rapidly dividing body tissues, such as blood cells, hair follicles, and the entire lining of the gastrointestinal tract, are the most vulnerable to radiation-induced damage. The normal tissues included in the area of treatment react at a given dose of radiation. Any part of the digestive system included in the treatment field is likely to be affected, with subsequent development of eating problems.

The type of cancer and the patient's individual sensitivity also influence the likelihood of side effects experienced during radiation therapy treatments. In addition to the predictable side effects determined by the site of treatment, most patients also experience generalized fatigue, anorexia, and emotional stress. Most radiation therapy–induced nutrition difficulties are transient and subside about 2 weeks after treatments are finished.

## NUTRITION SUCCESS

Nutrition success in managing radiation therapy patients depends on many factors. The obvious, imperative factor is the dietitian. The dietitian needs to be knowledgeable about side effects that are common with the various types of radiation treatments and be in tune with the appropriate management for these effects. Also, there must be a manageable number of patients per dietitian.

Ideally an initial dietitian consultation should take place a few days after patients start their treatments. The first days are usually inappropriate times for consultation because of lengthy treatment planning procedures, patient discussions with the oncologists regarding benefits and risks of radiation therapy, possible additional diagnostic tests, and high patient anxiety. The physical presence of the dietitian in the radiation therapy department is immensely reassuring to patients and families.

Providing patients access to a dietitian by giving them a listed telephone number or by directing them to another area of the hospital for nutrition counseling greatly diminishes the success of nutrition interventions. It is less likely that patients or their families will bother to contact a dietitian for any problem when the dietitian is not readily available in the radiation therapy department. In the oncology environment all nutrition difficulties need immediate attention; otherwise they can blossom into major eating problems.

## NUTRITION PROBLEMS ASSOCIATED WITH SPECIFIC RADIATION TREATMENT SITES

### Head and Neck

Patients with head and neck cancer who are receiving radiation therapy typically pose the greatest challenge to the dietitian. These patients often present in a malnourished state and have a long history of dietary indiscretions. Often, head and neck cancer patients are alcohol and tobacco abusers. Patients are advised not to smoke or consume alcohol during treatments. These substances exacerbate oral pain and dysphagia. Many head and neck cancer patients receive irradiation in a postoperative setting. Eating impairment secondary to radical surgery and possible adjustment to new chewing and swallowing techniques often result in significant weight loss and slow recovery.

Radiation therapy side effects compound the nutrition risks of these patients. The lining of the mouth and throat is particularly sensitive and reactive to radiation. Frequent complications experienced by head and neck cancer patients who receive radiation are stomatitis and esophagitis, which are due to the breakdown or ulceration of the mucosa. The loss of oral mucosal integrity may allow microorganisms to enter the systemic circulation, which leads to life-threatening infection in immunocompromised patients (Himmelberg & Christen, 1989).

Changes in oral mucosa may be accompanied by altered saliva production as a result of fibrosis and the high sensitivity of the salivary glands to radiation. The saliva becomes quite thick and tenacious. Viscous saliva compounds dysphagia and poor oral intake. The patient eventually progresses to a marked dry mouth (xerostomia). Permanent deficit in salivary flow may result. Normal saliva contains important lubricating proteins, antimicrobial factors, and enzymes (Himmelberg & Christen, 1989). Because the treatments decrease salivary flow, there is a loss of some of these important factors. In addition, there is a decrease in intraoral $pH$, alterations in the oral flora, and loss of salivary buffering capacity, which all contribute to a high incidence of dental caries. Many patients have a past history of poor oral hygiene and poor dentition, which accentuates their risk for oral complications.

Most patients with head and neck cancer who are undergoing radiation therapy contract superimposed oral infections that accentuate oral pain. Eighty-five percent of patients experience colonization and progressively invasive oropharyngeal-esophageal yeast infections. The incidence of secondary bacterial infections approaches 100% in these patients. The pathogenicity varies from mild to brisk mucositis. There is a direct correlation between the degree of mucositis and the degree of xerostomia. The risk of viral infection is also great in head and neck cancer patients. Viral lesions occur in 30% to 50% of this population (Poland, 1989).

The diagnosis and differentiation of oral infections is a complex process, especially given the prevalence of concurrent yeast, bacterial, and viral infections. The patient's ability to achieve satisfactory nutrition often depends on the prompt identification and treatment of oral infections. The regional pain associated with head and neck infections can be severe, which greatly compromises the patient's ability to eat. Nutrition care of these patients should be intense to mount a maximal immune response.

Food intake is further adversely affected by impairment of the sense of smell and by profound taste abnormalities. Radiation damage can cause both heightened and suppressed sensations of taste and odor. Taste abnormalities vary greatly among patients. The most common complaint is hypogeusia, which is simply a deterioration in taste perception. With hypogeusia, patients complain of a generalized loss of flavor and describe food as tasting flat or like cardboard.

Dysgeusia, an altered sense of taste, is also prevalent during head and neck irradiation. Patients with dysgeusia often describe foods as tasting rancid, bitter, or metallic. These patients seem to experience the most severe taste distortion with meats, coffee, chocolate-flavored foods, and sometimes plain water. Hypogeusia and dysgeusia are larger barriers to eating than most patients ever anticipate. Taste acuity may not return to normal for several months after the completion of radiation therapy.

Counseling early in a patient's course of treatment is imperative. The importance of maintaining good nutrition, curtailing further weight loss, and frankly discussing anticipated eating difficulties should all be reviewed with the patient and family. Generally the alterations in taste perception or saliva production and any oral discomfort do not occur to any great degree for the first 2 weeks of treatment. The dietitian should use this time to educate and motivate the patient in an aggressive fashion.

Most patients understand the risks and side effects of radiation treatment. They psychologically brace themselves for a few weeks of uncomfortable or forced eating. Most patients depend on high-calorie, high-protein beverages and commercial nutrition supplements. They often can manage bland, moist, soft, nonacidic, and nonabrasive foods such as omelettes, soups, ice creams, puddings, certain casseroles, mild yogurts, and cold tuna or meat salads creamed with mayonnaise. The limited number of foods tolerated during radiation-induced complications results in monotony in the diet. This, along with pain or lack of enjoyment while eating, greatly interferes with adequate oral intake (Hearne et al., 1985). Only motivation can override such obstacles to eating.

Even with ongoing, intense nutrition counseling, most patients struggle to minimize weight loss. Drastic weight loss seems to be inevitable given the major obstacles to achieving adequate oral intake. Most patients, however, are able to keep weight loss to less than 10 lb with persistent nutrition guidance and motivation. Motivation is derived from patients' courage and longing to regain their health in addition to inspirational counseling skills on the part of the dietitian.

Those patients who are unable to approach adequate oral caloric intake and who steadily lose weight should be considered candidates for nutrition support. Their eating problems are mechanical in nature because they normally have a functional gut. Therefore, enteral nutrition should be the support of choice. Most radiation therapy patients are outpatients, so that percutaneous endoscopic gastrostomy feeding tubes are a simple, reasonable, and socially acceptable solution to delivering nutrition. Patients usually express great relief and satisfaction with gastrostomy feedings after a losing struggle with eating and weight loss.

### Thorax

Radiation fields that include the mediastinum are common with lung cancers, esophageal cancers, Hodgkin's disease, and breast cancer treatments that include the internal mammary lymph nodes. Patients usually experience problems with dysphagia due to esophagitis. This is often described as a sore, irritated throat or as a lump in the throat. These symptoms have also been noted in patients receiving radiation to their thoracic spine as a result of exit radiation dose effect to the esophagus. Other symptoms reported with mediastinal radiation include indigestion and early satiety. Nausea is not a common side effect.

In severe cases, patients express a fear of choking on both liquids and solids, and food seems to stick in the esophagus. Dysphagia may well be present before radiation treatments begin as a result of intrinsic or extrinsic tumor compression. This is especially true with esophageal cancers because of the constricting nature of the neoplasm. Other mediastinal masses can cause symptoms of dysphagia as a result of partial obstruction. Such patients often report relief from their dysphagia as their radiation therapy treatments shrink their tumors, thereby lessening the obstruction.

Patients with Hodgkin's disease and most of those with breast cancer on the whole maintain a good appetite throughout radiation therapy. They tend to manage their eating well and to maintain their weight. Generally, their dysphagia is intermittent, mild to moderate, and manageable.

Lung cancer patients are at great nutrition risk because of symptoms associated with the disease itself. These patients frequently experience problems with weight loss, anorexia, pain, hypogeusia, weakness, fatigue, recurring infections, coughing, and shortness of breath. These symptoms are often present even before radiation therapy treatments begin and may continue throughout the course of treatment. Lung cancer patients also demonstrate marked emotional distress, including depression and frustration over their symptoms and poor prognosis. Many patients grapple with feelings of guilt, anger, and denial over past lifestyles, namely their smoking history and its contribution to their lung cancer.

Dietary counseling for patients receiving mediastinal radiation includes general good nutrition, avoidance of weight loss, and guidelines for dysphagia. These guidelines review eating slowly; chewing food well; eating soft, moist foods during periods of dysphagia; and relaxing while eating. Most radiation therapy departments have a lidocaine-antacid solution to medicate patients with dysphagia. Those patients with more severe symptoms require intense nutrition counseling. Introduction of high-calorie, high-protein beverages and supplements is often necessary. Patients with esophageal cancer who demonstrate progressive symptoms of obstruction usually require a bypass feeding tube.

## Abdomen and Pelvis

The gastrointestinal tract is responsible for nutrition sequelae of irradiation of the abdomen and pelvis (Donaldson, 1984). There is a broad range of patient tolerance to abdominal irradiation from severe nausea and vomiting to complete absence of symptoms. Patients may experience mild nausea for approximately 2 hours after a radiation treatment. Such patients adapt well to eating lightly before and after treatments until nausea subsides. Patients then resume normal eating with an emphasis on extra calories and protein to preserve their nutrition status.

Patients who experience treatment-related emesis and nausea usually respond well to antiemetics. If emesis continues despite medication, the radiation oncologist may reduce the daily treatment dose in an attempt to alleviate symptoms. Nausea and vomiting may be caused by factors other than radiation, such as hypercalcemia or metastatic disease to the liver or brain, that would necessitate immediate attention.

Dietary concerns are understandably great in patients who experience nausea and vomiting. There is often reluctance to eat; fear of eating, treatments, and loss of control; and heightened anxiety. The dietitian must approach these patients with sensitivity and specifics. Brevity and discretion should be used when inquiring about food tolerances. A gradual progression from clear liquids to plain, regular foods should be instituted in accordance with changes in symptoms, food tolerances, and response to antiemetics. Integrating clear liquid supplemental feedings into flavored ices, gelatins, and clear beverages has frequently been a successful part of nutrition support.

Family members are often at a loss as to how to nourish the patient who has emesis. Usually, family members are eager to accept guidance and education about dietary management. Family members tend to respect specific instructions, but the nauseated patient may find that discussions about food may accentuate symptoms. Therefore, dietary management discussions may be more effective without the nauseated patient's presence.

Abdominal and pelvic radiation decreases the absorptive capacity of the gastrointestinal tract and causes morphologic changes. Chronic bowel damage from radiation is now rare, occurring only in about 5% of patients. This is attributed to modern treatment techniques and sophisticated treatment planning that limit daily radiation dose fractions and total treatment doses.

Most patients receiving pelvic radiation therapy report symptoms after 2 to 3 weeks of treatment. Most patients experience problems with diarrhea, bloating, and flatulence. Some patients exhibit symptoms of mild lactose intolerance, with poor tolerance to large quantities of milk. A few patients experience problems with nausea. When symptoms of diarrhea begin, patients are instructed to reduce their intake of insoluble fiber–rich foods, gas-forming foods, and high-bacteria foods such as raw vegetables and fruits. Milk intake should also be limited, especially if the patient reports gassy cramps. Should diarrhea continue, antidiarrheals are prescribed. As with other sites of treatment, symptoms vary from patient to patient. Overall, however, diarrhea can be well controlled in patients receiving abdominal radiation therapy. Symptoms usually subside 2 to 3 weeks after the completion of radiation therapy. Most patients are able gradually to resume normal eating when their symptoms subside.

### Central Nervous System

Patients with cancers of the brain often experience symptoms of headaches, seizures, altered mentation, nausea, and vomiting. Most patients who have a primary brain cancer or metastatic disease to the brain experience acute weight loss secondary to their symptoms. Symptoms and weight loss typically subside with administration of high-dose steroids.

About 20% of patients experience persistent anorexia or nausea (or both) throughout their treatment. Some patients note changes in taste perception, food cravings, and increased sensitivity to all types of odors. A few patients may have problems with sporadic incidents of vomiting without any sensation of nausea. More than 80% of patients on steroids contract invasive yeast infections, which cause oral pain or dysphagia.

During cranial irradiation, most patients fare well in terms of nutrition despite their symptoms. Most patients experience a stimulated appetite from steroid medication. Often patients report a voracious appetite and are quite concerned about their inability to feel satiety regardless of their volume of intake. Fluid retention and weight gain are common.

Patients with high-grade brain malignancies experience more anorexia and eating difficulties than those with low-grade brain malignancies. Changes in appetite, tolerance of food odors, taste perceptions, and changes in food likes and dislikes are probably a combined result of tumor location in the brain, tumor grade, steroid usage, and irradiation. Elevated blood glucose levels are not uncommon in patients on steroid preparations. Diabetic patients are particularly at risk in this regard. Blood glucose monitoring should be done periodically throughout the course of treatment.

Patients who are receiving concurrent craniospinal irradiation are at a high risk for nutrition difficulties. These patients often experience nausea, vomiting, and anorexia leading to progressive weight loss. With partial spinal irradiation, such as that for discreet metastatic areas, there is an exit radiation dose effect on the gastrointestinal tract in that area. For example, patients receiving cervical spine irradiation may experience dysphagia, and lumbar spinal irradiation may cause diarrhea.

## NUTRITION EDUCATION

Initial nutrition consultations can range from 20 to 60 minutes depending on the patient's symptoms, degree of risk, and capacity to exchange and retain information. Initial nutrition consultations should commence with a height and weight check. A comprehensive nutrition history should follow in a pleasant office setting.

After the nutrition history is obtained, the education process proceeds with an explanation of the role of nutrition during radiation therapy. A positive approach should focus on the benefits of improved or preserved nutrition rather than on the negative aspects of malnutrition. Nutrition education should be delivered in a straightforward, sensitive, and motivating manner.

A positive attitude and a hope-filled approach to confronting barriers to eating nurtures motivation and an active, informed role on the part of the patient. During the initial consultation, the patient should be guided about ways to manage present eating problems and encouraged to discuss eating difficulties during anticipated radiation side effects. Nutrition education should involve not only the patient but the family and significant others as well.

All patients should receive the *Eating Hints* booklet from the National Cancer Institute (1989) in addition to any other educational materials that are deemed suitable. It is beneficial to have concise supplemental education materials available that are directed at management of specific side effects and specific symptoms. Patients should be encouraged to post a summary sheet in a highly visible location in the home, such as the refrigerator, for quick reference. A nutrition education bulletin board in the radiation therapy department's patient waiting area is another successful method to spread the nutrition message that eating well should be a complement to radiation treatments.

Experience has shown that displaying education materials about nutrition's role in cancer prevention is not appropriate in cancer therapy departments. Although data support nutrition's role in cancer prevention, such materials may set off feelings of guilt and anxiety among patients who already have cancer. Nutrition and cancer-prevention literature often cause confusion because the patient and family may erroneously conclude that it is advantageous to attempt weight loss and to cut back on calorie and protein intake, as are sometimes advised in such materials as cancer-prevention strategies.

Monitoring of weight, food intake, treatment side effects, and nutrition education should be ongoing. Weight checks and inquiries about eating, appetite, and symptoms should be done weekly for all patients. High-risk patients, those taking nutrition supplements, and those who are symptomatic require close and frequent monitoring, guidance, and encouragement. Detailed nutrition care plan cards should be maintained for all patients. These should include a diet history; radiation therapy prescription; age; sex; weight history and ongoing weight measurements; operative, medical, and social histories; and dietitian recommendations.

Periodic staff education about the role of nutrition and cancer therapy is a professional responsibility of the radiation therapy dietitian. The oncologists and staff play a supportive role in encouraging patients to eat well during treatment and should be trained to be attentive to patient concerns over nutrition and to notify the dietitian if the patient verbalizes a problem. Regardless of the size of the department, the dietitian should provide ongoing updates to the radiation oncologists and oncology nurses about the nutrition progress of patients.

A resourceful dietitian uses other support personnel such as nurses, chaplains, and social workers in dealing with cancer patients. Working together as a team provides holistic, quality care. Oncology health care providers share a unique bond to one another by the nature of cancer care's intense emotional demands.

## CONCLUSION

Patients of all ages and all walks of life are susceptible to the nutrition difficulties imposed by cancer and its treatments. All radiation therapy patients are subject to anorexia and eating problems. With some diseases, such as lung cancer and oropharyngeal cancers, profound problems with poor nutrition are predictable and require strict attention. Minimizing weight loss and preserving nutrition status result in patients with fewer infections, better self-esteem and sense of well-being, better overall food tolerance, and faster recovery after the completion of radiation therapy. Good nutrition during radiation therapy is also advantageous to the patient who requires any further cancer therapy.

**REFERENCES**

Donaldson, S.S. (1984). Nutritional support as an adjunct to radiation therapy. *Journal of Parenteral and Enteral Nutrition, 8*(3), 302–310.

Hearne, B.E., Dunaj, J.M., Daly, J.M., Strong, E.W., Vikram, B., LePorte, B.J., & DeCosse, J.J. (1985). Enteral nutrition support in head and neck cancer: Tube vs.

oral feeding during radiation therapy. *Journal of the American Dietetic Association, 85*(6), 669–677.

Himmelberg, C., & Christen, C. (1989). Management of stomatitis. *Michigan Drug Letter, 37*(9).

National Cancer Institute. (1989). *Eating hints.* Bethesda, MD: Author.

Poland, J.M. (1989). *Oropharyngeal-esophageal fungal infections during head and neck radiotherapy.* Paper presented at the International Workshop on Oral and Gastrointestinal Candidosis: From Pathology to Therapy, May 27, 1989, Munich, Germany.

Chapter 18

# Impact of Radiation Therapy on the Nutrition Status of the Cancer Patient: Acute and Chronic Complications

*Jeanne A. Darbinian and Ann M. Coulston*

Radiation therapy is a primary treatment modality for various malignant diseases. Ionizing radiation, administered in doses that eradicate tumor cells, may also damage normal, surrounding tissues lying in the therapeutic field. The severity and extent of injury are contingent on the total volume of irradiated tissue, tumor site, regions irradiated, duration of treatment, and total radiation dose administered (Donaldson, 1977, 1984; Kokal, 1985; Coulston & Darbinian, 1986).

Deleterious effects of radiation therapy on normal host tissue may occur acutely, during treatment, or long after therapy is completed. Early consequences of radiation therapy are generally transient and resolve several weeks after discontinuation of treatment. Chronic manifestations, however, may not occur for months to years after treatment and are frequently irreversible (Donaldson, 1977, 1984; Kokal, 1985). Direct radiation effects on normal tissue may have profound nutrition sequelae if resultant damage interferes significantly with food intake or utilization. Adverse nutrition consequences of radiation therapy may be particularly devastating to patients who present for treatment in a malnourished state, have previously undergone debilitating surgery, or will receive concomitant chemotherapy (Donaldson, 1977, 1982, 1984; Kokal, 1985; Donaldson & Lenon, 1979; McAnena & Daly, 1986).

Areas of the body typically affected by radiation therapy may be identified regionally as (1) the central nervous system, (2) the head and neck, (3) the thorax (esophagus, lungs, and mediastinum), and (4) the abdomen and pelvis (Donaldson, 1984; Donaldson & Lenon, 1979). This chapter delineates the nutrition consequences of radiation therapy in relation to the site of radiation-induced injury. Both acute and chronic complications are discussed in conjunction with appropriate nutrition interventions employed in the management of patients who develop these sequelae. An overall summary is given in Appendix 18-A.

## CENTRAL NERVOUS SYSTEM

Tumors located in the central nervous system by themselves may lead to diminished oral intake by producing lethargy, irritability, somnolence, and confusion. Frequently, there is increased intracranial pressure with resultant headache, nausea, and vomiting. Altered food and fluid intake patterns and electrolyte derangements may ensue from malignancies involving the hypothalamus or pituitary gland. Cranial irradiation may alleviate some symptoms while exacerbating others, especially if cerebral edema supervenes. Moreover, craniospinal radiation therapy may itself induce nausea, vomiting, and

181

anorexia by its direct action on the central nervous system as well as on peripheral tissues (i.e., pharynx and gastrointestinal tract) (Donaldson, 1984; Donaldson & Lenon, 1979).

Corticosteroid therapy may alleviate untoward symptoms by reducing cerebral edema (Donaldson & Lenon, 1979). Tumor or therapy affecting the hypothalamic-pituitary axis may precipitate the syndrome of inappropriate antidiuretic hormone with resultant hyponatremia. This may acutely entail severe fluid restriction until electrolyte abnormalities have resolved. Intake is frequently limited to dry meals during this period with allowed fluid provided as visible water or liquid. Underlying anorexia may be exacerbated by a regimen that often prohibits foods that patients most prefer. Effort must be directed toward increasing the caloric and nutrient density of permitted items during this period. This can be accomplished with the use of added fats, glucose polymers, and protein modules in powdered form. Whenever possible, consumption of liquid nutrition supplements should be encouraged.

Severe nausea and vomiting can lead to weight loss, dehydration, and electrolyte imbalances. Although the underlying cause of these symptoms (e.g., cerebral edema and increased intracranial pressure) can often be effectively treated anorexia may be slow to resolve, and further nutrition deficits may ensue. If efforts to optimize oral nutrient and fluid intake are unsuccessful, alternative nutrition support modalities should be considered. Nasogastric tube feeding may be useful provided that the risk of aspiration is minimal and that nausea and vomiting have sufficiently subsided. Small-bore, flexible feeding tubes may be passed transpylorically (distal to the ligament of Treitz), but tip location should be periodically confirmed because proximal movement into the stomach may occur. Intravenous fluid and electrolyte replacement may be indicated for the short term; long-term support is usually unnecessary, however. Total parenteral nutrition (TPN) is rarely utilized except in cases of severe malnutrition with concomitant gastrointestinal losses for which enteral or peripheral venous support may be inadequate to reverse the deficiency state.

## HEAD AND NECK

Radiation therapy to the oropharynx, nasopharynx, and hypopharynx can result in significant mucosal injury, which is a function of the administered radiation dosage and volume of tissue treated (Donaldson, 1977). Mucositis or stomatitis may occur within the first week of treatment and persist for its duration (Coulston & Darbinian, 1986). Pseudomembrane formation, superficial ulceration, and bleeding may result from progressive denudation of oropharyngeal epithelia (Donaldson, 1977, 1984; Donaldson & Lenon, 1979). In most cases, recovery may be expected 2 to 3 weeks after therapy is discontinued (McAnena & Daly, 1986). Occasionally, however, chronic radiation ulcers develop (Donaldson, 1977, 1984). Inflamed or ulcerated tissues can result in severe oral pain and odynophagia, which in turn can lead to a marked reduction in nutrient intake and subsequent weight loss.

Oropharyngeal irradiation may damage the microvilli of taste cells and their surfaces with resultant alterations in taste sensation (Donaldson, 1984; Donaldson & Lenon, 1979; McAnena & Daly, 1986). Both hypogeusia (with "mouth blindness") and dysgeusia may occur. Manifestations of the latter may include heightened or lowered thresholds for sweet, salty, bitter, and, to a lesser extent, sour taste sensations. Protein-rich foods such as meats, eggs, and dairy products may especially be perceived as abnormal tasting and avoided by patients with radiation-induced dysgeusia (Chencharick & Mossman, 1983; Mossman, Shatzman, & Chencharick, 1982). In contrast, sugar intake may be increased to compensate for a diminished sweet taste acuity (Chencharick & Mossman, 1983). Interestingly, before receiving treatment some cancer patients experience alterations in taste sensation, which may be related to the tumor-bearing state (Enig, Petersen, Smith, & Larsen, 1987). Subsequent therapy that further impairs taste perception can lead to significant changes in food selection with the attendant risk of caloric and nutrient deficiencies.

Radiation-induced impairment of taste function may occur by the second week of therapy

(Chencharick & Mossman, 1983; Mossman et al., 1982). Although taste sensation usually returns to pretreatment acuity by 1 year after cessation of therapy, recovery may be seen in some patients within a few months. Moreover, long-term effects of radiation therapy on taste function have been reported. These findings suggest that there is a small subset of patients whose treatment-induced changes in taste perception may never completely resolve (Mossman et al., 1982). The practitioner must identify persistently offending foods and replace them with acceptable items containing essential nutrients. For example, meat may continue to have a bitter or metallic taste; thus poultry, fish, *tofu* (soybean curd), legumes, eggs, cheeses, and other protein-rich foods should be offered.

Altered sense of smell (dysosmia) may be another sequela of radiation therapy to the head and neck region. This complication results from damage to the peripheral olfactory apparatus located in the nasopharynx (Donaldson, 1984; Donaldson & Lenon, 1979). If the radiation field includes the oropharynx and nasopharynx, there is the potential for impairment of both taste and smell perception. Patients so affected may find eating to be an unpleasant, even dreaded experience. Not infrequently, patients develop learned food aversions as an additional consequence of altered gustatory and olfactory sensation (Kokal, 1985; McAnena & Daly, 1986; Chencharick & Mossman, 1983). Food groups may be avoided (e.g., milk and dairy products or red meats), so that overall intake becomes inadequate to maintain body weight and nutrient reserves (Chencharick & Mossman, 1983).

Salivary glands included in the irradiated field also incur significant damage. Changes in the volume and quality of secretions ensue, which may have serious nutrition consequences. A marked decrease in salivary flow rate has been observed after the first week of treatment, with continued diminution throughout the period of radiation exposure (Chencharick & Mossman, 1983; Mossman et al., 1982). By the completion of therapy many patients experience severe xerostomia, which creates chewing and swallowing difficulties and leads to depressed oral intake. Diminished salivary flow may persist for more

than 5 years after radiation. Partial recovery of gland function has been observed to occur as early as 2 to 6 months after cessation of treatment. Major determinants include patient age, radiation dosage, and field of exposure (Makkonen & Nordman, 1987).

Radiation-induced damage to major salivary glands also alters the character of saliva. Secretions change from clear, watery, and neutral to viscous, acidic, and semiopaque as the result of the presence of abnormally large quantities of organic material (Donaldson, 1977, 1984). Dysphagia commonly ensues and in turn leads to a marked reduction in oral intake (Donaldson, 1984; Kokal, 1985; Donaldson & Lenon, 1979). Mucosal injury to surrounding tissues, alterations in the quantity and quality of saliva, and an accompanying increase in oral bacteria with its high cariogenic potential accelerate the formation of dental caries (Donaldson, 1977, 1984; Donaldson & Lenon, 1979). No longer protected by the inherent cleansing mechanism that saliva affords, teeth become covered by a tenacious material that is particularly vulnerable to bacterial attack. Additional sequelae that further promote formation of caries are lowered intraoral *p*H levels and decreased quantities of salivary immunoglobulins and protective enzymes (Donaldson, 1977, 1984; Donaldson & Lenon, 1979; McAnena & Daly, 1986). Radiation may affect developing teeth by inflicting direct cellular damage as well as altering cell replication. Once formed, teeth may undergo structural changes if radiation denatures or disrupts organic components that make up the tooth matrix. Resultant symptoms are typically enhanced sensitivity to heat, cold, or concentrated sweets (Donaldson, 1977; Donaldson & Lenon, 1979). To avoid significant interference with energy and nutrient intake foods and beverages should be offered at room temperature, and specific foods identified as inducing dental pain should be avoided.

Late-onset effects of head and neck radiation therapy include chronic mucosal ulceration, radiation-induced osteonecrosis, and trismus (Donaldson, 1977; Kokal, 1985; Donaldson & Lenon, 1979; McAnena & Daly, 1986). Each of these complications can result in suboptimal nutrient intake from attendant pain or mechanical impairment. Osteonecrosis involves the mandible in the vast majority of cases, and a significant number of patients require a partial mandibulectomy (Kokal, 1985; McAnena & Daly, 1986). Associated problems with mastication and deglutition are common and adversely affect food intake. Trismus or tetany of the jaw, resulting from tumor infiltration or postradiation fibrosis of primary mastication muscles, may preclude intake completely in severe cases (Donaldson, 1977).

Consistent oral hygiene is imperative to prevent or reduce the incidence of infection. Sterile dilute sodium bicarbonate solutions soothe inflamed tissue, normalize intraoral $pH$ levels, and effectively clear the mouth of viscous salivary secretions (Donaldson, 1977; Donaldson & Lenon, 1979). Thrice-daily rinses with chlorhexidine (0.12% or diluted 1:1 with sterile water) may afford further antiseptic protection and alleviation of pain. Use of neutral sodium fluoride solutions is recommended during treatment to minimize the risk of or to prevent dental decay (Donaldson, 1977; Donaldson & Lenon, 1979). After completion of therapy, topical fluoride treatments with gel or mouth wash should continue on a daily basis. Commercial mouth washes, rather than alleviating symptoms, may produce further tissue irritation or disrupt the balance of oral flora with resultant mycotic superinfection (Donaldson, 1977). Gentle but effective brushing and flossing of teeth and gums should be an integral component of the daily regimen and should proceed after appropriate technique has been demonstrated by the patient. The extent of mucosal injury is the primary factor limiting the frequency with which these procedures may be performed.

Oropharyngeal mucositis and associated pain may preclude ingestion of adequate food and fluid intake. Alterations in diet consistency and texture toward foods that are soft and nonirritating as well as augmentation of caloric and nutrient density may be useful temporizing measures. Alcohol, tobacco, caffeine, and foods that may be chemically or thermally irritating (e.g., hot or spicy) should be excluded (Chencharick & Mossman, 1983). In many cases, weight loss inevitably supervenes unless aggressive efforts are directed toward the patient's nutrition support. Nasogastric or orogastric tube feeding may be indicated to provide nutrient and fluid requirements for patients with intact gastrointestinal function (Hearne et al., 1985). If the osmolality can be tolerated, highly calorie-dense formulas may be the more appropriate choice, especially in volume-sensitive individuals or if a cyclic or nocturnal regimen is desired. Such formulas should be initiated at half strength but increased to full strength before volume is significantly advanced if patient tolerance permits. Careful, consistent monitoring is essential to avoid or minimize potential complications and to foster patient compliance.

Xerostomia can create chewing and swallowing difficulties and render unprotected oral mucosa vulnerable to chemical, thermal, and mechanical irritants. Symptoms may be relieved by use of synthetic saliva substitutes and salivary stimulants such as citric acid–containing beverages, sugarless gum, and lemon drops (Donaldson, 1977; Chencharick & Mossman, 1983). Dietary texture and consistency modifications (e.g., soft, room temperature, bland, and not too salty) are often necessary to minimize discomfort. Although increased liquid consumption may offer patients symptomatic relief, water, unlike salivary mucin, has no lubricating and hence no protective properties (Chencharick & Mossman, 1983). For this reason use of sauces and gravies, especially those with a high-fat content, should be encouraged for their lubricating effects and high calorie content (Hearne et al., 1985).

Radiation-induced alterations in taste and smell may have a profound impact on the patient's nutrition status. Once-favorite foods may suddenly be perceived as tasteless or intolerably sweet, bitter, or salty. Learned food aversions are a natural consequence of dysgeusia, and it is not unusual for patients to avoid many protein-rich and calorically dense items (Chencharick & Mossman, 1983). Furthermore, taste fatigue may result from what is frequently a monotonous dietary regimen (Hearne, 1985). Eating can thus become such an anxiety ridden, repugnant experience that anorexia emerges as a major problem. These adverse consequences may necessitate interim use of tube feeding to avert further weight loss in patients whose nutrition status is already severely compromised. For other individuals, redirection of food toward stimulation of other, more intact senses (i.e., olfaction, vision, taction, and audition) may result in improved appetite and hence improved intake (Chencharick & Mossman, 1983). Food should be presented in an attractive manner with attention to color combination, portion sizes, and texture.

Effective nutrition management of radiation therapy patients with altered perceptions of taste or smell entails ongoing identification of food preferences and aversions as well as evaluation of appetite and food intake and utilization. This approach enables appropriate dietary modifications and substitutions to be made without frustrating efforts to maximize nutrient intake. Use of oral zinc (as zinc sulfate) supplements to ameliorate taste function has met with variable patient response (Chencharick & Mossman, 1983). As is the case with any patient, actual or potential nutrient deficiencies should be identified and corrected throughout that individual's treatment course. Unless a specific pharmacologic effect has been documented and is desired, supplementation (in the absence of underlying deficiency) of one essential nutrient to the exclusion of others may create toxicities or imbalances.

Patients with head and neck cancer are frequently malnourished at the outset of radiation therapy. Contributing factors include predisposing behavior patterns as well as physical effects of the tumor on food intake and utilization. Subsequent therapy may result in further nutrition sequelae, leaving the patient in such a debilitated and depleted state that wound healing is impaired, immune function is compromised, and tolerance to therapy is diminished. Use of nutrition support in such patients is justified because the effects of treatment can be expected to preclude adequate nutrient intake. Selecting the appropriate modality is governed largely by gastrointestinal function and the ability of the regimen nutritionally to rehabilitate or at least to maintain the patient during radiation therapy (Donaldson, 1984). Enteral support by means of nasogastric or gastrostomy feeding tube may be effective in achieving the desired outcome; gas-

trointestinal tolerance may be a limiting factor, however, especially in the face of antecedent malnutrition. On the other hand, for patients who develop chronic complications of head and neck radiation therapy tube feeding is likely to be the most appropriate choice. TPN should be considered for malnourished patients who are undergoing a protracted course of radiation therapy and for whom enteral nutrition support is either contraindicated or has been ineffective in reversing weight loss.

Regardless of the route of administration, it must be emphasized that nutrition rehabilitation should be approached carefully, with gradual increments in caloric and nutrient support as patient tolerance is demonstrated. Overly zealous attempts at repletion can precipitate metabolic abnormalities or hepatic dysfunction and may result in undesirable or disproportionate weight gain (i.e., excessive adipose tissue deposition without improvement in visceral protein reserves or skeletal muscle mass) (Sax & Bower, 1988; Solomons, 1985; Weinsier & Krumdieck, 1981; Askanazi, Elwyn, Silverberg, Rosenbaum, & Kinney, 1980). Individual patient response to nutrition support should be consistently monitored so that appropriate adjustments in the regimen can be made.

## THORAX

Irradiation of thoracic malignancies commonly produces esophagitis. Consequently, patients may complain of dysphagia 2 to 3 weeks after initiation of therapy. Symptoms may persist for the duration of and for several weeks after the completion of therapy (Donaldson, 1977; Donaldson & Lenon, 1979). Food intake may be significantly reduced during this period, with ensuing weight loss. Protracted radiation exposure of the esophagus and pharynx may result acutely in epithelial denudement and submucosal edema. Chronic manifestations of radiation injury include fibrosis, stenosis, and, in cases involving an esophageal malignancy, fistula formation, ulceration, and perforation. These complications are attributable to local tumor necrosis and the lower radiation tolerance of the diseased esophagus relative to its normal counterpart (Donaldson, 1977, 1984; Donaldson & Lenon, 1979).

Radiation injury to the esophagus may be intensified by concomitant or even subsequent administration of certain chemotherapeutic agents (Donaldson, 1977, 1982; Donaldson & Lenon, 1979; McAnena & Daly, 1986). The mechanism of enhancement is either an additive toxic effect (e.g., with vinblastine, hydroxyurea, and procarbazine) or a synergistic effect (e.g., with dactinomycin and doxorubicin) (Donaldson, 1982; McDonald & Tirumali, 1984; Mitchell & Schein, 1982). Moreover, dactinomycin and doxorubicin may elicit a recall phenomenon, which manifests as recurrent injury to a previously irradiated area after drug administration. This reactivation may occur weeks to months after radiation therapy (Mitchell & Schein, 1982).

The mucosal insult observed with combined therapies may be quite severe, making adequate oral intake impossible during the acute period of injury. Symptoms usually resolve, however, although in some cases esophageal stricture may develop and necessitate medical intervention to prevent starvation (Donaldson, 1977; Donaldson & Lenon, 1979). Mucosal inflammation may be subsequently associated with abnormal motility, which leads to impaired acid clearing from the esophagus (McDonald & Tirumali, 1984). This problem may be exacerbated by concomitant xerostomia (induced by chemotherapy or oropharyngeal irradiation) because saliva also plays an important role in neutralizing refluxed acid in the esophagus. Consequently peptic esophagitis may be yet another complication, creating more pain and dysphagia. Fungal or viral superinfection may follow the immunosuppressive effects of combination chemotherapy and irradiation. The severity of symptoms is variable and can be quite pronounced (McDonald & Tirumali, 1984; Mitchell & Schein, 1982).

In mild cases of radiation-induced esophagitis, appropriate dietary modifications may enable the patient to meet fluid and nutrient requirements by oral intake alone. Soft, bland foods (e.g., cooked cereal, custard, and canned or stewed fruit) served at a temperature acceptable to the patient are often well tolerated. Removal of alcohol, caffeine, and other chemical irritants from the diet helps minimize pain associated with food ingestion. Topical anesthetic agents (e.g., viscous lidocaine) and analgesics applied or taken before meals may alleviate dysphagia and pain and thus facilitate eating (Donaldson, 1977; Donaldson & Lenon, 1979). In cases of suspected or documented peptic esophagitis, antireflux measures and antacid therapy may be efficacious (McDonald & Tirumali, 1984).

Nutrition care should be directed toward augmenting the caloric and nutrient density of acceptable foods. Generous use of fat and glucose polymers, within the constraints of patient tolerance, is recommended to increase calorie intake. Addition of enteral protein modules and dry milk solids to appropriate beverages and predominantly liquid foods (e.g., soups) are practical ways to enhance protein intake. Significant problems with deglutition may necessitate conversion to a predominantly liquid diet, which can be optimized by use of the more palatable commercial nutrition supplements. Such regimens, however, may quickly become monotonous and lead to taste fatigue and, ultimately, rejection by the patient. Regular counseling and encouragement may provide some amelioration, especially if current intake-associated problems are accurately identified. Creative manipulation of dietary components within narrow tolerance constraints may be difficult but is usually feasible barring severe pain, obstruction, or poor patient compliance. Examples of well-tolerated and accepted foods include fruit-flavored milk shakes made with yogurt, ice cream, sherbet, or nondairy frozen dessert; peanut butter malted milk, and moist casseroles seasoned with mild herbs that enhance flavor without inducing oral pain.

Tube feeding may be necessary for patients who cannot maintain body weight or who presented for therapy with malnutrition. In cases of esophageal fistula or stricture gastrostomy tube feeding is required, either permanently or until the anatomic or physiologic problem is corrected or attenuated. The choice of appropriate formula and administration regimen varies with individual patient tolerance, nutrition status, and lifestyle. Consistent follow-up to assess improvement in nutrition status and to identify any problems that the patient may have with respect to formula or regimen tolerance or administration is key to a successful outcome.

## ABDOMEN AND PELVIS

Low-dose irradiation of the stomach may result in diminished secretion of free hydrochloric acid and pepsin. Supervening anorexia and nausea may occur but are usually mild and self-limited and thus have a minimal impact on food intake. With high-dose gastric irradiation, however, ulcers may subsequently develop and induce severe epigastric pain, vomiting, bleeding, and progressive weight loss (Donaldson, 1977, 1984; Donaldson & Lenon, 1979). Surgical resection may be ultimately required for mitigation of symptoms (Donaldson, 1984; Donaldson & Lenon, 1979).

Acute effects of radiation therapy to the small and large intestine include nausea, vomiting, and diarrhea. These symptoms may occur soon after initiation of treatment (nausea and vomiting usually have an immediate onset; diarrhea may present after 1 week of therapy) and persist throughout its duration (McAnena & Daly, 1986). Although resolution is usually seen within several weeks of completion of therapy, patients may incur significant nutrition insult. Acute radiation-induced enteritis is characterized by reduced mitotic activity of intestinal epithelial cells and shortening of villi, both of which are histologic abnormalities caused by direct mucosal injury by ionizing radiation. This disruption of the normal intestinal architecture can result in malabsorption of fat, protein, and carbohydrates as well as severe fluid imbalance and electrolyte derangements (Donaldson, 1977, 1984; Donaldson & Lenon, 1979). The extent and severity of radiation injury and associated nutrition sequelae are related to the dose and treatment volume of administered radiation, the type of neoplasm, prior surgical history, concurrent use of chemotherapeutic agents, and overall performance status of the patient (Donaldson, 1984). Antecedent small vessel disease, such as that observed in hypertension and diabetes, has been identified as an important

predisposing factor (Donaldson, 1984; Donaldson & Lenon, 1979; McAnena & Daly, 1986). Moreover, (gastrointestinal) bacteria, which are known to flourish in the aftermath of early tissue destruction, may contribute to the pathogenesis of radiation injury (Donaldson, 1984; Donaldson & Lenon, 1979).

The malabsorption syndrome may encompass a protein-losing enteropathy, disaccharide (lactose) and protein maldigestion or malabsorption, steatorrhea, and trace element, vitamin, and electrolyte deficiencies (Donaldson, 1984; Kokal, 1985). Intake may be significantly limited by the discomfort associated with diarrhea and abdominal cramping. What is ingested may be poorly (if at all) utilized or further exacerbate symptoms. Dehydration, severe electrolyte imbalances, and significant weight loss can ensue if the diarrhea does not remit or if losses are not adequately replaced.

Delayed effects of radiation-induced intestinal injury may not present for months to years after completion of therapy (Kokal, 1985; Galland & Spencer, 1985). Associated complications include chronic enteritis or colitis, ulceration, fistula formation, fibrosis, stricture formation, partial or complete bowel obstruction, hemorrhage, and perforation (Donaldson, 1977; Donaldson & Lenon, 1979). Concomitant use of certain chemotherapeutic agents may enhance the risk of late stricture formation or small bowel obstruction by an additive or synergistic toxic effect (Donaldson, 1982; Mitchell & Schein, 1982). Many patients who incur these sequelae have also sustained severe acute radiation enteritis, which suggests that early injury presages late-onset complications.

Patients with chronic radiation enteritis may incur significant to severe malabsorption, which is clinically manifested as protein-calorie malnutrition. Adipose tissue reserves and skeletal muscle mass may be severely depleted, with the patient appearing to be wasted and even cachectic. Visceral protein stores may also be compromised secondary to intercurrent infection; moreover, hypoalbuminemia may reflect enteric protein losses. Intermittent obstructive episodes may entirely preclude oral or enteral intake for significant periods of time. Resulting weight loss may be extremely debilitating to the patient when it is superimposed on a preexisting state of chronic undernutrition.

In some cases, surgical resection is possible if radiation-induced injury is limited to a small portion of the small or large intestine (Pezner & Archambeau, 1985). Although removal of the involved segment may ameliorate symptoms, nutrient deficiencies may arise de novo if the remaining small bowel cannot assume the absorptive functions of the resected area. For example, the distal ileum is the site of absorption of bile salts, vitamin $B_{12}$, and, to a lesser extent, zinc. Surgical resection of this segment can result in malabsorption of fat and fat-soluble vitamins with attendant steatorrhea, vitamin $B_{12}$, and zinc deficiencies, especially if the remaining ileum has sustained radiation damage. The jejunum is not able to acquire the absorptive physiology of the distal small bowel. Thus, to avert deficiencies, specific nutrients must be administered by the appropriate route or in the most utilizable form (e.g., intramuscular vitamin $B_{12}$ injections and water-miscible, fat-soluble vitamins). When the radiation field has included an extensive area small bowel surgery is usually infeasible, and the patient may experience no remission of symptoms. Chronic radiation enteritis can be progressive, with new developments carrying a high probability of compounding existing nutrition deficits (Galland & Spencer, 1985; Beer, Fan, & Halsted, 1985). Patients with initial presentation of fistula, perforation, and (to a lesser degree) stricture may be especially at increased risk of developing new lesions that may necessitate surgical or medical intervention (Galland & Spencer, 1985).

A sound knowledge of gastrointestinal physiology, digestion, and absorption is imperative if potential nutrient intake and utilization problems are to be anticipated and deficiencies effectively prevented or minimized. Management of acute effects of gastrointestinal irradiation should be initially aimed at alleviating symptoms, replacing fluid and electrolyte losses, and correcting any overt nutrient deficiencies. Administration of antiemetics, antispasmodic or anticholinergic agents, and antidiarrheal drugs may provide effective, temporary relief (Donaldson, 1977; Donaldson & Lenon, 1979). Withholding food at least 2 hours before and after treatments may

significantly reduce the incidence of nausea and vomiting and potentially minimize subsequent development of learned food aversions (Coulston & Darbinian, 1986). Fluid, electrolyte (including magnesium, phosphorus, and calcium), and acid-base balances must be monitored carefully; intravenous replacement is required if attempts at enteral repletion exacerbate diarrhea or result in dehydration.

Antacid therapy and small, frequent meals (devoid of alcohol and caffeine) may attenuate gastric irritation. Specific foods to be avoided are usually determined on a highly individual basis. Therefore, accurate identification of patient preferences and tolerances must be made by the practitioner. Such an approach is more responsible and efficacious than merely restricting traditionally irritating foods (e.g., spicy, hot foods and raw vegetables), a measure that may result in unnecessarily depriving the patient of eating-associated pleasure without conferring any therapeutic benefit. If significant weight loss ensued from preoperative vomiting, pain, and anorexia, postoperative jejunostomy tube feedings should be considered for patients with intact gastrointestinal tracts; TPN should be considered for those without an adequately functioning bowel. Nutrition support can be tapered as oral intake is tolerated and after weight loss has been clearly reversed or halted.

After surgery, depending on the location of the ulcer and the area resected, patients may develop minimal to significant nutrition-related complications. Potential problems include vitamin $B_{12}$ deficiency (from lack of intrinsic factor), delayed gastric emptying, or dumping syndrome (if there was vagus nerve involvement). Appropriate adjustments in meal composition (e.g., meals with little or no concentrated sweets, including juices, and high in fat and protein; liquids administered between meals in small volumes), size, and frequency may be necessary to alleviate symptoms and to avert weight loss. Periodic intramuscular injections of vitamin $B_{12}$ obviate deficiency in this essential nutrient.

Radiation enteritis frequently requires dietary modification to avoid exacerbating malabsorption and its attendant symptoms. A secondary lactose intolerance, resulting from radiation-induced injury to the intestinal brush border, frequently occurs and is best managed by provisionally removing this disaccharide from the patient's diet. This need not result in complete exclusion of dairy products and hence of an excellent source of calories, protein, and essential minerals. Lactose-reduced milk and milk products (e.g., LactAid) are now commercially available and may be substituted for milk.

Enzyme activity can usually be expected to return once mucosal damage resolves and normal histology is restored (Welsh, 1981). Low-residue foods are easily digested and may help reduce fecal output. Empirical restriction of fat in the presence of malabsorption and steatorrhea is common clinical practice, but symptomatic relief and overall nutrition benefit may be variable (Beer et al., 1985; Woolf, Miller, Kurian, & Jeejeebhoy, 1983). Initially, it is advisable at least moderately to restrict fat and subsequently to increase the amount in the diet by graded increments as patient tolerance permits. Judicious use of medium-chain triglycerides may provide a concentrated source of calories without further exacerbating the diarrhea. Attention to fat-soluble vitamin status is essential to prevent deficiencies and associated physiologic sequelae. Aqueous preparations of vitamins A, D, E, and K are available; in severe cases of malabsorption, high-risk patients may require intramuscular or parenteral administration of vitamins. Some clinicians advocate the use of cholestyramine to bind unabsorbed bile salts, thus preventing their deleterious effects on colonic mucosa (Kokal, 1985). This treatment may cause significant nausea and abdominal distention, however. Alterations in microbial flora, intestinal motility, and villous morphology may lead to small bowel bacterial overgrowth, as mentioned above (Donaldson, 1977, 1984). Resultant fermentation of unabsorbed carbohydrate and deconjugation of bile salts can aggravate underlying malabsorption. This potential development should be ruled out and appropriately treated if diagnosed before stringent dietary restrictions are imposed.

Specific diet therapy has been associated with histologic reversal of delayed radiation enteritis with small bowel obstruction. Five children who developed these complications were treated with a low-fat, low-residue regimen free of gluten, milk and milk products, and lactose for periods ranging from 1 to 2 years (Donaldson et al., 1977). In each of the patients, radiographic and histologic reversal of severe intestinal injury was observed coincident with the diet. Furthermore no subsequent episode of small bowel obstruction occurred, and gradual resumption of a normal diet was successfully achieved. Physicians affiliated with the institute where this study was performed (Institut Gustave-Roussy in Villejuif, France) have since utilized this regimen prophylactically for children undergoing combination high-dose hemiabdominal or whole abdominal irradiation and chemotherapy. Reportedly, there have been no cases of either severe acute or delayed enteritis since this supportive measure has been employed (Donaldson, 1982, 1984). Routine use of such a restricted regimen may be limited by the low feasibility of patient compliance. Nonetheless, the possibility that preventive diet therapy may obviate or minimize radiation-induced enteritis is intriguing and warrants further investigation.

Use of liquid elemental or defined-formula diets may benefit patients who have significantly impaired intestinal digestive and absorptive capacities in the absence of bowel obstruction. Oral administration is frequently limited by characteristic unpalatability of the formulas. Such formulas are compositionally hyperosmolar, low in residue and fat, and lactose free. Protein sources range from free amino acids to hydrolysates with various proportions of dipeptides, tripeptides, and polypeptides. Typically carbohydrate, which constitutes the major percentage of calories, is in the form of glucose oligosaccharides or hydrolysis products of corn starch.

Tube feeding by the most appropriate route may be indicated for patients who, though unable orally to consume adequate volumes of elemental formula, still have sufficient intestinal function remaining to permit enteral nourishment. Regimens should be initiated with diluted formula (i.e., at no greater than 300 mOsm/kg) and subsequently advanced, according to patient tolerance, by volume (if the fluid is required) or by strength (if hydration status is intact). Finally, there will be a cohort of patients undergoing curative radiation therapy for abdominopelvic malignancies whose malnutrition cannot be effectively reversed with enteral nutrition support. For these individuals, TPN should be instituted and continued until improvement in nutrition status is achieved and successful transition to oral or enteral support has occurred.

There is an ongoing controversy regarding the relative benefits of bowel rest compared to bowel use to reduce radiation injury during a course of therapy. The rationale for provisionally bypassing the intestine is that mucosal injury will not be further exacerbated by pancreatic secretions and bile flow and thus will heal more readily and effectively. On the other hand, it has been argued that the functional capacity of the intestinal mucosa is contingent on enteral provision of appropriate trophic factors that preserve villous architecture (Donaldson, 1984). These issues should be included in the decision-making process employed to select the most appropriate mode of nutrition support.

The morbidity associated with chronic radiation-induced enteritis may necessitate the long-term use of nutrition support in the form of gastrostomy or jejunostomy tube feeding or TPN. Patients receiving such regimens frequently do so on a nocturnal or cyclic basis to allow an 8- to 12-hour unencumbered period during the day. Barring cases of severe complications (e.g., bowel obstruction, stricture or fistula formation, or perforation), oral intake may be permitted to afford some pleasure and partially to restore normalcy to the patient's lifestyle. Often, dietary modifications are necessary because of intestinal damage resulting in lactase deficiency or disaccharide intolerance, bile salt and fat malabsorption, and bezoar formation, among others. These sequelae may be observed in many patients with late presenting effects of abdominopelvic irradiation (Beer et al., 1985). Nutrition management substantially parallels that employed in cases of acute radiation enteritis. A major divergent focus, however, is helping the patient develop appropriate strategies for coping with chronic disease and illness (e.g., learning to take one day at a time; establishing a routine, such as a regular meal pattern; and varying daily activities).

## CONCLUSION

With the emergence of radiation therapy as a major oncologic treatment modality has been an accompanying recognition of its secondary complications. Normal tissues lying in the designated therapeutic field may be subject to a vast spectrum of injury of variable onset, intensity, and duration. Concomitant nutrition sequelae may be equally diverse and associated with significant morbidity. Although curative doses of radiation inevitably produce some degree of untoward effects, careful planning of the treatment regimen may partially spare normal tissue and preserve function without diminishing therapeutic efficacy. The extent of salivary dysfunction, for example, directly correlates with the volume of major glands irradiated. If part of the parotid or submandibular glands may be shielded from the radiation beam, mild rather than severe xerostomia may result (Makkonen & Nordman, 1987). Similarly, the risk of radiation-induced enteritis may be minimized by close attention to the time, dose, and fractionation of administered radiation. Excessive normal tissue damage may be prevented by use of lead shielding or beam-shaping devices (Donaldson, 1977; Donaldson & Lenon, 1979).

In a collateral fashion, anticipation of untoward nutrition consequences of radiation therapy may forestall or attenuate weight loss or malabsorption. Whether this is achieved by prophylactic dietary modifications, aggressive counseling aimed especially at maximizing intake during therapy-free periods, or a combination thereof is contingent on individual patient considerations and response as well as the experience of the involved nutrition professional. Initial nutrition evaluation should concur with the inception of radiation therapy. Malnourished patients or those at increased risk of becoming so early in the treatment course can thus be identified and appropriate interventional measures taken. Throughout treatment, close attention to subjective complaints as well as serial monitoring of nutrition assessment parameters are crucial to effective patient management. Response, as measured by anthropometric changes, nitrogen balance data, and metabolic indices, and tolerance to nutrition support must be carefully and consistently assessed so that appropriate modifications can be made in individual regimens. Follow-up and support should continue after completion of therapy until problems with food intake and utilization are resolved and nutrition restoration effected.

There remains a paucity of data demonstrating the favorable impact of nutrition support on tolerance and response to radiation therapy, decreased incidence of treatment-associated complications, and overall survival. Nevertheless, improving or maintaining the patient's nutrition status may at the very least provide an increased sense of well-being and thus enhance the quality of life regardless of the ultimate prognosis.

## REFERENCES

Askanazi, J., Elwyn, D.H., Silverberg, P.A., Rosenbaum, S.H., & Kinney, J.M. (1980). Respiratory distress secondary to a high carbohydrate load: A case report. *Surgery, 87,* 596–598.

Beer, W.H., Fan, A., & Halsted, C.H. (1985). Clinical and nutritional implications of radiation enteritis. *American Journal of Clinical Nutrition, 41,* 85–91.

Chencharick, J.D., & Mossman, K.L. (1983). Nutritional consequences of the radiotherapy of head and neck cancer. *Cancer, 51,* 811–815.

Coulston, A.M., & Darbinian, J.D. (1986). Nutrition management of patients with cancer. *Topics in Clinical Nutrition, 1,* 26–36.

Donaldson, S.S. (1977). Nutritional consequences of radiotherapy. *Cancer Research 37,* 2407–2413.

Donaldson, S.S. (1982). Effects of therapy on nutritional status of the pediatric cancer patient. *Cancer Research, 42* (Suppl.), 729s–736s.

Donaldson, S.S. (1984). Nutritional support as an adjunct to radiation therapy. *Journal of Parenteral and Enteral Nutrition, 8,* 302–310.

Donaldson, S.S., Jundt, S., Ricour, C., Sarrazin, D., Lemerle, J., & Schweisguth, O. (1977). Radiation enteritis in children: A retrospective review, clinicopathologic correlation, and dietary management. *Cancer, 35,* 1167–1178.

Donaldson, S.S., & Lenon, R.A. (1979). Alterations of nutritional status: Impact of chemotherapy and radiation therapy. *Cancer, 43,* 2036–2052.

Enig, B., Petersen, H.N., Smith, D.F., & Larsen, B. (1987). Food preferences, nutrient intake and nutritional status in cancer patients. *Acta Oncologia, 26,* 301–305.

Galland, R.B., & Spencer, J. (1985). The natural history of clinically established radiation enteritis. *Lancet, 1,* 1257–1258.

Hearne, B.E., Dunaj, J.M., Daly, J.M., Strong, E.W., Vikram, B., LePorte, B.J., & DeCrosse, J.J. (1985). Enteral nutrition support in head and neck cancer: Tube vs. oral feeding during radiation therapy. *Journal of the American Dietetic Association, 85,* 669–677.

Kokal, W.A. (1985). The impact of antitumor therapy on nutrition. *Cancer, 55,* 273–278.

Makkonen, T.A., & Nordman, E. (1987). Estimation of long-term salivary gland damage induced by radiotherapy. *Acta Oncologia, 26,* 307–312.

McAnena, O.J., & Daly, J.M. (1986). Impact of antitumor therapy on nutrition. *Surgical Clinics of North America, 66,* 1213–1228.

McDonald, G.B., & Tirumali, N. (1984). Intestinal and liver toxicity of antineoplastic drugs. *Western Journal of Medicine, 140,* 250–259.

Mitchell, E.P., & Schein, P.S. (1982). Gastrointestinal toxicity of chemotherapeutic agents. *Seminars in Oncology, 9,* 52–64.

Mossman, K., Shatzman, A., & Chencharick, J. (1982). Long-term effects of radiotherapy on taste and salivary function in man. *International Journal of Radiation Oncology/Biology/Physics, 8,* 991–997.

Pezner, R., & Archambeau, J.O. (1985). Critical evaluation of the role of nutritional support for radiation therapy patients. *Cancer, 55,* 263–267.

Sax, H.C., & Bower, R.H. (1988). Hepatic complications of total parenteral nutrition. *Journal of Parenteral and Enteral Nutrition, 12,* 615–618.

Solomons, N.W. (1985). Rehabilitating the severely malnourished infant and child. *Journal of the American Dietetic Association, 85,* 28–39.

Weinsier, R.L., & Krumdieck, C.L. (1981). Death resulting from overzealous total parenteral nutrition: The refeeding syndrome revisited. *American Journal of Clinical Nutrition, 34,* 393–399.

Welsh, J.D. (1981). Causes of isolated low lactase levels and lactose intolerance. In D.M. Paige & T.M. Bayless (Eds.), *Lactose digestion: Clinical and nutritional implications* (pp. 69–79). Baltimore: Johns Hopkins University Press.

Woolf, G.M., Miller, C., Kurian, R., & Jeejeebhoy, K.N. (1983). Diet for patients with a short bowel: High fat or high carbohydrate? *Gastroenterology, 84,* 823–828.

# Acute and Chronic Effects of Radiation Therapy: Nutrition Sequelae and Recommended Management

| Radiation-Induced Complication | Corresponding Field of Radiation Administered | Nutrition Consequences | Suggested Intervention(s) |
|---|---|---|---|
| Nausea and vomiting* | Central nervous system, abdomen and pelvis | Decreased oral intake, weight loss | Have the patient refrain from food and fluid consumption 2 hours before and after treatment. Do not offer favorite or new foods during the most acute phase of nausea and vomiting. Identify specific foods and odors (e.g., fish and cruciferous vegetables) that exacerbate symptoms, and avoid or remove them. Encourage small, frequent meals. Alternate liquid and dry items. Avoid excessively sweet, spicy, and fatty or fried foods. Emphasize easily digested foods that are cold, cool, or at room temperature (e.g., ginger ale, flavored ices, nonacidic juices; dry cereal and bread products; rice; boiled potato). Maintain adequate ventilation. |
| | | Dehydration, electrolyte imbalances | Consider intravenous support if efforts to replace fluid and electrolyte losses enterally are unsuccessful. |
| Anorexia* | Central nervous system, head and neck, abdomen and pelvis | Weight loss | Encourage small, frequent meals. Augment caloric density of foods by means of generous use of fats (e.g., butter, margarine, vegetable oil, mayonnaise, cream), canned fruits in heavy syrup, dried fruits, glucose polymers. Encourage high-protein foods (e.g., eggs, poultry, fish, soybean curd), or enhance protein content of diet by |

*Primarily acute.
†May be both acute and chronic.
‡Primarily chronic.

| Radiation-Induced Complication | Corresponding Field of Radiation Administered | Nutrition Consequences | Suggested Intervention(s) |
|---|---|---|---|
| | | | adding dry milk solids to appropriate liquids, chopped meats to soups or casseroles, shredded cheese to sauces and vegetables, powdered protein modules to liquids or moist solids and by spreading peanut butter on crackers, vegetable sticks, fruit slices. Encourage liquids between meals. Emphasize liquids of high nutrient and caloric density (e.g., milk shakes, liquid nutrition supplements) rather than noncaloric beverages or those composed primarily of carbohydrate. Create a mealtime ambience that is relaxed, nonthreatening, unhurried. Present food in an attractive manner. Encourage exercise, increased activity as tolerated to stimulate appetite. |
| Mucositis or stomatitis,* odynophagia,* oropharyngeal ulceration† | Head and neck | Suboptimal caloric and nutrient intake, weight loss | Encourage daily mouth care with sterile, dilute sodium bicarbonate solution. Offer foods that are cool or at room temperature initially. Avoid hot, highly spiced or salty, coarse, dry, acidic foods; emphasize instead smooth or well-blended, bland foods that are moist or liquid at room temperature (e.g., custard, puddings, milk shakes, cream soups, pureed meats and vegetables, soft cooked eggs, cooked cereal, mashed potatoes). Avoid alcohol, tobacco, and caffeine. Consider tube feeding in severe cases in which oral intake is virtually precluded but a feeding tube can be physically tolerated by the patient. |
| Dysgeusia† | Head and neck | Suboptimal caloric and nutrient intake due largely to exclusion of many protein-rich foods, weight loss | Identify specific taste sensations that are altered and to what extent they are altered; correlate findings with specific foods and modify (by appropriate spicing or serving at an acceptable temperature) or substitute with items of comparable nutrient content and composition (e.g., fish, poultry, legumes, cheese, eggs for red meats). Serve food in an attractive manner, placing emphasis on color, texture, and feeling in the mouth. |
| Hypogeusia† | Head and neck | Suboptimal caloric and nutrient intake, weight loss | Identify which taste sensations are particularly blunted or diminished so that effective modifications can be made (e.g., by use of appropriate seasonings, marinade, herbs, spices or selection of saltier or sweeter foods). Determine the temperature (usually warm) at which food is rendered most flavorful or acceptable to the patient. Vary the diet as much as possible to minimize taste fatigue. |

| Radiation-Induced Complication | Corresponding Field of Radiation Administered | Nutrition Consequences | Suggested Intervention(s) |
|---|---|---|---|
| Dysosmia* | Head and neck | Inadequate nutrient intake with resultant weight loss | Ascertain which odors are offensive or favorable to the patient so that they may be eliminated or enhanced. Emphasize visual and tactile aspects of food. |
| Xerostomia† | Head and neck | Chewing and swallowing difficulties, inadequate nutrient intake, eventual weight loss, peptic esophagitis or dysphagia, dental caries (long term) | Encourage daily mouth care and frequent rinsing. Avoid alcohol and tobacco. Increase consumption of citric acid–containing beverages (e.g., lemonade, orange-flavored soft drinks, citrus-flavored juice bars or ices). Consider use of artificial saliva. Offer sugar-free gum or lemon drops. Increase moisture content and lubricating quality of food by use of sauces, gravy, melted butter or margarine, mayonnaise, salad dressings, broths or cream soups. Encourage adequate liquid consumption with meals and throughout the day. |
| Dental caries‡ | Head and neck | Oral pain causing problems with mastication, hence suboptimal caloric and nutrient intake; increased sensitivity to heat, cold, and concentrated sweets; eventual interference with oral intake | Encourage daily mouth care, including rinses with neutral sodium fluoride solution during therapy and use of topical fluoride gel or mouth washes after treatment is completed. Offer foods at room temperature (avoid extremes). Identify and exclude foods that induce dental pain. |
| Radiation-induced osteonecrosis‡ | Head and neck | Impaired ability to chew and swallow with supervening weight loss and malnutrition | Convert to a predominantly liquid or pureed diet. Encourage liquid nutrition supplements of high caloric and nutrient density. Institute tube feeding in cases in which oral intake is severely compromised or precluded. |
| Trismus‡ | Head and neck | Inanition resulting from inability to consume food and fluids | Administer tube feedings to prevent further weight loss and eventually to promote nutrition restoration. |
| Esophagitis and dysphagia* | Thorax | Significant reduction in food intake with eventual weight loss | Modify texture, consistency, and temperature of foods toward mechanically soft (e.g., pureed), nonirritating (i.e., mildly seasoned to bland), smooth, moist. Augment caloric and nutrient density of acceptable foods by use of added fat, glucose polymers, dry milk solids, powdered protein modules. Use commercial liquid nutrition supplements to optimize caloric and nutrient intake. Remove alcohol, caffeine, tobacco, and other chemical irritants (e.g., pepper). Vary the flavor of blended, pureed, and soft foods as tolerated to enhance patient acceptability and to minimize taste fatigue (e.g., try fruit-flavored milk shakes, peanut butter malted milks, |

| Radiation-Induced Complication | Corresponding Field of Radiation Administered | Nutrition Consequences | Suggested Intervention(s) |
|---|---|---|---|
| | | | moist casseroles or pureed meats and vegetables seasoned with mild, nonirritating herbs). Encourage use of viscous lidocaine or analgesics before meals as a temporizing measure. Employ anti-reflux measures and antacid therapy. Consider tube feeding in severe cases in which oral intake is suboptimal despite conversion to a full liquid diet. |
| Esophageal fibrosis, stenosis, stricture formation, fistula formation‡ | Thorax | Severe weight loss and protein-energy malnutrition | Institute gastrostomy tube feedings to maintain or restore nutrition status. |
| Gastrointestinal ulceration† | Abdomen and pelvis | Decreased oral intake with eventual significant to severe weight loss | Encourage small, frequent meals. Institute jejunostomy tube feedings if oral intake is limited, if weight loss ensues, and if the patient has intact intestinal function. In severe cases of gastric ulceration, necessitating surgical resection, consider TPN if bowel is dysfunctional. Identify specific foods that exacerbate symptoms, and provisionally exclude them. |
| | | Delayed gastric emptying | Encourage small, frequent meals. Use fat in moderation initially; increase as tolerated. |
| | | Dumping syndrome | Emphasize small, frequent meals. Limit or exclude concentrated sweets and simple sugars. Provide a diet that is relatively high in fat and protein balanced with complex carbohydrates. Have the patient consume liquids in small volumes between meals. |
| | | Vitamin $B_{12}$ deficiency | Administer periodic intramuscular injections of vitamin $B_{12}$. |
| Diarrhea† | Abdomen and pelvis | Fluid and electrolyte imbalances | Attempt to replace losses enterally by means of oral or tube feeding. Provide intravenous support if above efforts are unsuccessful. |
| Malabsorption,† enteritis† | Abdomen and pelvis | Significant to severe weight loss, protein-calorie malnutrition | Determine the most appropriate route of providing nutrition support on the basis of current gastrointestinal physiology. Offer low-residue or easily digested foods such as refined grains, breads, cereal products; cooked root vegetables; strained applesauce, bananas; boiled and skinned potatoes. Avoid foods that tend to produce flatulence (e.g., cruciferous vegetables, legumes). Exclude whole grains, nuts, seeds, raw vegetables, dried and fresh fruits (except as above). Avoid caffeine. Minimize or avoid spicy foods. Offer elemental or defined-formula diet if the above regimen or intact enteral formula is not tolerated by the patient; administer as tube feeding if formula is unpalatable but intestinal tract |

| Radiation-Induced Complication | Corresponding Field of Radiation Administered | Nutrition Consequences | Suggested Intervention(s) |
|---|---|---|---|
| | | | can still be utilized. Institute TPN if intestinal function is so impaired as to prohibit enteral provision of nutrients or if severe malnutrition cannot be effectively reversed by enteral nutrition support. |
| | | Protein-losing enteropathy | Try to provide adequate dietary protein in the form of foods that are easily digested (e.g., baked or broiled skinless poultry, fish, lean red meats, soft cooked eggs). |
| | | Protein maldigestion or malabsorption | Use liquid elemental or defined formulas that contain protein in the form of free amino acids or dipeptides and tripeptides. Provide protein (and calories) parenterally if the above efforts do not replace losses and reverse nutrient deficiencies. |
| | | Disaccharidase deficiency or carbohydrate malabsorption (lactose intolerance) | Limit or provisionally exclude lactose from the diet. Substitute lactose-free nondairy products or milk and dairy products that have been treated with commercially available lactase enzyme. Offer yogurt with active cultures or cheeses aged more than 90 days in small quantities (initially) as patient tolerance permits. |
| | | Steatorrhea or fat malabsorption | Monitor calcium and magnesium status closely (unabsorbed fatty acids in the intestinal lumen can form insoluble complexes with these divalent cations, thus creating deficiencies). Exclude greasy, fried, and highly fatty foods. Begin with a moderate dietary fat restriction, and augment gingerly as tolerance permits. Consider use of medium-chain triglyceride oil to increase calories without exacerbating symptoms. |
| | | Fat-soluble vitamin deficiencies | Try water-miscible forms of vitamins A, D, E, and K; use intramuscular injections if these are ineffective. |
| | | Vitamin $B_{12}$ deficiency | Administer periodic intramuscular injections. |
| | | Trace element deficiencies (e.g., zinc, copper, selenium). | Monitor serum levels closely. Replace losses or deficits by the most appropriate route (i.e., enteral or parenteral). |
| | | Bile salt malabsorption, which can result in fat malabsorption and fat-soluble vitamin deficiencies | See above discussion. |
| | | Choleretic enteropathy | Consider a trial of cholestyramine, which binds unabsorbed bile salts and thus prevents or alleviates their deleterious effects on colonic mucosa. |

| Radiation-Induced Complication | Corresponding Field of Radiation Administered | Nutrition Consequences | Suggested Intervention(s) |
|---|---|---|---|
| Colitis† | Abdomen and pelvis | Fluid and electrolyte imbalances | Monitor fluid and electrolyte status closely, and replace losses promptly by means of the most appropriate and effective route. |
| Intestinal fistula formation, fibrosis stricture formation, obstruction, perforation, hemorrhage‡ | Abdomen and pelvis | Severe protein-calorie malnutrition, potential starvation if appropriate surgical or medical interventional measures not taken | Attempt to support or rehabilitate enterally if feasible. Choose appropriate formulas (e.g., elemental, predigested, low residue, lactose free); administer as tube feeding (by the most appropriate route, i.e., bypassing ulcerated, obstructed, or fibrotic areas) if patient is unable to take sufficient volume orally. Institute TPN if intestinal lesion precludes enteral delivery of nutrients. Allow home TPN patients with chronic radiation enteritis to eat small amounts of tolerated foods during the day to promote a normal lifestyle. |

# Chapter 19

# Bone Marrow Transplantation: Nutrition Support and Monitoring

*Saundra N. Aker*

## INTRODUCTION TO BONE MARROW TRANSPLANTATION: TREATMENT BACKGROUND

Bone marrow transplantation is now an accepted form of therapy for many hematologic disorders, including aplastic anemia, genetically determined diseases such as thalassemia, and malignant diseases such as leukemia. This procedure is used to restore marrow function in patients given intensive chemotherapy and radiation therapy for malignant disease (Thomas 1987a, 1987b). Marrow transplants have been successful in patients ranging in age from younger than 1 year to almost 60 years, with the best results being obtained in those younger than 30 years (Beatty et al., 1987). Survival rates vary considerably depending on a patient's disease type, such as aplastic anemia or leukemia, remission or relapse, identical or nonidentical human leukocyte antigen (HLA) donor matching; previous treatment for the disease; clinical condition at time of transplant; and age. Survival rates approach 90% in patients with aplastic anemia receiving a marrow transplant early in the

Preparation of this chapter was supported in part by grants CA18029, CA38552, HL36444, and DK35816 from the National Cancer Institute, National Heart, Lung and Blood Institute, and the Clinical Nutrition Research Unit, Department of Health and Human Services.

course of their disease. Patients with acute lymphoblastic leukemia receiving a transplant in second or subsequent remission have a survival rate of 25% to 40%. Patients with acute non-lymphoblastic leukemia in remission have survival rates ranging from 45% to 70%. Survival ranges from 60% to 90% in patients receiving a transplant during the chronic phase of chronic granulocytic leukemia.

Intensive chemotherapy, frequently in conjunction with total body irradiation (TBI), is used to suppress the patient's immune system to destroy diseased marrow and to facilitate engraftment with donor marrow. The therapy is followed by an intravenous infusion of bone marrow from a suitable donor, who is usually a family member but can be an unrelated person (allogeneic transplant), from an identical twin (syngeneic transplant), or from the patient himself or herself (autologous transplant). Donor selection is based on HLA tissue typing, and the National Marrow Donor Registry may be used to identify a matched donor if a suitable family member is not available (Thomas, 1987a). Complications of marrow transplantation include marrow graft rejection, graft-versus-host disease (GVHD), infections, and recurrence of the leukemia.

This chapter discusses the nutrition sequelae of acute and long-term complications of marrow transplantation and current nutrition intervention strategies. Guidelines for nutrition assessment and support modalities are presented.

## ACUTE AND LONG-TERM COMPLICATIONS

### Conditioning Treatment Toxicities

Acute toxic reactions, including nausea, vomiting, cystitis, cardiac toxicity, and diarrhea, occur with the administration of cytotoxic chemotherapy and TBI. After high-dose chemotherapy alone, the patient's hematologic function is in most cases temporarily impaired. Chemotherapy coupled with TBI results in total destruction of marrow function and requires donor marrow for restoration of marrow function. High-dose therapy causes more severe and prolonged symptoms than normal-dose chemotherapy (Wolford & McDonald, 1988). Oropharyngeal mucositis may last for several weeks, but nausea and diarrhea from chemotherapy and TBI seldom persist beyond day 15 (day 0 is the day of marrow infusion).

Patients typically eat little during the conditioning period and the first 30 days after transplant and require aggressive support measures such as total parenteral nutrition (TPN) to maintain body weight. When TPN is initiated during the preparative regimen, it appears favorably to influence long-term survival (Weisdorf et al., 1987). During many types of high-dose chemotherapy infusions, such as those with cyclophosphamide, or during single-dose TBI eating is negligible, with cold, clear liquids including carbonated and fruit-ade beverages being the primary foods requested. If irradiation is given in daily morning fractions appetite may resume by late afternoon, although actual intake averages 50% or less of recommended calorie requirements. If a patient is able to eat in the early transplant period, TPN can be adjusted so as not to exceed nutrient requirements. Among patients with aplastic anemia whose preparative regimen includes only cyclophosphamide, a larger percentage are able to maintain a reasonable level of oral intake than patients with leukemia whose regimen includes TBI (Figs. 19-1 and 19-2).

### Venocclusive Disease

Hepatic venocclusive disease (VOD) is a clinical and histologic process characterized by occlusion of small hepatic veins, damaged hepatocytes, fluid retention, hepatomegaly, and jaundice. It is associated with high-dose conditioning therapy, second marrow transplants, hepatitis before conditioning, and possibly older age and female sex (Jones et al., 1987; McDonald, Sharma, Matthews, Shulman, & Thomas, 1985; Wolford & McDonald, 1988). VOD most commonly occurs in patients with leukemia. The incidence of VOD among patients receiving marrow transplant for malignancy is approximately 20% but may approach 50% in a high-risk patient population. Although nearly one-third of these cases are progressive and fatal, in about 15% VOD persists but does not directly contribute to death, and approximately half the cases resolve spontaneously.

Insidious weight gain is the first sign of VOD and is followed shortly by jaundice. Clinical symptoms typically develop 1 to 3 weeks after transplant and may include hyperbilirubinemia (often substantial and with disproportionately low liver enzyme elevations), right upper quadrant pain, hepatomegaly, fluid and sodium retention, significant weight gain, and, in half the patients, ascites. If VOD progresses more severe symptoms of liver failure occur, including encephalopathy and coagulopathy (Jones et al., 1987; McDonald et al., 1985), and often terminate in multiorgan failure. Derangements in fluid balance may result in significant intravascular volume depletion, diminished renal blood flow, and azotemia requiring hemodialysis. It is unclear whether these secondary renal effects of VOD are due to VOD alone or are produced by other factors, including amphotericin or cyclosporine administration.

There are currently no methods shown to prevent VOD other than judicious patient selection for marrow transplantation. There is no known specific treatment for VOD, but about half the affected patients resolve their jaundice and fluid accumulation by day 35 after transplant (Jones et al., 1987). Nutrition and fluid management is complicated. The therapeutic goal is to facilitate a reversal of the intravascular fluid and elec-

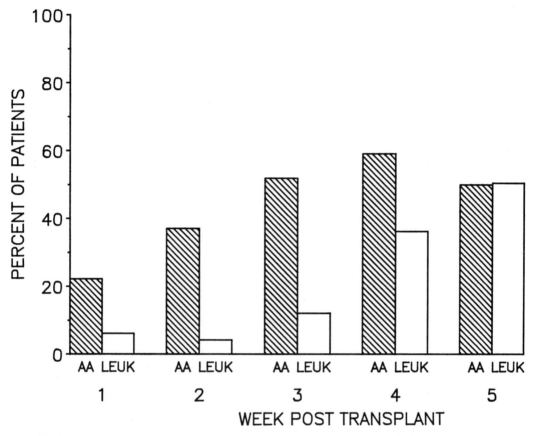

**Figure 19-1** Percentage of Patients with an Average Daily Oral Energy Intake of 30% of Baseline Requirements or More (Harris & Benedict, 1919) among Patients with Aplastic Anemia (AA, $n = 27$) and Leukemia (LEUK, $n = 421$) at Weeks 1 to 5 after Transplant.

trolyte losses. Because no specific study has assessed the efficacy of interventions in marrow transplant patients, appropriate treatment is controversial and can have undesirable effects on other organ systems. For example, limitation of intravenous fluids, including TPN formulas, in an attempt to minimize edema and ascites is frequently complicated by intravascular volume depletion and deterioration of renal function. Conversely, repleting the intravascular space with intravenous solutions often results in pulmonary edema and massive ascites.

Daily monitoring of weight gain, abdominal girth, and blood chemistry values such as serum sodium, bilirubin, creatinine, blood urea nitrogen (BUN), and albumin levels helps alert the clinician to early developing VOD (Darbinian & Schubert, 1985). Also monitored is the total sodium load from all sources including TPN,

intravenous fluids, antibiotics, food, and albumin infusions. Restriction of sodium and use of spironolactone help promote negative sodium balance, and the reduction of total fluid input may decelerate fluid accumulation. Extremes of fluid excess and intravascular volume depletion need to be avoided.

Intravenous lipids may be provided as a 20% solution and dextrose as a 70% solution if renal perfusion is adequate. Autopsies of marrow transplant recipients with VOD have revealed no evidence of hepatocyte fatty infiltration (Shulman, McDonald, & Matthews, 1980), suggesting tolerance of concentrated dextrose solutions. Administration of intravenous fat emulsions during VOD requires monitoring of lipid utilization, particularly in patients with serum bilirubin elevations. Suggested monitoring methods include nephelometry testing

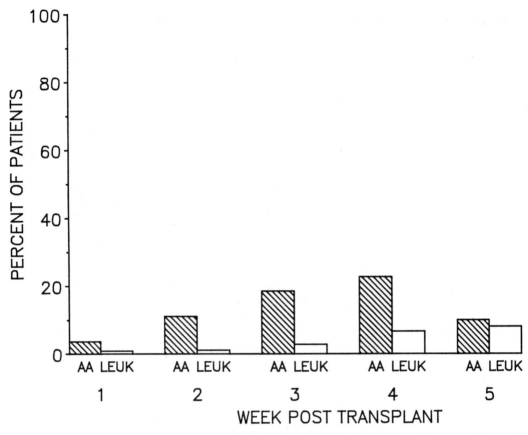

**Figure 19-2** Percentage of Patients with an Average Daily Oral Protein Intake of 0.50 g/kg or More among Patients with Aplastic Anemia (AA, $n = 27$) and Leukemia (LEUK, $n = 421$) at Weeks 1 to 5 after Transplant.

(Carlson & Rossner, 1972), which permits evaluation of the patient's capacity to eliminate from the blood stream exogenously administered lipids.

Some patients with VOD consume large volumes of oral fluids; this may require restriction. Red blood cell transfusions are used to maintain the hematocrit at 40% to 45% during times when fluid balance is critical. Further in VOD as in other obstructive liver diseases, a dynamic circulation of albumin exists between the extravascular and intravascular spaces. Serum albumin infusions contribute significantly to the colloid osmotic pressure in the intravascular system (Rothschild, Oratz, & Schreiber, 1988). Some investigators hold that hypoalbuminemia leads to capillary leak syndrome. In symptomatic VOD patients, administration of intravenous albumin (e.g., 12.6 g every 6 to 12 hours for serum albumin levels less than

3.0 g/dL) may be beneficial in mobilizing extravascular fluid into the intravascular lumen. This therapy is controversial; the disadvantages include high cost and risk of albumin accumulation in the extravascular space, resulting in increased osmotic pressure on the wrong side of the vascular membrane. This approach has not been studied in marrow transplant patients, but in nontransplant patients it has been beneficial in preserving renal blood flow.

Some patients with VOD may develop hepatic encephalopathy with symptoms of confusion, disorientation, agitation, or asterixis that can proceed to coma. If liver failure is suspected as a primary or coexisting cause for encephalopathy, a plasma amino acid profile may be helpful in determining whether hepatic failure amino acid solutions should be considered for use (discussed below). Serum ammonia levels do not correlate well with the presence of hepatic encephalopathy and are generally not helpful. Patients who have minimal oral intake or are receiving oral or intravenous antibiotics may not generate ammonia in their gastrointestinal tract. Twice normal values for serum phenylalanine, tyrosine, tryptophan, or methionine may warrant the use of Hepatamine. The use of ratios of branched chain amino acids to aromatic amino acids is not appropriate in this population because the ratios are usually decreased, even in patients with VOD. As mental function improves or worsens, subsequent amino acid profiles assist in assessing tolerance of the intravenous protein solution support.

A small, blind, randomized study of marrow transplant patients with VOD-induced encephalopathy ($n = 9$) compared standard amino acid therapy, modified amino acid therapy (Hepatamine), and withdrawal of protein (Lenssen, Spencer, & McDonald, 1987). The results showed no evidence that the composition or withdrawal of intravenous amino acids affected acute hepatic coma. Because of the small study size, however, some degree of clinical benefit for Hepatamine cannot be ruled out. It is recommended that patients with encephalopathy continue on protein support to reduce muscle breakdown and endogenous protein contribution to the urea pool.

## Renal Disease

Patients are subject to compromised vascular integrity throughout the early course of marrow transplantation, which may result in a capillary leak syndrome. Conventional fluid balance practices may therefore result in extracellular fluid volume excess, intravascular volume depletion, and organ hypoperfusion. Inadequate renal perfusion, volume depletion, and the use of nephrotoxic drugs all may contribute to renal complications. Renal complications are best managed by maintaining sufficient intravascular volume, correcting electrolyte imbalances, and reducing drug dosages. Renal damage is suspected when the serum creatinine level increases to twice the pretransplant baseline level. The serum BUN level is a clinically useful index of renal function, but an increased level can reflect increased protein intake, gastrointestinal bleeding, hypercatabolism, or steroid therapy. Restriction of protein intake to minimize the increase in BUN levels should be avoided to ensure that adequate calorie and protein support are provided to the catabolic patient.

Acute renal failure is characterized by a progressive azotemia caused by a reduction or cessation of glomerular filtration and is defined by a serum creatinine level of 3.0 mg/dL or a BUN level of 80 mg/dL or greater. Primary causes of acute renal failure include nephrotoxins such as antimicrobials, antifungals, cyclosporine, and possibly antivirals; hypotension secondary to severe intravascular volume depletion as a result of third spacing, capillary leak syndrome, severe gastrointestinal fluid losses, septic shock, abdominal emergencies, anesthesia, and severe hemorrhage; and hepatorenal syndrome. Complications of acute renal failure include fluid and electrolyte disorders, pulmonary edema, acidosis, and uremia. As kidney function deteriorates and uremic symptoms worsen, hemodialysis is required. General indications for hemodialysis are to control extracellular fluid volume expansion, acidemia, hyperkalemia, and azotemia.

Management of renal complications includes maintaining sufficient intravascular volume and correcting electrolyte imbalances. Water load is monitored by assessing intake and output, twice daily weights, and serum electrolyte concentration. The large fluid load necessitated by TPN presents a problem for the oliguric patient and may have to be manipulated on a daily basis depending on urine output and clinical signs of fluid overload. Sodium may be deleted from TPN solutions depending on quantities provided by antibiotics, albumin infusions, and other medications. Hypervolemic hyponatremia is treated with water restriction to prevent congestive heart failure. Potassium status requires close monitoring. Hyperkalemia and acidemia often coexist and may be lethal.

The primary goal of nutrition therapy in acute renal failure is to minimize uremic toxicity and other metabolic derangements while preventing malnutrition. The urea nitrogen appearance (UNA) equation can be used to ascertain protein needs of the marrow transplant patient with acute renal failure because of the rapidly progressive nature of the disease. The UNA equation is a useful means of estimating the degree of net catabolism and amino acid requirements (Kopple, 1981). Because of severe fluid restrictions in the renal failure patient, actual volumes of intravenous protein support infused are often less than what would be tolerated. Protein levels generally administered to adults approximate 0.6 g per kilogram ideal body weight per day. During dialysis, protein intake may be increased to 1.0 to 1.2 g per kilogram ideal body weight per day or more according to UNA calculations unless contraindicated by controlled azotemia or encephalopathy due to worsening hepatic dysfunction. Amino acid losses during hemodialysis average approximately 2 to 3 g/hour, or 6 to 8 g lost during one treatment. Intravenous renal failure amino acid solutions such as Nephramine are not recommended because of their high concentration of aromatic amino acids, which are usually contraindicated because of concomitant liver disease.

Hypertonic dextrose solutions (i.e., 35% or more) are recommended to increase the caloric density of limited volume infusates. Glucose losses during hemodialysis with a glucose-free dialysate approximate 20 to 50 g (68 to 170 kcal) per dialysis and should be figured into estimated energy requirements. For the oliguric patient, intravenous lipid emulsions provide a concentrated source of nonprotein calories. Current recommendations are to provide 25% to 30% of the total calories as intravenous lipids. Monitoring of lipid tolerance could include nephelometry testing to assess lipid clearance (Carlson & Rossner, 1972), particularly in the septic patient on dialysis.

Intravenous ascorbic acid supplementation may require modification to avoid secondary oxalosis in patients with acute renal failure (Freidman et al., 1983). Oxalic acid is produced by metabolism of ascorbic acid, which may lead to the formation of calcium oxalate renal calculi.

## Infection and Pulmonary Disease

Opportunistic infections result from the effects of the conditioning regimens and from immunosuppressive drugs such as methotrexate, cyclosporine, and prednisone used after the marrow transplant to prevent and treat complications (Meyers & Thomas, 1988). A period of pancytopenia (usually 2 to 4 weeks) follows a marrow graft. Bacterial infections, particularly by Gram-negative organisms, are likely to occur. With current antibiotic therapy or ultraisolation techniques (or both), however, bacterial infections now account for less than 10% of deaths. Viral, fungal, and protozoan infections constitute a much more grave threat, particularly from cytomegalovirus (CMV). About half the pneumonia cases are associated with CMV infections. For a patient and donor who are both CMV antibody negative, the administration of blood products from CMV-negative donors has significantly reduced the incidence of CMV infection. Prevention of CMV infection among patients who are CMV antibody positive involves the use of immunoglobulins, antiviral agents such as acyclovir and gancicylovir, and possibly leukocyte-poor blood products.

The nutrition support of the septic patient is dependent on the patient's general clinical state, including metabolic and volume status and the type and degree of organ dysfunction. Although the need for adequate nutrition support is unequivocal, the proportion of individual nutrient substrates that should be prescribed remains less well defined. Conflicting studies have been reported regarding the effect of lipid emulsions on immunologic impairment such as antibody formation, neutrophil chemotaxis, phagocytosis, and reticuloendothelial function (Skeie et al., 1988; Wolfe & Ney, 1986). Lipids are cleared from the bloodstream by lipoprotein lipase; when this enzyme is saturated, the reticuloendothelial system removes excess lipid. Circulating neutrophils may become lipid laden and exhibit impaired function. No studies in humans at doses routinely used in clinical practice have demonstrated an adverse impact of intravenous lipids on infectious morbidity or mortality (Wolfe & Ney, 1986). Even so, this potential concern for the effect of lipids on immunity underscores the importance of monitoring lipid levels in the critically ill marrow transplant patient.

The malnourished patient with chronic pulmonary disease is not typically seen in the marrow transplant setting because of eligibility criteria that exclude such patients. Patients are subject to various acute pulmonary complications that affect nutrition support, however, including interstitial pulmonary edema, airway obstruction, pneumonia, and emboli.

Pulmonary edema can be associated with rapid and significant weight gain. The pathogenesis is attributed to capillary permeability changes caused by various clinical occurrences and medical intervention, including chemotherapy and radiation therapy damage compounded by iatrogenic fluid overloading. Management of pulmonary edema includes reducing total sodium from primary sources including oral intake, intravenous fluids, and medications. TPN formulas can be concentrated to decrease the total fluid volume administered while providing optimum caloric support. Serum electrolytes and renal function must be closely monitored, particularly if the patient is diuresed.

During ventilator dependency, nutrition support should be provided at energy substrate levels adequate to reduce muscle breakdown. The initial goal is to provide estimated baseline energy requirements on the basis of the basal energy expenditure (BEE) (1.3 to 1.5 × BEE) (Harris & Benedict, 1919). If this support level is well tolerated and if additional support is clinically indicated because of infection and trauma, estimated stress energy requirements (1.7 to 1.9 × BEE) should be prescribed. Protein intake should be maintained at a minimum level of 1.5 g per kilogram ideal body weight for adults and modified by age for children. It is recommended that mixed-substrate TPN formulas be administered with approximately 50% of the total calories as carbohydrate, 25% to 30% as lipids, and 20% to 25% as protein.

Marrow transplant patients generally have complex ventilatory perfusion abnormalities. The carbohydrate concentration of the TPN solution need not be adjusted unless a transplant patient demonstrates problems with ventilation associated with increased carbon dioxide production. Currently, there are no conclusive data to suggest that intravenous lipid emulsions are contraindicated or should be used sparingly in the transplant patient with pulmonary dysfunction. Tolerance to lipid emulsions, however, should be monitored by assessment of daily serum turbidity, serum triglyceride levels, and a lipid clearance test as clinically indicated (Carlson & Rossner, 1972), particularly in the septic patient. If lipid clearance is abnormal, lipid infusion times may be increased (e.g., over 12 to 18 hours per 24 hours) in conjunction with a decrease in the total lipid dose. In these cases lipid levels should not exceed 50% of the total calories. If lipids are withheld, they should be reinstituted as soon as possible.

### Acute Graft-Versus-Host Disease

Approximately two-thirds of patients receiving a transplant from a matched sibling develop some evidence of GVHD within 10 to 80 days after transplant. GVHD may be minimal, with only a slight skin rash, or it may become life threatening, with skin, liver, or gut involvement (or all three) (McDonald, Shulman, Sullivan, & Spencer, 1986). A skin rash is usually the first sign of GVHD and may progress to severe desquamation and bullae reminiscent of second-degree burns.

In acute gastrointestinal GVHD voluminous diarrhea is a prominent manifestation, with the volume corresponding to the extent of mucosal damage (Wolford & McDonald, 1988). Diarrhea volume can range from 500 mL, which is considered the least severe level, to as high as 10 to 15 L daily. The diarrheal fluid is green and watery with ropy strands of mucus, protein, and cellular debris and often contains occult blood. Protein content is high, as evidenced by falling plasma protein levels or by measuring α-1-antitrypsin in fecal water (Weisdorf, Salati, Longsdorf, Ramsay, & Sharp, 1985). Associated symptoms include anorexia, nausea, vomiting, and crampy abdominal pain that is partially relieved by passing diarrheal stools. Abdominal pain may be related to food ingestion or may occur spontaneously as a result of an edematous intestine, which causes large volumes of fluid to pass through the intestine.

Acute liver GVHD is characterized by abnormal liver function tests, jaundice and mild hepatomegaly, ascites, and, in severe cases, encephalopathy. Liver GVHD is clinically staged by increases in bilirubin (>2.0 mg/dL). Histopathologic features are severe cholangiolar-hepatocellular cholestasis, portal vein inflammation, and significant bile duct abnormalities including periportal bile thrombi, lymphocytic infiltration, and individual cell necrosis and destruction. Hepatic synthesis and enterohepatic circulation of bile salts may be diminished or inhibited, resulting in steatorrhea.

About one-third of patients who develop moderate to severe GVHD die of the disease or its complications. The primary complication is infection due to the severe immunologic deficiency that accompanies GVHD. Prophylactic immunosuppression with methotrexate immediately after marrow infusion combined with a long course of cyclosporine (Storb et al., 1986) has been shown to reduce the incidence and severity of GVHD. Other treatment agents include prednisone and antithymocyte globulin. T-Cell depletion of donor marrow and monoclonal antibodies capable of modulating T-cell function are also being explored as methods to prevent GVHD. Treatment of GVHD remains an area of intensive research because current therapeutic regimens are unsatisfactory.

Adequate nutrition support is a vital adjunct to immunosuppressive drug therapy in the treatment of acute GVHD. In severe skin GVHD, energy and protein requirements may exceed stress levels if total body surface involvement is greater than 50%. Protein needs may also be significantly increased. Fluid losses may be substantial, so that adequate fluid replacement is imperative.

In liver GVHD, nutrition management is contingent on the degree of hepatic involvement. The composition of the energy substrate should parallel that for VOD. If encephalopathy develops, a plasma amino acid profile can be used to determine whether elevated aromatic amino acid and methionine levels are contributing to the observed encephalopathy. If the levels of these specific amino acids are elevated to two or three times their normal values, a trial of a hepatic failure amino acid formulation (Hepatamine) is clinically indicated. If the amino acid profile is within normal limits, no TPN protein solution

change is required. The use of Hepatamine in severe liver GVHD has not been systematically evaluated.

In gastrointestinal GVHD, TPN is generally required until the intestinal tract has healed sufficiently for the patient to tolerate oral feedings. Patients with severe gastrointestinal GVHD require TPN and total gut rest until abdominal pain subsides and stool volume is diminished. Limiting oral intake is the only way to diminish diarrheal volume (Wolford & McDonald, 1988). Total gut rest is defined as restriction of all foods and fluids, including free water and ice chips. If required for patient cooperation, medications may be taken with 30 mL of a fruit-ade beverage. After large-volume diarrhea and pain resolve, oral liquid supplements are begun to stimulate intestinal regeneration and to assess intestinal absorption (Darbinian & Schubert, 1985; Gauvreau et al., 1981). As long as the patient remains symptom free, foods are gradually introduced and TPN reduced. Guidelines for the introduction of oral intake have been empirically derived (Table 19-1) and use a five-phase regimen emphasizing foods low in lactose, fat, fiber, and total acidity (Aker, Lenssen, Darbinian, Cheney, & Cunningham, 1983; Darbinian & Schubert, 1985; Gauvreau et al., 1981; Weisdorf et al., 1985).

## Chronic Graft-Versus-Host Disease and Other Late Complications

Approximately 25% to 50% of patients surviving longer than 100 days develop some form of chronic GVHD (Nims & Strom, 1988). Of patients without a prior history of acute GVHD, 20% develop chronic GVHD de novo. Symptoms of chronic GVHD can include keratoconjunctivitis, sclerodermalike skin disease, buccal mucositis, esophageal strictures, gut involvement, pulmonary insufficiency, chronic liver disease, and general wasting syndrome. Bacterial infections are common. Oral involvement, which occurs in 80% of patients, includes reduced keratinization and saliva flow, increasing the risk of dental caries. Although 80% of patients may respond to treatment with cyclosporine, azathioprine, or steroids, treatment may

**Table 19-1** Gastrointestinal GVHD Diet Progression

| Phase | Clinical Symptoms | Diet | Clinical Symptoms of Diet Intolerance |
|---|---|---|---|
| 1. Bowel rest | Gastrointestinal (GI) cramping, large volumes of watery diarrhea, depressed serum albumin level, severely reduced transit time, small bowel obstruction or diminished bowel sounds, nausea and vomiting | Oral: nothing by mouth<br>Intravenous (IV): stress energy and protein requirements | |
| 2. Introduction of oral feeding | Minimal GI cramping, diarrhea less than 500 mL/day, guaiac-negative stools, improved transit time (minimum, 1.5 hours), infrequent nausea and vomiting | Oral: isosmotic, low-residue, low-lactose beverages, initially 60 mL every 2 to 3 hours, for several days<br>IV: as for phase 1. | Increased stool volume or diarrhea, increased emesis, increased abdominal cramping |
| 3. Introduction of solids | Minimal or no GI cramping, formed stool | Oral: allow introduction of solid food, once every 3 to 4 hours: minimal lactose,* low fiber, low fat (20 to 40 g/day),† low total acidity, no gastric irritants<br>IV: as for phase 1. | As in phase 2 |
| 4. Expansion of diet | Minimal or no GI cramping, formed stool | Oral: minimal lactose,* low fiber, low total acidity, no gastric irritants; if stools indicate fat malabsorption: low fat†<br>IV: as needed to meet nutrition requirements | As in phase 2 |
| 5. Resumption of regular diet | No GI cramping, normal stool, normal transit time, normal serum albumin level | Oral: progress to regular diet by introducing one restricted food per day: acid foods with meals, fiber-containing foods, lactose-containing foods; order of addition will vary, depending on individual tolerances and preferences; slowly liberalize fat restriction in patients with resolved steatorrhea.<br>IV: discontinue when oral nutrition intake meets estimated requirements | As in phase 2 |

*Lactase is one of the last disaccharide-splitting enzymes to return after villous atrophy. Commercially prepared lactase liquid or tablets (LactAid) are used to reduce the lactose content of milk by more than 90%. LactAid milk (70% lactose free) is also commercially available.

†Additional calories may be provided by commercially available medium-chain triglycerides, which do not exacerbate symptoms.

*Source:* From *Nutritional Assessment and Management during Marrow Transplantation: A Resource Manual* (pp. 63–80) by P. Lenssen and S. Aker (Eds.), 1986, Seattle, Washington: Fred Hutchinson Cancer Research Center. Adapted by permission.

be required for as long as 1 to 2 years. If not treated early serious contractures may develop, and pulmonary insufficiency may become life threatening (Sullivan, 1986; Sullivan et al., 1988).

Late complications are primarily due to the effects of chemotherapy and TBI and the problems related to chronic GVHD. Sterility as a result of TBI is probable in almost all patients, including children. Cataracts occur within 1 to 3 years in approximately 80% of patients given single-exposure TBI and in 25% of patients given fractionated TBI. Restrictive and obstructive chronic pulmonary disease occurs in 5% to 15% of patients who develop chronic GVHD. Studies of growth and development show that most children with aplastic anemia who were prepared by cyclophosphamide alone have normal growth. Those with leukemia and particularly those with chronic GVHD, almost all of whom had received prior chemotherapy and prophylactic cranial irradiation, who were prepared with cyclophosphamide and TBI before grafting have delayed growth and development (Sanders et al., 1986).

Nutrition support is dependent on the severity and organ involvement of the chronic GVHD (Darbinian & Schubert, 1985). With mild oral involvement, patients complain that acid foods burn their mouths; in more severe cases only bland liquids and soft foods may be tolerated. Complete nutrition supplements should be prescribed if weight loss or poor intake continue. The calorie level of well-tolerated foods can be enhanced by using carbohydrate polymers such as Polycose. Esophageal abnormalities such as webbing or constricture can result in severe nutrition depletion because of inability to swallow. If oral intake remains insufficient, tube feedings and esophageal dilation should be considered. TPN is rarely used.

With chronic liver GVHD, dietary management includes provision of calories adequate for weight maintenance or gain and a high protein level (twice normal needs). A moderate fat restriction (50 to 70 g/day in adults) may be necessary if steatorrhea is present. Medium-chain triglyceride (MCT) oil can be an additional caloric source because bile salts are not required for its absorption. Because steatorrhea is associated with losses of fat-soluble vitamins and minerals (primarily potassium, magnesium, and calcium), supplementation of these nutrients is usually indicated, especially if corticosteroid therapy is prescribed. Magnesium supplementation is frequently required in patients receiving cyclosporine therapy. Water-soluble preparations of fat-soluble vitamins are available and should be considered. Stool volume and quantity, weight changes, and gastrointestinal symptoms should be monitored closely.

Chronic GVHD on rare occasions may affect the gastrointestinal tract and is characterized by severe diarrhea, steatorrhea, panmalabsorption, crampy abdominal pain, and pronounced malnutrition (Shulman, Sullivan, et al., 1980). Before diagnosis, infection, microbial overgrowth, and lactase deficiency should be ruled out. Dietary management parallels that employed in malabsorption syndrome, with

requirements being similar to those delineated for chronic GVHD of the liver. Of particular concern is the patient's level of fat tolerance and vitamin and mineral deficit.

Pulmonary insufficiency may increase metabolic requirements and interfere with oral intake of adequate calories and nutrients. Some patients demonstrate normal intake but are unable to meet the imposed hypercaloric needs required to prevent weight loss and debilitation. The use of nutrition supplements and small, frequent, calorie-dense meals helps increase the nutrient content of the diet. If pulmonary problems persist or worsen, use of enteral feedings should be considered.

Corticosteroids are used to reduce the morbidity and mortality associated with chronic GVHD (Sullivan et al., 1981). Steroids may induce sodium and fluid retention, an increase in adipose tissue, diminished insulin sensitivity, glucose intolerance, skeletal muscle catabolism, hypokalemia, osteoporosis, hypertriglyceridemia, peptic ulceration, and growth retardation in children (Darbinian & Schubert, 1985). Nutrition recommendations include a high-protein (twice the recommended dietary allowance [RDA]), sodium-restricted (level contingent on the degree of fluid retention) diet with adequate levels of vitamin D and increased levels of calcium (1.5 times the RDA). Calcium-rich antacids (Tums or Rolaids) may be used to alleviate gastrointestinal symptoms. Finally, regular exercise is essential to minimize or reduce bone mineral and skeletal muscle mass depletion. For many patients, the most frustrating effect of steroid therapy is the rapid weight gain resulting from insatiable appetite and fluid retention.

## Economic and Psychosocial Implications

The marrow transplant procedure has a significant impact on the economic and psychosocial status of the patient and family. The entire family's quality of life is compromised while they struggle physically and mentally with therapy and the disruption of their lives (Nims & Strom, 1988). The tempo of patient recovery and coping with fear occupies much of their adaptive energies. Fatigue is common. Medical problems take precedence, occasionally to the exclusion of psychologic needs. Guilt, relief, anger, anxiety, and fear are the most common emotions. Added to the emotional issues is the economic impact of the transplant. In the first month after transplant, 10% of patient families become economically destitute because of the expenses of the transplant and relocation living costs. This can emotionally affect patients, particularly if they were the wage earners or parents of children.

Financially strained transplant patients and their families may require financial and food supply support. Transplant outpatients occasionally sacrifice food supplies that they require to feed their children. The dietitian can detect such problems through routine nutrition counseling sessions. Emergency and continuing assistance can be obtained by referring these problems to the social worker. Families may be eligible for welfare or community support such as local food banks. Some transplant centers, through money and food contributions, establish an emergency food supply to assist families. Utilizing other members of the health care team (i.e., nursing staff, social workers, and psychologists) helps give the family unit more comprehensive support.

## TRANSPLANT COMPLICATIONS AFFECTING ORAL INTAKE

### Nausea and Vomiting

Nausea and vomiting present as acute and delayed reactions for a multitude of reasons. The etiology of persistent nausea is frequently difficult to diagnose, and eating ability may be impaired for a long period of time (Spencer et al., 1986). Before the transplant, severe nausea and vomiting accompany the chemotherapy and TBI but rarely persist beyond day 15. Nausea and occasionally vomiting accompany the use of many drugs, including cyclosporine, narcotics, trimethoprim-sulfamethoxazole, interferon, interleukin-2, and intravenous and oral nonabsorbable antibiotics (Wolford & McDonald, 1988). Lipid infusions and high

serum glucose or amino acid levels are also associated with nausea, although these associations have not been studied in the marrow transplant population. Dehydration and electrolyte imbalances, mucositis, and gastrointestinal GVHD may also induce nausea. Nausea and vomiting are also prominent symptoms of CMV and herpes simplex virus (HSV) infections, particularly in the esophagus and gastrointestinal tract (Spencer et al., 1986). Nausea and vomiting have been seen as presenting manifestations of peptic esophagitis, encephalitis, spontaneous subdural hematomas, septicemia, and adrenal insufficiency as well as with intra-abdominal processes such as cholecystitis, pancreatitis, and infiltrative liver disease (Spencer et al., 1986).

During nausea accompanied by severe vomiting, oral intake is minimized because of the risk of aspiration (Aker & Lenssen, 1988). Clear liquids, salty foods, and fruits such as watermelon are occasionally tolerated. Overly sweet and greasy foods may increase the discomfort, as can strong odors. Drinking liquids rapidly, eating too fast, or moving suddenly can stimulate vomiting. Fluid status needs to be monitored with excessive vomiting. Antiemetics are almost always required to control severe nausea with or without vomiting.

### Oral Mucositis, Esophagitis, and Oral Infections

Inflammation or breakdown of the mucous membranes of the mouth and oropharynx may be present in varying degrees of severity. The primary contributors to mucosal damage are chemotherapy and radiation therapy regimens and opportunistic oral infection. Cyclophosphamide causes mucosal atrophy and, rarely, ulceration. TBI causes mucosal atrophy, ulceration, and vasculitis. Methotrexate causes thinning and ulceration of the mucosal epithelium. The severity of the mucositis is increased in patients treated with methotrexate as prophylaxis for GVHD. Patients frequently cannot initiate a swallow because of pain. Mouth rinsing with physiologic saline helps alleviate soreness, but narcotics are frequently required for pain control. The mucosal ulcerations generally develop 4 to 10 days after the preparative chemotherapy and several days after the first doses of TBI. Healing begins with marrow engraftment and the return of circulating neutrophils. Complete healing can be seen as early as 20 days after transplant, whereas with acute and chronic GVHD lesions can persist for up to 6 to 8 months after transplant. Mucositis appears to be more severe and to persist longer in adults than in children.

From day 30 to day 75, acid-peptic esophagitis is the most common cause of dysphagia. Spencer et al. (1986) found no organisms in about half the marrow transplant patients who had gross esophagitis at endoscopy and assumed that esophagitis in those cases was caused by reflux of gastric juices. Factors relating to reflux include gastric stasis, esophageal dysmotility caused by inflammation, and poor salivary flow related to mucositis and GVHD. Most of the esophageal pain may also be related more to the reflux of gastric juices than to infections. Sucralfate, antacids, and intraesophageal antacid drips are used to control symptoms. Approximately 10% of patients with extensive chronic GVHD have esophageal involvement, presenting with dysphagia, retrosternal pain, insidious weight loss, and aspiration (Sullivan et al., 1981).

Mucositis and decreased saliva predispose patients to oral infections that can be painful and potentially lethal if they seed a systemic infection. The oral cavity can often be implicated as the source of organisms recovered from blood cultures. Oral colonization with *Candida* organisms is common and is a source of concern because the risk of systemic fungal infection is high. Oral antifungals are necessary to prevent candidal colonization.

Herpetic infections can present orally and may be difficult to differentiate visually from chemotherapy-induced or radiation therapy–induced mucositis. Prophylactic administration of acyclovir decreases the incidence of virus reactivation; therapeutic administration results in rapid healing of HSV lesions.

Mucosal and esophageal lesions are the primary reason that most transplant patients are not able to eat for upward of 1 month after transplant and require TPN support. If oral and esophageal soreness and general tenderness develop, a soft,

nonirritating diet will be best tolerated (Aker & Lenssen, 1988). Foods that are rough, raw, acid, or spicy should be avoided. Some patients complain that salty foods burn their mouths. If symptoms are severe, the diet may need to be liquid or semiliquid for extended periods. Foods to avoid include meat, spicy entrees, grainy cereals and breads, juices, fresh raw fruits and vegetables, bananas, highly salted foods, and crunchy snacks. Also to be avoided are hot spices, alcoholic beverages, caffeine, and extreme hot and cold food temperatures.

## Xerostomia

Xerostomia occurs after TBI but is also associated with the use of antiemetics (Schubert & Izutsu, 1987). Saliva production returns to normal within 2 to 3 months after transplant, but some degree of xerostomia can be permanent, particularly in patients with chronic GVHD. In the absence of the antimicrobial effects of saliva, good mouth care is vital. Oral care includes plaque control by means of soft toothbrushes, atraumatic flossing, fluoride and other bland rinses (0.9% saline), and saliva substitutes.

A lack of saliva makes it difficult to chew and swallow many foods such as meat and bread products (Aker & Lenssen, 1988), but the fluid content of foods can be increased with the use of gravy, broths, or sauces. It is suggested that liquids be served with meals and that total daily fluid intake be kept high. If the salivary glands are functioning but at minimum levels, citric acid, as found in lemonade or sugarless lemon drops, stimulates saliva production. Foods to avoid are plain meats, bread products, crackers, bananas, dry cake, alcohol, and excessively hot foods. Artificial saliva formulas have occasionally been helpful when the mouth is dry. Drugs such as pilocarpine and bethanechol, which directly stimulate the salivary glands, can also be tried. These drugs can produce side effects, however, such as stomach cramping, sweating, flushing, and heart flutters.

## Thick, Viscous Mucus Production

A thick, viscous saliva, which is caused by the high sensitivity to radiation of the mucus glands, can develop after TBI. Saliva may be slightly thickened and require removal by suctioning or so thick that intubation is necessary to maintain an open airway. Mucus that is swallowed can cause nausea and vomiting. The thick saliva generally persists for only 2 to 3 weeks after TBI and resolves with engraftment and healing of the oral mucosa. Recurrence of a sticky, bothersome saliva can be precipitated by dehydration or medications.

When chewing and swallowing foods becomes difficult because of thick and sticky saliva, switching temporarily to a liquid diet may be beneficial (Aker & Lenssen, 1988). Patients report that club soda, hot tea with lemon, or sour lemon drops help break up the mucus. A high fluid intake also helps loosen the mucus. Foods to avoid include meats that require chewing, bread products, gelatin desserts, oily foods, thick cream soups, drinks, nectars, juices, desserts, and hot cereals. Dense liquids such as milk products are sometimes hard to swallow, but no studies have demonstrated an association between milk products and mucus thickness. Recommended foods include soft cooked fish and chicken, broth-based soups, well-thinned cereals, diluted juices, "blenderized" fruits or vegetables diluted to a thin consistency, and fruit-ade beverages.

## Dysgeusia

Dysgeusia and hypogeusia, which refer to alterations in taste perception, are primarily an effect of TBI. Drugs such as morphine, antibiotics, and possibly cyclophosphamide and other chemotherapeutic agents may also alter taste. The taste loss is temporary, with recovery occurring between 45 and 60 days after transplant (Barale, Aker, & Martinsen, 1982). Sweet is the first taste to recover and is followed by bitter, sour, and finally salty. Taste changes are individual and somewhat less severe in children than adults. The temporary taste alterations compound the lack of desire for food.

Up to day 25 after transplant, the inability to detect the normal flavor of foods is a major determent to eating (Barale et al., 1982). This is particularly so for children, who often do not understand the problem or its temporary nature.

Bland foods, such as mashed potatoes or vanilla milk shakes, may have no flavor at all. Before and after the conditioning regimen, patients need counseling and information regarding forthcoming changes in taste thresholds. To counteract the negative impact of the dysgeusia yet encourage oral intake, meal trays and food need to be attractively presented. Aroma, which does not appear to be impaired after marrow transplantation, can be used to stimulate appetite (Aker & Lenssen, 1988). Strongly flavored foods such as chocolate, lasagna, spaghetti, or barbequed foods, whose taste may be better detected, are recommended, particularly for patients with minimal or no mucositis. Foods to be avoided are bland casseroles, custards and puddings, unsalted chips and crackers, overcooked vegetables, and plain meats, fish, poultry, and milk shakes.

## Diarrhea and Steatorrhea

Diarrhea can result from pretransplant chemotherapy and TBI, delayed mucosal damage induced by radiation therapy, drugs such as oral nonabsorbable antibiotics, gastrointestinal GVHD, and intestinal infections. Acute and chronic liver GVHD as well as acute gastrointestinal GVHD involving the ileum may produce fat malabsorption.

Oral nonabsorbable antibiotics cause mild diarrhea in the fasting state and more diarrhea when food is ingested (malabsorbed dietary carbohydrate causes osmotic diarrhea when the colon flora cannot metabolize carbohydrate) (Wolford & McDonald, 1988). Similarly, patients receiving oral or parenteral antibiotics may experience diarrhea with or without overgrowth of *Clostridium difficile*. Other diarrhea-causing drugs in this setting include magnesium salts, metoclopramide, and methotrexate.

Secretory diarrhea is a prominent manifestation of intestinal involvement in acute gastrointestinal GVHD. Viral, fungal, parasitic, and bacterial infections can produce diarrheal illness that is similar to gastrointestinal GVHD, but they more commonly coexist with or complicate acute GVHD (McDonald et al., 1986).

Adequate hydration is of paramount importance with diarrhea. Diet modifications, such as avoidance of foods that contain roughage or bulk or are high in fat, are recommended. Lactose-containing foods may require treatment with LactAid enzyme, which is available in both liquid and tablet form. Some grocery stores carry LactAid pretreated milk products. Foods to avoid include untreated milk and milk products, dried beans and legumes, nuts, fried foods, whole grain breads and cereals, fruits with skin and seeds, dried fruits, raw vegetables, gas-forming vegetables, fried snack foods, and rich gravies, sauces, and desserts. The addition of MCT oil to the diet has been successful in patients with documented steatorrhea.

### Anorexia and Failure To Thrive

Loss of appetite may stem from the disease, delayed chemotherapy or TBI effects, drug toxicities, infections, fluid and electrolyte imbalance, and psychologic and environmental factors. Anorexia and failure to thrive are frequently the reasons that children require prolonged TPN after transplant (Lenssen, Moe, Cheney, Aker, & Deeg, 1983). The etiology of anorexia is often difficult to define, so that the condition is difficult to correct. The patient may be afraid to eat for fear of vomiting or pain. Eating is also the one function over which patients maintain power, so that the refusal to eat becomes an attempt to gain control of their environment. Occasionally, patients with post-transplant anorexia have had a history of poor oral intake or were characterized as being "picky eaters" before admission for transplantation.

Diagnosis by the dietitian in consultation with the clinical team as to the etiology of the eating impairment is of paramount importance. Counseling and intervention strategies can then be formulated to prevent further debilitation and wasting. Approaches may include recommending that the patient initiate a moderate exercise program, such as walking, or increase his or her level of self-care, such as preparing some meals. Patients and families may respond to suggestions concerning food preparation or modified approaches to food presentation. If the eating impairment appears to be primarily psychologic, intervention on the part of the social worker or psychologist is recommended.

## NUTRITION ASSESSMENT AND MONITORING

The goals of nutrition assessment are (1) to identify potential risk factors, (2) to determine nutrient requirements, and (3) to evaluate the success of nutrition support in maintaining or improving nutrition status (Dickson & Barale, 1985). Nutrition assessment begins before transplant and continues through the hospitalization period of acute stress and neutropenia, the ambulatory period of stabilization and recovery after engraftment, and the long-term period until the patient demonstrates absence of chronic GVHD activity and is independent of medications. The focus of monitoring varies in each period and depends on the nutrition support required and other nutrition-related problems (Table 19-2).

### Before Transplant: Admission Work-Up

Prospective transplant patients usually undergo an initial prehospitalization medical work-up for the purpose of gathering baseline medical and laboratory data and to confirm histocompatibility typing. An essential part of the work-up is the nutrition evaluation and screening by the dietitian.

Routine anthropometric data can include height, weight, triceps skin fold, arm circumference, elbow breadth, and distance from the elbow to the midpoint of the arm to provide a landmark for serial measurements. Accurate height measurements to assess later growth are important; thus a wall-mounted stadiometer and, in children younger than 2 years old, an infant measuring table are recommended. Ideal body weight, body surface area, and arm muscle and arm fat areas are calculated and recorded. These measurements are used by the medical staff to determine chemotherapy and other drug dosages. Historical information includes current appetite, gastrointestinal or other complaints interfering with oral intake, food allergies or intolerances, recent activity level, usual weight, recent voluntary or involuntary weight changes, special diets, recent growth in children and adolescents, age of onset of menarche in female adolescents, recent or current medications, and

**Table 19-2** Nutrition Assessment, Support, and Monitoring of the Marrow Transplant Patient: Preadmission through Long-Term Follow-Up

| Phase of Treatment | Focus of Intervention |
|---|---|
| Pretransplant | Nutrition assessment work-up: baseline anthropometric and biochemical measurements, diet and weight histories |
| Chemotherapy and irradiation | Start calorie (TPN, IV, and oral) counts; assessment of TPN and oral tolerance and delivery |
| Days 0 to 20 | Assess TPN, renal, oral toxicities |
| Days 15 to 20 | Assess oral tolerance; provide diet counseling |
| Day 20+ | Assess GVHD, infection, and renal, pulmonary, liver toxicities; taper TPN with increasing oral intake |
| Day 25+ | Hospital discharge teaching; nutrition inpatient discharge summary; weekly outpatient counseling with outpatient department dietitian; daily calorie counts for outpatients on TPN, hydration, special diet or with weight loss; body weight checks daily or three times per week |
| Day 40 | Complete nutrition assessment, repeat anthropometry |
| Day 60+ | Assess oral intake, weight |
| Day 100 | Nutrition work-up and summary on departure from transplant center: nutrition risk factors (infection, chronic GVHD), current diet, nutrition course during 100 days, nutrition recommendations; repeat anthropometry |
| Day 100+ | Screen for nutrition problems, especially in patients with chronic GVHD |

family history of chronic diseases. The dietitian also notes any pertinent data from available past medical records.

Pretransplant counseling includes patient introduction to the nutrition problems associated with marrow transplantation and the concept of enteral and parenteral nutrition. Patients with significant weight loss or active problems interfering with adequate nutrient intake require nutrition counseling and follow-up if they are not admitted immediately to the hospital. Follow-up includes prescribing nutrition supplements, recommending nutrition intervention such as TPN, additional laboratory monitoring, and weight checks.

**Posttransplant (Hospitalization) Evaluation and Monitoring**

A complete nutrition assessment is charted for all transplant patients, including a record of the preadmission work-up data (history, anthropometry, and biochemistry), on their admission to the hospital. Exhibit 19-1 is a sample admission nutrition assessment form used for marrow transplant patients.

High-dose chemotherapy, TBI, fever, infection, major organ dysfunction or failure, and GVHD make the nutrition response of transplant patients similar to that of trauma patients and those experiencing other stress states. The transplant procedure has been associated with prolonged negative nitrogen balance (Lenssen et al., 1984; Szeluga, Stuart, Brookmeyer, Utermohlen, & Santos, 1985), loss of muscle mass (Layton, Gallucci, & Aker, 1981), and a gender difference in terms of metabolic response to stress. Cheney, Lenssen, et al. (1987) studied sex differences in nitrogen balance in 40 adults and suggested higher per-kilogram nutrient requirements in men during stressful episodes after marrow transplantation.

Calorie needs are calculated to compensate for increased requirements due to chemotherapy and radiation therapy and the sequelae of marrow transplantation in the first 30 to 50 days after transplant (Dickson & Barale, 1985). The basis for calculating energy needs is the BEE equation (Harris & Benedict, 1919). For infants and children less than 21 kg, the basal metabolic rates derived by the Food and Agriculture Organization–World Health Organization (FAO-WHO) are recommended (Joint FAO-WHO Ad Hoc Expert Committee, 1973). Basal energy requirements are increased by 70% to 90% (stress energy levels, 1.7 to 1.8 × BEE in adults, 1.8 to 1.9 × BEE for children) immediately after transplant and account for the stress of the conditioning regimen, fever and infection

**Exhibit 19-1** Sample Form for Charting Admission Nutrition Assessment and Recommendations

| DATE | INTERDISCIPLINARY NOTE |
|---|---|
| | *NUTRITIONAL ASSESSMENT AND RECOMMENDATIONS* |

S-  CLINICAL SYMPTOMS/PROBLEMS:

Weight Hx:

Food Allergies:                                    Activity Level:

Other:

O-  ANTHROPOMETRY:                              BIOCHEMISTRY:

Ht:_____cm_____%tile NCHS grids                 Prealbumin: _____ mg/dl

Wt:_____kg_____%tile NCHS grids/%IBW            Albumin: _____ gm/dl

Usual BW:_____kg  BSA:_____M²

IBW:_____kg  Wt-for-Ht:_____%tile NCHS          DRUGS (affecting nutritional status):

Arm Muscle Area:_____cm²_____%tile

Arm Fat Area:_____cm²_____%tile

ESTIMATED ANABOLIC REQUIREMENTS:

|  | Baseline | Stress |
|---|---|---|
| Kcal/24⁰ | | |
| Gm Protein/24⁰ | | |

Catheter/Tube: _____

Maintenance Fluid/24⁰:_____

Other Factors Added in Estimate:

A-  OVERALL NUTRITIONAL STATUS:

VERY POOR     POOR     FAIR     GOOD     EXCELLENT

P-  TPN RECOMMENDATIONS:

a. _____ ml _____% lipid emulsion.  Infuse _____ml/hr  for  first _____.

If tolerated then progress to _____ml/hr over _____hours.

b. _____ ml _____ % dextrose-amino acids _____ % to run at _____ml/hr.

Advance second _____ ml to _____% dextrose-amino acids _____% to run at _____ml/hr.

Total infusion over _____hours = _____ml.

c. Standard additives per Marrow Transplant TPN Guidelines.

*Source:* Courtesy of Fred Hutchinson Cancer Research Center, Seattle, Washington.

(60%), bedrest or light activity (10% to 20%), weight gain in undernourished patients (10%), and growth in children and adolescents (10%). The calorie recommendations refer to total calories from all energy sources (i.e., protein, fat, and carbohydrate), not just from nonprotein calorie sources. Patients with open wounds, severe skin GVHD, or relatively high activity levels may have requirements beyond these recommended levels.

Protein requirements (adults, 1.5 to 2.0 g per kilogram ideal body weight; obese adults, 1.5 to 2.0 g per kilogram adjusted ideal body weight; children and adolescents, 1.8 to 3.0 g per kilogram ideal body weight) are related to age, body size, organ function, and catabolic corticosteroid therapy. During steroid therapy, protein levels of 1.5 to 2.0 g/kg ideal body weight may be required in adults. Protein needs are modified depending on hepatic, renal, and neurologic function. Maintenance fluid requirements are based on body surface area or weight. Additional fluid is required during fever and diarrhea and other gastrointestinal losses. Less than maintenance fluid levels may be utilized during hepatic, renal, or cardiac dysfunction.

Baseline and stress nutrient requirements as well as specific volumes, concentrations, and rates of parenteral and enteral nutrition support are stated in the admission patient chart note. Subsequent nutrition monitoring and charting should occur weekly at a minimum but with more frequency depending on the patient's clinical course. A complete reassessment including anthropometric measurements at day 40 after transplant is recommended, particularly in patients who remain hospitalized.

Routine daily monitoring includes laboratory and hematologic data, daily weight, total intake and output, diarrhea volume and consistency (every 24 hours and by 8-hour shift), emesis volume, oral fluid volume (every 24 hours), oral and intravenous (TPN and dextrose-containing hydration solutions) nutrient intake levels, and type of food selected (Table 19-3). The daily oral and intravenous nutrient intake levels as calculated for all inpatients are crucial to successful and timely patient assessment. This patient population is especially sensitive to overfeeding and overhydration from all sources, so that these levels not only enable the dietitian to monitor oral intake and tolerance but to manage the total contribution of nutrition support from all sources, including fluids such as those used for intravenous hydration. Following actual infused levels every 24 hours is of crucial importance because TPN support is frequently supplied at volumes less than and occasionally greater than those ordered, so that TPN rate and

concentration adjustments are often required as a result of line interference by other solutions (Lenssen, 1989; Sanders et al., 1982). It is also helpful for the dietitian to maintain individual patient records of the total daily sodium load from TPN, oral intake, antibiotics, hydration solutions, and albumin infusions. Total sodium from these combined sources can occasionally exceed patient electrolyte requirements and tolerance. Laboratory data in conjunction with clinical and nutrition observations constitute the background information required for comprehensive evaluation and medical charting.

Nutrient requirements are scaled downward as patients are prepared for discharge. Baseline energy requirements (1.3 to 1.4 times BEE in adults, 1.3 to 1.5 times BEE in children) are the approximation of energy requirements for patients on bedrest, off antibiotics, with hematologic evidence of engraftment, without fever, and without complications such as GVHD. Patients are counseled to achieve baseline requirements during preparation for hospital discharge. TPN is reduced in proportion to increasing oral intake, with intravenous lipids being stopped first. To facilitate early hospital discharge, patients who have achieved 30% to 50% of their baseline requirements by oral intake receive partial parenteral nutrition (1 to 1.5 L of dextrose and amino acids daily) at night in the home setting. Continued daily monitoring of oral and intravenous intake facilitates timely discontinuation of intravenous support. In some patients, attaining required oral fluid levels is the limiting factor for hospital discharge. Patients can be discharged on 1 to 2 L of intravenous hydration fluids, again being infused by family members in the home setting. Hydration status is crucial especially in patients receiving cyclosporine. The use of home parenteral nutrition or hydration support depends on the individual institution's parenteral nutrition teaching and support program, the availability of infusion equipment, patient and family dynamics and understanding, and a clinical structure for patient monitoring.

## Outpatient Counseling and Monitoring

Patients are discharged from the hospital once they are hematologically and clinically stable

**Table 19-3** Nutrition Monitoring of the Hospitalized Marrow Transplant Patient

| Measure | Interval | Comments |
|---|---|---|
| **Anthropometric** | | |
| Arm muscle area (AMA), arm fat area (AFA) | Pretransplant and day 40 | Falsely elevated arm circumference with overhydration, and vice versa; elevated AFA with corticosteroid therapy; AMA may be favorably affected by resistive exercise program (Cunningham et al., 1986) |
| Body weight | Daily | Reflects hydration status; twice daily measurements recommended in small children and patients with fluid problems |
| **Biochemical** | | |
| Albumin | Twice per week | Falsely low with overhydration, and vice versa; decreased with hepatic dysfunction; increased with exogenous albumin infusions |
| Prealbumin | Variable | Measure of visceral protein status; decreased by corticosteroid therapy, fever; increased with protein intake; may indicate metabolic stress; may not be useful as visceral protein indicator before initial engraftment |
| Electrolytes | Daily | Many drugs as well as the patient's clinical status may adversely affect electrolyte status |
| Glucose (serum and urine) | Daily | Increased by concentrated dextrose solutions, corticosteroid therapy, sepsis |
| BUN and creatinine | Daily | Increased with nephrotoxic agents, catabolism, dehydration; aids in assessment of substrate tolerance and fluid status |
| Serum turbidity | Daily | Assess clearance of IV fat emulsions |
| Liver function tests | Twice per week | Increased secondary to VOD, GVHD, drug toxicities, hepatitis; increases due to TPN are mild and transient; when grossly elevated, tolerance of TPN substrates requires monitoring |
| Magnesium, calcium, potassium | Weekly | Magnesium and potassium frequently decrease, so that extra supplementation is required; calcium decreases by 0.8 mg/dL for each 0.1 g/dL drop in serum albumin |
| Triglycerides | As clinically indicated | May be increased with decreased lipid clearance, renal or hepatic dysfunction, steroid or cyclosporine therapy, sepsis; level at which IV lipids are contraindicated is unknown |
| Lipid clearance test (nephelometry) | Variable | To be performed when serum is turbid; IV lipid utilization decreased during sepsis or with hepatic, pulmonary, or renal dysfunction (Carlson & Rossner, 1972) |
| Copper, zinc | Variable | Early supplementation required; increased needs with excessive GI losses |
| Creatinine excretion | Variable | 24-Hour urine collection for 3 days preferable; index of muscle mass, can be standardized to height; increased early after transplant probably because of fever, excess catabolism; decreased with renal dysfunction; collections complicated by mixing of stool and urine |
| Nitrogen balance | Variable | 24-Hour urine collection for total urinary nitrogen over a 3-day period preferable; measures adequacy of nutrient support; requires correction for urea pool (Kopple, 1981); collections complicated by mixing of stool and urine; in patients requiring dialysis, urea generation rate indicates nitrogen balance |
| Plasma amino acid profile | Variable | Increased phenylalanine levels seen after transplant; if accompanied by encephalopathy, may indicate need for altered amino acid solution |
| Fecal fat test | Variable | 72-Hour stool collection; used to diagnose or quantitate fat malabsorption during recovery from ileal or liver GVHD |

**Table 19-3** continued

| Measure | Interval | Comments |
|---|---|---|
| Nutrient intake | | |
| Oral and TPN energy, protein, and fluid intake | Daily | Provides documentation of oral, TPN, and fluid support provided; IV hydration, blood products, drugs may interfere with TPN prescription; TPN can be reduced or increased with oral intake changes; daily measurement prevents overfeeding and underfeeding |
| Clinical | | |
| Total intake and output per 24 hours | Daily | Assesses hydration status |
| Stool and emesis volume | Daily | Signals changing GI function, clinical response to GVHD treatment |
| Temperature | Daily | Assesses nutrient and fluid requirements |

*Source:* From *Nutritional Assessment and Management during Marrow Transplantation: A Resource Manual* (pp. 5–14) by P. Lenssen and S. Aker (Eds.), 1986, Seattle, Washington: Fred Hutchinson Cancer Research Center. Adapted by permission.

and independent of intravenous medications. If daily calorie counts are to be continued, the patient and family are instructed by the dietitian regarding maintenance of food and fluid records. Discharge teaching includes provision of education materials, food intake sheets, directions for recording food intake and daily weight, and samples of nutrition supplements. Exhibit 19-2 provides a comprehensive review of the patient's nutrition course; anthropometric measurement and weight changes; laboratory values; current clinical problems and medications; TPN and hydration fluid volumes; oral calorie, protein, and fluid levels; and outpatient support recommendations. All outpatients are prescribed a daily oral multivitamin supplement, which is continued for 1 year after transplant.

Patients remain at risk for developing numerous complications until 100 days after transplant or longer. At a minimum, weekly monitoring of blood counts, GVHD status, and tolerance to oral medications, including those for GVHD prophylaxis or treatment, is recommended. Nutrition status is frequently not stable during this period; even if it is apparently stable, a minimum of once-weekly monitoring by the dietitian is suggested (Table 19-4). Assessments should include nutrient requirements and daily intakes, daily fluid intake, periodic weights, laboratory values, parenteral nutrition and hydration levels, and changes in clinical condition. Patients on prophylactic trimethoprim-sul-

famethoxazole (Bactrim or Septra), which is a broad-spectrum antibiotic, may experience nausea, vomiting, anorexia, glossitis, stomatitis, abdominal pain, and diarrhea with consequent impaired oral intake. As outpatients become more physically active, energy needs are increased accordingly. It is important to rely on growth parameters to assess actual baseline energy needs for children. Children without fluid balance disturbances should not lose weight.

## Evaluation at Day 100 and Yearly after Transplant

Ongoing nutrition assessment may be required for an extended period, especially in patients with chronic GVHD. An assessment of nutrition-related posttransplant problems and current recommendations helps alert the referring (home) physician to patients who may need continued nutrition counseling or intervention (see Table 19-2).

The aims of nutrition assessment after day 100 are to identify nutrition problems that are amenable to dietary intervention as associated with chronic GVHD or its therapy and, less commonly, with non–GVHD-related infectious complications; to assess growth in children; and to identify any nutrient deficiencies that are contrary to the promotion of good health. Nutrition screening should include anthropometric meas-

**Exhibit 19-2** Sample Form for Charting Final Discharge Summary of Nutrition Course and Recommendations for Follow-Up

---

### MARROW TRANSPLANT NUTRITIONAL DISCHARGE SUMMARY

PATIENT NAME_____ DISCHARGE DATE_____

AGE_____ SEX_____ DIAGNOSIS _____ ADMISSION DATE _____

ANTHROPOMETRY:                                          LABORATORY:
                                                                            Other:

| | Weight (kg) | Height (cm) | Arm Muscle Area (cm²) | Arm Fat Area (cm²) | | | Albumin | | |
|---|---|---|---|---|---|---|---|---|---|
| Admit | | | | | | Admit | | | |
| Discharge | | | | | | Discharge | | | |

Ideal Body Weight: _____kg
Minimum Acceptable Body Weight:  _____kg
Weight for Height: _____%tile NCHS

DIET:                                          CURRENT DRUGS AFFECTING
Daily Requirements:                      NUTRITIONAL STATUS:
Fluid _____ml/24⁰           _____
Kcal_____Protein_____grams   _____
Current Diet: _____      _____
_____        _____
Nutritional Supplements: _____      _____
_____        _____

Activity Level: _____
MAJOR NUTRITIONAL PROBLEMS:
Ongoing:    _____
Resolved:   _____

RECOMMENDATIONS:

General
1.  Multivitamin supplement with folate for one year after transplant.
2.  Follow weight at clinic visits. If weight falls below minimum acceptable weight, physical status may be impaired and enteral supplementation is urged. FHCRC research dietitians would appreciate a consult.
3.  Daily exercise to maintain or restore muscle mass.

During Steroid Therapy
1.  High calcium diet (1800 mg for adolescents; 1200 mg for adults and children) with 400 IU Vitamin D from the multivitamin to counteract osteoporosis.
2.  High protein diet to counteract muscle wasting.
3.  Reduction of sodium intake if fluid retention or rapid weight gain occur.
4.  Daily exercise to counteract osteoporosis, muscle wasting and cushingnoid appearance.
5.  Monitor serum potassium.

COMMENTS:

Prepared by: _____  Date: _____

Signature_____

*Source:* Courtesy of Fred Hutchinson Cancer Research Center, Seattle, Washington.

---

urements, weight history, estimation of activity level, biochemical and biophysical measurements such as fecal fat quantitation and pulmonary function tests, and medications. The diet history should include oral and gastrointestinal symptoms, changes in dietary preferences, and an estimation of average calorie, protein, major vitamin, and mineral intake.

**Table 19-4** Outpatient Nutrition Assessment

| Measure | Interval | Comments |
|---|---|---|
| **Anthropometric** | | |
| Weight | Daily or three times per week | Reflects body composition changes in patients off IV fluids and steroids; weight loss frequently seen after hospital discharge as a result of resolving VOD or cessation of IV fluids |
| AMA, AFA | Day 40 and day 100 | For ongoing assessment of body composition changes |
| Height | Every 3 months in children | For growth assessment |
| **Biochemical** | | |
| Albumin | Weekly | Depressed albumin levels seen with hepatic dysfunction; most likely to reflect altered nutrition status in outpatients |
| Electrolytes, BUN, creatinine | Two to three times per week | Many drug therapies continue adversely to affect fluid and electrolyte status |
| Liver function tests | Weekly | Increases due to drugs, infections, GVHD may depress appetite; if accompanied by unexplained weight loss or symptoms of steatorrhea, may indicate need for malabsorption work-up |
| Magnesium | Weekly | May require oral or parenteral supplementation, especially during cyclosporine therapy |
| **Nutrient intake** | | |
| Calories, protein, fluid | Daily until stable and patient is off TPN, hydration, diet modifications | Necessary for weight and hydration assessment |
| Fat | Variable | Requires monitoring when malabsorption is present |
| **Clinical** | | |
| Temperature | Twice per day | Requires monitoring because fevers increase fluid and calorie needs |
| GI symptoms | Variable | Changes in nutrition status may reflect common complaints of nausea, vomiting, anorexia, increases in stool volume, changes in stool consistency |

*Source:* From *Nutritional Assessment and Management during Marrow Transplantation: A Resource Manual* (pp. 5–14) by P. Lenssen and S. Aker (Eds.), 1986, Seattle, Washington: Fred Hutchinson Cancer Research Center. Adapted by permission.

## NUTRITION SUPPORT MODALITIES

### Promoting Oral Intake

Oral intake is severely depressed during the first month after transplant. In a comparison of the frequency of poor oral intake in patients with leukemia and those with aplastic anemia in the first 5 weeks after transplant (see Fig. 19-1), few of the patients with leukemia were able to consume at least 30% of their baseline energy requirements during this time, although the proportion of patients doing so increased by week 4 after transplant. A larger proportion of patients with aplastic anemia were able to eat at this minimal level earlier in the posttransplant course, presumably because of the effects of TBI on the patients with leukemia. Even with increasing energy intake, protein intake remained inadequate throughout the acute posttransplant period (see Fig. 19-2). Figure 19-3 compares oral energy intake in children, adolescents, and adults. Regardless of age, few patients were able to consume 30% of baseline energy needs until weeks 4 and 5 after transplant, at which time a larger percentage of adults and adolescents were able to eat at this level than children.

Because most patients eat poorly for a prolonged period, nutrition counseling by the dietitian during the early transplant period is crucial. Patients are provided with information about treatment and transplant complications that interfere with eating. Suggestions of better-tolerated foods are provided if the patient is able and willing to eat. Food is not forced on patients. The acute transplant complications coupled with resistance to or fear of eating only create a negative atmosphere and prevent successful refeeding. During this period many patients consume only water or ice chips. When the patient is clinically stable and when hospital discharge is anticipated, counseling is initiated for a gradual increase in tolerated food and fluid volumes.

In determining food service requirements for marrow transplant patients being prepared for

first hospital discharge, Gauvreau-Stern, Cheney, Aker, and Lenssen (1989) reported that per-patient meal orders increased from 2.6 to 5.3 per day and that the mean number of food items ordered per day increased from 4.9 to 12.4 at 14 days compared to 1 day before discharge (Fig. 19-4). Beverages were the most frequently requested item and were followed by bread products and cooked fruits and vegetables. Patients consumed an average of approximately 60% of total calories from oral intake 1 day before discharge. The food service for this patient population must be designed to provide a variety of foods at frequent intervals to meet patient tolerance and thereby to reduce dependence on TPN (Aker, 1979; Driedger & Burstall, 1987; Gauvreau-Stern et al., 1989; Moe, Aker, & Schubert, 1985).

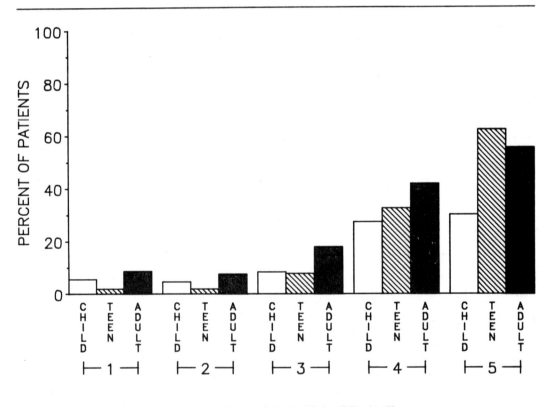

**Figure 19-3** Percentage of Patients with Average Daily Oral Energy Intake of 30% of Baseline Requirements or More (Harris & Benedict, 1919) in Children (12 Years of Age or Younger, $n = 107$), Adolescents (13 to 18 Years of Age, $n = 51$), and Adults (19 Years of Age or Older, $n = 290$) at Weeks 1 to 5 after Transplant.

## Nutrition Supplements

Patient tolerance of nutrition supplements during the acute posttransplant period is poor. Glucose polymers are most acceptable and can be combined with fruit-ade beverages and served frozen as slushes when patients experience mucosal ulceration, thick viscous saliva, nausea, or anorexia. Patients with acute gastrointestinal GVHD or diarrhea from other causes require low-osmolar, low-lactose formulas.

After hospital discharge, various nutritionally complete supplements such as Ensure Plus, Instant Breakfast, and Sustacal are well tolerated. The flavor of a given supplement is impor-

tant to patients once their sense of taste starts to recover after the acute hospitalization period (Barale et al., 1982). Supplements are used effectively by individuals who are unable to maintain or gain weight and occasionally by those with dysgeusia or oral mucositis.

## Tube Feedings

The use of tube feedings has been minimally attempted in marrow transplant patients, primarily because of the universal placement of the multipurpose central venous catheters that facilitate the use of parenteral feedings. The risks associated with tube feeding vary depending on

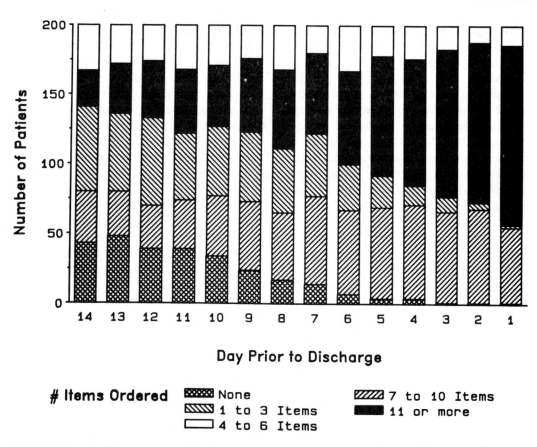

**Figure 19-4** Frequency and Number of Food Items Ordered Daily per Marrow Transplant Patient during the 14 Days before First Hospital Discharge. *Source:* From J.M. Gauvreau-Stern, C.L. Cheney, S.N. Aker, and P. Lenssen, "Food Intake Patterns and Foodservice Requirements on a Marrow Transplant Unit." Copyright The American Dietetic Association. Reprinted by permission from *Journal of the American Dietetic Association*, Vol. 89: 367–372, 1989.

the severity of mucosal and esophageal ulceration, nausea and vomiting, mucositis and local infection of the mouth and esophagus, low platelet counts and the attendant risk of gastrointestinal bleeding, and the risk of aspiration and pneumonia. Institutions that have extensive experience with tube feedings and competent, trained clinical staff for preparation, administration, and monitoring of the feedings may be comfortable using this feeding modality.

Szeluga, Stuart, Brookmeyer, Utermohlen, and Santos (1987) performed a randomized study of 57 adult and pediatric marrow transplant patients with leukemia, aplastic anemia, lymphoma, and other malignancies on an enteral feeding program compared to TPN for the first month after transplant. The results showed better maintenance of body composition in the TPN group but no differences for time to engraftment, sepsis, length of hospitalization, and short-term survival. Of the patients receiving enteral feeding, 73% required parenteral amino acid supplementation for an average of 1 week during the first month after transplant. Additionally, 25% of the patients receiving enteral feedings were unable to continue because of nausea, vomiting, and diarrhea and were placed on prolonged TPN support. The estimated energy requirements were not achieved by the enteral route alone, and total calorie and protein intake levels in the enterally fed patients were half those of patients receiving TPN. In the enterally fed patients no adverse complications associated with nasoenteric feeding were reported, but the extent to which tube feedings were actually used was unclear. There was a cost difference, with enteral nutrition representing a lower cost to the patient than TPN. Nutrition department staffing levels were increased to provide additional staff who worked to get patients to eat as well as monitored the enteral feedings, but such a food service is beyond the capabilities of many institutions.

**Parenteral Nutrition Support**

The patient's clinical course after marrow transplantation is characterized by acute symptoms that inhibit oral intake for prolonged periods after transplant (Aker et al., 1982). The delayed complications and severe metabolic stress also adversely affect patients' nutrition status (Layton et al., 1981; Reed, Halpin, Herzig, & Gross, 1981; Schmidt, Blume, & Gross, 1980) and result in profound nitrogen losses during the acute phase (Cheney, Abson, et al., 1987; Cheney, Lenssen, et al., 1987; Cunningham et al., 1986; Lenssen et al., 1984; Lenssen, Cheney, et al., 1987; Weisdorf, Hofland, & Sharp, 1984). Standard supportive care includes TPN (Aker et al., 1982; Van Lint et al., 1986; Yamanaka, Tilmont, & Aker, 1984), and many patients rely on TPN to some degree even after their discharge from the hospital (Lenssen et al., 1983).

In deciding when and whether to begin TPN several issues need to be considered, including initial nutrition status, age and possible long-term effects of inadequate nutrition on growth, use of toxic cytoreductive regimens such as TBI and intensive chemotherapy, and risk of early GVHD or other organ complications. Certainly some low-risk patients do not require TPN, but it is difficult to identify such patients before transplant. Furthermore it appears that most marrow transplant patients need some form of TPN during their posttransplant course, as suggested by studies attempting to define the benefits and risks of TPN (Szeluga et al., 1987; Weisdorf et al., 1987).

Weisdorf et al. (1987) performed a randomized study of 137 marrow transplant patients receiving either prophylactic TPN or dextrose hydration supplemented with vitamins, minerals, and electrolytes (control population) during the first month after transplant. Although the control patients were encouraged to eat and were offered oral nutrition supplements, their enteral intake was inadequate; most (40 of 66) required TPN for nutrition repletion. There were no differences between groups for time to engraftment, duration of hospitalization, or incidence of GVHD and bacteremia. Overall survival, time to relapse, and disease-free survival times were significantly improved in patients receiving prophylactic TPN. Prophylactic nutrition therapy appears to be indicated even for well-nourished transplant patients.

Parenteral nutrition or hydration (or both) can be used successfully to facilitate early hospital discharge and to reduce costs for clinically stable patients who are unable to attain baseline levels of nutrient (calories and protein) and fluid requirements while they are hospitalized. Lenssen et al. (1983) reported that 65% of marrow transplant patients discharged to an outpatient setting received partial parenteral nutrition support for a median of 2 weeks. Patients with leukemia required TPN substantially more frequently and for longer periods than patients with aplastic anemia. Adults required TPN most often for stomatitis, whereas in children no specific complaint could be found to account for appetite loss. Some patients were orally attaining sufficient calorie and protein levels to allow for discontinuation of TPN at the time of hospital discharge but were unable to attain required fluid levels, which is particularly important for patients taking cyclosporine.

The key to outpatient nutrition support is weekly counseling by the dietitian, daily or three times weekly weight checks, daily calorie counts and fluid intake documentation, and clinical monitoring of TPN tolerance.

## REFERENCES

Aker, S.N. (1979). Oral feedings in the cancer patient. *Cancer, 43,* 2103–2107.

Aker, S.N., Cheney, C., Sanders, J.E., Lenssen, P., Hickman, R.O., & Thomas, E.D. (1982). Nutritional support in marrow graft recipients with single versus double lumen right atrial catheters. *Experimental Hematology, 10,* 732–737.

Aker, S.N., & Lenssen, P. (1988). *A guide to good nutrition during and after chemotherapy and radiation* (3rd ed.). Seattle, WA: Fred Hutchinson Cancer Research Center.

Aker, S.N., Lenssen, P., Darbinian, J., Cheney, C.L., & Cunningham, B.A. (1983). Nutritional assessment in the marrow transplant patient. *Nutritional Support Services, 3,* 22–27.

Barale, K., Aker, S.N., & Martinsen, C.S. (1982). Primary taste thresholds in children with leukemia undergoing marrow transplantation. *Journal of Parenteral and Enteral Nutrition, 6,* 287–290.

Beatty, P.G., Witherspoon, R.P., Sullivan, K.M., Martin, P.J., Sanders, J.E., Appelbaum, F.R., Buckner, C.D., Storb, R., & Thomas, E.D. (1987). Long term results of bone marrow transplantation: The Seattle experience. In J.L. Touraine (Ed.), *Transplantation and clinical immunology, proceedings of the 19th international course* (pp. 203–216). New York: Excerpta Medica.

Carlson, L.A., & Rossner, S. (1972). A methodological study of an intravenous fat tolerance test with Intralipid emulsion. *Scandinavian Journal of Clinical Laboratory Investigation, 29,* 271–280.

Cheney, C.L., Abson, K.G., Aker, S.N., Lenssen, P., Cunningham, B.A., Buergel, N.S., & Thomas, E.D. (1987). Body composition changes in marrow transplant recipients receiving total parenteral nutrition. *Cancer, 59,* 1515–1519.

Cheney, C.L., Lenssen, P., Aker, S.N., Cunningham, B.A., Gauvreau, J.M., Darbinian, J., & Barale, K.V. (1987). Sex differences in nitrogen balance following marrow grafting for leukemia. *Journal of the American College of Nutrition, 6,* 223–230.

Cunningham, B.A., Morris, F., Cheney, C.L., Buergel, N.S., Aker, S.N., & Lenssen, P. (1986). Effects of resistive exercise on skeletal muscle in marrow transplant recipients receiving total parenteral nutrition. *Journal of Parenteral and Enteral Nutrition, 10,* 558–563.

Darbinian, J., & Schubert, M.M. (1985). Special management problems. In P. Lenssen & S.N. Aker (Eds.), *Nutritional assessment and management during marrow transplantation: A resource manual* (pp. 63–80). Seattle, WA: Fred Hutchinson Cancer Research Center.

Dickson, B., & Barale, K.V. (1985). Nutritional assessment. In P. Lenssen & S.N. Aker (Eds.), *Nutritional assessment and management during marrow transplantation: A resource manual* (pp. 5–14). Seattle, WA: Fred Hutchinson Cancer Research Center.

Driedger, L., & Burstall, C.D. (1987). Bone marrow transplantation: Dietitians' experience and perspective. *Journal of the American Dietetic Association, 87,* 1387–1388.

Freidman, A.L., Chesney, R.W., Gilbert, E.F., Gilchrist, K.W., Latorrac, R., & Segar, W.E. (1983). Secondary oxalosis as a complication of parenteral alimentation in acute renal failure. *American Journal of Nephrology, 3,* 248–252.

Gauvreau, J.M., Lenssen, P., Cheney, C., Aker, S.N., Hutchinson, M., & Barale, K.V. (1981). Nutritional management of patients with acute gastrointestinal graft-versus-host disease. *Journal of the American Dietetic Association, 79,* 673–677.

Gauvreau-Stern, J.M., Cheney, C.L., Aker, S.N., & Lenssen, P. (1989). Food intake patterns and food service requirements on a marrow transplant unit. *Journal of the American Dietetic Association, 89,* 367–372.

Harris, J.A., & Benedict, F.G. (1919). *Biometric studies of basal metabolism in man* (Publication no. 279). Washington, DC: Carnegie Institution of Washington.

Joint Food and Agriculture Organization—World Health Organization Ad Hoc Expert Committee Report (1973). *Energy and protein requirements.* Rome: Food and Agriculture Organization of the United Nations.

Jones, R.J., Lee, K.S.K., Beschorner, W.E., Vogel, V.G., Grochow, L.B., Braine, H.G., Vogelsang, G.B., Sensenbrenner, L.L., Santos, G.W., & Saral, R. (1987). Venoocclusive disease of the liver following bone marrow transplantation. *Transplantation, 44,* 778–783.

Kopple, J.D. (1981). *Profiles in nutritional management: The renal patient* (Abbott Laboratories Monograph). Chicago: Medical Directions.

Layton, P., Gallucci, B., & Aker, S.N. (1981). Nutritional assessment of allogeneic bone marrow recipients. *Cancer Nursing, 4,* 127–135.

Lenssen, P. (1989). Monitoring and complications of parenteral nutrition. In A.L. Skipper (Ed.), *The dietitian's handbook of enteral and parenteral nutrition* (pp. 347–373). Rockville, MD: Aspen.

Lenssen, P., Cheney, C.L., Aker, S.N., Cunningham, B.A., Darbinian, J., Gauvreau, J.M., & Barale, K.V. (1987). Intravenous branched chain amino acid trial in marrow transplant recipients. *Journal of Parenteral and Enteral Nutrition, 11,* 112–118.

Lenssen, P., Cheney, C., Flournoy, N., Aker, S., Barale, K., & Gauvreau, J. (1984). Nitrogen losses associated with marrow transplantation. *Clinical Nutrition, 4*(Special Supplement). Abstract No. P.28.

Lenssen, P., Moe, G.L., Cheney, C.L., Aker, S.N., & Deeg, H.J. (1983). Parenteral nutrition in marrow transplant recipients after discharge from the hospital. *Experimental Hematology, 11,* 974–981.

Lenssen, P., Spencer, G.D., & McDonald, G.B. (1987). A randomized trial of Freamine vs. Hepatamine vs. placebo in acute hepatic coma. *Gastroenterology, 92,* 1749.

McDonald, G.B., Sharma, P., Matthews, D.E., Shulman, H.M., & Thomas, E.D. (1985). The clinical course of 53 patients with venoocclusive disease of the liver after marrow transplantation. *Transplantation, 39,* 603–608.

McDonald, G.B., Shulman, H.M., Sullivan, K.M., & Spencer, G.D. (1986). Intestinal and hepatic complications of human bone marrow transplantation (Parts I and II). *Gastroenterology, 90,* 460–477.

Meyers, J.D., & Thomas, E.D. (1988). Infection complicating bone marrow transplantation. In R.H. Rubin & L.S. Young (Eds.), *Clinical approach to infection in the compromised host* (pp. 525–556). New York: Plenum.

Moe, G., Aker, S.N., & Schubert, M.M. (1985). Enteral nutrition. In P. Lenssen & S.N. Aker (Eds.), *Nutritional assessment and management during marrow transplantation: A resource manual* (pp. 31–44). Seattle, WA: Fred Hutchinson Cancer Research Center.

Nims, J.W., & Strom, S. (1988). Late complications of bone marrow transplant recipients: Nursing care issues. *Seminars in Oncology Nursing, 4,* 47–54.

Reed, M.D., Halpin, T.C., Herzig, R.H., & Gross, S. (1981). Cyclic parenteral nutrition during allogeneic bone marrow transplantation. *Journal of Parenteral and Enteral Nutrition, 5,* 37–39.

Rothschild, M.A, Oratz, M., & Schreiber, S.S. (1988). Serum albumin. *Hepatology, 8,* 385–401.

Sanders, J.E., Hickman, R.O., Aker, S.N., Hersman, J., Buckner, C.D., & Thomas, E.D. (1982). Experience with double lumen right atrial catheters. *Journal of Parenteral and Enteral Nutrition, 6,* 95–99.

Sanders, J.E., Pritchard, S., Mahoney, P., Amos, D., Buckner, C.D., Witherspoon, R.P., Deeg, H.J., Doney, K.C., Sullivan, K.M., Appelbaum, F.R., Storb, R., & Thomas, E.D. (1986). Growth and development following marrow transplant for leukemia. *Blood, 68,* 1129–1135.

Schmidt, G.M., Blume, K.G., & Gross, K.J. (1980). Parenteral nutrition in bone marrow transplant recipients. *Experimental Hematology, 8,* 506–511.

Schubert, M.M., & Izutsu, K.T. (1987). Iatrogenic causes of salivary gland dysfunction. *Journal of Dental Research, 66,* 680–688.

Shulman, H.M., McDonald, G.B., & Matthews, D.E. (1980). An analysis of hepatic venocclusive disease and centrilobular hepatic degeneration following bone marrow transplantation. *Gastroenterology, 79,* 1178–1191.

Shulman, H.M., Sullivan, K.M., Weiden, P.L., McDonald, G.B., Striker, G.E., Sale, G.E., Hackman, R., Tsoi, M.S., Storb, R., & Thomas, E.D. (1980). Chronic graft-versus-host syndrome in man: A long-term clinico-pathologic study of 20 Seattle patients. *American Journal of Medicine, 69,* 204–217.

Skeie, B., Askanazi, J., Rothkopf, M.M., Rosenbaum, S.H., Kvetan, V., & Thomashow, B. (1988). Intravenous fat emulsions and lung function: A review. *Critical Care Medicine, 16,* 183–194.

Spencer, G.D., Hackman, R.C., McDonald, G.B., Amos, D.E., Cunningham, B.A., Meyers, J.D., & Thomas, E.D. (1986). A prospective study of unexplained nausea and vomiting after marrow transplantation. *Transplantation, 42,* 602–607.

Storb, R., Deeg, H.J., Whitehead, J., Appelbaum, F., Beatty, P., Bensinger, W., Buckner, C.D., Clift, R., Doney, K., Farewell, V., Hansen, J., Hill, R., Lum, L., Martin, P., McGuffin, R., Sanders, J., Stewart, P., Sullivan, K., Witherspoon, R., Yee, G., & Thomas, E.D. (1986). Methotrexate and cyclosporine compared with cyclosporine alone for prophylaxis of acute graft versus host disease after marrow transplantation for leukemia. *New England Journal of Medicine, 314,* 729–735.

Sullivan, K.M. (1986). Acute and chronic graft-versus-host disease in man. *International Journal of Cell Cloning, 4*(Suppl. 1), 42–93.

Sullivan, K.M., Shulman, H.M., Storb, R., Weiden, P.L., Witherspoon, R.P., McDonald, G.B., Schubert, M.M., Atkinson, K., & Thomas, E.D. (1981). Chronic graft-versus-host disease in 52 patients: Adverse natural course and successful treatment with combination immunosuppression. *Blood, 57,* 267–276.

Sullivan, K.M., Witherspoon, R.P., Storb, R., Weiden, P., Flournoy, N., Dahlberg, S., Deeg, H.J., Sanders, J.E., Doney, K.D., Appelbaum, F.R., McGuffin, R., McDonald, G.B., Meyers, J., Schubert, M.M., Gauvreau, J., Shulman, H.M., Sale, G.E., Anasetti, C., Loughran, T.P., Strom, S., Nims, J., & Thomas, E.D. (1988). Prednisone and azathioprine compared with prednisone and placebo for treatment of chronic graft-v-host disease: Prognostic influence of prolonged thrombocytopenia after allogeneic marrow transplantation. *Blood, 72,* 546–554.

Szeluga, D.J., Stuart, R.K., Brookmeyer, R., Utermohlen, V., & Santos, G.W. (1985). Energy requirements of parenterally fed bone marrow transplant recipients. *Journal of Parenteral and Enteral Nutrition, 9,* 139–143.

Szeluga, D.J., Stuart, R.K., Brookmeyer, R., Utermohlen, V., & Santos, G.W. (1987). Nutritional support of bone marrow transplant recipients: A prospective randomized clinical trial comparing total parenteral nutrition to an enteral feeding program. *Cancer Research, 47,* 3309–3316.

Thomas, E.D. (1987a). Bone marrow transplantation. *CA— A Cancer Journal for Clinicians, 37,* 291–301.

Thomas, E.D. (1987b). Bone marrow transplantation in hematologic malignancies. *Hospital Practice* (February 15), 77–91.

Van Lint, M.T., Zunino, P., Mansuino, P., Pittaluga, P.A., Occhini, D., Peralvo, J., Bacigalupo, A.M., & Marmont, A.M. (1986). Total parenteral nutrition following BMT. *Bone Marrow Transplantation, 1*(Suppl. 1), 222–223.

Weisdorf, S., Hofland, C., & Sharp, H.L. (1984). Total parenteral nutrition in bone marrow transplantation: A clinical evaluation. *Journal of Pediatric Gastroenterology and Nutrition, 3,* 95–100.

Weisdorf, S., Lysne, J., Wind, D., Haake, R.J., Sharp, H.L., Goldman, A., Schissel, K., McGlave, P.B., Ramsay, N.K., & Kersey, J.H. (1987). Positive effect of prophylactic total parenteral nutrition on long term outcome of bone marrow transplantation. *Transplantation, 43,* 833–838.

Weisdorf, S.A., Salati, L.M., Longsdorf, J.A., Ramsay, N.K., & Sharp, H.L. (1985). Graft-versus-host disease of the intestine: A protein losing enteropathy characterized by fecal α-1-antitrypsin. *Gastroenterology, 85,* 1076–1081.

Wolfe, B.M., & Ney, D.M. (1986). Lipid metabolism in parenteral nutrition. In J.L. Rombeau & M.D. Caldwell (Eds.), *Clinical nutrition: Vol. 2. Parenteral nutrition* (pp. 72–99). Philadelphia: Saunders.

Wolford, J.L., & McDonald, G.B. (1988). A problem-oriented approach to intestinal and liver disease after marrow transplantation. *Journal of Clinical Gastroenterology, 10,* 419–433.

Yamanaka, W.K., Tilmont, G., & Aker, S.N. (1984). Plasma fatty acids of marrow transplant recipients on fat-supplemented parenteral nutrition. *American Journal of Clinical Nutrition, 39,* 607–611.

# Part IV

# Methods of Management

Page 15

# Chapter 20

# Encouraging Oral Intake

*Marcia L. Nahikian-Nelms*

Encouraging and maintaining adequate oral intake for cancer patients is one of the most difficult jobs for the clinical dietitian. It is extremely time consuming and often frustrating, but it can also be one of the most rewarding experiences in patient care. Through identifying feeding problems, instituting appropriate interventions, and providing individual education, the clinical dietitian can promote adequate oral intake in these patients. The dietitian is the key figure for orchestrating the nutrition support program, but its success requires the full support and cooperation of the health care team. Kelly (1986) notes that key factors to success are early intervention and continued observation and encouragement. These form the framework for encouraging oral intake.

## PATIENT INTERVIEW: ASSESSING THE PROBLEM

The patient interview is one of the most important parts of the nutrition assessment. During the patient interview, the dietitian elicits the information that helps identify the adequacy of current oral intake as well as any potential problems preventing adequate nutrition. The success of this interview depends on the dietitian's professional competence, interviewing skills, and bedside manner. This interview also lays the groundwork for a continued professional relationship with the patient. If a patient feels comfortable with the dietitian and trusts him or her, there is a great opportunity for accomplishing nutrition interventions.

The following list of interview questions may assist a dietitian in eliciting accurate information about the patient's ability to obtain oral nutrition:

1. How would you describe your appetite?
2. Has it changed recently?
3. Are you eating differently than you have most of your life?
4. Do you usually eat three meals each day? Has this changed recently?
5. Are you nauseated or experiencing vomiting? Is this food related or medication related? How long have you been experiencing this? How often do you have emesis?
6. Do you have a bowel movement every day? Has this changed?
7. Do you have diarrhea? If so, do you think this may be food related?
8. Do food smells or cooking odors bother you?
9. Do you have difficulty chewing?
10. Do your dentures (if any) fit? Do you wear them?

11. Do you have difficulty swallowing?
12. Is your mouth dry? Does your saliva seem to be different? Is it thicker or decreased in amounts?
13. Do you find it easier to drink liquids than to eat solid food?
14. What were you able to eat yesterday? (Obtain a brief 24-hour dietary recall.)
15. Are there certain foods that you are unable to eat right now?
16. Do some foods taste differently to you? Can you give an example?
17. Have you ever taken any high-calorie, high-protein supplements? When? What kind? How often? Were you able to tolerate them?
18. Do you take a multivitamin supplement?
19. Do you have any food allergies or intolerances? Are these new, or have you always experienced these intolerances?
20. Do you prepare your own meals? If so, do you ever feel too tired to prepare something to eat?

A successful patient interview is illustrated by the case of Mrs. C. During the patient interview, Mrs. C. related to the dietitian that generally her appetite seemed to be good but that it perhaps was slightly decreased recently. She had always eaten three meals every day, but often lunchtime passed without her knowing it. Breakfast seemed to fill her up for a much longer time than before. Mrs. C. was not experiencing nausea, vomiting, or diarrhea. She had a full set of dentures, but they did not fit "exactly right." Mrs. C. said that food just didn't interest her very much and that things just didn't taste as good as they used to. She lived with her husband and generally prepared most of the meals, although she admitted to being more tired and that food preparation was limited to "quick and easy meals."

This discussion provided the dietitian with significant data. The patient was experiencing a decreased oral intake even though she initially described her appetite as good. She was experiencing anorexia, dysgeusia, and early satiety. A decreased energy level contributed to difficulty in meal preparation. There seemed to be a definite change in oral intake that clinically correlated with a significant weight loss.

Other information related to a patient's social environment, emotional status, or medical status often comes out during a patient interview, as illustrated above. A skilled practitioner can then begin to formulate an appropriate nutrition care plan from the information received.

To assess the adequacy of a patient's diet, the clinician needs to determine what the optimal intake is for that patient. The patient's recommended energy and protein requirements should be determined so that an optimal goal can be established. The clinician then uses these parameters as a comparison with the patient's assessed intake. The Harris-Benedict equation (below) is the favored method for calculating basal energy expenditure (BEE) (Harris & Benedict, 1919). This equation has proved to be as good as more costly methods of estimating energy requirements, such as indirect calorimetry. The equation utilizes height, age, weight, and sex rather than just weight, as other methods do.

Men: BEE = 66 + (13.7 × weight [in kg]) + (5 × height [in cm]) − (6.8 × age [in years])

Women: BEE = 655 + (9.6 × weight [in kg]) + (1.7 × height [in cm]) − (4.7 × age [in years])

Other factors that should be considered in determining energy requirements include activity level, weight maintenance, weight gain, and the presence of other stress factors such as fever or infection.

The metabolic requirements of the cancer patient are controversial, and the practitioner can only estimate the stress that disease and treatment place on the patient. It seems that most practitioners utilize 150% to 160% of the BEE as a starting point for establishing caloric requirements (Teasley, Shronts, Lysne, Nuwer, & Cerra, 1983; Blackburn & Bistrian, 1976; Selig, 1979). Adjustments can then be made in the caloric goal depending on the patient's progress (i.e., weight gain or loss).

Blackburn and Bistrian (1976) recommend that at least 16% of the calculated caloric requirements be provided by protein. The remaining calories should be from nonprotein sources to attain a nitrogen-to-calorie ratio of 1:150. Lerebours et al. (1988) investigated the energy and protein status of adult patients with acute leukemia who were undergoing induction chemotherapy. They determined all patients to be hypermetabolic before initiation of chemotherapy (34% ± 6% more than the theoretical resting energy expenditure). This finding is in agreement with recent work by Merritt et al. (1981) and Klein and Camitta (1987), who found increases in BEE of 136% and 150% (±34%), respectively. This research included only leukemia patients. Research continues in this area to support the daily clinical decisions that must be made by the practicing dietitian.

It is helpful to include the patient in setting calorie and protein goals. Patients need to be invested in these goals to meet them. Most patients do not understand a simple caloric total, so that it is helpful to provide a simple guideline of calorie and protein values of common foods. One patient who effectively used this information added up his own intake after the evening meal every day. If he fell short of his goal, he would eat the remaining amounts before bedtime.

For the obese cancer patient, weight loss is contraindicated during periods of treatment. It is recommended that caloric requirements be established to maintain weight.

## INTERVENTIONS

With problems identified and nutrition requirements established, interventions must then be determined to assist in reaching the goal of optimal intake. From the initial meeting with the patient, it is essential to establish the importance of adequate nutrition. This may be easier said than done, however. Motivation can be difficult for the health care provider to elicit when the patient does not realize the importance of nutrition. An initial education session with a patient, therefore, is indicated to outline the basic physical requirements for adequate calorie and protein intake. The dietitian can then elucidate the stress placed on the body by disease, treatment, and infection and the additional requirements for nutrition support.

The patient may be too emotionally upset at first to focus on nutrition. Patients often describe feeling a loss of control when initiating medical treatment such as chemotherapy or radiation therapy. The nutrition care plan, however, is one area of the overall treatment plan over which the patient can exert some degree of control, and this fact ought to be stressed. If the nutrition support goals can be presented in this manner to the patient, he or she may be more willing to comply with planned interventions. For example, the dietitian could say to the patient "Meeting your nutrition needs every day is something you can do to help yourself. It will keep your energy levels up and allow you to continue your daily activities as much as possible." The dietitian should not allow the patient to believe that adequate oral intake can change the prognosis of the diease, however.

Maximizing oral intake for the hospitalized patient is certainly a challenge. The hospital environment often encourages nutrient deficits and is not always conducive to nutrition rehabilitation. Different eating styles, lack of access to favorite foods, and isolation are just a few of the problems that the cancer patient must face while trying to eat in the hospital. Again, the oncology dietitian, as the patient's nutrition advocate, can play a significant role in preventing and treating these deficits.

After performing a thorough nutrition assessment and patient interview in which deficits and problems are identified, the dietitian must begin to initiate interventions. At Ohio State University Hospitals, one of the first steps in assisting in increasing oral intake is teaching the patient to select appropriately from the menu. A menu selection guide was developed to help patients receive the most nutrition from their daily menu choices (Exhibit 20-1). These basic meal modifications also begin to teach the patient possible interventions for home use. If a patient is experiencing significant anorexia, however, the simple process of menu selection can be overwhelming. In such a case, a dietetic technician or dietitian may assist the patient in making appropriate food choices. Not only does this allow for meal selection, but daily visitation with the patient provides a consistent source of feedback regarding his or her ability to eat.

The variety of foods that each individual patient may request is not always possible to provide. Oncology patients often have lengthy hospital stays and frequent readmissions. Food intake is often negatively associated with disease, treatment, and pain. Learned food aver-

**Exhibit 20-1** Hints from Your Oncology Dietitian: How To Get the Best Nutrition Value from Your Meals

---

Why do I need "the *best* nutrition?"

1. To rebuild tissues
2. To stabilize or gain weight
3. To increase strength and energy

1. Always select three meals. Even when you're not sure you will eat it—ORDER IT! You won't have the choice to eat it if it isn't served.
2. Try to order a good variety of foods from all food groups if at all possible.
3. *But* if there are certain foods you cannot eat (for whatever reason), stay away from them. Concentrate on the types of foods you can tolerate. For example, it is O.K. to choose soup and ice cream at every meal.
4. If food smells bother you, ask your nurse or dietary clerk to remove the cover from the tray before it is brought to you. This will allow the food odor to decrease before you even have the chance to smell it! You may also want to concentrate on cold foods such as cheese, fruits, custard, etc. that have less smell to them.
5. If you have problems chewing or swallowing, you should have a "MODIFIED" menu. This will give you the choice of soft foods that are easy to chew and swallow. If you don't have this, ask your dietitian.
6. "I can only eat two or three bites"—sound familiar? If you get full easily, we can try small, frequent meals. Order "HALF PORTIONS" on your menu by writing it in. We can make up your calories by adding between-meal supplements and snacks.
7. Use your write-in list to add additional foods not available on the standard menu. This should help on days when only a soup and sandwich sounds good.
8. Add calories and protein wherever possible. High-protein foods include meats, poultry, cheese, eggs, peanut butter, milk, yogurt, eggnog, and milk shakes.

> Always order two to three pats of butter or margarine and add them to your food selections. Three pats of butter will add 135 calories to your meal.
>
> Drink whole milk at every meal if possible. This is one of your best protein sources.
>
> Do not deny yourself your sweet tooth—order dessert, ice cream, pudding, or custard, and add sugar to your beverages (unless your physician advises otherwise).

9. Make the "most" of your between-meal supplements. Even when we are not used to snacking, it is often easy to drink something between meals. This can be a quick way to boost your nutrition. Our dietetic technicians and dietitian will ask you for your choices of these supplements. We want to make the best choices for you. If you are having difficulty, let us know. We can easily set a "supplement taste test" designed just for you!
10. The important thing to remember—it is O.K. for your preferences and tastes to change! We can and will make those changes!

*Source:* Courtesy of Marcia Nahikian-Nelms, Department of Nutrition and Dietetics, The Ohio State University Hospitals.

---

sions are common, and hospital food service is a frequent target of these food aversions. It is always helpful to have alternative meal choices available as well as to encourage family members to bring favorite foods from home if possible.

Other nutrition interventions should be planned for each specific eating problem. Making changes in mechanical consistency and timing of meals, increasing nutrient density of foods, and using high-calorie, high-protein supplements are all examples of specific interventions that may be required for the patient.

Hoffman (1979) describes a nutrition care plan that makes use of a behavior modification model:

1. Determine the problem.
2. Produce an intervention to change the problem.
3. Educate the patient.
4. Achieve the goal by taking one step at a time.
5. Quantify the behavior, and record feedback.
6. Evaluate the intervention.

The following two examples show how nutrition goals can be achieved in this manner.

1. Mrs. K. was experiencing nausea associated with food odors. This problem was discovered by the dietitian during the initial interview. The dietitian instructed Mrs. K. to choose specific foods that tend to have minimal odors, such as cold plates, soups, yogurt, and cottage cheese. The dietitian and the dietetic technician assisted the patient with menu selection daily as well. The food service clerks who delivered Mrs. K.'s trays also were requested to remove the lids from the trays in the hall so that most odors were gone before the trays were brought into the room. Calorie counts were obtained to evaluate the adequacy of Mrs. K.'s oral intake.

2. A 17-year-old bone marrow transplant patient was experiencing significant anorexia 2 years after his transplant. His diet was extremely low in protein, and he complained of getting full quickly. His problems were identified as anorexia and early satiety resulting in inadequate calorie and protein intake with subsequent weight loss. Initial interventions included an individualized feeding schedule with six to eight small meals per day. The dietitian helped the patient determine foods high in protein that he liked. He agreed to choose one of those foods at each small feeding. A calorie goal was established, and the patient kept a food diary and calorie counter at his bedside. The dietitian met with him daily to evaluate his intake and to give positive reinforcement and suggestions. Weights were taken daily, as were calculated calorie counts to measure the effectiveness of the dietary interventions.

Evaluation tools to measure the effectiveness of nutrition intervention methods can include daily calorie counts, body weight measurements, and meal rounds. Consistent follow-up is absolutely necessary when working with cancer patients because symptoms can change quickly. For example, a patient may develop mucositis overnight, necessitating a change in the texture of the diet. A patient may develop nausea and vomiting with a chemotherapy regimen and be unable to participate in the nutrition plan. Thus interventions made yesterday may be inappropriate today.

Much can be said about the dietitian's role in encouraging oral intake for the cancer patient. This role requires a caring, positive attitude and persistent daily contact with patients. Successful nutrition support also requires input from all health care team members.

Nursing can be of great assistance with the encouragement of oral intake. Grant (1986) offers suggestions for nursing's role in assisting with nutrition problems. Nurses can prepare for mealtimes by assisting patients with daily oral and hygiene care. They can make the environment more conducive to eating by taking away unnecessary equipment and ensuring that unpleasant odors are removed from the patient's environment. Simple assistance with the tray can be a great help. Patients with limited energy have trouble opening milk cartons or cutting meats. It also is helpful to have company during mealtimes. This is a time when patients feel isolated. If family members are not available or not supportive, a volunteer or health team member may provide that needed social encouragement (Grant, 1986).

The physician can also be an important source of encouragement for nutrition support by reiterating the importance of oral nutrition and giving positive reinforcement.

Administration of antiemetics and pain control medications should be scheduled to assist with oral intake. Administration of antiemetics should not be scheduled so that they end up being given to the patient after meals. It is also difficult for the anorexic patient to take multiple medications and then attempt to eat a meal; there simply is not "enough room."

The entire health care team's involvement in providing positive reinforcement and encouragement can make a big difference in the success of a nutrition care plan. A clinician's acknowledgment of a patient's weight gain or ability to complete a meal can smooth the way for continued nutrition accomplishments.

**REFERENCES**

Blackburn, G.L., & Bistrian, B.R. (1976). Nutritional care of the injured and/or septic patient. *Surgical Clinics of North America, 56,* 1195–1224.

Grant, M. (1986). Nutritional interventions: Increasing oral intake. *Seminars in Oncology Nursing, 2*, 36–43.

Harris, J.A., & Benedict, F.G. (1919). *A biometric study of basal metabolism in man* (Carnegie Institution of Washington Publ. No. 279). Washington, DC: Carnegie Institution of Washington.

Hoffmann, P.K. (1979). Nutrition rehabilitation: A modality of behavior modification. In J. Wollard (Ed.), *Nutritional management of the cancer patient* (pp. 167–177). New York: Raven.

Kelly, K. (1986). An overview of how to nourish the cancer patient by mouth. *Cancer, 58*, 1897–1901.

Klein, C.L., & Camitta, B.M. (1987). Close association of accelerated rates of whole body turnover (synthesis and breakdown) and energy expenditure in children with newly diagnosed acute lymphocytic leukemia. *Journal of Parenteral and Enteral Nutrition, 11*, 129–134.

Lerebours, E., Tilly, H., Rinbert, A., Delarue, J., Piquet, H., & Colin, R. (1988). Change in energy and protein status during chemotherapy in patients with acute leukemia. *Cancer, 61*, 2412–2417.

Merritt, R.J., Ashley, J.M., Siegel, S.E., Sinatra, F., Thomas, D.W., & Hays, D.M. (1981). Calorie and protein requirements of pediatric patients with acute nonlymphocytic leukemia. *Journal of Parenteral and Enteral Nutrition, 5*, 20–23.

Selig, D.E. (1979). Nutritional supplementation. In J. Wollard (Ed.), *Nutritional management of the cancer patient* (pp. 179–200). New York: Raven.

Teasley, K.M., Shronts, E.P., Lysne, J., Nuwer, N., & Cerra, F.B. (1983). Nutritional metabolic support: Parenteral and enteral. In D.J. Higby (Ed.), *Supportive care in cancer therapy* (pp. 93–123). Boston: Martinus Nijhoff.

# Chapter 21

# Use of Supplements: Types of Supplements

*Marcia L. Nahikian-Nelms*

The common nutrition-related symptoms that cancer patients experience, such as anorexia and early satiety, necessitate interventions that make use of high-calorie, high-protein nutrition supplements. These supplements concentrate the largest amounts of nutrients in the smallest volume, which is one goal of nutrition education of cancer patients and their families. Patients are usually more willing to consume these nutrient-dense liquids than to eat large amounts of solid food. When experiencing anorexia, for example, patients often find it overwhelming to face a large meal. One cup of supplement may not seem as intimidating to such patients.

Supplements can be divided in three categories:

1. commercial supplements
2. homemade or readily available supplements
3. modular supplements (commercial and readily available varieties)

Most clinicians are aware of certain commercial supplements (e.g., Ensure and Sustacal) that are available in most hospital and other clinical environments. These supplements are typically well tolerated by patients, but it is important to remember that use of supplements should be individualized for each patient. Cancer patients may experience various symptoms that alter their tolerance to oral intake, and the dietitian must take into account these individual symptoms when designing a supplement program for each patient.

The patient's involvement in his or her nutrition care plan can ensure its success. The same principle applies to a supplement program. Patients should be involved in the choice of supplements. At Ohio State University Hospitals, patients are routinely offered samples of five or six supplements and allowed to determine which products they prefer. Often the patient starts with small quantities, and together with the patient the nutrition staff set goals for the quantities that ultimately need to be ingested. Individual patients may also require scheduling of supplements as medications, which involves the entire health care team's commitment to the nutrition care plan. This involvement on the part of the team may be needed to convince the patient of the importance of adequate nutrition.

Variety is essential when choosing supplements for a cancer population (Parkinson et al., 1987). Individual tolerance, including taste preference and physiologic tolerance, varies widely among these patients. The use of one or two supplements does not supply a sufficient variety. Also, those supplements that a general population might not choose are often the ones that are tolerated by a cancer population.

## COMMERCIAL SUPPLEMENTS

In general, commercial supplements are nutritionally complete. They can be used as meal replacements, if necessary. The prescribed amount meets 100% of the recommended daily allowance of vitamins and minerals as well as 100% of energy and protein needs. These products are suitable for oral intake and are available in various flavors. Their use demands little or no preparation, which is an advantage for some patients. Their cost can make them prohibitive, however, and for some patients their taste may be unacceptable.

When determining product selection, nutrient composition should be analyzed. Commercial supplements can be further divided into three general categories on this basis.

### Supplements Containing Whole Protein and Lactose

Supplements containing whole protein and lactose (Table 21-1) should be utilized for patients with a normal digestive tract who have no lactose intolerance.

### Lactose-Free Supplements Containing Whole or Hydrolyzed Protein

Lactose-free supplements that contain whole or hydrolyzed protein (Table 21-2) should be used for patients with lactose intolerance.

### Defined-Formula Diets

Defined-formula diets (Table 21-3) contain both medium-chain and long-chain triglycerides, dipeptides and tripeptides, whole protein, and single amino acids; they are low in residue and lactose free. These formulas should be used for patients with malabsorptive conditions such as short bowel syndrome, radiation enteritis, or graft-versus-host disease involving the gastrointestinal tract. They are designed primarily for

use as tube feedings because of their poor taste, but there has been success with oral feedings with various flavor combinations (Exhibit 21-1). These flavor combinations can also be applied to any commercial supplement to enhance patient acceptance and variety.

## HOMEMADE OR READILY AVAILABLE SUPPLEMENTS

Homemade supplements can be prepared at home from items that can be purchased from a grocery store. Their advantages include low cost, large variety, and increased patient and family involvement in their preparation (Selig, 1979). Disadvantages include the preparation time and the need for adequate kitchen facilities (Selig, 19⁻ ). The usual kitchen items that are needed include a refrigerator, a freezer, and a blender. Homemade or readily available supplements include instant breakfast mixes, milk shakes, and eggnogs. At Ohio State University Hospitals, a recipe booklet is used to teach patients and families how to utilize homemade supplements (Exhibit 21-2).

The patient who is experiencing a decreased taste threshold for sweets or who does not like milk or milk shakes makes the use of these supplement suggestions difficult. For such patients fruit juice–based concoctions, the addition of lemon juice, or the use of buttermilk as an ingredient may be useful (Exhibit 21-2).

## MODULAR SUPPLEMENTS

Modular supplements (Table 21-4) consist of one nutrient: protein, carbohydrate, or fat. They can be utilized as additions to liquid supplements or specific foods (Campbell, Garza, Groziak, Mellen, & Nahikian-Nelms, 1987). The use of modular supplements in the feeding of the cancer patient allows the nutrient density of a food or supplement to be increased. Disadvantages include the need for individual preparation, differences in product consistency, taste acceptance, and cost (Selig, 1979). The patient may

*(continues on page 263)*

**Table 21-1** Commercial Nutrition Supplements Containing Whole Protein and Lactose (Amounts are per 1,000 kcal)

| | Biocare Shake Mix† Food Science Corp. | C.I.B.*† Carnation | Compleat Regular‡ Sandoz | Compleat Modified‡ Sandoz |
|---|---|---|---|---|
| Protein, g (% total kcal) | 56.1 (22%) | 55.2 (22%) | 40.0 (16%) | 40.0 (16%) |
| Source | Whey | Nonfat milk | Beef | Beef |
| | Ca caseinate | Soy protein | Nonfat milk | Ca casenate |
| | Na caseinate | Na caseinate | | |
| Fat, g (% total kcal) | 36.3 (32%) | 29.4 (26%) | 40.0 (36%) | 34.2 (55%) |
| Source | Soy oil | Milk fat | Corn oil | Corn oil |
| | | | Beef fat | Beef fat |
| Carbohydrate, g (% total kcal) | 111.2 (44%) | 128.4 (51%) | 120.0 (48%) | 132.5 (55%) |
| Source | Sucrose | Sucrose | Hydrolyzed cereal solids | Hydrolyzed cereal solids |
| | Corn syrup solids } 51.7 (21%) | Corn syrup solids (34%) } 44.4 (18%) | Maltodextrins | Vegetables |
| | Lactose, 59.5 (23%) | Lactose, 84.0 | Vegetables | Peaches |
| | | | Fruits, Orange juice | Orange juice |
| | | | Lactose, 24.4 (10%) | |
| Lactose, g | 59.5 | 84.0 | 24.4 | 0 |
| Volume for 1,000 kcal (mL) | 891.0 | 880 | 935 | 935 |
| Minerals | | | | |
| Calcium, mg | 1,485.0 | 1,435.0 | 625.0 | 625.0 |
| Phosphorus, mg | 1,155.0 | 1,387.3 | 1,250.0 | 875.0 |
| Magnesium, mg | 391.9 | 414.7 | 250.0 | 250.0 |
| Iron, mg | 114.8 | 16.9 | 11.3 | 11.3 |
| Iodine, µg | 123.8 | 176.2 | 93.8 | 93.8 |
| Copper, mg | 2.5 | 1.9 | 1.3 | 1.3 |
| Manganese, mg | N/A§ | N/A | 2.5 | 2.5 |
| Zinc, mg | 12.4 | 14.3 | 9.4 | 9.4 |
| Chromium, µg | N/A | N/A | 93.8 | 93.8 |
| Selenium, µg | N/A | N/A | 62.5 | 62.5 |
| Molybdenum, µg | N/A | N/A | 187.5 | 187.5 |
| Sodium, mEq | 39.4 | 42.6 | 51.6 | 27.2 |
| Potassium, mEq | 48.0 | 70.8 | 33.6 | 33.6 |
| Chloride, mEq | N/A | N/A | 22.9 | 12.3 |
| mOsm/kg | N/A | 700 | 405 | 300.0 |
| Volume to provide 100% RDAs (mL)# | 1,000 | 1,060 | 1,500 | 1,500 |

*continues*

**Table 21-1 continued**

| | Meritene Liquid* Sandoz | Meritene*† Sandoz | NutriCare† Advanced Health Care | Nutrimed Robard |
|---|---|---|---|---|
| Protein, g (% total kcal) | 60.0 (24%) | 64.8 (26%) | 57.1 (23%) | 150.0 (60%) |
| Source | Concentrated skim milk<br>Na caseinate | Nonfat milk<br>Whole milk<br>Ca caseinate | Whey<br>Whole milk | Egg white solids<br>Nonfat milk |
| Fat, g (% total kcal) | 33.3 (30%) | 32.4 (29%) | 33.3 (30%) | 0 |
| Source | Corn oil<br>Mono-, diglycerides | Milk fat | Milk fat | |
| Carbohydrate, g (% total kcal) | 115.0 (46%) | 111.6 (45%) | 117.8 (47%) | 100.0 (40%) |
| Source | Corn syrup solids, Sucrose } 58.3 (23%)<br>Lactose, 56.7 (23%) | Corn syrup solids, 14.4 (6%)<br>Sucrose, 17.2 (7%)<br>Lactose, 80.0 (32%) | Sucrose<br>Maltodextrin<br>Lactose | Sucrose, 83.3 (33%)<br>Lactose, 16.7 (7%) |
| Lactose, g | 56.7 | 80.0 | N/A | 16.7 |
| Volume for 1,000 kcal (mL) | 1,042 | 1,000 | 1,000 | 2,000 |
| **Minerals** | | | | |
| Calcium, mg | 1,250.0 | 2,070.0 | 1,667.9 | 2,004.0 |
| Phosphorus, mg | 1,250.0 | 1,820.0 | 1,249.5 | 1,167.0 |
| Magnesium, mg | 333.3 | 364.0 | 499.8 | 500.0 |
| Iron, mg | 15.0 | 16.0 | 22.5 | 60.1 |
| Iodine, µg | 125.0 | 138.0 | 185.6 | 501.0 |
| Copper, mg | 1.7 | 1.8 | 2.5 | 6.7 |
| Manganese, mg | 3.3 | 3.6 | 4.6 | 13.3 |
| Zinc, mg | 12.5 | 14.0 | 18.9 | 50.0 |
| Chromium, µg | N/A | N/A | N/A | N/A |
| Selenium, µg | N/A | N/A | N/A | N/A |
| Molybdenum, µg | N/A | N/A | N/A | N/A |
| Sodium, mEq | 39.8 | 44.0 | 40.4 | 130.0 |
| Potassium, mEq | 42.7 | 68.0 | 58.6 | 71.6 |
| Chloride, mEq | 47.0 | 58.5 | N/A | N/A |
| mOsm/kg | 505 | 690 | 840 | 600 |
| Volume to provide 100% RDAs (mL)# | 1,250 | 1,040 | N/A | N/A |

| | Nutrimed 420*<br>Robard | Sustacal + Milk**†<br>Mead Johnson | Sustagen + Water*<br>Mead Johnson | Vitaneed‡<br>Sherwood Medical |
|---|---|---|---|---|
| Protein, g (% total kcal) | 166.6 (67%) | 60.3 (24%) | 61.0 (24%) | 35.0 (14%) |
| Source | Egg white solids<br>Ca, Na caseinate<br>Nonfat milk | Nonfat milk<br>Whole milk | Nonfat milk<br>Whole milk<br>Ca caseinate | Beef<br>Na, Ca caseinate |
| Fat, g (% total kcal) | 2.4 (2%) | 24.4 (22%) | 9.1 (8%) | 40.0 (36%) |
| Source | | Milk fat | Milk fat | Soy oil |
| Carbohydrate, g (% total kcal) | 76.2 (30%) | 134.4 (54%) | 171.0 (68%) | 125.0 (50%) |
| Source | Sucrose<br>Fructose } 60.3 (24%)<br>Lactose, 15.9 (6%) | Sucrose, 36.2 (14%)<br>Corn syrup solids, 11.8 (5%)<br>Lactose, 85.8 (34%) | Corn syrup solids, 101.4 (40%)<br>Sucrose, 8.0 (3%)<br>Lactose, 61.6 (25%) | Maltodextrin<br>Vegetables<br>Peaches |
| Lactose, g | 15.9 | 85.8 | 61.6 | 0 |
| Volume for 1,000 kcal (mL) | 1,420 | 750 | 549 | 1,000 |
| Minerals | | | | |
| Calcium, mg | 2,380 | 1,612.4 | 1,824.0 | 500.0 |
| Phosphorus, mg | 1,475.6 | 1,334.4 | 1,368.0 | 500.0 |
| Magnesium, mg | 952.0 | 375.3 | 228.0 | 200.0 |
| Iron, mg | 42.8 | 16.7 | 10.3 | 9.0 |
| Iodine, μg | 357.0 | 138.9 | 85.5 | 75.0 |
| Copper, mg | 4.8 | 1.9 | 1.1 | 1.0 |
| Manganese, mg | 9.5 | 2.8 | 2.9 | 2.5 |
| Zinc, mg | 35.7 | 13.9 | 11.4 | 15.0 |
| Chromium, μg | 357.0 | N/A | N/A | N/A |
| Selenium, μg | 357.0 | N/A | N/A | N/A |
| Molybdenum, μg | 714.0 | N/A | N/A | N/A |
| Sodium, mEq | 98.3 | 39.8 | 29.8 | 21.7 |
| Potassium, mEq | 61.0 | 64.8 | 46.7 | 32.0 |
| Chloride, mEq | N/A | 37.6 | 43.3 | 23.9 |
| mOsm/kg | N/A | 899 | 1,100 | 375 |
| Volume to provide 100% RDAs (mL)# | 600 | 800 | 960 | 2,000 |

*Vanilla.
†Value includes whole milk.
‡With residue.
§N/A = Value not available.
#Including vitamins.

Appreciation is expressed to Mindy Hermann-Zaidins, RD, Memorial Sloan-Kettering Cancer Center, Clinical Nutrition Support Kitchen, for revision of this table, originally prepared by A.S. Bloch and M.E. Shils in the 6th Edition of Modern Nutrition in Health and Disease.

Source: From *Modern Nutrition in Health and Disease* (pp. 1607–1609) by M.E. Shils and V.R. Young (Eds.), 1988, Philadelphia: Lea & Febiger. Copyright 1988 by Lea & Febiger. Reprinted by permission.

**Table 21-2** Commercial Lactose-Free Nutrition Supplements Containing Whole or Hydrolyzed Protein (Amounts are per 1,000 kcal)

| | Enrich† Ross | Ensure* Ross | Ensure HN Ross | Ensure Plus* Ross |
|---|---|---|---|---|
| Protein, g (% total kcal) | 36.1 (14%) | 35.2 (14%) | 42.0 (17%) | 36.6 (15%) |
| Source | Na, Ca caseinate Soy protein | Na, Ca caseinate Soy protein isolate | Na, Ca caseinate Soy protein isolate | Na, Ca caseinate Soy protein isolate |
| Fat, g (% total kcal) | 33.8 (30%) | 35.2 (31%) | 33.6 (30%) | 35.5 (15%) |
| Source | Corn oil | Corn oil | Corn oil | Corn oil |
| Carbohydrate, g (% total kcal) | 147.2 (56%) | 137.2 (55%) | 133.6 (53%) | 133.2 (53%) |
| Source | Hydrolyzed cornstarch Sucrose Soy polysaccharide | Hydrolyzed cornstarch Sucrose | Hydrolyzed cornstarch Sucrose | Hydrolyzed cornstarch Sucrose |
| Lactose, g | 0 | 0 | 0 | 0 |
| Volume for 1,000 kcal (mL) | 909 | 946 | 960 | 666 |
| Minerals | | | | |
| Calcium, mg | 654.5 | 520.0 | 720.0 | 423.0 |
| Phosphorus, mg | 654.5 | 520.0 | 720.0 | 423.0 |
| Magnesium, mg | 260.9 | 200.0 | 288.0 | 211.0 |
| Iron, mg | 11.9 | 9.0 | 13.2 | 9.5 |
| Iodine, µg | 100.0 | 76.0 | 108.0 | 70.4 |
| Copper, mg | 1.3 | 1.0 | 1.4 | 1.1 |
| Manganese, mg | 3.2 | 2.0 | 3.6 | 1.4 |
| Zinc, mg | 14.6 | 15.0 | 16.4 | 15.9 |
| Chromium, µg | N/A‡ | N/A | N/A | N/A |
| Selenium, µg | N/A | N/A | N/A | N/A |
| Molybdenum, µg | N/A | N/A | N/A | N/A |
| Sodium, mEq | 33.6 | 34.8 | 38.3 | 33.1 |
| Potassium, mEq | 36.3 | 37.8 | 38.0 | 39.6 |
| Chloride, mEq | 36.9 | 38.4 | 38.3 | 37.3 |
| mOsm/kg | 480 | 450 | 470 | 600 |
| Volume to provide 100% RDAs (mL)§ | 1,530 | 1,892 | 1,400 | 2,000 |

| | Ensure Plus HN<br>Ross | Entralife<br>Navaco | Entrition<br>Biosearch | Fortical<br>Sherwood Medical |
|---|---|---|---|---|
| Protein, g (% total kcal) | 41.1 (17%) | 33.2 (14%) | 35.0 (14%) | 40.0 (16%) |
| Source | Na, Ca caseinate<br>Soy protein isolate | Whey<br>Isolated soy protein | Na, Ca caseinate | Na, Ca caseinate |
| Fat, g (% total kcal) | 32.8 (30%) | 33.2 (32%) | 35.0 (32%) | 40.0 (36%) |
| Source | Corn oil | Corn oil | Corn oil | Corn oil<br>Lecithin |
| Carbohydrate, g (% total kcal) | 131.5 (53%) | 129.4 (54%) | 136.0 (54%) | 120.0 (48%) |
| Source | Hydrolyzed cornstarch<br>Sucrose | Hydrolyzed cornstarch<br>Sucrose | Maltodextrin | Maltodextrin |
| Lactose, g | 0 | 0 | 0 | 0 |
| Volume for 1,000 kcal (mL) | 667 | 943 | 1,000 | 667 |
| Minerals | | | | |
| Calcium, mg | 695.0 | 471.6 | 500.0 | 625.0 |
| Phosphorus, mg | 695.0 | 471.6 | 500.0 | 625.0 |
| Magnesium, mg | 278.0 | 188.4 | 200.0 | 250.0 |
| Iron, mg | 12.5 | 8.4 | 9.0 | 11.2 |
| Iodine, µg | 105.6 | 70.8 | 75.0 | 100.0 |
| Copper, mg | 1.4 | 0.8 | 1.0 | 1.5 |
| Manganese, mg | 1.4 | 2.4 | 2.0 | 2.5 |
| Zinc, mg | 10.6 | 14.0 | 7.5 | 15.0 |
| Chromium, µg | N/A | 339.6 | N/A | N/A |
| Selenium, µg | N/A | 45.2 | N/A | N/A |
| Molybdenum, µg | N/A | 716.8 | N/A | N/A |
| Sodium, mEq | 33.8 | 32.8 | 30.5 | 29.6 |
| Potassium, mEq | 30.6 | 35.6 | 30.7 | 29.5 |
| Chloride, mEq | 29.8 | 36.0 | 28.2 | 29.9 |
| mOsm/kg | 650 | 450 | 300 | 410 |
| Volume to provide 100% RDAs (mL)§ | 1,420 | 2,000 | 2,000 | 1,060 |

*continues*

**Table 21-2** continued

| | Fortison Sherwood Medical | Fortison, L.S. Sherwood Medical | Isocal Mead Johnson | Isocal HCN Mead Johnson |
|---|---|---|---|---|
| Protein, g (% total kcal) | 40.0 (16%) | 40.0 (16%) | 32.5 (13%) | 37.5 (15%) |
| Source | Na, Ca caseinate | Ca, K caseinate | Na caseinate Soy protein isolate | Na, Ca caseinate |
| Fat, g (% total kcal) | 40.0 (36%) | 40.0 (36%) | 42.0 (37%) | 51.0 (45%) |
| Source | Corn oil Lecithin | Corn oil Lecithin | Soy oil, 33.6 (30%) MCT oil, 8.4 (7%) | Soy oil, 34.0 (31%) MCT oil, 14.5 (12%) Lecithin, 2.5 (2%) |
| Carbohydrate, g (% total kcal) | 120.0 (48%) | 120.0 (48%) | 126.0 (50%) | 100.0 (40%) |
| Source | Maltodextrin | Maltodextrin | Glucose oligosaccharides | Corn syrup solids |
| Lactose, g | 0 | 0 | 0 | 0 |
| Volume for 1,000 kcal (mL) | 1,000 | 1,000 | 960 | 500 |
| Minerals | | | | |
| Calcium, mg | 625.0 | 625.0 | 600.0 | 500.0 |
| Phosphorus, mg | 625.0 | 625.0 | 500.0 | 500.0 |
| Magnesium, mg | 250.0 | 250.0 | 200.0 | 200.0 |
| Iron, mg | 11.2 | 11.2 | 9.0 | 9.0 |
| Iodine, µg | 100.0 | 100.0 | 75.0 | 75.0 |
| Copper, mg | 1.5 | 1.5 | 1.0 | 1.5 |
| Manganese, mg | 2.5 | 2.5 | 2.5 | 1.7 |
| Zinc, mg | 15.0 | 15.0 | 10.0 | 15.0 |
| Chromium, µg | N/A | N/A | N/A | N/A |
| Selenium, µg | N/A | N/A | N/A | N/A |
| Molybdenum, µg | N/A | N/A | N/A | N/A |
| Sodium, mEq | 29.6 | 8.7 | 21.5 | 17.5 |
| Potassium, mEq | 29.5 | 29.5 | 32.1 | 21.5 |
| Chloride, mEq | 29.9 | 7.0 | 28.2 | 17.0 |
| mOsm/kg | 300 | 240 | 300 | 690 |
| Volume to provide 100% RDAs (mL)§ | 1,600 | 1,600 | 1,920 | 1,000 |

|  | *Isolife*<br>*Navaco* | *Isotein HN*<br>*Sandoz* | *Magnacal*<br>*Sherwood Medical* | *Newtrition*<br>*Knight Medical* |
|---|---|---|---|---|
| Protein, g (% total kcal)<br>Source | 42.5 (15%)<br>Whey (processed)<br>Soy protein | 57.1 (23%)<br>Lactalbumin<br>Na caseinate | 35.0 (14%)<br>Na, Ca caseinate | 33.3 (13%)<br>Na, Ca caseinate<br>Soy protein isolate |
| Fat, g (% total kcal)<br>Source | 33.6 (30%)<br>Corn oil, 23.3 (21%)<br>MCT oil, 10.3 (9%) | 28.6 (25%)<br>Soy oil, 21.1 (19%)<br>MCT oil, 7.5 (6%)<br>Mono-, diglycerides | 40.0 (36%)<br>Soy oil<br>Mono-, diglycerides<br>Lecithin | 37.0 (33%)<br>Corn oil |
| Carbohydrate, g (% total kcal)<br>Source | 137.6 (55%)<br>Hydrolyzed cornstarch | 131.4 (53%)<br>Maltodextrin<br>Monosaccharides | 125.0 (50%)<br>Maltodextrin<br>Corn syrup solids<br>Sucrose | 129.6 (53%)<br>Maltodextrin<br>Sucrose<br>Glucose solids |
| Lactose, g | Trace | 0 | 0 | 0 |
| Volume for 1,000 kcal (mL) | 1,000 | 843 | 500 | 926 |
| *Minerals* |  |  |  |  |
| Calcium, mg | 520.8 | 476.2 | 500.0 | 555.5 |
| Phosphorus, mg | 520.8 | 476.2 | 500.0 | 555.5 |
| Magnesium, mg | 183.3 | 190.5 | 200.0 | 222.2 |
| Iron, mg | 10.4 | 8.6 | 9.0 | 10.0 |
| Iodine, µg | 79.2 | 71.4 | 75.0 | 55.6 |
| Copper, mg | 1.0 | 1.0 | 1.0 | 1.1 |
| Manganese, mg | 1.0 | 1.9 | 2.5 | 1.9 |
| Zinc, mg | 7.9 | 7.1 | 15.0 | 8.3 |
| Chromium, µg | 104.1 | 71.4 | N/A | N/A |
| Selenium, µg | 104.1 | 71.4 | N/A | N/A |
| Molybdenum, µg | 26.0 | 142.8 | N/A | N/A |
| Sodium, mEq | 23.2 | 22.8 | 21.8 | 24.2 |
| Potassium, mEq | 26.7 | 23.2 | 16.0 | 23.7 |
| Chloride, mEq | 40.5 | 22.8 | 13.4 | 15.6 |
| mOsm/kg | 300 | 300 | 590 | 450 |
| Volume to provide 100% RDAs (mL)§ | 1,000 | 1,770 | 1,000 | 1,667 |

NUTRITION MANAGEMENT OF THE CANCER PATIENT

**Table 21-2** continued

| | Newtrition High Nitrogen Knight Medical | Newtrition Isotonic Knight Medical | Nutrex Besure Nutrex | Nutrex Drink Nutrex |
|---|---|---|---|---|
| Protein, g (% total kcal) | 50.0 (20%) | 34.0 (14%) | 35.2 (14%) | 52.5 (20%) |
| Source | Na, Ca caseinate Soy protein isolate | Na, Ca caseinate Soy protein isolate | Na, Ca caseinate Soy protein isolate | Egg white solids |
| Fat, g (% total kcal) | 33.3 (28%) | 34.0 (30%) | 35.2 (32%) | 0.7 (0.6%) |
| Source | Corn oil, 16.7 (15%) MCT oil, 16.6 (13%) Mono-, diglycerides | Corn oil MCT oil Mono-, diglycerides | Vegetable oil Mono-, diglycerides Lecithin | Mono-, diglycerides |
| Carbohydrate, g (% total kcal) | 133.2 (53%) | 139.6 (56%) | 137.2 (55%) | 198.8 (80%) |
| Source | Maltodextrin | Maltodextrin | Maltodextrin Sucrose | Corn syrup solids Sucrose |
| Lactose, g | 0 | 0 | 0 | 0 |
| Volume for 1,000 kcal (mL) | 832 | 943 | 960.0 | 1,408 |
| *Minerals* | | | | |
| Calcium, mg | 666.0 | 566.0 | 520.0 | 1,126.4 |
| Phosphorus, mg | 666.0 | 566.0 | 520.0 | 1,126.4 |
| Magnesium, mg | 266.4 | 188.7 | 200.0 | 475.9 |
| Iron, mg | 12.0 | 8.5 | 9.0 | 26.8 |
| Iodine, µg | 99.9 | 56.6 | 76.0 | 178.8 |
| Copper, mg | 1.3 | 0.9 | 1.0 | 2.4 |
| Manganese, mg | 1.7 | 0.2 | 2.0 | 3.0 |
| Zinc, mg | 10.0 | 7.1 | 15.0 | 17.9 |
| Chromium, µg | N/A | N/A | N/A | N/A |
| Selenium, µg | N/A | N/A | N/A | N/A |
| Molybdenum, µg | N/A | N/A | N/A | N/A |
| Sodium, mEq | 21.7 | 24.6 | 34.8 | 36.7 |
| Potassium, mEq | 21.3 | 24.2 | 37.9 | 57.8 |
| Chloride, mEq | 16.4 | 18.6 | 38.3 | 24.7 |
| mOsm/kg | 300 | 300 | 450 | 450 |
| Volume to provide 100% RDAs (mL)§ | 1,250 | 2,000 | 1,920 | 1,200 |

| | Nutrex Encaret Nutrex | Nutrex Protamin Nutrex | Osmolite Ross | Osmolite HN Ross |
|---|---|---|---|---|
| Protein, g (% total kcal) | 26.8 (11%) | 31.3 (12%) | 35.2 (14%) | 41.9 (17%) |
| Source | Na, Ca caseinate Egg white solids | Na, Ca caseinate Soy protein | Na, Ca caseinate Soy protein isolate | Na, Ca caseinate Soy protein isolate |
| Fat, g (% total kcal) | 125.7 (23%) | 29.9 (27%) | 36.4 (31%) | 34.7 (30%) |
| Source | Soy oil | Corn oil Lecithin | MCT oil, 17.2 (14%) Corn oil Soy oil, 19.2 (17%) | MCT oil, 18.3 (15%) Corn oil, 13.5 (12%) Soy oil, 3.4 (3%) |
| Carbohydrate, g (% total kcal) | 162.2 (65%) | 149.8 (60%) | 137.2 (55%) | 133.0 (53%) |
| Source | Corn syrup solids Sucrose Fiber | Corn syrup solids Sucrose | Hydrolyzed cornstarch | Hydrolyzed cornstarch |
| Lactose, g | 0 | 0 | 0 | 0 |
| Volume for 1,000 kcal (mL) | 676 | 799 | 946 | 946 |
| Minerals | | | | |
| Calcium, mg | 540.8 | 666.0 | 498.1 | 714.0 |
| Phosphorus, mg | 540.8 | 666.0 | 498.1 | 714.0 |
| Magnesium, mg | 228.5 | 266.4 | 199.0 | 284.9 |
| Iron, mg | 10.3 | 12.0 | 9.0 | 12.8 |
| Iodine, µg | 85.5 | 99.9 | 74.5 | 106.6 |
| Copper, mg | 1.1 | 1.3 | 1.0 | 1.4 |
| Manganese, mg | 2.2 | 2.5 | 2.4 | 3.6 |
| Zinc, mg | 8.6 | 10.0 | 11.2 | 16.0 |
| Chromium, µg | N/A | N/A | N/A | N/A |
| Selenium, µg | N/A | N/A | N/A | N/A |
| Molybdenum, µg | N/A | N/A | N/A | N/A |
| Sodium, mEq | 2.9 | 5.8 | 26.0 | 38.2 |
| Potassium, mEq | 29.5 | 34.1 | 24.4 | 37.7 |
| Chloride, mEq | 15.2 | 16.9 | 22.4 | 38.2 |
| mOsm/kg | 460 | 450 | 300 | 300 |
| Volume to provide 100% RDAs (mL)§ | 1,200 | 1,200 | 1,887 | 1,321 |

*continues*

**Table 21-2 continued**

| | Portagen Mead Johnson | Precision HN Sandoz | Precision Isotonic Sandoz | Precision LR Sandoz |
|---|---|---|---|---|
| Protein, g (% total kcal) | 35.0 (14%) | 41.7 (17%) | 30.0 (12%) | 23.6 (10%) |
| Source | Na caseinate | Egg white solids | Egg white solids | Egg white solids |
| Fat, g (% total kcal) | 47.7 (40%) | 1.2 (1%) | 31.3 (28%) | 1.4 (1%) |
| Source | MCT oil, 41.0 (34%) | Soy oil | Soy oil | Soy oil |
| | Corn oil, 5.5 (5%) | | | |
| | Lecithin, 1.3 (1%) | | | |
| Carbohydrate, g (% total kcal) | 115.0 (46%) | 205.7 (82%) | 150.0 (60%) | 225.4 (89%) |
| Source | Corn syrup solids, 85.3 (34%) | Maltodextrin | Maltodextrin | Maltodextrin |
| | Sucrose, 29.1 (12%) | Sucrose | Sucrose | Sucrose |
| Lactose, g | 0 | 0 | 0 | 0 |
| Volume for 1,000 kcal (mL) | 1,000 | 952 | 1,000 | 909 |
| Minerals | | | | |
| Calcium, mg | 936.0 | 333.3 | 640.0 | 527.3 |
| Phosphorus, mg | 702.0 | 333.3 | 640.0 | 527.3 |
| Magnesium, mg | 208.0 | 133.3 | 256.0 | 212.7 |
| Iron, mg | 18.7 | 6.0 | 11.5 | 9.5 |
| Iodine, µg | 72.9 | 50.0 | 96.2 | 80.0 |
| Copper, mg | 1.6 | 0.7 | 1.3 | 1.1 |
| Manganese, mg | 1.2 | 1.3 | 2.7 | 2.2 |
| Zinc, mg | 9.4 | 5.0 | 9.6 | 8.0 |
| Chromium, µg | N/A | 50.5 | 96.0 | 79.7 |
| Selenium, µg | N/A | 58.1 | 64.0 | 53.2 |
| Molybdenum, µg | N/A | 100.0 | 192.0 | 159.1 |
| Sodium, mEq | 20.8 | 40.6 | 33.5 | 27.6 |
| Potassium, mEq | 32.2 | 22.2 | 24.6 | 20.5 |
| Chloride, mEq | 23.9 | 32.0 | 29.0 | 28.2 |
| mOsm/kg | 320 | 525 | 300 | 480 |
| Volume to provide 100% RDAs (mL)§ | 960 | 2,850 | 1,560 | 1,710 |

*continues*

| | *Pre-Fortison*<br>**Sherwood Medical** | *Resource*<br>**Sandoz** | *Ross SLD*<br>**Ross** |
|---|---|---|---|
| Protein, g (% total kcal) | 40.0  (16%) | 34.9  (14%) | 53.6  (21%) |
| Source | Na, Ca caseinate | Na, Ca caseinate<br>Soy protein isolate | Egg white solids |
| Fat, g (% total kcal) | 40.0  (36%) | 34.9  (32%) | 0.7  (1%) |
| Source | Corn oil<br>Lecithin | Soy oil<br>Mono-, diglycerides | |
| Carbohydrate, g (% total kcal) | 120.0  (48%) | 135.9  (55%) | 195.6  (78%) |
| Source | Maltodextrin | Maltodextrin<br>Sucrose | Sucrose<br>Hydrolyzed cornstarch |
| Lactose, g | 0 | 0 | 0 |
| Volume for 1,000 kcal (mL) | 2,000 | 943 | 1,428 |
| Minerals | | | |
| Calcium, mg | 625.0 | 515.5 | 1,192.3 |
| Phosphorus, mg | 625.0 | 515.5 | 1,192.3 |
| Magnesium, mg | 500.0 | 197.8 | 478.4 |
| Iron, mg | 22.5 | 8.9 | 21.4 |
| Iodine, µg | 200.0 | 75.0 | 178.5 |
| Copper, mg | 3.0 | 1.0 | 2.4 |
| Manganese, mg | 5.0 | 2.0 | 6.0 |
| Zinc, mg | 30.0 | 14.9 | 27.1 |
| Chromium, µg | N/A | N/A | N/A |
| Selenium, µg | N/A | N/A | N/A |
| Molybdenum, µg | N/A | N/A | N/A |
| Sodium, mEq | 29.6 | 34.6 | 51.7 |
| Potassium, mEq | 29.5 | 37.5 | 30.5 |
| Chloride, mEq | 29.9 | 37.0 | 40.2 |
| mOsm/kg | 150 | 450 | 545 |
| Volume to provide 100% RDAs (mL)§ | 1,600 | 1,896 | 1,200 |

**Table 21-2 continued**

| | Susta II† Mead Johnson | Sustacal Liquid Mead Johnson | Sustacal HC Mead Johnson | Travasorb Liquid Travenol |
|---|---|---|---|---|
| Protein, g (% total kcal) | 43.2 (17%) | 60.1 (24%) | 40.0 (16%) | 35.0 (14%) |
| Source | Na caseinate Soy protein isolate | Na, Ca caseinate Soy protein | Na, Ca caseinate | Na, Ca caseinate Soy protein isolate |
| Fat, g (% total kcal) | 33.2 (30%) | 23.1 (21%) | 37.8 (34%) | 35.0 (31%) |
| Source | Corn oil | Soy oil | Soy oil Lecithin | Corn oil Soy oil |
| Carbohydrate, g (% total kcal) | 132.0 (53%) | 137.8 (55%) | 122.2 (49%) | 136.4 (55%) |
| Source | Corn syrup solids Sucrose Soy polysaccharide | Sucrose, 97.0 (39%) Corn syrup solids, 40.8 (16%) | Corn syrup solids Sucrose | Sucrose Corn syrup solids |
| Lactose, g | 0 | 0 | 0 | 0 |
| Volume for 1,000 kcal (mL) | 960 | 980 | 667 | 1,000 |
| *Minerals* | | | | |
| Calcium, mg | 800.0 | 1,000.0 | 555.6 | 500.0 |
| Phosphorus, mg | 668.0 | 925.9 | 555.6 | 500.0 |
| Magnesium, mg | 268.0 | 375.0 | 222.3 | 200.0 |
| Iron, mg | 12.0 | 16.7 | 10.0 | 9.0 |
| Iodine, μg | 100.0 | 138.9 | 83.3 | 75.0 |
| Copper, mg | 1.3 | 1.9 | 1.1 | 1.0 |
| Manganese, mg | 1.7 | 2.8 | 1.7 | 2.0 |
| Zinc, mg | 13.2 | 13.9 | 8.3 | 15.0 |
| Chromium, μg | N/A | N/A | N/A | N/A |
| Selenium, μg | N/A | N/A | N/A | N/A |
| Molybdenum, μg | N/A | N/A | N/A | N/A |
| Sodium, mEq | 29.0 | 39.8 | 24.2 | 30.4 |
| Potassium, mEq | 33.8 | 51.9 | 24.7 | 30.8 |
| Chloride, mEq | 37.2 | 43.5 | 23.6 | 28.4 |
| mOsm/kg | N/A | 620* | 650 | 488 |
| Volume to provide 100% RDAs (mL)§ | 1,420 | 1,060 | 1,200 | 2,000 |

| | Travasorb MCT Travenol | TwoCal HN Ross |
|---|---|---|
| **Protein, g (% total kcal)** | 49.0 (20%) | 41.8 (17%) |
| Source | Lactalbumin | Na, Ca caseinate |
| **Fat, g (% total kcal)** | 32.9 (31%) | 45.4 (40%) |
| Source | MCT oil (25%) | Corn oil |
| | Sunflower oil (6%) | MCT oil |
| **Carbohydrate, g (% total kcal)** | 122.8 (49%) | 108.5 (43%) |
| Source | Corn syrup solids | Hydrolyzed cornstarch |
| | | Sucrose |
| Lactose, g | 0 | 0 |
| Volume for 1,000 kcal (mL) | 500 | 500 |
| **Minerals** | | |
| Calcium, mg | 500.0 | 528.5 |
| Phosphorus, mg | 500.0 | 528.5 |
| Magnesium, mg | 200.0 | 211.5 |
| Iron, mg | 9.0 | 9.5 |
| Iodine, µg | 75.0 | 79.5 |
| Copper, mg | 1.0 | 1.0 |
| Manganese, mg | 2.0 | 2.6 |
| Zinc, mg | 15.0 | 12.9 |
| Chromium, µg | N/A | N/A |
| Selenium, µg | N/A | N/A |
| Molybdenum, µg | N/A | N/A |
| Sodium, mEq | 15.2 | 23.0 |
| Potassium, mEq | 44.6 | 29.8 |
| Chloride, mEq | 34.7 | 22.0 |
| mOsm/kg | 312 | 690 |
| Volume to provide 100% RDAs (mL)§ | 2,000 | 947 |

*Vanilla.
†Contains fiber.
‡N/A = Not available.
§Including vitamins.

Appreciation is expressed to Mindy Hermann-Zaidins, RD, Memorial Sloan-Kettering Cancer Center, Clinical Nutrition Support Kitchen, for revision of this table, originally prepared by A.S. Bloch and M.E. Shils in the 6th Edition of *Modern Nutrition in Health and Disease*.

Source: From *Modern Nutrition in Health and Disease* (pp. 1610–1619) by M.E. Shils and V.R. Young (Eds.), 1988, Philadelphia: Lea & Febiger. Copyright 1988 by Lea & Febiger. Reprinted by permission.

**Table 21-3** Defined-Formula Diets (Amounts are per 1,000 kcal)

| | Criticare HN Mead Johnson | Nutrex Aminex Nutrex | Pepti 2000 Sherwood Medical | Reabilan Roussel |
|---|---|---|---|---|
| Protein, g (% total kcal) | 36.0 (14%) | 38.2 (15%) | 40.0 (16%) | 31.5 (13%) |
| Source | Casein hydrolysate | Crystalline amino acids | Hydrolyzed lactalbumin | Wheat peptides Casein peptides |
| Fat, g (% total kcal) | 3.0 (3%) | 2.8 (3%) | 10.0 (9%) | 38.9 (34%) |
| Source | Sunflower oil | Safflower oil | MCT oil, 5.0 (4%) Corn oil, 5.0 (5%) | MCT oil, 15.5 (12%) Oenothera biennis oil Soy oil Lecithin |
| Carbohydrate, g (% total kcal) | 210.0 (83%) | 205.7 (82%) | 188.8 (76%) | 131.5 (53%) |
| Source | Maltodextrin | Maltodextrin Modified starch | Maltodextrin | Maltodextrin Tapioca starch |
| Lactose, g | 0 | 0 | 0 | 0 |
| Volume for 1,000 kcal (mL) | 946 | 1,000 | 1,000 | 1,000 |
| Minerals | | | | |
| Calcium, mg | 500.0 | 499.5 | 625.0 | 498.7 |
| Phosphorus, mg | 500.0 | 499.5 | 625.0 | 498.7 |
| Magnesium, mg | 200.0 | 199.8 | 250.0 | 250.7 |
| Iron, mg | 9.0 | 9.0 | 11.3 | 10.0 |
| Iodine, µg | 75.0 | 74.9 | 100.0 | 74.7 |
| Copper, mg | 1.0 | 1.0 | 1.5 | 1.6 |
| Manganese, mg | 2.5 | 1.0 | 2.5 | 2.0 |
| Zinc, mg | 10.0 | 10.0 | 15.0 | 10.0 |
| Chromium, µg | N/A* | 16.6 | N/A | N/A |
| Selenium, µg | N/A | 50.0 | N/A | 50.7 |
| Molybdenum, µg | N/A | 50.0 | N/A | N/A |
| Sodium, mEq | 26.0 | 20.0 | 29.6 | 30.4 |
| Potassium, mEq | 32.0 | 20.1 | 29.5 | 32.1 |
| Chloride, mEq | 28.0 | 23.1 | 29.9 | 56.3 |
| mOsm/kg | 650 | 600 | 490 | 350 |
| Volume to provide 100% RDAs (mL)† | 1,892 | 2,000 | 1,600 | 2,000 |

| | Reabilan HN Roussel | Travasorb STD Travenol | Travasorb HN Travenol |
|---|---|---|---|
| Protein, g (% total kcal) | 43.6 (17%) | 30.0 (12%) | 45.0 (18%) |
| Source | Whey peptides<br>Casein peptides | Hydrolyzed lactalbumin | Hydrolyzed lactalbumin |
| Fat, g (% total kcal) | 39.0 (36%) | 13.4 (11%) | 13.4 (11%) |
| Source | MCT oil<br>Oenothera biennis oil<br>Soy oil<br>Lecithin | MCT oil, 9.0 (7%)<br>Sunflower oil, 4.4 (4%) | MCT oil, 9.0 (7%)<br>Sunflower oil, 4.4 (4%) |
| Carbohydrate, g (% total kcal) | 118.6 (47%) | 190.0 (76%) | 175.0 (70%) |
| Source | Maltodextrin<br>Tapioca starch | Glucose oligosaccharides | Glucose oligosaccharides |
| Lactose, g | 0 | 0 | 0 |
| Volume for 1,000 kcal (mL) | 750 | 1,000 | 1,000 |
| Minerals | | | |
| Calcium, mg | 338.0 | 500.0 | 500.0 |
| Phosphorus, mg | 376.0 | 500.0 | 500.0 |
| Magnesium, mg | 248.0 | 200.0 | 200.0 |
| Iron, mg | 10.0 | 9.0 | 9.0 |
| Iodine, µg | 76.0 | 75.0 | 75.0 |
| Copper, mg | 1.0 | 1.0 | 1.0 |
| Manganese, mg | 2.0 | 1.3 | 1.3 |
| Zinc, mg | 10.0 | 7.5 | 7.5 |
| Chromium, µg | 62.0 | N/A | N/A |
| Selenium, µg | 50.0 | N/A | N/A |
| Molybdenum, µg | N/A | N/A | N/A |
| Sodium, mEq | 32.6 | 40.0 | 40.0 |
| Potassium, mEq | 31.9 | 30.0 | 30.0 |
| Chloride, mEq | 52.8 | 42.9 | 39.0 |
| mOsm/kg | 490 | 560* | 560 |
| Volume to provide 100% RDAs (mL)† | 2,000 | 2,000 | 2,000 |

*continues*

**Table 21-3 continued**

| | Vital HN Ross | Vivonex Norwich Eaton |
|---|---|---|
| Protein, g (% total kcal) | 41.7 (17%) | 21.8 (9%) |
| Source | Partially hydrolyzed whey, meat, and soy | Crystalline amino acids |
| Fat, g (% total kcal) | 10.8 (8%) | 1.4 (1%) |
| Source | Safflower oil, 5.9 (5%) MCT oil, 4.9 (3%) | Safflower oil |
| Carbohydrate, g (% total kcal) | 188.3 (75%) | 230.6 (90%) |
| Source | Hydrolyzed cornstarch Glucose | Glucose oligosaccharides |
| Lactose, g | 0.83 | 0 |
| Volume for 1,000 kcal (mL) | 1,000 | 1,000 |
| Minerals | | |
| Calcium, mg | 667.0 | 550.0 |
| Phosphorus, mg | 667.0 | 550.0 |
| Magnesium, mg | 267.0 | 222.2 |
| Iron, mg | 12.0 | 10.0 |
| Iodine, µg | 100.0 | 83.3 |
| Copper, mg | 1.3 | 1.1 |
| Manganese, mg | 2.5 | 1.6 |
| Zinc, mg | 10.0 | 8.3 |
| Chromium, µg | N/A | 27.8 |
| Selenium, µg | N/A | 83.0 |
| Molybdenum, µg | N/A | 83.0 |
| Sodium, mEq | 16.7 | 20.4 |
| Potassium, mEq | 29.8 | 30.0 |
| Chloride, mEq | 18.8 | 20.4 |
| mOsm/kg | 460 | 550 |
| Volume to provide 100% RDAs (mL)† | 1,500 | 1,800 |

| | Vivonex HN Norwich Eaton | Vivonex T.E.N. Norwich Eaton |
|---|---|---|
| Protein, g (% total kcal) | 44.4  (17%) | 38.2  (15%) |
| Source | Crystalline amino acids | Crystalline amino acids (33% BCAA) |
| Fat, g (% total kcal) | 0.9  (1%) | 2.8  (2%) |
| Source | Safflower oil | Safflower oil |
| Carbohydrate, g (% total kcal) | 210.0  (82%) | 205.6  (82%) |
| Source | Glucose oligosaccharides | Maltodextrin Modified starch |
| Lactose, g | 0 | 0 |
| Volume for 1,000 kcal (mL) | 1,000 | 1,000 |
| *Minerals* | | |
| Calcium, mg | 330.0 | 500.0 |
| Phosphorus, mg | 330.0 | 500.0 |
| Magnesium, mg | 133.0 | 200.0 |
| Iron, mg | 6.0 | 9.0 |
| Iodine, µg | 50.0 | 75.0 |
| Copper, mg | 0.7 | 1.0 |
| Manganese, mg | 0.9 | 0.9 |
| Zinc, mg | 5.0 | 10.0 |
| Chromium, µg | 16.7 | 17.0 |
| Selenium, µg | 50.0 | 50.0 |
| Molybdenum, µg | 50.0 | 50.0 |
| Sodium, mEq | 23.0 | 20.0 |
| Potassium, mEq | 30.0 | 20.0 |
| Chloride, mEq | 23.1 | 25.0 |
| mOsm/kg | 810 | 630 |
| Volume to provide 100% RDAs (mL)† | 3,000 | 2,000 |

*N/A = Value not available.
†Including vitamins.

Appreciation is expressed to Mindy Hermann-Zaidins, RD, Memorial Sloan-Kettering Cancer Center, Clinical Nutrition Support Kitchen, for revision of this table, originally prepared by A.S. Bloch and M.E. Shils in the 6th Edition of *Modern Nutrition in Health and Disease.*

Source: From *Modern Nutrition in Health and Disease* (pp. 1620–1623) by M.E. Shils and V.R. Young (Eds.), 1988, Philadelphia: Lea & Febiger. Copyright 1988 by Lea & Febiger. Reprinted by permission.

**Exhibit 21-1** Flavoring Suggestions for Commercially Available Supplements for Use in Oral Feedings

The types of flavoring used should be determined by individual tastes and physiologic tolerance.

*Chocolate*—Add one heaping teaspoon or more to taste. Examples of brands: Hershey's Instant, Nestle's Quik, Swiss Miss Sugar-Free* Chocolate Milk Maker

*Extracts**—Add a few drops to taste of vanilla, almond, lemon, orange, or other extract. These are available in the spice section of the grocery store. Different types and brands vary in strength.

*Coffee*—For the coffee lover, add one level teaspoon instant coffee to a small amount of supplement; add this mixture to the rest of the supplement and mix well. Decaffeinated coffee can be used as well.

*Mocha*—Add instant coffee and chocolate flavorings.

*Butterscotch*—Add butterscotch syrup (1 tsp) or butterscotch powdered pudding mix (1 tbsp).

*Peanut Butter*—For patients with no fat restrictions, add 1 tsp of peanut butter to an 8-oz cup of formula and mix in a blender.

*Other Ideas**—Add dry powdered drink mix or gelatin mix (regular or sugar free) to provide an excellent variety of fruit flavors. One teaspoon of powder added to 8 oz of formula is appropriate.

*These suggestions are appropriate for use in a defined-formula diet.

**Exhibit 21-2** Recipe Suggestions

## MEAL IN A GLASS

MAKES: 1 serving          CALORIES: 320          PROTEIN: 15 g

1 cup milk
1 envelope (1.22 ounces) strawberry-flavored instant breakfast drink
1/4 cup crushed pineapple

Blend 5 to 10 seconds on high speed.

---

MAKES: 1 serving          CALORIES: 385          PROTEIN: 15 g

1 cup milk
1 envelope (1.22 ounces) vanilla-flavored instant breakfast drink
1 jar (4 1/2 ounces) pureed fruit (baby food) or 6 canned apricot halves

Blend 5 to 10 seconds on high speed.

---

MAKES: 1 serving          CALORIES: 345          PROTEIN: 15 g

1 cup milk
1 envelope (1.22 ounces) vanilla-flavored instant breakfast drink
1/4 cup frozen raspberries, strawberries, or blueberries

Blend 5 to 10 seconds on high speed.

---

MAKES: 1 serving          CALORIES: 390          PROTEIN: 16 g

1 cup milk
1 envelope (1.22 ounces) chocolate-flavored instant breakfast drink
1 small banana, cut up

Blend 5 to 10 seconds on high speed.

---

**Exhibit 21-2** continued

### BLENDER BANANA

MAKES: 1 serving          CALORIES: 630          PROTEIN: 8 g

1 cup light cream (20%)                              1 small banana, cut up
1 tbsp honey

Place all ingredients in blender. Blend on high speed until smooth, about 10 seconds. Serve immediately or freeze for a dessert.

---

### HIGH-PROTEIN SMOOTHIES

MAKES: 3 servings          CALORIES: 158/serving          PROTEIN: 14 g/serving

These smoothies are like milk shakes, thin or thick, depending on the temperature.

Blend until smooth:

1 cup cottage cheese
1 cup yogurt

Add one of the following:

1 banana + some strawberries + 1 tsp vanilla + honey to taste
1 peach + some strawberries + 1 tsp vanilla + honey to taste
1 banana + 2 tsp peanut butter + 1 tsp vanilla + honey to taste

VARIATIONS: Substitute your favorite fruit or jam. Substitute chocolate or other flavoring for vanilla. If you want it thinner, add milk or more yogurt. If you want it colder, blend with a cracked ice cube.

---

### VERY HIGH–CALORIE MILK SHAKE

MAKES: 1 serving          CALORIES: 780          PROTEIN: 5 g

1/2 cup ice cream (any flavor)
1/2 cup whipping cream (unwhipped)
1/4 cup Karo syrup
1 tsp vanilla flavoring

Mix all ingredients together in blender.

---

### CHOCOLATE PEANUT BUTTER MILK SHAKE

MAKES: 2 servings          CALORIES: 491/serving          PROTEIN: 12 g/serving

2 cups ice cream                                     1/3 cup half and half
2 1/2 tbsp peanut butter                             1 tsp vanilla flavoring
3 tbsp chocolate syrup

Blend together.

---

*continues*

**Exhibit 21-2** continued

---

### FROZEN FRUIT SLUSH

MAKES: 4 servings          CALORIES: 130/serving          PROTEIN: 1 g/serving

The slushy consistency of this dessert makes it easy to swallow.

1 6-oz can frozen fruit juice concentrate          4 tbsp sugar
3 cups crushed ice

Put all ingredients in blender and blend to desired consistency. Spoon into dishes and serve.

---

### EASY BLENDER FRUIT WHIP

MAKES: 4 servings          CALORIES: 91/serving          PROTEIN: 3 g/serving

1 10-oz package frozen fruit, cut into small pieces          2 tbsp lemon juice
1 tbsp gelatin powder          1/2 cup boiling water
2 unbeaten egg whites

Blend gelatin, lemon juice, and boiling water for 40 seconds. Add egg white and blend 10 seconds. Continue to blend while adding frozen fruit, one piece at a time. When mixture is blended, pour into a wet mold and chill at least 4 hours before serving.

---

### EGG CUSTARD

MAKES: 6 servings          CALORIES: 140/serving          PROTEIN: 6 g/serving

3 eggs          dash of salt
1/4 cup sugar          2 1/2 cups scalded milk
1 tsp vanilla

Blend eggs, sugar, salt, and vanilla. Gradually add scalded milk. Pour into 6 custard cups. Place cups in pan of hot water 1/2 in deep. Bake at 350° until set, approximately 45 minutes.

VARIATION: Make a caramel sauce by putting 1 tbsp brown sugar at the bottom of each cup before filling.

---

### STRAWBERRY FROST

MAKES: 1 serving          CALORIES: 220          PROTEIN: 6 g

2 tsp sugar          1 tbsp apple juice
2/3 cup strawberries          1/4 cup + 2 tbsp strawberry yogurt
3 oz orange juice

Combine ingredients in a blender and whip 10 seconds.

---

### SHERBET SHAKE

MAKES: 1 serving          CALORIES: 325          PROTEIN: 8 g

This is a lighter shake than the milk shake and is a good snack for a fat-restricted diet.

3/4 cup nonfat milk          1 cup sherbet, any flavor

Combine ingredients in a blender and blend to desired thickness.

---

**Exhibit 21-2** continued

### ORANGE FREEZE

MAKES: 1 serving                CALORIES: 340                PROTEIN: 3 g

3/4 cup orange juice                                1 cup orange sherbet
1 tbsp lemon juice

Combine ingredients in a blender and blend to desired thickness.

---

### PEACH YOGURT SHAKE

MAKES: 2 servings            CALORIES: 268/serving        PROTEIN: 10 g/serving

1 cup sliced peaches                                1 cup skim milk
1 cup plain yogurt                                  1 tbsp honey

Combine ingredients in a blender and blend until smooth.

VARIATIONS:  Instead of peaches, use 1 cup sliced bananas, fruit cocktail, strawberries, raspberries, or blackberries. If you use raspberries or blackberries, strain after blending to remove seeds.

---

### STRAWBERRY-BLUEBERRY SMOOTHIE

MAKES: 1 serving                CALORIES: 260                PROTEIN: 11 g

3/4 cup blueberry yogurt                            3 tbsp skim milk
1/3 cup strawberries                                2 tsp sugar

Combine ingredients in a blender and whip to desired thickness.

---

### TART TROPICAL FIZZ

MAKES: 1 serving                CALORIES: 230                PROTEIN: 2 g

1 cup grapefruit juice, chilled                     3/4 cup club soda, chilled
1/2 cup orange juice, chilled                       1 cup lime sherbet
1/4 cup pineapple juice, chilled                    Mint leaves

Mix fruit juices and club soda. Serve in glasses with ice cubes or crushed ice, and top each serving with a scoop of lime sherbet. Garnish with mint leaves.

NOTE:  If you do not have fresh mint, substitute a thin slice of orange, lemon, or lime.

---

### CRANBERRY DELIGHT

MAKES: 2 servings            CALORIES: 230/serving        PROTEIN: 3 g/serving

1 cup cranberry juice                   1 cup vanilla ice cream, slightly softened
1/4 cup orange juice

Measure all ingredients into blender container. Cover and blend until smooth. Pour into glasses and serve with straws.

*continues*

Exhibit 21-2 continued

## EGGNOG ("GUGGLE MUGGLE")

MAKES: 1 serving         CALORIES: 235         PROTEIN: 15 g

1/4 cup egg substitute          2 to 3 tsp sugar
1 cup milk          1/2 tsp vanilla

Combine all ingredients in a blender and blend until smooth.

NOTE: Egg substitutes are available in the frozen food or dairy section of your supermarket.

## PEACH EGGNOG

MAKES: 1 serving         CALORIES: 290         PROTEIN: 15 g

1/4 cup egg substitute          1 tbsp thawed frozen orange juice concentrate
1 cup milk
1/2 cup sliced peaches

Combine all ingredients in a blender and blend until smooth.

VARIATION: Instead of peaches, use 1/2 ripe banana, sliced.

NOTE: Egg substitutes are available in the frozen food or dairy section of your supermarket.

## BREAKFAST IN A GLASS

MAKES: 1 serving         CALORIES: 370         PROTEIN: 16 g

1 medium banana          1 tsp wheat germ
1/2 cup egg substitute          1 tsp honey
1/3 cup water          Dash salt
1 1/2 tbsp frozen orange juice concentrate (thawed)

Slice banana into blender; add remaining ingredients. Blend on high speed until smooth, about 1 minute.

NOTE: Egg substitutes are available in the frozen food or dairy section of your supermarket.

## BREAKFAST SHAKE

MAKES: 1 serving         CALORIES: 315         PROTEIN: 14 g

3/4 cup milk or half and half          1 banana, cut up
1/4 cup egg substitute          1/2 tsp vanilla

Place all ingredients in blender container. Cover and blend until smooth. Pour into large glass.

VARIATIONS: Substitute 1 peach (peeled, pitted, and cut up), 1 cup strawberries, or 1 cup blueberries for the banana.

NOTE: Egg substitutes are available in the frozen food or dairy section of your supermarket.

**Exhibit 21-2** continued

## STRAWBERRY-BANANA YOGURT COOLER

MAKES: 2 servings          CALORIES: 260/serving          PROTEIN: 9 g/serving

1/2 cup plain yogurt
1/2 cup light cream (20%) or milk
1/2 cup strawberries

1/2 banana
1/4 cup egg substitute
1 tbsp sugar

Measure all ingredients into blender. Blend on high speed until smooth, about 30 seconds. Pour into tall glass.

NOTE: Egg substitutes are available in the frozen food or dairy section of your supermarket.

## BUTTERMILK SHAKE

MAKES: 1 serving     CALORIES: 685 (without egg)     PROTEIN: 16 g (without egg)
                              760 (with egg)                       23 g (with egg)

1/2 cup buttermilk
1/2 cup lemonade
1 1/2 cup ice cream (3 to 4 scoops)
1/4 cup instant nonfat dry milk powder
1 egg (raw, no cracks), optional

Combine all ingredients in blender and blend until smooth.

## JUICE SHAKE

MAKES: 1 serving     CALORIES: 645 (without egg)     PROTEIN: 11 g (without egg)
                              720 (with egg)                       18 g (with egg)

3/4 cup fruit juice
1 1/2 cup ice cream (3 to 4 scoops)
1/4 cup instant nonfat dry milk powder
1 egg (raw, no cracks), optional

Combine all ingredients in blender and blend until smooth.

*Sources:* (1) From *Nutrition and the Cancer Patient* by J.D. Margie and A.S. Bloch, 1983, Radnor, PA: Chilton Book Company. Copyright 1983 by Chilton Book Company; (2) Courtesy of the Department of Nutrition and Dietetics, The Ohio State University Hospitals.

**Table 21-4** Modular Nutrition Supplements (Amounts are per 1,000 kcal)

| | Biocare Pudding Mix Food Sciences Corp.† | Biomed Pudding Robard‡ | Cal-Plus Henkel | Casec Mead Johnson | Citrotein Sandoz |
|---|---|---|---|---|---|
| Protein, g | 39.0 (14%) | 187.5 (75%) | 0 | 237.8 (95%) | 60.5 (24%) |
| Fat, g | 36.0 (32%) | <10.0 | 0 | 5.4 (5%) | 2.6 (2%) |
| Carbohydrate, g | 132.0 (53%) | 125.0# (25%) | 250.0 (100%) | 0 | 184.2 (74%) |
| Sodium, mEq | 43.8 § | N/A | 12.77 | 17.6 | 45.8 |
| Potassium, mEq | 40.51§ | N/A | 0.48 | 20.0 | 26.8 |
| Amount needed to give 1,000 kcal | 227.0 g dry weight | 322.0 g dry weight | 266.0 g dry weight | 270.3 g dry weight | 263.4 g dry weight |
| TYPE | Nutritional supplement | Protein, carbohydrate source | Carbohydrate source | Protein source | Protein, vitamin, mineral supplement |

| | Controlyte Sandoz | Forta Pudding Ross | High MCT Navaco | High Protein Gelatin Delmark | Hycal Beecham-Massengill |
|---|---|---|---|---|---|
| Protein, g | Trace | 27.2 (11%) | 0 | 119.7 (48%) | 0.1 |
| Fat, g | 48.0 (43%) | 38.8 (35%) | 77.4 (70%) | 1.4 (1%) | 0.1 |
| Carbohydrate, g | 143.0 (57%) | 136.0 (54%) | 66.6 (30%) | 126.7 (51%) | 244.7 (100%) |
| Sodium, mEq | 0.85 | 38.3 | 12.8 | 76.5 | 1.48 |
| Potassium, mEq | 0.20 | 30.7 | 36.4 | 37.9 | 0.07 |
| Amount needed to give 1,000 kcal | 198.0 g dry weight | 568.0 g dry weight | 163.0 g dry weight | 266.1 g dry weight | 407.0 ml liquid |
| TYPE | Low-protein, low-electrolyte calorie source | Nutritional supplement | Fat, carbohydrate source | Protein, calorie supplement | Carbohydrate source |

| | L.C. Navaco | Lipomul-Oral Upjohn | Lipomul-Oral Saccharine-Free Upjohn | Lonalac Mead Johnson |
|---|---|---|---|---|
| Protein, g | 0 | 0 | 0 | 53.1 (21%) |
| Fat, g | 0 | 111.1 (100%) | 106.5 (97%) | 54.7 (49%) |
| Carbohydrate, g | 250.0 (100%) | 0 | 8.0 (3) | 75.0 (30%) |
| Sodium, mEq | 10.0 | 1.2 | 0.73 | 1.7 |
| Potassium, mEq | 2.0 | 0 | 0 | 48.10 |
| Amount needed to give 1,000 kcal | 400.0 ml liquid | 166.7 ml liquid | 159.7 ml liquid | 1,478.0 ml standard dilution or 197 g dry weight |
| TYPE | Carbohydrate source | Fat source | Fat source | Low-sodium, high-protein source |

| | Lytren *Mead Johnson* | MCT Oil *Mead Johnson* | Microlipid *Sherwood Medical* | Moducal *Mead Johnson* | Nutrex Broth *Nutrex* |
|---|---|---|---|---|---|
| Protein, g | 0 | 0 | 0 | 0 | 30.8 (46%) |
| Fat, g | 0 | 120.5 (100%) | 111.0 (100%) | 0 | 0 |
| Carbohydrate, g | 253.0 (100%) | 0 | 0 | 250.0 (100%) | 216.0 |
| Sodium, mEq | 97.2 | 0 | 0 | 7.9 | 12.17 |
| Potassium, mEq | 83.3 | 0 | 0 | 0.3 | 19.48 |
| Amount needed to give 1,000 kcal | 268.0 g dry weight or 3,286 ml standard dilution | 120.5 g liquid | 222.0 ml liquid | 263.2 g dry weight | 261.3 g dry weight |
| TYPE | Calorie and electrolyte source | Medium-chain triglycerides | Fat source | Carbohydrate source | Protein, carbohydrate source |

| | Nutrex CLD *Nutrex* | Nutrex ProMax *Nutrex* | Nutrisource—Amino Acids *Sandoz* | Nutrisource Amino Acids—High Branched Chain *Sandoz* | Nutrisource Carbohydrate *Sandoz* | Nutrisource Lipid—Long Chain Triglycerides *Sandoz* | Nutrisource Lipid—Medium Chain Triglycerides *Sandoz* |
|---|---|---|---|---|---|---|---|
| Protein, g | 114.3 (46%) | 178.6 (71%) | 250.0 (100%) | 250.0 (100%) | 0 | 0 | 0 |
| Fat, g | 0 | 21.4 (19%) | 0 | 0 | 0 | 111.1 (100%) | 61.0 (90% MCT) |
| Carbohydrate, g | 128.5 (51%) | 23.8 (10%) | 0 | 0 | 250.0 (100%) | 0 | 0 |
| Sodium, mEq | 62.3 | 20.35 | 0 | 0 | 0.27 | 0 | 0 |
| Potassium, mEq | 40.6 | 59.28 | 0 | 0 | 0.10 | 0 | 0 |
| Amount needed to give 1,000 kcal | 243.7 g dry weight | 235.7 g dry weight | 256.0 g dry weight | 256.0 g dry weight | 312.5 ml liquid | 455.2 ml liquid | 490.2 ml liquid |
| TYPE | Protein, calorie supplement | Protein source | Protein module | Protein module | Carbohydrate module | Fat module | Fat module |

*continues*

**Table 21-4 continued**

| | Nutrisource-Protein Sandoz | P.C. Navaco | Pedialyte Ross | Polycose Ross | Pro-Mix Navaco |
|---|---|---|---|---|---|
| Protein, g | 187.5 (75%) | 0 | 0 | 0 | 213.0 (85%) |
| Fat, g | 17.5 (16%) | 0 | 0 | 0 | 10.6 (10%) |
| Carbohydrate, g | 21.2 (8%) | 250.0 (100%) | 250.0 (100%) | 250.0 (100%) | 13.3 (5%) |
| Sodium, mEq | 28.75 | 1.62 | 150.0 | 12.50 | 17.47 |
| Potassium, mEq | 36.25 | 0 | 100.0 | 2.50 | 91.16 |
| Amount needed to give 1,000 kcal | 248.0 g dry weight | 259.1 g dry weight | 500.0 ml liquid | 263.0 g dry weight | 266.2 g dry weight |
| TYPE | Protein module | Carbohydrate source | Calorie and electrolyte source | Oligosaccharides | Protein source |

| | ProMod Ross | Propac Sherwood Medical | Sumacal Sherwood Medical | Sustacal Pudding Mead Johnson |
|---|---|---|---|---|
| Protein, g | 178.6 (71%) | 192.3 (77%) | 0 | 28.3 (11%) |
| Fat, g | 21.4 (19%) | 20.5 (18%) | 0 | 39.6 (36%) |
| Carbohydrate, g | 23.9 (10%) | 12.8 (5%) | 250.0 (100%) | 133.3 (53%) |
| Sodium, mEq | 20.35 | 25.08 | 14.13 | 21.7 |
| Potassium, mEq | 59.28 | 32.87 | 1.0 | 34.2 |
| Amount needed to give 1,000 kcal | 235.7 g dry weight | 250.0 g dry weight | 500.0 ml liquid | 590.6 g dry weight |
| TYPE | Protein source | Protein source | Carbohydrate source | Nutritional supplement |

Individual items in this table may be used in appropriate amounts and combinations to prepare modular-type diets for patient needs.
†Cereal and soup available.
‡High-protein cocoa, soup, beverage, and gelatin available.
§Vanilla flavored.
#Part polydextrose, at 1 cal/g.

Appreciation is expressed to Mindy Hermann-Zaidins, RD, Memorial Sloan-Kettering Cancer Center, Clinical Nutrition Support Kitchen, for revision of this table, originally prepared by A.S. Bloch and M.E. Shils in the 6th Edition of *Modern Nutrition in Health and Disease.*

*Source:* From *Modern Nutrition in Health and Disease* (pp. 1624–1626) by M.E. Shils and V.R. Young (Eds.), 1988. Philadelphia: Lea & Febiger. Copyright 1988 by Lea & Febiger. Reprinted by permission.

want to test various products in commonly used foods and supplements to determine their acceptability and consistency.

The concept of modular supplementation also works well with foods that the patient may have at home. The use of modular supplements with dry milk powder, margarine, or butter is commonly recommended in nutrition education for the cancer patient. It should not be taken for granted, however, that patients and families know how to prepare these foods with supplements. It is probably wise to go over sample meal plans and to instruct patients about the use of modular supplementation in their regular diets. Patients who routinely used skim milk and avoided fried foods and margarine before their illness may not realize the added caloric benefit of utilizing whole milk or half-and-half and of adding margarine to their foods.

## CONCLUSION

The use of supplements can be an integral part of the cancer patient's nutrition care plan. Variety, individualization, patient involvement, and support from the health care team all help ensure the success of this nutrition intervention.

### REFERENCES

Campbell, S.M., Garza, R., Groziak, P., Mellen, C., & Nahikian-Nelms, M. (1987). *Modular enteral feeding.* Chicago: American Dietetic Association.

Parkinson, S.A., Lewis, J., Morris, R., Allbright, A., Plant, H., & Slerin, M.L. (1987). Oral protein and energy supplements in cancer patients. *Human Nutrition: Applied Nutrition, 41A*, 233–243.

Selig, D.E. (1979). Nutritional supplementation. In J. Wollard (Ed.), *Nutritional management of the cancer patient* (pp. 179–200). New York: Raven.

# Chapter 22

# Use of Supplements: Practical Suggestions

*Debbie Zibell-Frisk*

Finding a nutrition supplement that is acceptable to an oncology patient is one of the most challenging tasks to a clinical dietitian. Many of the commercial supplements are found to be too sweet to most oncology patients, so that asking them to consume two to four cans per day results in defeat from the outset. Another frequent complaint is that drinking the supplements prevents them from having sufficient appetite at mealtime. The patient and dietitian need patience and an agreement to work together to find the right combination of taste, temperature, and texture.

## TASTE

Patients often show taste fatigue and need various flavors to maintain adequate intake. Preferences for taste can also vary frequently, sometimes even from day to day. The dietitian may encounter patients who make frequent requests for sour flavors and who express a dislike for sweets; lemon, lime, and marguerita-type flavorings may help with such patients. Diluting supplements with milk helps reduce sweetness without sacrificing calories and protein. If lactose needs to be avoided, using a nonflavored supplement such as Osmolite or Isocal will achieve the same purpose. Flavoring supplements and drinks with instant coffee also helps cut down on sweetness.

If tolerance to sweetness is not a problem, supplements can be flavored by adding ice cream or sherbet and blending into a milk shake. Supplements can also be blended with fresh or canned fruit to give them a fresher taste. Strawberries, raspberries, bananas, and peaches are the most popular. Adding ice cream and a small amount of liqueur such as amaretto, creme de cacao, or khalua (if alcohol does not conflict with current medications) is another way of enhancing the flavor of supplements. Recipes that make use of the supplements are available in booklet form from most manufacturers. If milk is tolerated, homemade milk shakes, instant breakfast mixes, and other milk-based drinks are usually better accepted for taste and may be less expensive than commercial supplements.

## ODOR

For patients who have difficulty with the sight or smell of the supplements, use of a covered cup with a straw inserted into the cover (like a take-out beverage) may improve acceptability.

*Note:* Portions of this chapter were adapted with permission from "Nutritional Care of the Individual with Cancer" by J. Kouba, 1988, *Nutrition in Clinical Practice, 3,* pp. 175–182. Copyright 1988 by Williams & Wilkins Company.

## TEXTURE AND TEMPERATURE

The texture of supplements can be altered in several ways. The supplement can be frozen in a small dish or paper cup and served as a sorbet with a spoon, or it can be frozen as individual ice cubes for the patient to suck on. Ice cream or sherbet can be added to achieve the consistency of a milk shake. Supplements in pudding form can be offered to break the monotony of the liquid consistency if milk is tolerated. Adding cooked rice or tapioca also helps vary the texture of the supplement.

Most oncology patients, especially during chemotherapy and radiation therapy, prefer foods (including supplements) that are chilled.

## ENHANCING NUTRITION VALUE AND INTAKE

If oral intake is inadequate, it is necessary to concentrate calories and protein in whatever small amount of food the patient can consume.

Working out a feeding schedule with five to six small snacks sometimes results in better intake than trying to use the supplements and three meals per day. The dietitian should set easily reachable goals with the patient, such as improving intake by 100 to 200 kcal/day, and give support and encouragement. A goal of 1,800 to 2,000 kcal/day is overwhelming when current intake is poor.

The following suggestions can result in increased protein intake:

1. add nonfat dry milk (2 g of protein per tbsp) or a powdered protein module (3 g/tbsp) to soups, casseroles, drinks, hot cereals, pancake or waffle mix, and baked products
2. add dry or frozen pasteurized egg whites or egg substitutes (7 g of protein per ¼ c) to milk shakes, supplements, casseroles, or meat loaves

3. add chopped or pureed meats to soups
4. add shredded cheese to soups and sauces, or use it to top vegetables
5. encourage snacking with high-protein items
   - cheese
   - cottage cheese
   - peanut butter
   - chicken, egg, or tuna salad
   - eggnog
   - cereal with milk
   - creamed soups made with milk
   - milk shakes
   - yogurt

Calorie intake can be increased in the following ways:

1. add butter or margarine to soups, vegetables, hot cereals, and bread
2. spread nut butters or cream cheese on raw vegetables or crackers
3. use cream instead of milk in coffee, soups, and cereals
4. use mayonnaise on sandwiches
5. add whipped cream to fruit or gelatin desserts
6. add a glucose polymer (30 kcal/tbsp) to beverages, juices, or toppings for ice cream
7. use jams, jellies, or preserves as a spread or topping
8. use canned fruits packed in heavy syrup (syrup should be consumed)
9. add brown sugar, honey, or syrup to hot cereals, pancakes, and waffles
10. add chocolate or other syrups to milk, ice cream, and milk shakes
11. add a scoop of sherbet to a glass of ginger ale or milk
12. use sour cream and salad dressings as flavorful toppings for potatoes and cooked vegetables

# Chapter 23

# Tube Feeding: Overview

*Sheila M. Campbell*

Enteral feeding has been defined as the provision of liquid formula diets into the gastrointestinal tract orally or by means of feeding tubes (American Society for Parenteral and Enteral Nutrition [ASPEN], 1987). Delivery of nutritive liquids into the upper gastrointestinal tract was reported as early as 1598 (Randall, 1984). Until recently, however, health care professionals have not regarded enteral tube feeding as sophisticated, and they considered it less desirable than parenteral nutrition support during the 1970s and early 1980s.

In the last several years tube feeding has undergone a resurgence because of a number of factors. Enteral nutrition costs less than other methods of specialized nutrition support (McArdle, Palmason, Morency, & Brown, 1981) and has relatively few complications (Cataldi-Betcher, Seltzer, Slocum, & Jones, 1983). In addition, the development of sophisticated enteral formulas and feeding devices plus continuing improvements in techniques have facilitated enteral feeding of many patients who previously would not have been candidates.

In 1979, Heymsfield, Bethel, Ansley, Nixon, and Rudman described tube feeding as being more physiologic than parenteral feeding. Since that time, investigators have accumulated evidence demonstrating that intraluminal delivery of nutrients confers some benefits not seen with parenterally administered nutrients (Roche,

1988). Enterally administered nutrients enhance development of the immature gut and digestive enzymes (Castillo, Pittler, & Costa, 1988), help maintain gastrointestinal mass and function, minimize secretion of catabolic hormones (Mochizuki et al., 1984; Saito et al., 1987), attenuate stress-induced elevations in resting metabolic expenditure (McArdle, Palmason, Brown, Brown, & Williams, 1983; Mochizuki et al., 1984), and help maintain immunocompetence (McArdle et al., 1983; Mochizuki et al., 1984; Saito et al., 1987). McArdle, Reid, Laplante, and Freeman (1986) demonstrated a specific benefit of enteral feeding to some cancer patients by showing that feeding an elemental diet to patients with bladder cancer before abdominal radiation therapy provided prophylaxis against radiation enteritis.

Clinicians were initially enthusiastic about the ability of nutrition support to improve tumor response to therapy, to reduce treatment toxicity, and to enhance patient survival. Results of subsequent studies, however (Levine et al., 1982; Mohler & Flanigan, 1987; van Eys, 1982), have caused clinicians to temper their excitement over earlier claims for the benefits of intensive nutrition support. Currently, health care professionals take a moderate view regarding the role of nutrition therapy of cancer patients. Maillet (1987) stated that the goals of nutrition support are maintenance or improvement of nutrition status and preservation of strength.

## CANDIDATES FOR TUBE FEEDING

Patients may experience numerous problems associated with oncologic disease, antineoplastic therapy, and related complications that interfere with their ability to ingest adequate oral diets. Tube feeding has been shown to prevent weight loss and hypoalbuminemia in patients with cancer who are unable to maintain sufficient food intake (de Vries, Mulder, Houwen, & de Vries-Hospers, 1982).

Tube feeding is the preferred method of nutrition support for cancer patients who have functional gastrointestinal tracts but who are unable to maintain sufficient oral intake. Enteral nutrition support by tube has been recommended for patients experiencing anorexia and mild gastric discomfort as a consequence of radiation therapy or chemotherapy. Conversely, clinicians do not view enteral feeding by tube as desirable for patients with radiation enteritis, intractable vomiting, or severe diarrhea induced by antineoplastic therapy because of the increased potential for gastrointestinal intolerance (ASPEN, 1986). Furthermore, patients with extreme short bowel syndrome, severe malabsorption, total obstruction of the gastrointestinal tract or fistula in the distal small intestine or individuals requiring bowel rest may need parenteral nutrition.

Some individuals cannot be safely intubated. Patients who are not candidates for enteral feeding include those with altered levels of consciousness, which puts them at particular risk of aspiration of gastric contents, and individuals with edematous or friable bowel, which precludes surgical or percutaneous placement of feeding tubes. Ideally for patients with cancer, nasally placed tubes should be positioned before blood counts fall and impairment of immunocompetence related to antineoplastic therapy occurs because of the potential for minor trauma and bleeding during insertion of nasoenteric feeding tubes (Meguid, Eldar, & Wahba, 1985), Myelosuppressed patients with mucositis and esophagitis due to therapy or herpetic and fungal

infections may not tolerate passage of nasoenteric feeding tubes. These patients may benefit from the use of an alternative enteral feeding site.

## ENTERAL FEEDING SITES

Selection of the most appropriate enteral feeding site depends on gastrointestinal tract function and anticipated duration of tube feeding and on whether patients can tolerate surgical or percutaneous tube placement. Figure 23-1 depicts a logical method for considering these factors when choosing feeding sites to meet specific patient needs.

After the physician has evaluated the gastrointestinal tract and the health care team has determined that enteral feeding is the nutrition support method of choice, the next step is to select the most appropriate feeding site. Before the development of small-bore tubes specifically designed for nasoenteric tube feeding, clinicians had no alternatives for rubber or plastic, large-caliber, nasogastric suction tubes. They found these tubes to be unsatisfactory because of their size and material. Relatively long-term use of large-bore tubes causes mechanical complications such as pharyngitis, esophagitis, otitis, and erosion of nasolabial tissue (Bernard & Forlaw, 1984). Health care professionals have discovered that large tubes also compromise the lower esophageal sphincter, increasing the risk of gastric reflux. Health care professionals should take every step to prevent pulmonary aspiration of gastric contents because this is a potentially lethal complication. For this reason, patients benefit from the use of small-bore feeding tubes whenever possible because small tubes cause less compromise of the lower esophageal sphincter, thereby reducing the chance of aspiration (Treloar & Stechmiller, 1984).

Further, rubber and plastic nasogastric tubes harden and crack in the presence of gastric juices, making them undesirable for long-term use. Feeding tubes made of biocompatible materials, such as silicone or polyurethane, remain soft and pliable during use, obviating the need for frequent replacement. Most clinicians prefer feeding by enterostomy tube when the expected

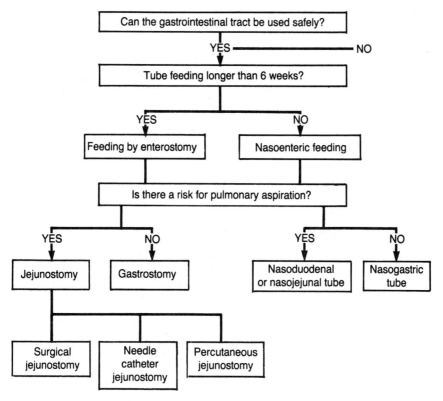

**Figure 23-1** Decision-Making Algorithm for Selection of Enteral Feeding Sites. *Source:* From *Clinical Nutrition: Enteral and Tube Feeding* (p. 263) by J.L. Rombeau and M.D. Caldwell (Eds.), 1984, Philadelphia: W.B. Saunders Company. Copyright 1984 by W.B. Saunders Company. Adapted by permission.

duration of tube feeding extends beyond 6 weeks, however, because of the association between prolonged use of nasally placed tubes and physical (Meguid et al., 1985) and psychologic distress (Padilla et al., 1979).

Surgeons sometimes create feeding esophagostomies during resection of tumors in the head and neck area. Depending on the technique used to construct the esophagostomy and to secure the feeding tube, patients may be able to remove the feeding tube between feedings.

More than 30 surgical techniques exist for the creation of tube enterostomies. Physicians frequently use Latex bulbous catheters (e.g., Foley catheters) or mushroom-tip catheters (e.g., de Pezzar catheters). Problems associated with these feeding gastrostomies include the need for relatively frequent replacement of catheters made of nonbiocompatible materials, leakage of gastric contents, tube migration resulting in gastric outlet obstruction, tube dislodgement, and

the need for initial surgical placement (Gauderer & Stellato, 1986).

Tubes specifically developed for gastrostomy feeding have features designed to reduce or alleviate the difficulties frequently encountered when Foley or de Pezzar catheters are used. These silicone gastrostomy tubes incorporate antireflux valves to prevent gastric backflow and proximal retention devices to maintain tube position. Because of their shorter length and lower profile, such tubes are less likely to be inadvertently removed than Foley or de Pezzar catheters. Figure 23-2 illustrates the features of these tubes that make them less obvious than other tubes when they are in place, contributing to enhanced physical and psychologic comfort.

Patients who are not surgical candidates may benefit from percutaneous insertion of gastrostomy feeding tubes (van Sonneberg et al., 1986). Foutch, Haynes, Bellapravalu, and Sanowski (1986) described a technique for

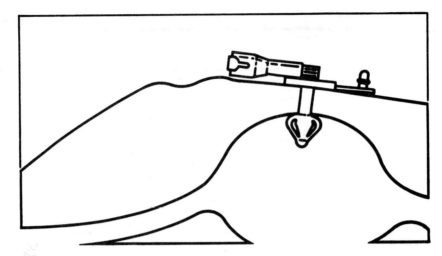

**Figure 23-2** Features of Tubes Especially Designed for Gastrostomy Feeding. Some biocompatible gastrostomy tubes incorporate short-length lumens, right-angle feeding adapters, and other features that make them less apparent and more comfortable than other catheters that are frequently used for gastrostomy feeding. *Source:* Reprinted with permission of Ross Laboratories, Columbus, Ohio, 1988.

placement of percutaneous gastrostomy tubes under endoscopic control (PEG tubes), which is a nonsurgical method for creating feeding gastrostomies. Physicians have found PEG to be especially useful in facilitating enteral nutrition support of critically ill patients after head and neck cancer surgery (Kelly et al., 1988). Use of PEG obviates the need for general anesthesia and laparotomy; this may make PEG placement less expensive than creation of surgical gastrostomies.

Pulmonary aspiration of stomach contents has been identified as a relatively frequent and extremely serious complication of enteral feeding (Schlichtig & Ayres, 1988). Obtunded or critically ill patients; individuals with impaired gag reflexes, gastrointestinal dysmotility, neuromuscular disease, or anatomic abnormalities; and persons with endotracheal tubes have increased potential for pulmonary aspiration of gastric contents. Certain maneuvers, such as elevating the head of the bed during and after feeding, routinely monitoring gastric residuals, and using enteral feeding pumps to control formula delivery, may reduce the risk of aspiration (Heitkemper & Williams, 1985). Placement of feeding tubes in the duodenum or jejunum may further decrease the chance of pulmonary aspiration of gastric contents (Thurlow, 1986).

Many brands of nasoduodenal and nasojejunal feeding tubes feature distal weights as placement aids, but clinicians have found initial tube placement and maintenance of proper tube position to be difficult (Keohane, Attrill, & Silk, 1986). Clinicians may find maintenance of tube position to be especially difficult in cancer patients who are experiencing vomiting and abnormal peristaltic action due to antineoplastic therapy. Moreover, the presence of tumors in the esophagus, stomach, and upper small intestine may prevent transnasal feeding tube placement. Because of the difficulties encountered during insertion of nasoenteric tubes, some physicians advocate the use of endoscopic or fluoroscopic assistance during transpyloric tube placement (Rees, Payne-James, & Silk, 1988).

Surgical or percutaneous enterostomies are used more frequently than transnasal tubes when jejunostomy feeding is desired. Surgeons usually create feeding jejunostomies in conjunction with abdominal surgery. Needle catheter jejunostomies (NCJ), which represent an alternate method of obtaining jejunal access, are created by threading an extremely small–caliber tube through a submucosal tunnel in the antimesenteric border of the jejunum. Because of their small caliber NCJ tubes cause little trauma to the bowel lumen, but formula choice may be limited because viscous formulas may not readily flow through the small internal lumen. Conditions present in some cancer patients, such as edematous or friable bowel tissue (as in radiation enteritis) or profound immunosuppression, may contraindicate NCJ placement because of the increased opportunity for complications (Ryan & Page, 1984).

Percutaneous jejunostomies can be created through preexisting gastrostomies by a number of techniques (Lambiase, Dorfman, Cronan, Paolella, & Caldwell, 1988). The advantages of percutaneous jejunostomies include gaining jejunal access through an existing gastrostomy while maintaining the gastrostomy tube for drainage and decompression, if necessary, and the opportunity to use a relatively large-caliber tube for jejunal feeding. Specialty tubes, which incorporate lumina for decompression and jejunal feeding in a single tube, facilitate both enteral feeding and gastric decompression (Rombeau, 1986).

## ENTERAL FORMULAS

Clinicians must consider nutrient needs and medical condition when selecting appropriate formulas for cancer patients. Each patient requires careful evaluation because nutrient needs vary among individuals. Some persons do not experience changes in caloric requirements as a result of disease, whereas others exhibit increased or decreased needs (Hoerr & Young, 1987). Moreover, the patient's medical condition or feeding method may require alteration of standard protocols. Some cancer patients may experience malabsorption, dumping syndrome, or intolerance to specific nutrient sources as a result of the effects of antineoplastic therapy. In these cases, condition-specific formulas may be appropriate. Patients experiencing malabsorption, for example, may benefit from formulas that are low in fat and residue. Postgastrectomy patients may need formulas that contain relatively long-chain carbohydrates. After pancreatectomy, patients may require formulas low in fat and short-chain carbohydrates (Kouba, 1988).

Patients who have normal digestive and absorptive function can be maintained on standard formulas. Standard formulas contain amino acid profiles similar to the profile of casein: protein contributes 12% to 20% of calories, carbohydrates provide 45% to 60% of calories and fat provides 30% to 40% of calories. The caloric density of standard formulas ranges from 1 to 2 kcal/mL (Skipper, 1986). Heimburger and Weinsier (1985) developed general criteria for categorizing standard formulas into therapeutically equivalent groups. Most commercially available meal replacement formulas can be grouped by use of the method shown in Table 23-1 on the basis of major characteristics such as protein content, caloric density, osmolality, degree of digestion required, and route of administration.

Although Heimburger and Weinsier (1985) consider formula residue, vitamin, mineral, and electrolyte content inconsequential, these constituents take on greater importance during enteral nutrition support of cancer patients. Kyle

**Table 23-1** Categorization of Standard Formulas

| Caloric Density of Formula | Isotonic | | | | Hypertonic | | | |
|---|---|---|---|---|---|---|---|---|
| | Standard Protein | | High Protein | | Standard Protein | | High Protein | |
| | Unflavored | Flavored | Unflavored | Flavored | Unflavored | Flavored | Unflavored | Flavored |
| 1.0 kcal/mL | | | | | | | | |
| 1.5 kcal/mL | | | | | | | | |
| 2.0 kcal/mL | | | | | | | | |

*Source:* From "An Overview of Commercially Available Enteral Formulas" by S.M. Campbell, 1986, *Pharmacy Practice News, 3,* p. 13. Copyright 1986 by McMahon Publishing Company. Adapted by permission.

and Bradford (1988) found that fiber-supplemented formulas normalize bowel function in patients with head and neck cancer who are receiving intermittent tube feedings. Other investigators have reported that patients on long-term tube feeding exhibit reduced serum levels of certain trace minerals (Feller et al., 1987). Therefore, cancer patients receiving long-term tube feedings may benefit from the use of formulas supplemented with trace minerals. The fluid and electrolyte contribution of formulas provided to cancer patients requires attention because many cancer patients exhibit conditions (e.g., diarrhea, gastric and small bowel fluid losses, and impaired renal reabsorption due to drug therapy) that may cause excessive fluid losses and mineral deficiencies (e.g., hypochloremia due to diuretic or antibiotic therapies and reduced potassium, sodium, magnesium, or bicarbonate serum levels secondary to fluid losses from the gastrointestinal tract) (Mirtallo, 1987).

As research in enteral nutrition continues, more new enteral formulations will probably become commercially available. Currently, there are more than 60 enteral products formulated for adults. Hui (1988) and Shils and Young (1988) have compiled compendia of enteral formulas that clinicians may find useful in selecting an appropriate product.

## DELIVERY SYSTEMS

Enteral delivery systems typically include a formula reservoir, administration tubing, and possibly an enteral feeding pump. Until the early 1970s, health care professionals commonly used syringes to deliver relatively large volumes of "blenderized" food mixtures as intermittent feedings. With the advent of homogenous, relatively low-viscosity, commercially prepared feedings, containers and tubing used to administer parenteral fluids were adapted for enteral feeding. Since that time, manufacturers of enteral products have developed various flexible and semirigid administration containers specifically designed for enteral feedings.

Feeding containers range in size from 500 to 1,500 mL. Eight–fluid ounce, prefilled bottles are useful when small-volume feedings are given intermittently. Care givers may find large-volume containers to be more convenient than small containers, however, because more formula can be hung. Large-volume containers must be used carefully because they facilitate longer formula "hangtime" than small-volume containers. If the formula is initially contaminated, long hangtimes can promote significant microbial proliferation (Schroeder, Fisher, Volz, & Paloucek, 1983).

The deleterious effects of feeding microbially contaminated enteral formulas include diarrhea (Anderson, Norris, Godfrey, Avent, & Butterworth, 1984) and the potential for sepsis due to translocation of microbes from the gut. Maintenance of the microbiologic quality of enteral feeding solutions is of particular importance for cancer patients whose immune system is impaired as a result of disease and therapy. Recently, large-volume, prefilled formula containers have been introduced commercially. Nurses find them beneficial because they reduce the time associated with administration of tube feedings (Pemberton, Lyman, Covinsky, Mandal, & Lander, 1985). Clinicians suggest that these containers are relatively impervious to microbial contamination (Crocker, Krey, Markovic, & Steffee, 1986; Vaughan, Manore, & Winston, 1988). Nevertheless, all enteral solutions can support microbial growth, regardless of container type. Therefore, care givers must apply meticulous handling techniques to all enteral delivery systems to avoid microbial contamination and proliferation. Use of sterile technique when handling enteral feedings is especially important when caring for immunosuppressed patients. Exhibit 23-1 gives suggested guidelines for safe handling of enteral feedings.

The type of tubing, or feeding set, used depends on the feeding method. There are specific sets available for gavage feeding and for use with enteral pumps. These types of tubing are not interchangeable. Additionally, feeding sets used with enteral feeding pumps are usually not interchangeable among pump brands. Although incompatibility of feeding sets among pump brands may be inconvenient, it does ensure accuracy of delivered volume because the tubing

**Exhibit 23-1** Suggested Guidelines for Administering Tube Feedings

1. Wash hands thoroughly with soap and water.
2. Use the least possible manipulation when preparing and administering formulas.
3. Carefully decant the formula into the feeding reservoir.
4. Attach the feeding set to the reservoir; avoid touching anything that will come in contact with the formula (e.g., the inside of the reservoir lid, the distal or proximal ends of the feeding set).
5. Limit hangtime to approximately 8 to 12 hours.
6. Discard any open, unused product within 24 hours.
7. Exchange feeding set and reservoir as needed or at least every 24 hours.
8. Never add a new supply of formula to a partially empty feeding reservoir.

is specifically calibrated for its intended pump. In the interest of reducing costs of supplies, care givers are often tempted to reuse feeding sets. Experts have suggested changing feeding reservoirs and sets every 24 hours in institution settings to reduce the chance of microbial contamination, although longer intervals may be permissible for stable patients in home settings (Guidelines, 1983). Health care professionals must carefully consider the risks of reusing disposable supplies for immunosuppressed patients.

Clinicians find enteral feeding pumps to be useful in situations in which patients need controlled delivery of formula. Such conditions include the need to maintain formula flow through extremely small-caliber feeding tubes (as in the case of NCJ tubes), the need for controlled formula flow to prevent gastrointestinal intolerance, and the need to prevent gastric pooling in patients who are prone to pulmonary aspiration of gastric contents.

The ideal enteral feeding pump has been described as inexpensive, safe, accurate, and easy to use (Forlaw & Chernoff, 1984). At least 20 different models of enteral feeding pumps are available. Enteral feeding pumps, which are electronic devices weighing 5 to 10 lb, control the delivery of formula by volume or peristalsis. Volumetric pumps measure infusion by volume; peristaltic pumps "count" the number of drops delivered per minute. Most pumps ensure accurate formula delivery within 5%.

Manufacturers have responded to the need for pumps that are useful in alternate care settings by developing pumps specially designed for outpatients. These pumps are lightweight, easy for patients or care givers to set up and operate, run on battery power, and feature carrying cases to facilitate ambulation. These features are a boon to cancer patients who receive outpatient antineoplastic therapies and need enteral nutrition support.

## SUMMARY

Health care professionals recognize enteral feeding as the preferred route of nutrition support. Most of the principles employed in caring for the general population of enterally fed patients are applicable to cancer patients. Feeding patients with cancer by tube, however, requires that clinicians pay special attention to the selection of appropriate feeding routes, formulas, and devices to ensure that these patients receive optimal nutrition support with minimal complications.

### REFERENCES

American Society for Parenteral and Enteral Nutrition Board of Directors. (1986). Guidelines for use of total parenteral nutrition in the hospitalized adult patient. *Journal of Parenteral and Enteral Nutrition, 10,* 441–445.

American Society for Parenteral and Enteral Nutrition Board of Directors. (1987). Guidelines for use of enteral nutrition in the adult patient. *Journal of Parenteral and Enteral Nutrition, 11,* 435–439.

Anderson, K.R., Norris, D.J., Godfrey, L.B., Avent, C.K., & Butterworth, E.C. (1984). Bacterial contamination of tube-feeding formulas. *Journal of Parenteral and Enteral Nutrition, 8,* 673–678.

Bernard, M., & Forlaw, L. (1984). Complications and their prevention. In J.L. Rombeau & M.D. Caldwell (Eds.), *Clinical nutrition: Vol. 1. Enteral and tube feeding* (pp. 542–569). Philadelphia: Saunders.

Castillo, R.O., Pittler, A., & Costa, R. (1988). Intestinal maturation in the rat: The role of enteral nutrients. *Journal of Parenteral and Enteral Nutrition, 12,* 490–495.

Cataldi-Betcher, E.L., Seltzer, M.H., Slocum, B.A., & Jones, K.W. (1983). Complications occurring during enteral nutrition support: A prospective study. *Journal of Parenteral and Enteral Nutrition, 7,* 546–552.

Crocker, K.S., Krey, S.H., Markovic, M., & Steffee, W.P. (1986). Microbial growth in clinically used enteral delivery systems. *American Journal of Infection Control, 14,* 250–256.

de Vries, E.G.E., Mulder, N.H., Houwen, B., & de Vries-Hospers, H.G. (1982). Enteral nutrition by nasogastric tube in adult patients treated with intensive chemotherapy for acute leukemia. *American Journal of Clinical Nutrition, 35,* 1490–1496.

Feller, A.G., Rudman, D., Erve, P.R., Johnson, R.C., Boswell, J., Jackson, D.L., & Mattson, D.E. (1987). Subnormal concentrations of serum selenium and plasma carnitine in chronically tube-fed patients. *American Journal of Clinical Nutrition, 34,* 476–483.

Forlaw, L., & Chernoff, R. (1984). Enteral delivery systems. In J.L. Rombeau & M.D. Caldwell (Eds.), *Clinical nutrition: Vol. 1. Enteral and tube feeding* (pp. 228–239). Philadelphia: Saunders.

Foutch, P.G., Haynes, W.C., Bellapravalu, S., & Sanowski, R.A. (1986). Percutaneous endoscopic gastrostomy (PEG): A new procedure comes of age. *Journal of Clinical Gastroenterology, 8,* 10–15.

Gauderer, M.W.L., & Stellato, T.A. (1986). Gastrostomies: Evolution, techniques, indications and complications. *Current Problems in Surgery, 23,* 661–719.

Guidelines for preventing contamination of enteral feeding. (1983). In *Report of the Ross workshop on contamination of enteral feeding products during clinical usage* (pp. 40–42). Columbus, OH: Ross Laboratories.

Heitkemper, M.M., & Williams, S. (1985). Prevent problems caused by enteral feeding (know about complications before they arise). *Journal of Gerontological Nursing, 11,* 25–30.

Heimburger, D.C., & Weinsier, R.L. (1985). Guidelines for evaluating and categorizing enteral feeding formulas according to therapeutic equivalence. *Journal of Parenteral and Enteral Nutrition, 9,* 61–67.

Heymsfield, S.B., Bethel, R.A., Ansley, J.D., Nixon, D.W., & Rudman, D. (1979). Enteral hyperalimentation: An alternative to central venous hyperalimentation. *Annals of Internal Medicine, 90,* 63–71.

Hoerr, R.A., & Young, V.R. (1987). Alterations in nutrient intake and utilization caused by disease. *Annals of the New York Academy of Sciences, 499,* 124–131.

Hui, Y.H. (1988). *Handbook of enteral and parenteral feedings.* New York: Wiley.

Kelly, K.M., Lewis, B., Gentili, D.R., Benjamin, E., Waye, J.D., & Iberti, T.J. (1988). Use of percutaneous gastrostomy in the intensive care patient. *Critical Care Medicine, 16,* 62–63.

Keohane, P.P., Attrill, H., & Silk, D.B.A. (1986). Clinical effectiveness of weighted and unweighted "fine bore" nasogastric feeding tubes in enteral nutrition: A controlled clinical trial. *Journal of Clinical Nutrition and Gastroenterology, 1,* 189–193.

Kouba, J. (1988). Nutritional care of the individual with cancer. *Nutrition in Clinical Practice, 3,* 175–182.

Kyle, U.G., & Bradford, K.B. (1988). *Use of fiber containing formula in bolus tube feedings for patients with head and neck (H&N) cancer who experience diarrhea.* Presented at the 71st annual meeting of the American Dietetic Association, October 6, 1988.

Lambiase, R.E., Dorfman, G.S., Cronan, J.J., Paolella, L.P., & Caldwell, M.E. (1988). Percutaneous alternatives in nutritional support: A radiologic perspective. *Journal of Parenteral and Enteral Nutrition, 12,* 513–520.

Levine, A.S., Brennan, M.V., Ramu, A., Fisher, R.I., Pizzo, P.A., & Glaubiger, D.L. (1982). Controlled clinical trials of nutritional intervention as an adjunct to chemotherapy, with a comment on nutrition and drug resistance. *Cancer Research, 42,* 774s–778s.

Maillet, J.O. (1987). The cancer patient. In C.E. Lang (Ed.), *Nutrition support in critical care* (pp. 243–264). Rockville, MD: Aspen.

McArdle, A.H., Palmason, C., Brown, R.A., Brown, H.C., & Williams, H.B. (1983). Protection from catabolism in major burns: A new formula for the immediate enteral feeding of burn patients. *Journal of Burn Care and Rehabilitation, 4,* 245–250.

McArdle, A.H., Palmason, C., Morency, I., & Brown, R.A. (1981). A rationale for enteral feeding as the preferable route for hyperalimentation. *Surgery, 90,* 613–623.

McArdle, A.H., Reid, E.C., Laplante, M.P., & Freeman, C.R. (1986). Prophylaxis against radiation injury. *Annals of Surgery, 121,* 879–885.

Meguid, M.M., Eldar, S., & Wahba, A. (1985). The delivery of nutritional support: A potpourri of new devices and methods. *Cancer, 55,* 279–289.

Mirtallo, J.M. (1987). Parenteral therapy. In C.E. Lang (Ed.), *Nutritional support in critical care* (pp. 113–130). Rockville, MD: Aspen.

Mochizuki, H., Trocki, O., Dominioni, L., Brackett, K.A., Joffee, S.N., & Alexander, J.W. (1984). Mechanism of prevention of postburn hypermetabolism and catabolism by early enteral feeding. *Annals of Surgery, 200,* 297–310.

Mohler, J.L., & Flanigan, R.C. (1987). The effect of nutritional status and support on morbidity and mortality of bladder cancer patients treated by radical cystectomy. *Journal of Urology, 137,* 404–407.

Padilla, G.V., Grant, M.M., Wong, H.L., Hansen, B., Hanson, R., Bergstrom, N., & Kubo, W. (1979). Subjective distress of nasogastric tube feeding. *Journal of Parenteral and Enteral Nutrition, 3,* 53–57.

Pemberton, L.B., Lyman, B., Covinsky, J., Mandal, J., & Lander, V. (1985). An evaluation of a closed enteral feeding system. *Nutrition Support Services, 5,* 36–42.

Randall, H.T. (1984). The history of enteral nutrition. In J.L. Rombeau & M.D. Caldwell (Eds.), *Clinical nutrition: Vol. 1. Enteral and tube feeding* (pp. 1–9). Philadelphia: Saunders.

Rees, R.G.P., Payne-James, J.J., & Silk, D.B.A. (1988). Spontaneous transpyloric passage and performance of "fine bore" polyurethane feeding tubes: A controlled clinical trial. *Journal of Parenteral and Enteral Nutrition, 12*, 469–472.

Roche, A.F. (Ed.). (1988). *The gastrointestinal response to injury, starvation, and enteral nutrition, report of the eighth Ross conference on medical research.* Columbus, OH: Ross Laboratories.

Rombeau, J.L. (1986). Enteral feeding into the jejunum with combined gastric decompression. *Nutrition in Clinical Practice, 1*, 205–208.

Ryan, J.A., & Page, C.P. (1984). Intrajejunal feeding: Development and current status. *Journal of Parenteral and Enteral Nutrition, 8*, 187–198.

Saito, H., Trocki, O., Alexander, J.W., Kopcha, R., Heyd, T., & Joffe, N.S. (1987). The effect of route of nutrient administration on the nutritional state, catabolic hormone secretion, and gut mucosal integrity after burn injury. *Journal of Parenteral and Enteral Nutrition, 11*, 1–7.

Schlichtig, R., & Ayres, S.M. (1988). Modes of delivery: Rationale, implementation, and mechanical complications. In R. Schlichtig & S.M. Ayres (Eds.), *Nutritional support of the critically ill* (pp. 143–168). Chicago: Year Book Medical.

Schroeder, P., Fisher, D., Volz, M., & Paloucek, J. (1983). Microbial contamination of enteral feeding solutions in a community hospital. *Journal of Parenteral and Enteral Nutrition, 7*, 364–368.

Shils, M.E., & Young, V.R. (Eds.). (1988). *Modern nutrition in health and disease* (7th ed., pp. 1607–1628). Philadelphia: Lea & Febiger.

Skipper, A. (1986). Specialized formulas for enteral nutrition support. *Journal of the American Dietetic Association, 86*, 654–658.

Thurlow, P.M. (1986). Bedside enteral feeding tube placement into duodenum and jejunum. *Journal of Parenteral and Enteral Nutrition, 10*, 104–105.

Treloar, D.M., & Stechmiller, J. (1984). Pulmonary aspiration in tube-fed patients with artificial airways. *Heart & Lung, 13*, 667–671.

van Eys, J. (1982). Effect of nutritional status on response to therapy. *Cancer Research, 42*, 747s–753s.

van Sonneberg, E., Wittich, G.R., Cabrera, O.A., Quinn, S.F., Casola, G., Lee, A.A., Princenthal, R.A., & Lyons, J.W. (1986). Percutaneous gastrostomy and gastroenterostomy: 2: Clinical experience. *American Journal of Radiology, 146*, 581–586.

Vaughan, L.A., Manore, M., & Winston, D.H. (1988). Bacterial safety of a closed-administration system for enteral nutrition solutions. *Journal of the American Dietetic Association, 88*, 35–37.

# Chapter 24

# Tube Feeding: Practical Suggestions

*Debbie Zibell-Frisk*

Patients who have a functional gastrointestinal tract but inadequate oral intake to meet nutrition requirements may benefit from tube feedings. The following guidelines for the use of enteral nutrition are adapted from "Guidelines for the Use of Enteral Nutrition in the Adult Patient" (American Society for Parenteral and Enteral Nutrition, 1987).

## INDICATIONS

### Anorexia from Chemotherapy or Radiation Therapy

Often as a result of prolonged illness or chemotherapy and radiation therapy, patients experience persistent poor appetite. When efforts to improve intake with the use of oral supplements, multiple small meals, and attention to individual food preferences and intolerances fail, insertion of a small-bore silicone elastomer feeding tube for enteral nutrition support should be considered. This method utilizes a functional gastrointestinal tract and often results in increased appetite and oral intake after enteral nutrition has improved overall nutrition status.

### Head and Neck Cancer: Dysphagia from Obstructing Tumors of the Larynx, Esophagus, and Stomach

Enteral nutrition should be considered if a tumor is present or if surgery of the head and neck area impairs or prevents swallowing. If the impairment is expected to resolve with surgery, chemotherapy, or radiation therapy, short-term enteral nutrition may be given through a small-bore nasogastric tube. If the impairment is permanent, however, placement of a gastrostomy or jejunostomy feeding tube makes long-term enteral nutrition more aesthetically pleasant to the patient and thus makes management easier, especially if self-care is intended. A tube exiting the abdomen is much easier for the patient to manipulate than a nasogastric tube and can be concealed underneath clothing, which enhances the patient's self-image. Also, an ostomy tube eliminates the need for checking tube placement before initiating feedings.

### Inadequate Oral Intake due to Brain Metastasis or Neurologic Injury

A patient who is not alert and is incapable of oral intake but who has a functional gastrointestinal tract is a good candidate for enteral nutrition support. The following provisions are necessary to decrease the risk of aspiration:

- elevate the head of the bed 30° or more during the feeding infusion
- gradually increase the flow rate by 20 to 30 mL/day until the goal rate is achieved
- use a small-bore (6F to 10F) silicone elastomer tube designed for use in enteral nutrition

## Transitional Support after Long-Term Parenteral Nutrition

Patients who have been maintained on parenteral nutrition for several weeks generally experience difficulty in resuming oral intake. Their appetite is usually poor, and some malabsorptive diarrhea is likely to occur as a result of atrophy of the small bowel surface area.

Thus parenteral nutrition should be continued until the patient demonstrates the ability to tolerate oral intake. The amount of parenteral nutrition can be decreased to help stimulate appetite. Nutrition supplements should be introduced and calorie counts begun in an effort to keep calorie and protein intake close to estimated needs. Parenteral nutrition is discontinued when the gstrointestinal tract has become functional (i.e., absence of vomiting, passage of flatus and stool, and improvement in diarrhea).

If persistent anorexia occurs during the transitional phase and if oral intake remains inadequate despite the use of nutrition supplements and multiple small meals, cyclic tube feeding should be considered. The purpose of a cyclic infusion schedule during transitional feeding is to provide supplemental nutrition but to allow and encourage the patient to eat. This is best accomplished by a nocturnal infusion schedule (e.g., 7:00 p.m. to 7:00 a.m.). When the infusion has been completed in the morning, the tube is flushed with water to maintain patency and then capped. The patient is encouraged to eat his or her meals during the day. Absence of the tube feedings during the day helps promote appetite and the return to a regular meal schedule. Calorie counts are continued to document the amount of

oral intake and to determine the amount of supplemental tube feedings needed at night. This schedule is continued until oral intake alone is adequate and the tube and tube feedings can be discontinued.

## CONTRAINDICATIONS

When parenteral nutrition is implemented, every effort should be made to convert to enteral nutrition if the gastrointestinal tract again becomes viable. If a functioning gastrointestinal tract is present, the enteral route is preferred because it is simpler, safer, and less expensive than the parenteral route. Enteral nutrition is also more physiologic because it maintains the structural and functional integrity of the small bowel and provides more efficient utilization of nutrients.

### Intestinal Obstruction

Patients with complete small or large bowel obstruction do not tolerate feeding into the gastrointestinal tract. Occasionally enteral nutrition may be administered if there is a partial obstruction, but it is safer to feed these patients parenterally until the obstruction resolves completely. Patients with obstruction of the small intestine may be fed through a surgically placed tube distal to the site of obstruction if there is sufficient length of nonobstructed bowel for adequate absorption.

### Ileus or Intestinal Hypomotility

Patients with ileus or intestinal hypomotility tolerate enteral nutrition poorly and are at increased risk of aspiration and infectious colitis. These patients should receive parenteral nutrition until normal gastrointestinal function returns.

### Severe Diarrhea

Patients with severe diarrhea from antineoplastic therapy who have not responded to pharmacologic therapy are difficult to feed enterally. The use of a fiber-enriched or chemically defined formula may help correct the diarrhea. If the diarrhea persists with no improvement, however, parenteral nutrition should be instituted for adequate hydration and to lessen irritation of the bowel to promote healing.

### High-Output Fistula

Patients with high-output (>500 mL/day) external fistulae usually have increased output when they are fed enterally. Enteric secretions are reduced and fistula closure is hastened when feeding is delivered parenterally rather than enterally in these patients. Once the fistula is closed, enteral nutrition can be resumed.

### Severe or Prolonged Vomiting due to Chemotherapy or Radiation Therapy

When a patient experiences prolonged vomiting, parenteral nutrition provides replacement fluid and maintains nutrition status until enteral nutrition can be resumed.

### Surgery Requiring Prolonged Periods of Receiving Nothing by Mouth

Parenteral therapy should always be considered when the period of receiving nothing by mouth exceeds, or is expected to exceed, 5 to 7 days. At this point a deficit in visceral protein status is evident, and wound healing and immune competence are likely to be impaired.

## FACTORS TO CONSIDER IN ENTERAL NUTRITION

### Route

Feeding jejunostomies and gastrostomies can be concealed between feeding times and may be more aesthetically acceptable to the patient than nasogastric tubes. Excoriation and infection are potential complications because the feeding tube penetrates the peritoneum. This potential problem can be minimized by using an appropriately sized tube. The tube should be large enough to accommodate commercial enteral formulas and medications but not so large that leakage is likely to occur around the insertion site. The ideal tube size for adults is 12F or 14F.

#### Nasal

Nasal intubation is the preferred route for short-term nutrition support. Small-bore silicone elastomer tubes are recommended to enhance the patient's comfort and to lessen the risk of aspiration.

#### Gastrostomy

Surgically placed and percutaneous endoscopic gastrostomy (PEG) tubes are indicated when obstruction makes insertion through the nares impossible, when long-term (76 weeks) feeding is anticipated, or when poor patient compliance makes it difficult to keep nasal tubes in place. The PEG is placed under endoscopic control, and the procedure does not require general anesthesia.

#### Jejunostomy

Jejunostomy tubes should be considered for the management of long-term nutrition in patients with chronic aspiration problems or gastric obstruction. Because jejunostomy feedings bypass the stomach, sterile water may need to be used for tube flushing and dilution of the formula, if needed, because the bactericidal effect of the hydrochloric acid is no longer intact. This may be significant for patients with compromised immune status or persistent diarrhea.

### Schedule

#### Continuous

Continuous 24-hour delivery of formula by enteral pump allows for the best patient tolerance. Bolus feedings are not recommended because the delivery of a large volume of formula in a few minutes may result in nausea, diarrhea, and aspiration.

For patients who are bed bound, those who have malabsorption or short bowel syndrome, or those whose fluid management is difficult, around-the-clock delivery is best. Once the continuous schedule is well tolerated and the patient is on an appropriate regimen to meet his or her full nutrition requirements, the feeding rate may be increased slightly to allow an 18-hour infusion. This will give the patient a temporary reprieve from the infusions, but it should not be attempted until tolerance of the continuous regimen has been achieved.

### Cyclic

Once tolerance of continuous feedings is achieved, cyclic feedings may be attempted to allow the patient freedom of movement between feedings. This is especially important in ambulatory patients. Cyclic feedings are usually administered nocturnally over 12 hours (7:00 p.m. to 7:00 a.m.). This allows normal daytime activity, accommodates radiation therapy and physical therapy schedules that the patient attends on a daily basis away from the hospital room, and facilitates oral intake of meals if possible. A cyclic schedule is ideal for home tube feeding. If the patient is hospitalized and unable to eat, a daytime schedule (7:00 a.m. to 7:00 p.m.) may be more desirable because of better staffing during those hours.

The formula infusion rate will eventually need to be doubled to allow the same volume of formula to be delivered in 12 hours as in 24 hours, but volume should be increased gradually. For example, if a patient needs 60 mL of a formula per hour to meet nutrition requirements, the regimen could be advanced in gradual steps as follows:

1. 60 mL/hour continuously
2. 75 mL/hour for 20 hours (7:00 p.m. to 3:00 p.m.)
3. 90 mL/hour for 16 hours (7:00 p.m. to 11:00 a.m.)
4. 120 mL/hour for 12 hours (7:00 p.m. to 7:00 a.m.)

If a rate other than 60 mL/hour is used the feeding time is simply reduced by 4 hours at each step, and the infusion rate is increased accordingly until a 12- to 14-hour schedule is achieved. The infusion rate is determined by dividing the volume of formula by the desired number of infusion hours.

*Example:* seven cans of formula (240 mL per can) = 1,680 mL

1. 1,680 mL/24 hours = 70 mL/hour
2. 1,680 mL/20 hours = 85 mL/hour
3. 1,680 mL/16 hours = 105 mL/hour
4. 1,680 mL/12 hours = 140 mL/hour

Most patients need 1 to 2 days at each level to adjust to the increased rate. Once tolerance is achieved, the next level can be attempted. It is important to monitor the patient closely and to observe for subjective complaints such as nausea, abdominal cramps, and diarrhea. Tolerance is highly individual and dictates how long it takes to achieve the 12-hour schedule. The infusion rate should not exceed 120 to 140 mL/hour to promote patient tolerance and to lessen the risk of aspiration.

If the patient is unable to tolerate the rate needed for a 12-hour schedule, decreasing the rate and infusing for 14 or 16 hours will still allow some off-time from the feedings. The exact time schedule for infusion of the feedings should be discussed with the patient and his or her care givers. The goal is for the patient to return to as normal a lifestyle as possible but still to receive adequate nutrition support.

The tube should be flushed with 50 to 100 mL of water before feedings are started and when they are finished to maintain patency. The tube is capped when not in use. Additional water flushes may be needed during the day depending on the patient's fluid needs and oral water intake or if medications are administered through the tube.

### Formula

The feeding schedule also helps determine the best formula. If a continuous schedule is found to be the most appropriate, a product that contains 1.0 kcal/mL will provide the most free water and meet most of the patient's nutrition needs, including vitamins, without having to add other modules separately. If a cyclic schedule is chosen, however, a more calorically dense product (1.5 kcal/mL) will allow provision of needed nutrition in a volume that is easily delivered over a 12-hour period. Patients who are volume sensitive or fluid restricted may do better with a product that contains 2.0 kcal/mL.

If a calorically dense (1.5 to 2.0 kcal/mL) product is used, careful attention must be paid to water balance. It is important to monitor closely the patient's daily intake and output of fluid to prevent dehydration. Often patients receive diuretic therapy along with fluid restrictions, so that dehydration may result. Monitoring the patient's blood chemistries for hypernatremia and elevated blood urea nitrogen (BUN) and creatinine levels enables early detection of dehydration. If dehydration is present, it may become necessary to change the enteral formula to provide more free water.

It should be remembered that enteral formulas are not 100% free water. The percentage of free water generally ranges from 60% to 85% depending on the caloric density. The least calorically dense products (1.0 kcal/mL) have the most free water, about 80% to 85%. The formulas containing 1.5 kcal/mL have about 70% free water, and those containing 2.0 kcal/mL have about 60%. It may be necessary to give the patient additional free water as flushes through the tube to meet full water needs.

Water requirements should be calculated on an individual basis, just as is done for calories and protein. Adolescent patients (11 to 18 years of age) require 40 to 50 mL of water per kilogram body weight, adults require 30 to 40 mL/kg, and elderly patients require 25 to 30 mL/kg. Additional water may also be required for patients with an elevated temperature or gastrointestinal fluid losses.

In any case, full consideration must be given to the completeness of the nutrition regimen. Supplementation of vitamins, free water, sodium, potassium, phosphorus, protein, and so forth may be necessary.

## Osmolality

The issue of osmolality and tolerance of an enteral formula is not as significant as was once thought. Iso-osmolar formulas are available, and

most other formulas have moderate osmolalities (400 to 600 mOsm), so that osmotic-induced diarrhea is not a frequent problem. The enteral products that contain protein in the free amino acid form generally have the highest osmolalities and thus should be diluted on initial administration. When diluting enteral formulas it is not necessary to dilute them to less than 300 mOsm, which is close to serum osmolarity (280 to 310 mOsm). Iso-osmolar formulas may be started at full strength. Diluting enteral formulas unnecessarily is apt to result in suboptimal nutrition regimens.

Keohane, Attrill, Love, Frost, and Silk (1984) performed a study of a large number of tube-fed patients and the relationship of osmolality to diarrhea. The incidence of diarrhea was found to be small and was not related to formula osmolality but to the administration of antibiotics.

## TUBE FEEDING COMPLICATIONS

The most frequently seen complications of tube feedings can be prevented through proper formula selection, proper administration, and careful patient monitoring.

### Fluid and Electrolyte Disturbances

Dehydration can result from excessive diarrhea, excessive protein intake, osmotic diuresis, or inadequate fluid intake. It is imperative to observe the water balance of patients receiving a calorically dense (1.5 to 2.0 kcal/mL) enteral formula and to monitor often electrolytes, BUN and creatinine levels, and input and output. A record of intake and output should be completed on a daily basis both in the hospital and at home for as long as the patient receives enteral nutrition. Electrolytes should be measured two to three times per week until the patient is stable, then once weekly while he or she is hospitalized, and finally once monthly after the patient is discharged to home and remains otherwise stable. BUN and creatinine levels should be measured weekly in the hospital and monthly at home, but the frequency ultimately depends on individual patient circumstances.

## Aspiration

Correct tube selection and placement are important precautionary measures. Small silicone elastomer tubes are recommended to reduce the risk of gastric reflux. The head of the bed should be elevated 30° to 45° during feedings. The nasogastric feeding tube must be checked for proper placement before enteral feedings are begun. In the hospital this is performed once per nursing shift and at home once daily. Infusion of the formula by continuous drip, either cyclically or around the clock, also helps lessen the risk of aspiration. As mentioned earlier, bolus feedings are not recommended because the delivery of a large volume in a few minutes is likely to result in nausea, vomiting, and aspiration. If chronic aspiration risk is evident, placement of a feeding jejunostomy tube may need to be considered.

## Diarrhea

Diarrhea can result from many causes.

### Bacterial Contamination

Bacterial contamination can be prevented by ensuring cleanliness during preparation, storage, and administration of feeding formulas.

*Preparation.* The area where the enteral products are prepared must be kept clean and away from the regular food preparation area. Mixing equipment such as blenders should be thoroughly cleansed after each use and used only for enteral product preparation, not shared with the kitchen staff.

If the product does not require mixing or preparation, it should be sent to the nursing unit unopened. The nursing staff can then open and pour the formula into the feeding bag or container just before administration to the patient. If dilution is required, the nurse can also do this and eliminate potential sources of contamination that may otherwise occur during transit from the preparation area.

*Storage.* Once opened, the formula should be covered, refrigerated, and used within 24 hours. To lessen wastage whole cans should be used as they are opened; partially filled cans are likely to be spilled or forgotten. If reconstituted products are used a 24-hour volume can be prepared, provided that it is labeled with the product name and date and is refrigerated in an unbreakable, air-tight container.

*Administration.* If formulas are begun slowly at isotonicity and their volume is gradually increased, diarrhea should not be a problem. Also, initial delivery by 24-hour continuous drip allows for the best patient tolerance.

The feeding bag and tubing should be thoroughly rinsed with water once each shift before more formula is added. This will prevent bacterial overgrowth (the sucrose-containing formula provides an excellent growth medium). Using a new feeding bag every 24 hours also helps eliminate bacterial growth.

### Hypoalbuminemia

Hypoalbuminemia, which is associated with poor water absorption by the colon, may also contribute to diarrhea. This is frequently seen in patients with edema and fluid overload. Changing the enteral formula to a more calorically dense product (1.5 to 2.0 kcal/mL) may help correct fluid balance by decreasing the patient's free water intake. In cases in which albumin levels are severely low (2.5 g/dL or less), parenteral albumin therapy may need to be considered to correct fluid balance and to enable protein repletion to occur.

### Fecal Impaction

Diarrhea may also be due to fecal impaction. Loose stool leaks around the site of impaction until the bowel is cleared. Patients who are bed bound or whose physical activity is restricted or limited frequently experience constipation and occasionally become impacted with stool. Patients with neurologic injuries or disorders may also experience this problem.

To prevent fecal impaction the following interventions are suggested:

- use fiber-containing formula to add bulk to the stool and to increase peristalsis
- ensure adequate water intake

- give liquid stool softeners one or two times daily (bolus by syringe through the feeding tube for maximal effect of the medication)
- provide routine enemas or suppositories if bowel movements do not occur

### Antacid Therapy

Antacid therapy is frequently the cause of diarrhea in patients receiving enteral feedings. The purpose of antacid therapy is to neutralize the acid content of the stomach and small bowel in patients with peptic ulcer disease or those at risk for stress ulcers after trauma, surgery, or cardiopulmonary arrest. The continuous administration of enteral nutrition achieves the same buffering effect, however, so that simultaneous antacid therapy is not needed. Discontinuing the antacids usually stops the diarrhea.

### Antibiotic Therapy

The diarrhea that occurs after tolerance to an enteral formula has been established may be due to bacterial overgrowth. This overgrowth is usually secondary to long-term antibiotic therapy. If this is suspected, a stool sample should be obtained to perform *Clostridium difficile* culture and toxin testing. If *C. difficile* is identified, oral vancomycin or metronidazole (Flagyl) therapy is indicated.

The use of a fiber-supplemented enteral formula has been successful in correcting loose stools. The fiber helps absorb water in the gastrointestinal tract, which promotes the production of formed stools. Stools usually begin to form within 48 to 72 hours of administration. If diarrhea persists, an antidiarrheal agent may be considered if there has been no improvement with the addition of fiber. Antidiarrheal medication must be used with caution, however, if there is a possibility of an infectious etiology because there is the potential for the development of a pseudo–intestinal obstruction or toxic megacolon (or both).

### Other Medications

Patients who are taking multiple medications may also have diarrhea. The physician should be consulted about eliminating as many medications as possible. Alternatively, it may be neces-

sary to change the brand or form of a particular medication. A pharmacist should also be consulted in this regard.

### Constipation

Because most commercial formulas are low in residue, decreased frequency of bowel movements is expected. Patients should have a rectal examination to rule out an impaction, however. Enemas or suppositories can be prescribed when necessary. A stool softener or additional fiber (or both) may be used for chronic constipation problems. Increasing water intake and physical activity may also help make stool elimination easier.

If bowels remain sluggish and if increased abdominal distention is noticed, it is necessary to evaluate the patient for the presence of a bowel obstruction or ileus. Bowel sounds should be monitored frequently and an abdominal radiograph obtained. If an obstruction or ileus is present, enteral nutrition should be stopped until bowel function returns.

### Other Gastrointestinal Problems

Common complaints include nausea, abdominal cramps, and distention. Generally these are avoided when appropriate formulas are given slowly by a continuous drip and are gradually increased as tolerated. If the patient experiences nausea the feeding should be stopped; relief may be obtained by stopping the feeding for 1 hour or by slowing the rate. Around-the-clock administration of antiemetics may also help. Ambulation may ease gastric distention. Gastric emptying may also be helped by the administration of metoclopramide (Reglan). Feedings should be discontinued if vomiting occurs.

### Tube Clogging

Frequently enteral feeding tubes become occluded, which prevents further administration of formula. When this occurs it is difficult to unclog the tube, and usually a new tube must be inserted. This results in interrupted administration of formula and creates an inconvenience for the patient and nursing staff. More important, if the patient is unable to swallow he or she will not receive necessary medications. Prevention of clogging is thus an essential component of daily feeding tube care. The following recommendations are helpful in this regard:

- Flush the feeding tube with 50 to 100 mL of water once per shift. If the patient needs additional free water, this may be done more often. If the patient is receiving cyclic tube feedings, use 100 mL of water before starting and stopping the infusion.
- Use medications in their liquid form. To achieve the maximal benefit of the medication, it is best to deliver it directly into the feeding tube. The one exception is potassium, which is hypertonic and irritating to the stomach and should be added to the feeding bag. If the medication is not available in liquid form, it should be crushed well and mixed with water to form a slurry before being delivered as a bolus into the tube. Always follow medication administration with 30 to 50 mL of water to ensure that the medication has been flushed from the feeding tube.
- If the tube is suspected of being clogged, try to inject a bolus of air (20 to 30 mL) to dislodge the clog. If this is unsuccessful it is doubtful that any water or liquid will be able to irrigate the tube, so that a new tube will have to be placed. If the air does seem to free the clog, however, follow it with 30 to 50 mL of warm water, cola, or cranberry juice to cleanse the tube. It should then be possible to resume the feedings.

## HOME ENTERAL NUTRITION

Home enteral nutrition helps promote the patient's emotional well-being by enabling him or her to be with family members in familiar surroundings. Also, allowing the family to participate in the patient's care decreases their sense of anxiety and helplessness, thus benefiting both the patient and family.

Despite its success, arranging home enteral nutrition is not quite as easy as it once was. Patients must meet specific criteria regarding diagnosis and reason for the intended therapy before they are eligible for home support. Medicare and other insurance providers no longer reimburse for home enteral therapy that is supplemental in nature. Without insurance coverage the cost of home enteral nutrition is prohibitive, averaging about $1,000 per month. It is thus important to explore the diagnosis, the anticipated length of therapy, and insurance coverage before approaching the patient and family about home therapy.

### REFERENCES

American Society of Parenteral and Enteral Nutrition Board of Directors. (1987). Guidelines for the use of enteral nutrition in the adult patient. *Journal of Parenteral and Enteral Nutrition, 11*, 435–439.

Keohane, P.P., Attrill, H., Love, M., Frost, P., & Silk, D.B.A. (1984). Relation between osmolality of diet and gastrointestinal side effects in enteral nutrition. *British Medical Journal, 288*, 678–680.

# Chapter 25

# Methods of Management: Parenteral Nutrition

*Monique D. Gelinas, Stacey J. Bell,*
*Paul Akerman, and George L. Blackburn*

Nutrition management of cancer patients is a rapidly evolving area in which concepts change frequently (Shanbhogue, Bistrian, & Blackburn, 1986). When total parenteral nutrition (TPN) therapy became safe and widely available and was shown to result in a positive nitrogen balance, numerous TPN studies were enthusiastically designed, and interest in enteral feeding waned. Because cancer cachexia and anorexia occur so commonly and adversely affect prognosis, no group of patients was more extensively studied than the tumor-bearing population (Shanbhogue et al., 1986; Lowry & Brennan, 1986; Souba & Copeland, 1988). Investigators tried to test the logical and intuitive idea that nutrition intervention by means of TPN might improve durable survival because of increased tolerance to aggressive tumor therapy. The clinical efficacy of and indications for TPN as well as nutrition requirements of cancer patients are discussed in this chapter.

## CLINICAL EFFICACY OF TOTAL PARENTERAL NUTRITION

Numerous uncontrolled, nonrandomized, and retrospective studies suggest that there are major benefits with the use of TPN in malnourished cancer patients (Schwartz, Greene, Bendon, Graham, & Blakemore, 1971; Dematteis & Her-

mann, 1973; Assa, Schramek, Barzilai, & Weisz, 1974; Copeland, MacFayden, & Dudrick, 1974, 1976; Copeland, MacFayden, Lanzotti, & Dudrick, 1975; Copeland, Mac-Fayden, MacComb, et al., 1975; Lanzotti, Copeland, George, Dudrick, & Samuels, 1975; Mullen, Buzby, Matthews, Smale, & Rosato, 1980; Daly et al., 1982; Bozzetti et al., 1987; Dempsey, Mullen, & Buzby, 1988):

- improved nutrition status (increase in body weight, nitrogen balance, and serum albumin, transferrin, and retinol-binding protein levels; improvement in triceps skin fold; reversal of skin anergy)
- reduced postoperative complications and mortality
- better tolerance of and response to antitumor therapy
- improved performance status

The positive impact of TPN on nutrition status has been confirmed by many prospective, randomized, and controlled studies as well (Holter, Rosen, & Fisher, 1977; Holter & Fisher, 1977; Moghissi, Hornshaw, Teasdale, & Dawes, 1977; Issel et al., 1978; Simms, Oliver, & Smith, 1980; Nixon et al., 1981; Burt, Stein, & Brennan, 1983; Drott, Unsgaard, Schersten, & Lundholm, 1988). Results, however, indicate that a certain metabolic block seems to exist with the progression of cancer that prevents exogenous nutrients from adequately restoring the lean body mass (Bozzetti et al., 1987; Copeland & Souba, 1988). Furthermore, results from randomized trials and from animal studies have raised doubts and controversies regarding the impact of TPN on morbidity and mortality as well as on patient tolerance to treatment (Kurzer & Mequid, 1986).

## Chemotherapy

Prospective, randomized, controlled clinical trials in cancer patients receiving chemotherapy (Table 25-1) have not demonstrated benefits of TPN (Chlebowski, 1986) compared to ad libitum oral feeding (no nutrition support) in survival and in delivery of the planned dosage of chemotherapy in both well and poorly nourished patients. On the contrary, as shown in Table 25-1, some studies have demonstrated increased complication rates and decreased survival associated with the use of central TPN (Chlebowski, 1986). This was also the conclusion of a meta-analysis of 12 chemotherapy and TPN trials (Klein, Simes, & Blackburn, 1986) (meta-analysis is a new discipline that critically reviews and statistically pools the data of previous research, especially the randomized, controlled trials because such trials are often too small to detect clinically important differences or tend inappropriately to reject the null hypothesis [Sacks, Berrier, Reitman, Ancona-Berk, & Chalmers, 1987]).

## Radiation Therapy

The utility of adjunctive parenteral nutrition in patients undergoing radiation has not been

**Table 25-1** Randomized Trials of TPN in Conjunction with Chemotherapy in Patients with Cancer

| Tumor Type | Number of Patients | Summary Results | Length of TPN (days) | Reference |
|---|---|---|---|---|
| Lung cancer Small cell | 119 | More febrile episodes on TPN | 30 | Clamon et al. (1985) |
| | 49 | No difference in outcome | 42 | Valdivieso et al. (1981) |
| | 19 | No difference in outcome | | Serrou et al. (1982) |
| Non small cell | 26 | Less myelosuppression on TPN | 10/21† | Issel et al. (1978) |
| | 65 | Decreased survival on TPN* | 10/25† | Jordan et al. (1981) |
| | 31 | No difference in outcome | 14 to 19 | Moghissi et al (1977) |
| | 27 | No difference in outcome | | Lanzotti et al. (1980) |
| Colon | 45 | Decreased survival on TPN* | 14 minimum | Nixon et al. (1981) |
| Lymphoma | 42 | No difference in outcome | 14 to 16 | Popp, Wagner, & Brito (1983) |
| Testicular | 30 | Trend to more infections on TPN | 18 to 48 | Samuels, Selig, Ogden, Grant, & Brown (1981) |
| Sarcoma | 27 | Increased relapse in patients on TPN* | | Shamberger et al. (1984) |
| Acute leukemia | 24 | No difference in outcome | 30 to 70 | Coquin, Maranichi, Gastant, & Carcassone (1981) |
| | 21 | More rapid bone marrow recovery on TPN | | Hays, Merritt, White, Ashley, & Siegel (1983) |
| Pediatric malignancies | 19 | No difference in outcome | 14 | van Eys et al. (1980) |

*Trials suggesting adverse effect of TPN in conjunction with chemotherapy.
†Before/after treatment.

*Sources:* (1) From "Nutritional Support for the Cancer Patient" by R.T. Chlebowski, 1986, *Clinics in Oncology, 5*(2), p. 366. Copyright 1986 by W.B. Saunders Company. (2) From *Parenteral Nutrition: Clinical Nutrition* vol. 2 (p. 463) by J.L. Rombeau and M.D. Caldwell (Eds.), 1986, Philadelphia: W.B. Saunders Company. Copyright 1986 by W.B. Saunders Company.

widely studied (Lowry & Brennan, 1986; Copeland & Souba, 1988). A number of investigators have prospectively evaluated the use of central TPN during abdominal and pelvic radiation for adults (Kinsella, Malcolm, Bothe, Valerio, & Blackburn, 1981; Valerio, Overett, Malcolm, & Blackburn, 1978; Solassol & Joyeux, 1979; Solassol, Joyeux, & Dubois, 1979; Bothe, Valerio, Bistrian, & Blackburn, 1979) or children (Donaldson et al., 1982; Ghavinsi, Shils, Scott, Brown, & Tamaroff, 1982). No obvious trends have emerged from these studies for either survival or treatment tolerance (Lowry & Brennan, 1986; Chlebowski, 1986; Klein et al., 1986). Some investigators have shown increased survival or tolerance, and others have shown decreased survival or no change with TPN. Nevertheless, because a large proportion of patients, especially children (25%), undergoing abdominal and pelvic radiation therapy in conjunction with chemotherapy can be expected to become malnourished during the course of treatment, a nutrition support regimen is essential in a therapeutic plan to reverse malnutrition (Donaldson et al., 1982). In adults and children who are not malnourished, the routine use of TPN is not supported by current evidence (Chlebowski, 1986). Additional prospective, randomized studies in this area are needed (Copeland & Souba, 1988).

### Cancer Surgery

The available data indicating that malnutrition is associated with poor outcome in surgical patients appear to be irrefutable (Dempsey et al., 1988; Buzby, Knox, et al., 1988). Several prospective, randomized studies have been performed with cancer patients undergoing gastrointestinal surgery (Table 25-2). These trials were designed to evaluate the impact of perioperative TPN on nutrition status as well as on morbidity and mortality. They were not limited to malnourished patients or to those who were unable to eat, however, so that their results created much confusion (Buzby, Knox, et al., 1988; Detsky, Baker, O'Rourke, & Goel, 1987).

Furthermore, patients who experienced severe weight loss (i.e., those who were truly

malnourished) were often excluded from randomization. Therefore, the subgroups that may have most benefited from TPN were not studied (Klein et al., 1986). Most of these studies demonstrated some improvement in patients receiving TPN in one or more nutrition parameters compared to those receiving no nutritional support. In most studies, there was a trend with TPN toward a decrease in complications (anastomotic leak, abdominal abscess, intestinal obstruction, peritonitis, prolonged ileus, and multiple wound complications). Only one of the studies (Müller et al., 1982) showed a statistical decrease in operative mortality for patients treated with TPN. According to two different meta-analyses (Klein et al., 1986; Detsky et al., 1987), in general the quality of the studies reviewed (Table 25-2) was poor. Nevertheless, the pooled results confirmed that TPN may be useful when used preoperatively in malnourished patients with gastrointestinal cancer in reducing major complications and operative mortality.

Important defects have been identified in the design of previous randomized studies (Bistrian, 1986; Buzby, 1988):

- inappropriate patient selection (absence of malnutrition, isolated marker for malnutrition, degree of malnutrition not assessed)
- defects in statistical design (sample size too small, inappropriate procedures for randomization)
- inappropriate treatment regimens (inadequate duration [<7 days] and intensity of TPN, use of forced feeding in control treatment not adequately standardized or individualized)
- inadequate definition of endpoint criteria

In an attempt to obviate these shortcomings, a large, randomized, multi-institutional clinical study (Veterans Administration cooperative trial) was carefully planned to assess the efficacy of perioperative TPN in malnourished surgical patients. Patients undergoing major, non-emergency intraperitoneal or intrathoracic surgery were eligible provided that they were malnourished as defined by objective measures of nutrition status and that they had no life-threatening complicating medical disorders (Buzby, Knox, et al., 1988). Two-thirds of the

**Table 25-2** Randomized Trials of TPN as Adjunct to Primary Surgical Therapy in Patients with Cancer

| Tumor Type | Patients Entered | Summary Results | Limited to Malnourished Patients | Duration of Preoperative TPN (days) | Reference |
|---|---|---|---|---|---|
| Upper gastrointestinal tract | 120 | Decreased surgical complications and operative mortality on TPN | No | 10 | Müller, Brenner, Dienst, & Pichlmaier (1982) |
| | 20 | Decreased surgical complications and operative mortality on TPN | Yes | 21 | Lim, Choa, Lam, Wong, & Ong (1981) |
| | 74 | Decreased wound infection on TPN | No | 7 to 10 | Heatley, Williams, & Lewis (1979) |
| | 48 | No difference in outcome | No | 7 to 10 | Williams, Heatley, Lewis, & Hughes (1976) |
| | 15 | Decreased wound infection on TPN | No | 5 to 7 | Moghissi et al. (1977) |
| | 20 | No difference in outcome | No | 7 to 10 | Simms et al. (1980) |
| Entire gastrointestinal tract | 26 | No difference in outcome | No | 3/10* | Holter & Fisher (1977) |
| | 55 | No difference in outcome | No | 2/10 | Holter et al. (1977) |
| Oropharyngeal | 60 | No difference in outcome | No | Variable | Sako et al. (1981) |

*Days preoperative/days postoperative.

*Sources:* (1) From "Nutritional Support for the Cancer Patient" by R.T. Chlebowski, 1986, *Clinics in Oncology*, 5(2), p. 370. Copyright 1986 by W.B. Saunders Company. (2) From *Parenteral Nutrition: Clinical Nutrition*, vol. 2 (p. 464) by J.L. Rombeau and M.D. Caldwell (Eds.), 1986, Philadelphia: W.B. Saunders Company. Copyright 1986 by W.B. Saunders Company.

patients had cancer. The background, rationale, and study protocol of that important study were well defined and were published in detail in 1988 (Dempsey et al., 1988; Buzby, 1988; Buzby, Williford, et al., 1988). As with any clinical trials, appropriate interpretation of the results depends on a good understanding of the study design and methodology. Review of this protocol also may be useful to other investigators who are planning future clinical nutrition intervention trials.

Although the results are not yet published, the data were examined and showed that perioperative TPN reduces surgical complications only in severely malnourished patients (Buzby, 1988). On the other hand, TPN increased infection rate and was deleterious to the relatively well-nourished patients; the view that a little preoperative TPN will not hurt is wrong. Essentially, TPN was administered for a minimum of 7 to 15 days preoperatively and a minimum of

3 days postoperatively at the established caloric and nitrogen goal, that is, 1,000 kcal/day in excess of the estimated energy expenditure by the Harris-Benedict formula (Harris & Benedict, 1919) multiplied by an appropriate stress factor; 550 kcal/day is provided as lipid and the remainder as dextrose (20% to 35%). Amino acids were given as Freamine III to yield a ratio of nonnitrogenous calories to nitrogen of 150:1 (that is, a total calorie-to-nitrogen ratio of 175) (Buzby, Knox, et al., 1988).

## Tumor Growth

The decreased patient survival seen in a few randomized, controlled studies (Nixon et al., 1981; Clamon et al., 1985; Jordan et al., 1981; Samuels et al., 1981; Valerio et al., 1978) raised concern that nutrition support could result in stimulation of cancer growth. In some animal tumor models with or without prior nutrition depletion, stimulation of tumor growth by prolonged TPN has been documented compared to controls with anorexia (Steiger, Oram-Smith, Miller, Kuo, & Vars, 1975; Cameron, Ackley, & Rogers, 1977; Oram-Smith, Stein, Wallace, & Mullen, 1977; Buzby et al., 1980; Cameron, 1981; Popp, Morrison, & Brennan, 1981; Fried et al., 1985; Grube, Gamelli, & Foster, 1985). Many investigators, however, have concluded that the relative benefit of TPN support is to the host (Oram-Smith et. al., 1977; Daly, Copeland, & Dudrick, 1978; Kishi, Iwasawa, Itoh, & Chibata, 1982; King et al., 1985). Others have found no increase in animal tumor growth with TPN or when intravenous carbohydrate calories were replaced with fat calories (Buzby et al., 1980; Enrione, Black, & Moore, 1985).

Most of these studies involved transplanted tumors of large bulk, whose sensitivity to nutrient supply may be markedly different from that of human tumors. Up to now, studies done in humans suggest that tumor growth is relatively insensitive to exogenous nutrient supply. There has been no unequivocal demonstration of enhanced tumor growth in humans due to TPN (Bozzetti et al., 1987; Chlebowski, 1986).

## ENTERAL COMPARED TO PARENTERAL FEEDING

Total parenteral nutrition is more expensive (>$200/day) and may subject patients to a greater number of technical and metabolic complications than tube feedings, such as increased risk of pneumothorax, arterial puncture, bleeding and hematoma formation, subclavian thrombosis, hyperglycemia (blood glucose concentrations greater than 200 mg/dL), rapid fall of magnesium and phosphorus levels, and infections (Brennan, 1981).

Feeding through the gastrointestinal tract seems to play a multifactoral role in reducing sepsis and enhancing the immune response. In fact, enteral feeding by tube or mouth:

- is safe and inexpensive
- is more physiologic than TPN (first-pass effect)

- protects the gut mucosal barrier and may reduce the incidence of bacterial translocation
- stimulates the natural immune response of the body
- improves everyday clinical practice (Andrassy, 1988)

It is important to remember that the best route for satisfying nutrition needs is the alimentary tract and that parenteral nutrition becomes necessary only when the gut is unusable or unable to accept adequate nutrition for long periods (Shanbhogue et al., 1986; Dudrick, Wilmore, Vars, & Rhoads, 1968). Various enteral supplements, tubes, and techniques are currently available. An experienced nutrition support service can be invaluable in encouraging patients to accept adequate oral or tube feeding diets.

Animal studies have shown that there is no nutritional advantage to parenteral alimentation over enteral feeding when gastrointestinal function is normal if there is isocaloric and isonitrogenous intake (Daly, Steiger, Vars, & Dudrick, 1974). Human studies (Burt et al., 1983; McArdle, Palmason, Morency, & Brown, 1981) tend to corroborate this, although weight gain, not necessarily lean body mass, has been reported to be superior and positive nitrogen balance to be attained more rapidly in malnourished cancer patients receiving TPN (Nixon et al., 1981; Lim et al., 1981).

### Objectives

*Ultimate Goals*

The ultimate goals of TPN support of cancer patients are to achieve a reduction in mortality and in postoperative or other treatment morbidity and, by implication, to reduce the length of hospitalization.

*Principal Goal*

The principal goal of TPN is to improve or maintain the patient's nutrition status, especially protein mass. The nutrition goals are:

- reduced weight loss
- improved nitrogen balance

- increased serum transport proteins
- increased creatinine-height index or mid-arm muscle area
- enhanced immune competence
- increased skinfold thickness or muscle fat area
- improved vitamin and mineral status

## Indications

The decision analysis for administering intra-venous nutrition in cancer patients is complex and depends on many variables, namely:

- nutrition assessment
- status of gastrointestinal function
- anticipated clinical course
- patient and family decision

Malnutrition is nearly always a prerequisite for initiating TPN, as is failure of the gastrointestinal tract (Copeland & Souba, 1988). Although TPN may sustain the life of the terminally ill cancer patient for brief periods, it must be regarded as a supportive modality (Lowry & Brennan, 1986; Bell, Coffey, & Blackburn, 1986).

Efforts to identify candidates for TPN should begin at the time of admission, and reassessment should be done periodically. It is wrong not to start TPN under the pretext that once TPN has been started it cannot be stopped.

Lowry and Brennan (1986) mentioned that, although the criteria are relatively arbitrary, intravenous feeding should be considered for any cancer patient for whom a hospital stay of at least 10 days will result in a therapeutic regimen of reasonable expectation for cure or palliation and in whom adequate nutrition cannot or will not be maintained by enteral means.

For cancer patients undergoing surgery, the following guidelines established by the American Society for Parenteral and Enteral Nutrition (1986) and published by the American College of Physicians (1987, p. 253) could be applied:

From the evidence actually available, perioperative parenteral nutrition should

be limited to selected groups of high-risk patients.

1. Perioperative use of parenteral nutrition is recommended for severely malnourished patients having major surgery, such as intra-abdominal or noncardiac intrathoracic surgery.
2. Postoperative use of parenteral nutrition is recommended for selected groups of moderately malnourished and previously well-nourished patients having surgery that usually results in prolonged periods (10 days or more) of inadequate nutritional intake (pancreaticoduodenectomy, esophagogastrectomy involving total gastric resection). Some of these patients may receive nutrients through a feeding jejunostomy tube instead of total parenteral nutrition.
3. Postoperative use of parenteral nutrition is recommended for previously well-nourished patients who develop postoperative complications that are expected to result in prolonged periods (10 days or more) of inadequate intake (e.g. peritonitis associated with small bowel resection).

The results of the Veterans Administration cooperative trial of perioperative TPN in malnourished surgical patients provide strong justification for the choice of the subgroup of patients described in the first recommendation (Buzby, 1988). The other recommendations are based on clinical judgment only (American College of Physicians, 1987).

## NUTRITION NEEDS

### Central Parenteral Nutrition

Central TPN is delivered through a large-diameter vein, usually the superior vena cava by way of the subclavian or internal jugular vein. The large diameter of the vein and consequently the large volume of blood flow facilitate rapid dilution of a hypertonic solution (up to

1,800 mOsm), which can satisfy the full nutrition needs of any patient (Shanbhogue et al., 1986).

Although malnutrition in the cancer patient does not appear to have the same metabolic pathways or etiologies as that in the stressed noncancer patient, actual guidelines for parenteral management are the same in cancer and noncancer patients.

Despite increasing knowledge of the factors leading to cachexia, little is known about methods to reverse or prevent it. Future research will probably lead to manipulation of amino acid profiles and caloric sources to ensure better individualization of TPN regimens for cancer patients. In fact, recent work has raised the question of whether, under the particular circumstances of TPN, some nonessential nutrients may be limiting or deficient. At least eight nitrogenous compounds have received particular attention in this regard and are now being investigated: tyrosine, glutamine, cysteine, taurine, choline, carnitine, nucleotides (Rudman & Williams, 1985), and arginine (Daly et al., 1988). There is also initial evidence that dipeptides, especially glycyl dipeptides and alanyl dipeptides, could optimize further the use of nitrogen in TPN.

### Macronutrients

*Energy, glucose, and proteins.* Providing adequate amounts of nonprotein calories is of paramount importance to induce and sustain protein synthesis in cancer patients (Lowry & Brennan, 1986). Limited data are available on the energy requirements of cancer patients, however. Negative energy balance is a well-known phenomenon in that group. It has been suggested that different tumors, stages of disease, and levels of TPN may exert different influences on the resting energy expenditures (REE) (Merrick, Long, Grecos, Dennis, & Blakemore, 1988). Variations in REE of $-10\%$ to $+120\%$ of normal have been reported (Young, 1977). As an example, Hodgkin's disease or leukemia induces a general increase in metabolism. Colorectal cancer patients with or without hepatic metastases appear to be normometabolic in the fasting and postabsorptive states. The energy requirements of a group of 21 homogeneous colorectal patients were measured by Merrick et al. (1988). The mean percentage change between predicted (from the Harris-Benedict equation) and measured (by indirect calorimetry) values was 3% (range, $-15\%$ to $+14\%$) when patients were fasting or receiving 5% dextrose intravenously. On a standard TPN solution, when calories were given at levels 1.5 to 2.7 times the patients' basal REE (2.7 times is excessive) a significant increase in postabsorptive REE (30% to 50%) was seen compared to the basal REE. As calories exceeded the basal REE, progressively greater increases in postabsorptive REE were seen. This confirms results in noncancer patients reported in other studies (Elwyn, Gump, Munro, Iles, & Kinney, 1979; Gil, Askanazi, Weissman, Elwyn, & Kinney, 1986). The increase in postabsorptive REE seen with TPN appears to be related to thermogenesis and to the energy cost of synthesis, as is seen in normal subjects whether they are receiving TPN or not (Merrick et al., 1988).

Ideally, energy requirements of malnourished cancer patients should be measured by indirect calorimetry, which measures REE including, of course, the stress factor (when present). In practice, maintenance energy and protein requirements may be satisfied in the great majority of hospitalized cancer patients with intakes of 25 to 35 kcal per kilogram current body weight and 1.2 to 1.5 g of protein per kilogram ideal body weight. For repletion purposes (primarily on discharge from the acute care setting), intakes of 35 to 40 kilogram current body weight and 1.0 to 1.5 g of protein per kilogram ideal body weight are sufficient.

A better individualization of energy requirements is obtained by the use of the Harris-Benedict equation, which factors in the patient's sex, weight, height, and age to estimate the REE. This is the method of choice when indirect calorimetry is not available.

It has been suggested that factors of activity and stress be included when estimating energy and protein needs (Long, Schaffel, Geiger, Schiller, & Blakemore, 1979; Geller, Blackburn, Glendon, Henneman, & Steffee, 1979). The application of these energy factors overestimates the energy requirements in most cancer patients receiving TPN, however. Therefore, low factors are recommended.

The total energy requirements for maintenance purposes are estimated by the Harris-Benedict equation, and the result is multiplied by an arbitrary factor of 1.3 g (Table 25-3) to take into account the cancer status (~10% above REE), the metabolic cost of nutrient metabolism (due to thermogenesis, ~10%), and a minimal level of activity (10%). For repletion purposes the REE is multiplied by 1.5, and adjustments are made according to the patient's response to TPN. With aggressive cancer treatment the energy expenses may indeed be much higher in certain patients, so that clinical judgment is essential.

Energy requirements for patients receiving TPN are often expressed as nonprotein calories, especially for repletion purposes. The same factors as for total calories are often applied, that is, 1.3 and 1.5 times the estimated REE for maintenance and repletion, respectively. Both methods (total calories or nonprotein calories) are acceptable because both are inherently imprecise. If the same constants are applied in both cases, the nonprotein method provides 6 kcal/kg more than the first method if 1.5 g of protein per kilogram is prescribed (1.25 g × 4 kcal/g = 6 kcal).

The advantage of calculating in terms of nonprotein calories is obvious; ignoring the caloric value of protein, the rationale is to be sure to calculate enough energy that the protein can serve for anabolic purposes and thus to be on the safe side. Both methods are easy to use; for practical purposes, the first method (protein included in the total calories) is preferred. Nevertheless, many clinicians working with TPN prefer to prescribe in terms of nonprotein calories, and both methods should be thoroughly understood by the dietitian.

Excessive calories given as glucose or fat (or both) must be avoided; this may induce hepatic steatosis, hypertriglyceridemia, increased oxygen consumption and carbon dioxide production, and respiratory dysfunction in patients with pulmonary disease or those under stress (Lowry & Brennan, 1986; Giner & Curtas, 1986; Chwals & Blackburn, 1986). Given the maximal oxidation rate of glucose, intake should be kept to less than 5 mg/kg/minute (7.2 g/kg/day).

*Lipids.* Lipids are given to provide an energy source and to prevent essential fatty acid deficiency (EFAD), which can be precipitated by a high glucose load in 10 days to 4 weeks of fat-

**Table 25-3** Maintenance Macronutrient Requirements of a Cancer Patient*

| Macronutrient | Amount† | Example |
|---|---|---|
| Calories (kcal) | Basal metabolism rate × 1.3 (Harris-Benedict equation) | 1,700 kcal × 1.3 = 2,210 kcal/day |
| Protein (amino acids) | 1.3 g × ideal body weight | 1.3 × 70 kg = 91 g of protein per day |
| Carbohydrate (dextrose) | 2.5 to 4.0 mg/kg/minute | 3.25 mg × 70 kg × 1,440 minute/day ÷ 1,000 mg/g = 328 g of carbohydrate per day |
| Fat (lipid emulsion)‡ | Make up remainder of total kilocalories after provision of carbohydrate and protein; total fat should be kept to less than 30% of total energy intake | 2,210 kcal − (364 kcal + 1,115 kcal carbohydrate) = 731 kcal fat or 33% of total energy |

*A 70-kg (154-lb) man at ideal body weight.
†For patients weighing less than ideal body weight, enter actual weight into Harris-Benedict equation to calculate calorie needs and use ideal body weight to determine complete protein needs.
‡Given the constraint on intravenous fat, total energy needs may not be met. If more calories are required, restrictions on carbohydrate and protein may be warranted.

*Source:* Adapted from "Use of Total Parenteral Nutrition in Cancer Patients" by S.J. Bell, L.M. Coffey, and G.L. Blackburn, 1986, *Topics in Clinical Nutrition, 1*(2), p. 43. Copyright 1986 by Aspen Publishers, Inc.

free TPN (Giner & Curtas, 1986). Administering at least 500 mL of a 10% lipid emulsion intravenously twice a week, or 3.2% of total caloric intake, prevents EFAD (Lowry & Brennan, 1986). Studies to date indicate that supplying all intravenous lipids as long-chain triglycerides may not be best for patients. Because of concerns that much of the infused long-chain triglycerides is not oxidized readily and that there may be some immune system impairment by preventing proper reticuloendothelial clearance (Hamawy et al., 1985; Jensen, Seidner, et al., 1988), the use of emulsions called structured lipids is being investigated. Structured lipids are triglycerides made from reesterified mixtures of medium-chain triglycerides and long-chain triglycerides (75% and 25%, respectively) (Babayan, 1987; Mascioli, Bistrian, Babayan, & Blackburn, 1987). They promise to become the preferred lipids because they combine the best features of medium-chain and long-chain triglycerides.

Until structured lipids become available, it is safest to try to limit the use of long-chain triglycerides to 30% or less of the nonprotein calorie intake (30% to 50% is currently used). Fat is contraindicated, except for the minimum essential fatty acids, when the concentration of serum triglycerides is more than 400 mg/dL (4.5 mmol/L), during continuous nutrition, and in hepatic dysfunction (Giner & Curtas, 1986). Moreover, giving lipid continuously may be preferable (Abbott, Grakauskas, Bistrian, Rose, & Blackburn, 1984).

Table 25-4 gives an example of a TPN regimen that meets the maintenance requirements described in Table 25-3. Substrates may be provided together in a three-in-one system (Driscoll, Bistrian, Baptista, Randall, & Blackburn, 1987) or with dextrose and amino acids in one bag and lipids administered separately.

## Fluids

The normal fluid requirement has been reported to be approximately 30 to 45 mL per kilogram ideal body weight, or 1 mL/kcal (unless the patient is on a low-calorie diet), or, more generally, 2,500 mL/day (Giner & Curtas, 1986; Phillips & Odgers, 1982; Schmitz, Ahnefeld, & Burn, 1983). For practical purposes, 30 mL/kg can be provided. Losses from fever, diarrhea, fistulas, prolonged nasogastric suction, and other sources should be considered and recorded. In the example given in Table 25-4, approximately 2,100 mL of fluid is required (70 kg × 30 mL/kg = 2,100 mL). Problems of excess fluid are more frequently encountered (Giner & Curtas, 1986; Chwals & Blackburn, 1986). If fluid must be restricted, maximally concentrated substrates (dextrose 70%, protein 15%, and fat 20%) should be used.

## Micronutrients

*Vitamins.* Multivitamin preparations for intravenous nutrition maintenance are an essential adjunct to daily TPN, especially for provision of water-soluble vitamins. Different tumors and drugs used in chemotherapy influence the vitamin status. Up to now, the recommendations for intravenous administration of vitamins from the American Medical Association (AMA) have been applied to cancer patients (AMA, Multivitamin preparations, 1979). A recent prospec-

**Table 25-4** Example of a Parenteral Regimen that Meets the Maintenance Macronutrient Requirements from Table 25-3

| Regimen | Amount of Solution (mL) | Protein (g) | Carbohydrate (g) | Lipid (g) | Calories (kcal) |
|---|---|---|---|---|---|
| Amino acids 10% | 1,000 | 100 | | | 400 |
| Dextrose 70%* | 500 | | 350 | | 1,190 |
| Lipid emulsion 10%† | 600 | | | 50 | 660 |
| Total | | 100 | 350 | 50 | 2,250 |

*1 g of intravenous dextrose yields 3.4 kcal/g.
†10% lipid emulsion yields 1.1 kcal/mL.

tive study in 43 cancer patients (Inculet et al., 1987) indicated that recommendations for intravenous doses of $B_1$, $B_2$, $B_6$, and niacin may be too low for patients undergoing cancer therapy. Because intravenous administration of these water-soluble vitamins is safe, increased daily doses (probably doubled) are recommended instead (Inculet et al., 1987). In fact, studies have shown that thiamine status seems to deteriorate with advanced breast cancer (Husami & Abumrad, 1986). Furthermore, breast and bladder cancer are known to affect pyridoxine status. According to Husami and Abumrad (1986), advanced cancer may also greatly increase requirements for vitamin C, especially with bone metastases from breast cancer. Further studies are needed on this important subject.

*Electrolytes.* A problem often encountered during TPN, especially in the absence of a nutrition team, is the omission of necessary electrolytes, which may be fatal. Close monitoring of electrolytes is mandatory. Except for patients who have excessive losses (due to diarrhea, fistulas, drainage, and the like) or organ failure, the need for electrolytes is the same for cancer patients and noncancer patients. Average daily recommendations are given in Table 25-5 and must be carefully individualized according to each patient's clinical and biochemical status (Giner & Curtas, 1986). It is also important to assess electrolyte intake (especially sodium)

from other sources (e.g., medications) and other intravenous solutions. The clinician must remember that 1 L of normal saline (0.9%) contains 154 mEq of sodium, that is, 3.5 g of sodium. Currently, the prescription of sodium when hypertension or edema is present is around 40 mEq (1 g).

*Trace elements.* The influence of cancer and TPN on micronutrients is not well known. Recommendations of the AMA (AMA, Guidelines, 1979) appear in Table 25-6. In 1988, new guidelines for the use of vitamins, trace elements, calcium, magnesium, and phosphorus in infants and children receiving TPN were published (Greene, Hambidge, Schanler, & Tsang, 1988).

**Table 25-5** Average Daily Recommendations for TPN Electrolytes for Adults

| Electrolyte | Amount |
| --- | --- |
| Sodium | 100 mEq |
| Potassium | 60 to 120 mEq |
| Phosphorus | 10 to 22 mmol |
| Magnesium | 8 to 20 mEq |
| Calcium | 10 to 15 mEq |
| Chloride | 100 mEq |

*Source:* "Use of Total Parenteral Nutrition in Cancer Patients" by S.J. Bell, L.M. Coffey, and G.L. Blackburn, 1986, *Topics in Clinical Nutrition,* 1(2), pp. 37–49. Copyright 1986 by Aspen Publishers, Inc.

**Table 25-6** Suggested Daily Intravenous Intake of Essential Trace Elements*

| Element | Stable Adult | Adult in Acute Catabolic State | Stable Adult with Intestinal Losses |
| --- | --- | --- | --- |
| Zinc | 2.5 to 4.0 mg | Additional 2.0 mg | Add 12.2 mg per liter of small bowel fluid lost; 17.1 mg per kilogram of stool or ileostomy output |
| Copper | 0.5 to 1.5 mg | | |
| Chromium | 10 to 15 μg | | 20 μg† |
| Manganese | 0.15 to 0.8 mg | | |

*Values derived by mathematical fitting of balance data from a 71–patient week study in 24 patients.
†Mean from balance study.

*Source:* From "Guidelines for Essential Trace Element Preparations for Parenteral Use" by the American Medical Association Department of Foods and Nutrition, 1979, *Journal of the American Medical Association,* 241, pp. 2051–2054. Copyright 1979 by American Medical Association. Adapted by permission.

### Peripheral Parenteral Nutrition

When TPN is required for a short period of time or when central TPN is needed but not possible, not clearly necessary, or being tapered down, parenteral nutrition may be delivered through a peripheral vein, usually in the hand or forearm. It presumes, as with central TPN, that the enteral route is not adequate or that, if the enteral route is viable, adequate intake cannot be achieved thereby. Peripheral nutrition is not usually applicable for extremely malnourished patients, those who are fluid restricted, or those with inadequate peripheral venous access (Shanbhogue et al., 1986).

Amino acid and dextrose solutions, alone or combined with a 10% or 20% lipid emulsion, may be administered to provide nutrition support by peripheral parenteral nutrition (Gazitua, Wilson, Bistrian, & Blackburn, 1979; Watters & Freeman, 1981). Because of the fragility of peripheral veins compared to large central veins, the tonicity of the solution that may be given (<600 mOsm/L) restricts the calories and necessitates a larger fluid volume than that with central TPN. To prolong peripheral venous access, heparin and hydrocortisone (1,000 U/L and 5 mg/L, respectively) may be administered together with the formula.

Two systems may be used: the lipid system or the protein-sparing system (Table 25-7). If full parenteral nutrition support is needed but central TPN is not possible, the lipid system will best approximate full energy and protein needs. In clinical studies, infusion of 1.3 g of lipid per kilogram body weight over 10 hours has been shown to suppress reticuloendothelial cell function (Seidner et al., in preparation). The same dose of lipid administered continuously over 24 hours has been shown not to adversely affect reticuloendothelial system function (Jensen et al., 1988). Interestingly, in these clinical studies there was not a statistically significant increase in reticuloendothelial system activity when infusions of medium-chain and long-chain triglyceride mixtures were supplied continuously over 24 hours (Jensen, Mascioli, Istfan, Domnitch, & Bistrian, 1988). Therefore, the recommended safe lipid infusion dose is no more than 1.3 g of lipid per kilogram or a total of 100 g of lipid per 24 hours.

In the lipid system, which uses 3 L, two options are available. If a three-in-one admixture is available, 3 L of 3% amino acids, 3% lipid, and 3% dextrose supplies 1,456 total kilocalories and 90 g of protein (Driscoll et al., 1987). If the three-in-one system is not available, a Y connection may be used to infuse a 10% lipid solution together with a 3.5% amino acid in 5% dextrose solution. Two doses of 500 mL (50 g) of 10% lipid, each administered over 8 to 10 hours, is acceptable; this supplies 70 g of protein and 1,520 total kilocalories. Both regimens meet a high proportion of energy and

**Table 25-7** Comparison of Parenteral Regimens

| Regimen (3 L/day) | Protein (g) | Total Calories (kcal) | Approximate Osmolality (mOsm/L) |
|---|---|---|---|
| 5% Dextrose | 0 | 510 | 253 |
| Peripheral parenteral nutrition | | | |
| Protein sparing: 3.5% amino acids in 5% dextrose | 105 | 630 | 555 |
| Lipid system | | | |
| 1. 3% Dextrose, 3% lipid, 3% amino acids | 90 | 1,476 | 540 |
| 2. 3.5% Amino acids and 5% dextrose (2 L) | 70 | 415 | 555 |
| plus 1 L (100 g) of 10% lipid | 0 | 900 | 300 |
| | | (total, 1,315) | |
| Central TPN: 4.25% amino acids in 25% dextrose (3 L) | 128 | 3,000 | 1,700 |

*Source:* From "Parenteral Nutrition by Peripheral Vein" by J.M. Watters and J.B. Freeman, 1981, *Surgical Clinics of North America, 61*(3), p. 596. Copyright 1981 by W.B. Saunders Company. Reprinted by permission.

protein requirements. The lipid system is not indicated in patients with severe liver dysfunction and is contraindicated in those with hypertriglyceridemia (Watters & Freeman, 1981).

Volume restriction may be the limiting factor in delivering adequate energy and protein by means of peripheral parenteral nutrition. Often cancer patients are receiving several antibiotics, which may require up to 1.5 to 2.0 additional liters of intravenous fluid per day. In addition, patients with renal and cardiac disease may not tolerate small changes in fluid status. The dangers of fluid overload must be weighed against the potential gain from a nutritionally replete regimen.

The protein-sparing system with amino acids and dextrose is indicated for short-term (5 to 10 days) peripheral nutrition, that is, until the patient is enterally receiving adequate intake, requires TPN, or weighs at least 50% more than his or her ideal body weight. Protein synthesis has been reported to be improved and muscle catabolism decreased with the protein system for delivery of peripheral parenteral nutrition.

## SUMMARY

Total parenteral nutrition, by allowing total control of exogenous nutrients, may be invaluable in the study of alternative nutrition therapies for cancer patients. Nevertheless, present evidence argues strongly against the routine use of TPN in unselected cancer patients. Whenever feasible, the alimentary tract should be used to feed patients. When the gut is unavailable, uncertain, or inadequate, however, TPN by central or peripheral routes can be useful. Prospective and retrospective studies have demonstrated that TPN can increase survival and reduce operative complications in severely malnourished patients. There may be deleterious effects in using TPN in well-nourished cancer patients. Insufficient information is available to evaluate adequately the use of TPN in conjunction with radiation therapy and chemotherapy. Sound clinical judgment should be exercised to identify candidates for TPN.

Provision of adequate energy and protein is of primary importance to retard cachexia, to improve immune function, and to prevent side effects of malnutrition. Periodic nutrition assessment should become an integral part of the therapeutic plan in cancer patients. Refinement of techniques suitable for use in a clinical setting is needed in this area.

## REFERENCES

Abbott, W.C., Grakauskas, A.M., Bistrian, B.R., Rose, R., & Blackburn, G.L. (1984). Metabolic and respiratory effects of continuous and discontinuous lipid infusion. *Archives of Surgery, 119,* 1367–1371.

American College of Physicians. (1987). Perioperative parenteral nutrition—Position paper. *Annals of Internal Medicine, 107,* 252–253.

American Medical Association Department of Foods and Nutrition. (1979). Guidelines for essential trace element preparations for parenteral use: A statement by an expert panel. *Journal of the American Medical Association, 241,* 2051–2054.

American Medical Association Department of Foods and Nutrition. (1979). Multivitamin preparations for parenteral use: A statement by the Nutrition Advisory Group. *Journal of Parenteral and Enteral Nutrition, 3,* 258–261.

American Society for Parenteral and Enteral Nutrition Board of Directors. (1986). Guidelines for use of total parenteral nutrition in the hospitalized patient. *Journal of Parenteral and Enteral Nutrition, 10,* 441–445.

Andrassy, R.J. (1988). Preserving the gut mucosal barrier and enhancing immune response. *Contemporary Surgery, 32*(2-A), 21–27.

Assa, J., Schramek, A., Barzilai, A., & Weisz, G.M. (1974). Intravenous hyperalimentation for the onco-surgical patient. *Journal of Surgical Oncology, 1,* 239–244.

Babayan, V.K. (1987). Medium chain triglycerides and structured lipids. *Lipids, 22*(6), 417–420.

Bell, S.J., Coffey, L.M., & Blackburn, G.L. (1986). Use of total parenteral nutrition in cancer patients. *Topics in Clinical Nutrition, 1*(2), 37–49.

Bistrian, B.R. (1986). Preoperative nutritional support. *Nutrition Reviews, 44,* 230–231.

Bothe, A. Jr., Valerio, D., Bistrian, B.R., & Blackburn, G.L. (1979). Randomized controlled trial of hospital nutritional support during abdominal radiotherapy (abstract). *Journal of Parenteral and Enteral Nutrition, 3,* 292.

Bozzetti, F., Ammatuna, M., Migliavacca, S., Bonalumi, M.G., Facchetti, M.A., Pupa, A., & Terno, G. (1987). Total parenteral nutrition prevents further nutritional deterioration in patients with cancer cachexia. *Annals of Surgery, 205*(5), 138–143.

Brennan, M.F. (1981). Total parenteral nutrition in the cancer patient. *New England Journal of Medicine, 305,* 375–382.

Burt, M.E., Stein, T.P., & Brennan, M.F. (1983). A controlled randomized trial evaluating the effects of enteral and parenteral nutrition on protein metabolism in cancer-bearing man. *Journal of Surgery Research, 34,* 303–314.

Buzby, G.P. (1988). Perioperative TPN. In G.L. Blackburn, A. Bothe, & B.R. Bistrian (Eds.), *Hyperalimentation: A practical approach* (conference presented for the course Advances in Hyperalimentation). Boston: Harvard Medical School.

Buzby, G.P., Knox, L.S., Crosby, L.O., Eisenberg, J.M., Haakenson, C.M., McNeal, G.E., Page, C.P., Peterson, O.L., Reinhardt, G.R., & Williford, W.O. (1988). Study protocol: A randomized clinical trial of parenteral nutrition in malnourished surgical patients. *American Journal of Clinical Nutrition, 47,* 366–381.

Buzby, G.P., Mullen, J.L., Stein, T.P., Miller, E.E., Hobbs, C.L., & Rosato, E.F. (1980). Host tumor interaction and nutrient supply. *Cancer, 45,* 2940–2948.

Buzby, G.P., Williford, W.O., Peterson, O.L., Crosby, L.O., Page, C.P., Reinhardt, G.R., & Mullen, J.L. (1988). A randomized clinical trial of total parenteral nutrition in malnourished surgical patients: The rationale and impact of previous clinical trials and pilot study on protocol design. *American Journal of Clinical Nutrition, 47,* 357–365.

Cameron, I.L. (1981). Effects of total parenteral nutrition on tumor-host responses in rats. *Cancer Treatment Reports, 65*(Suppl. 5), 93–99.

Cameron, I.L., Ackley, W.J., & Rogers, W. (1977). Responses of hematoma-bearing rats to total parenteral hyperalimentation and to ad libitum feeding. *Journal of Surgery Research, 23,* 189–195.

Chlebowski, R.T. (1986). Effect of nutritional support on the outcome of antineoplastic therapy. *Clinics in Oncology, 5,* 365–379.

Chwals, W.J., & Blackburn, G.L. (1986). Perioperative nutritional support in the cancer patient. *Surgical Clinics of North America, 66*(6), 1137–1165.

Clamon, G., Gardner, L., Pee, D., Stumbo, P., Feld, R., Evans, W., Weiner, R., Moran, E., Blum, R., Hoffman, F.A., & DeWys, W. (1985). The effect of intravenous hyperalimentation on the dietary intake of patients with small cell lung cancer: A randomized trial. *Cancer, 55,* 1572–1578.

Copeland, E.M., MacFayden, B.V., & Dudrick, S.J. (1974). Intravenous hyperalimentation in cancer patients. *Journal of Surgery Research, 16,* 241–247.

Copeland, E.M., MacFayden, B.V. Jr., & Dudrick, S.J. (1976). Effect of hyperalimentation on delayed hypersensitivity in the cancer patient. *Annals of Surgery, 184,* 60–64.

Copeland, E.M., MacFayden, B.V. Jr., Lanzotti, V.J., & Dudrick, S.J. (1975). Intravenous hyperalimentation as an adjunct to cancer chemotherapy. *American Journal of Surgery, 129,* 167–173.

Copeland, E.M., MacFayden, B.V. Jr., MacComb, W.S., Guillamondegui, O., Jesse, R.J., & Dudrick, S.J. (1975). Intravenous hyperalimentation in patients with head and neck cancer. *Cancer, 35,* 606–611.

Copeland, E.M., & Souba, W.W. (1988). Nutritional considerations in treatment of the cancer patient. *Nutrition in Clinical Practice, 3,* 173–174.

Coquin, J.Y., Maranichi, D., Gastant, J.A., & Carcassone, Y. (1981). Influence of parenteral nutrition on chemotherapy and survival of acute leukemias: Preliminary results of a randomized trial (abstract). *Journal of Parenteral and Enteral Nutrition, 5,* 357.

Daly, J.M., Copeland, E.M., & Dudrick, S.J. (1978). Effects of intravenous nutrition on tumor growth and host immunocompetence in malnourished animals. *Surgery, 84,* 655–658.

Daly, J.M., Massar, E., Giacco, G., Frazier, O.H., Mountain, C.F., Dudrick, S.J., & Copeland, E.M. (1982). Parenteral nutrition in esophageal cancer patients. *Annals of Surgery, 196*(2), 203–208.

Daly, J.M., Reynolds, J., Thom, A., Kinsley, L., Dietrick-Gallagher, M., Show, J., & Ruggieri, B. (1988). Immune and metabolic effects of arginine in the surgical patient. *Annals of Surgery, 208,* 522–523.

Daly, J.M., Steiger, E., Vars, H.M., & Dudrick, S.J. (1974). Postoperative oral and intravenous nutrition. *Annals of Surgery, 180,* 709–715.

Dematteis, R., & Hermann, R.E. (1973). Supplementary parenteral nutrition in patients with malignant disease: Guidelines to patient selection. *Cleveland Clinics, 40,* 139–145.

Dempsey, D.T., Mullen, J.L., & Buzby, G.P. (1988). The link between nutritional status and clinical outcome: Can nutritional intervention modify it? *American Journal of Clinical Nutrition, 47,* 352–356.

Detsky, A.S., Baker, J.P., O'Rourke, K., & Goel, V. (1987). Perioperative parenteral nutrition: A meta-analysis. *Annals of Internal Medicine, 107,* 195–203.

Donaldson, S.S., Wesley, M.N., Ghavinsi, F., Shils, M.E., Suskind, R.S., & DeWys, W. (1982). A prospective randomized clinical trial of total parenteral nutrition in children with cancer. *Medical and Pediatric Oncology, 10,* 129–139.

Driscoll, D.F., Bistrian, B.R., Baptista, R.J., Randall, S., & Blackburn, G.L. (1987). Base solution limitations and patient-specific TPN admixtures. *Nutrition in Clinical Practice, 2,* 160–163.

Drott, C., Unsgaard, B., Schersten, T., & Lundholm, K. (1988). Total parenteral nutrition as an adjuvant to patients undergoing chemotherapy for testicular carcinoma: Protection of body composition—A randomized, prospective study. *Surgery, 103*(5), 499–506.

Dudrick, S.J., Wilmore, D.W., Vars, H.M., & Rhoads, J.R. (1968). Long term total parenteral nutrition with growth, development and positive nitrogen balance. *Surgery, 64,* 134–142.

Elwyn, D.H., Gump, F.E., Munro, H.N., Iles, M., & Kinney, J.M. (1979). Changes in nitrogen balance of depleted patients with increasing infusions of glucose. *American Journal of Clinical Nutrition, 32,* 1597–1611.

Enrione, E.B., Black, C.D., & Moore, D.M. (1985). Response of tumor-bearing rats to high fat total parenteral nutrition. *Cancer, 56,* 2612–2616.

Fried, R.C., Mullen, J., Stein, T.P., Yuhas, J., Miller, E., & Buzby, G.P. (1985). The effects of glucose and amino acids on tumor and host DNA synthesis. *Journal of Surgery Research, 39*, 461–469.

Gazitua, R., Wilson, K., Bistrian, B.R., & Blackburn, G.L. (1979). Factors determining peripheral vein tolerance to amino acid infusions. *Archives of Surgery, 114*, 897–900.

Geller, R.J., Blackburn, S.A., Glendon, D.H., Henneman, W.H., & Steffee, W.P. (1979). Computer optimization of enteral hyperalimentation. *Journal of Parenteral and Enteral Nutrition, 3*, 79–83.

Ghavinsi, F., Shils, M.E., Scott, B.F., Brown, M., & Tamaroff, M. (1982). Comparison of morbidity in children requiring abdominal radiation and chemotherapy, with and without total parenteral nutrition. *Pediatrics, 101*, 530–533.

Gil, K.M., Askanazi, J., Weissman, C., Elwyn, D.H., & Kinney, J.M. (1986). Energy expenditure following infusions of glucose based parenteral nutrition (abstract). *Journal of Parenteral and Enteral Nutrition, 10*, 125.

Giner, M., & Curtas, S. (1986). Adverse metabolic consequences of nutritional support: Macronutrients. *Surgical Clinics of North America, 66*, 1025–1047.

Greene, H.L., Hambidge, K.M., Schanler, R., & Tsang, R.C. (1988). Guidelines for the use of vitamins, trace elements, calcium, magnesium, and phosphorus in infants and children receiving total parenteral nutrition: Report of the Subcommittee on Pediatric Parenteral Nutrition Requirements of the Committee on Clinical Practices Issues of the American Society for Clinical Nutrition. *American Journal of Clinical Nutrition, 48*, 1324–1342.

Grube, B.J., Gamelli, R.L., & Foster, R.S. (1985). Refeeding differentially affects tumor and host cell proliferation. *Journal of Surgery Research, 39*, 535–542.

Hamawy, K.J., Moldawer, L.L., Georgieff, M., Valicenti, A.J., Babayan, V.K., Bistrian, B.R., & Blackburn, G.L. (1985). The effect of emulsions on reticuloendothelial system function in the injured animal. *Journal of Parenteral and Enteral Nutrition, 9*, 559–565.

Harris, J.A., & Benedict, F.G. (1919). A biometric study of basal metabolism in man (Carnegie Institute Publication No. 279). Washington, DC: Carnegie Institution of Washington.

Hays, D.M., Merritt, R.J., White, L., Ashley, J., & Siegel, S.E. (1983). Effect of total parenteral nutrition on marrow recovery during induction therapy for acute non-lymphocytic leukemia in childhood. *Medical and Pediatric Oncology, 11*, 134–140.

Heatley, R.V., Williams, R.H.P., & Lewis, M.H. (1979). Preoperative intravenous feeding: A controlled trial. *Postgraduate Medical Journal, 55*, 541–545.

Holter, A.R., & Fisher, J.E. (1977). The effects of perioperative hyperalimentation on complications in patients with carcinoma and weight loss. *Journal of Surgery Research, 23*, 31–34.

Holter, A.R., Rosen, H.M., & Fisher, J.E. (1977). The effects of hyperalimentation on major surgery in patients with malignant disease: A prospective study. *Acta Chirurgica Scandinavica Supplementum (Stockholm), 466*, 86–87.

Husami, T., & Abumrad, N.N. (1986). Adverse metabolic consequences of nutritional support: Micronutrients. *Surgical Clinics of North America, 66*(5), 1049–1069.

Inculet, R.I., Norton, J.A., Nichoalds, G.E., Maher, M.M., White, D.E., & Brennan, M.F. (1987). Water-soluble vitamins in cancer patients on parenteral nutrition: A prospective study. *Journal of Parenteral and Enteral Nutrition, 11*, 243–249.

Issel, B.V., Valdivieso, M., Zaren, H.A., Dudrick, S.J., Freireich, E.J., Copeland, E.M., & Bodey, G.P. (1978). Protection against chemotherapy toxicity by IV hyperalimentation. *Cancer Treatment Reports, 62*, 1139–1143.

Jensen, G.L., Mascioli, E.A., Istfan, N.W., Domnitch, A., & Bistrian, B. (1988). Parenteral infusion of medium chain triglyceride and reticulendothelial system function in man (abstract). *American Journal of Clinical Nutrition, 47*, 786.

Jensen, G.L., Seidner, D.L., Mascioli, E.A., Istfan, F., Selleck, K., Blackburn, G., & Bistrian, B. (1988). Continuous infusion of long chain triglyceride emulsion and reticuloendothelial system function in man (abstract). *Journal of Parenteral and Enteral Nutrition, 12*, 45.

Jordan, W.M., Valdivieso, M., Frankmann, C., Gillespie, M., Issel, B.F., & Freireich, E.J. (1981). Treatment of advanced adenocarcinoma of the lung with ftorafur, doxorubicin, cyclophosphamide, and cisplatin (FACP) and intensive IV hyperalimentation. *Cancer Treatment Reports, 63*, 197–205.

King, W.W.K., Boelhouwer, R.U., Kingsnorth, A.N., Weening, J.J., Weber, G., Young, V.R., & Malt, R.A. (1985). Total parenteral nutrition with and without fat as a substrate for growth of rats and transplanted hepatocarcinoma. *Journal of Parenteral and Enteral Nutrition, 9*, 422–427.

Kinsella, T.J., Malcolm, A.W., Bothe, A., Valerio, D., & Blackburn, G.L. (1981). Prospective study of nutritional support during pelvic irradiation. *International Journal of Radiation Oncology/Biology/Physics, 7*, 543–548.

Kishi, T., Iwasawa, Y., Itoh, H., & Chibata, T. (1982). Nutritional responses of tumor-bearing rats to oral or intravenous feeding. *Journal of Parenteral and Enteral Nutrition, 6*, 295–300.

Klein, S., Simes, J., & Blackburn, G.L. (1986). Total parenteral nutrition and cancer trials. *Cancer, 58*, 1378–1386.

Kurzer, M.. & Mequid, M.M. (1986). Cancer and protein metabolism. *Surgical Clinics of North America, 66*(5), 969–1001.

Lanzotti, V., Copeland, E.M., Bhuchar, V., Wesley, M., Corriere, J., & Dudrick, S. (1980). A randomized trial of total parenteral nutrition with chemotherapy for non–oat cell lung cancer (abstract). *Proceedings of the American Association for Cancer Research, 21*, 377.

Lanzotti, V.J., Copeland, E.M., George, S.L., Dudrick, S.J., & Samuels, M.L. (1975). Cancer chemotherapeutic response and intravenous hyperalimentation. *Cancer Chemotherapy Reports, 59*, 437–439.

Lim, S.T.K., Choa, R.G., Lam, K.H., Wong, J., & Ong, G.B. (1981). Total parenteral nutrition vs. gastrostomy in the preoperative preparation of patients with carcinoma of the esophagus. *British Journal of Surgery, 68,* 69–72.

Long, C.L., Schaffel, N., Geiger, J.W., Schiller, W.R., & Blakemore, W.S. (1979). Metabolic response to injury and illness: Estimation of energy and protein needs for indirect calorimetry and nitrogen balance. *Journal of Parenteral and Enteral Nutrition, 3,* 452–456.

Lowry, S.F., & Brennan, M.F. (1986). Intravenous feeding of the cancer patient. In J.L. Rombeau & M.D. Caldwell (Eds.), *Parenteral nutrition, clinical nutrition* (Vol. 2, chap. 26). Philadelphia: Saunders.

Mascioli, E.A., Bistrian, B.R., Babayan, V.K., & Blackburn, G.L. (1987). Medium chain triglycerides and structured lipids as unique nonglucose energy sources in hyperalimentation. *Lipids, 22*(6), 421–423.

McArdle, A.H., Palmason, C., Morency, I., & Brown, R.A. (1981). A rationale for enteral feeding as the preferable route for hyperalimentation. *Surgery, 90*(4), 616–623.

Merrick, H.W., Long, C.L., Grecos, G.P., Dennis, R.S., & Blakemore, W.S. (1988). Energy requirements for cancer patients and the effect of total parenteral nutrition. *Journal of Parenteral and Enteral Nutrition, 12,* 8–14.

Moghissi, K., Hornshaw, J., Teasdale, P.R., & Dawes, E.A. (1977). Parenteral nutrition in carcinoma of the esophagus treated by surgery: Nitrogen balance and clinical studies. *British Journal of Surgery, 64,* 125–128.

Mullen, J.L., Buzby, G.P., Matthews, D.C., Smale, B.F., & Rosato, E.F. (1980). Reduction of operative morbidity and mortality by combined preoperative and postoperative nutritional support. *Annals of Surgery, 192*(5), 604–613.

Müller, J.M., Brenner, U., Dienst, C., & Pichlmaier, H. (1982). Preoperative parenteral feeding in patients with gastrointestinal carcinoma. *Lancet, 1,* 68–71.

Nixon, D.W., Lawson, D.H., Kutner, M., Amsley, J., Schwartz, M., Heymfield, S., Chawla, R., Cartwright, T.H., & Rudman, D. (1981). Hyperalimentation of the cancer patient with protein-calorie undernutrition. *Cancer Research, 41,* 2038–2045.

Oram-Smith, J.C., Stein, T.P., Wallace, H.W., & Mullen, J.L. (1977). Intravenous nutrition and tumor host protein metabolism. *Journal of Surgery Research, 22,* 499–503.

Phillips, G.D., & Odgers, C.L. (1982). Parenteral nutrition: Current status and concepts. *Drugs, 23,* 276.

Popp, M.B., Morrison, S.D., & Brennan, M.F. (1981). Total parenteral nutrition in a methylcholanthrene-induced rat sarcoma model. *Cancer Treatment Reports, 65*(Suppl. 5), 137–143.

Popp, M.B., Wagner, S.C., & Brito, O.J. (1983). Host and tumor responses to increasing levels of intravenous nutritional support. *Surgery, 92,* 300–307.

Rudman, D., & Williams, P.J. (1985). Nutrient deficiencies during total parenteral nutrition. *Nutrition Reviews, 43*(1), 1–13.

Sacks, H.S., Berrier, J., Reitman, D., Ancona-Berk, V.A., & Chalmers, T.C. (1987). Meta-analyses of randomized controlled trials. *New England Journal of Medicine, 316,* 450–455.

Sako, K., Lore, J.M., Kaufman, S., Razack, M.S., Bakamjian, V., & Reese, P. (1981). Parenteral hyperalimentation in surgical patients with head and neck cancer: A randomized study. *Journal of Surgical Oncology, 16,* 391–401.

Samuels, M.L., Selig, D.E., Ogden, S., Grant, C., & Brown, B. (1981). IV hyperalimentation and chemotherapy for stage II testicular cancer: A randomized study. *Cancer Treatment Reports, 68,* 615–627.

Schmitz, J.E., Ahnefeld, F.W., & Burn, C. (1983). Nutritional support of the multiple trauma patient. *World Journal of Surgery, 7,* 132.

Schwartz, G.F., Greene, H.L., Bendon, M.L., Graham, W.P., & Blakemore, W.S. (1971). Combined parenteral hyperalimentation and chemotherapy in the treatment of disseminated solid tumors. *American Journal of Surgery, 121,* 169–173.

Seidner, D.L., Mascioli, E.A., Istfan, N.W., et al. (In preparation). The effects of long chain triglyceride emulsions on reticuloendothelial system function in humans.

Serrou, B., Cupissol, D., Plagne, R., Boutin, P., Chollet, P., Carcassone, Y., and Michel, F.B. (1982). Follow-up of a randomized trial for oat cell carcinoma evaluating the efficacy of peripheral intravenous nutrition (PIVN) as adjunct treatment. *Recent Results in Cancer Research, 80,* 246–253.

Shamberger, R.C., Brennan, M.F., Goodgame, J.T. Jr., Lowry, S.F., Maher, M.M., & Pizzo, P.A. (1984). A prospective, randomized study of adjuvant parenteral nutrition in the treatment of sarcomas: Results of metabolic and survival studies. *Surgery, 96,* 1–13.

Shanbhogue, L.K.R., Bistrian, B.R., & Blackburn, G.L. (1986). Trends in enteral nutrition in the surgical patient. *Journal of the Royal College of Surgeons (Edinburgh), 31*(5), 267–273.

Simms, J.M., Oliver, E., & Smith, J.A.R. (1980). A study of total parenteral nutrition in major gastric and esophageal resection of neoplasia (abstract). *Journal of Parenteral and Enteral Nutrition, 4,* 422.

Solassol, C., & Joyeux, J. (1979). Artificial gut with complete nutritive mixtures as a major adjunctive therapy in cancer patients. *Acta Chirurgica Scandinavica Supplementum (Stockholm), 494,* 186–187.

Solassol, C., Joyeux, J., & Dubois, J.B. (1979). Total parenteral nutrition (TPN) with complete nutritive mixtures: An artificial gut in cancer patients. *Nutrition and Cancer, 1,* 13–18.

Souba, W.W., & Copeland, E.M. (1988). Parenteral nutrition and metabolic observations in cancer. *Nutrition in Clinical Practice, 3*(5), 191–197.

Steiger, E., Oram-Smith, J., Miller, E., Kuo, L., & Vars, H. (1975). Effects of nutrition on tumor growth and tolerance to chemotherapy. *Journal of Surgery Research, 18,* 455–461.

Valdivieso, M., Bodey, G.P., Benjamin, R.S., Barkley, H.T., Freeman, M.B., Ertel, M., Smith, T.L., & Mountain, C.F. (1981). Role of intravenous hyperalimentation as an adjunct to intensive chemotherapy for small cell bronchogenic carcinoma. *Cancer Treatment Reports, 5*(Suppl.), 145–150.

Valerio, D., Overett, L., Malcolm, A., & Blackburn, G.L. (1978). Nutritional support for cancer patients receiving abdominal and pelvic radiotherapy: A randomized prospective clinical experiment of intravenous versus oral feeding. *Surgery Forum, 29,* 145–148.

van Eys, J., Copeland, E.M., Cangir, A., Taylor, G., Teitell-Cohen, B., Carter, P., & Ortiz, C. (1980). A randomized controlled clinical trial of hyperalimentation in children with metastatic malignancies. *Medical and Pediatric Oncology, 8,* 63–73.

Watters, J.M., & Freeman, J.B. (1981). Parenteral nutrition by peripheral vein. *Surgical Clinics of North America, 61,* 593–604.

Williams, R.P.H., Heatley, R.V., Lewis, M.H., & Hughes, L.E. (1976). A randomized controlled trial of preoperative intravenous nutrition in patients with stomach cancer. *British Journal of Surgery, 63,* 667–671.

Young, V.R. (1977). Energy metabolism in requirements in the cancer patient. *Cancer Research, 37,* 2336–2347.

# Chapter 26

# Management Options: Food Service Facilities

*L. Charnette Norton*

Cancer patients present unique management challenges to food service facilities regardless of the number of patients served. During the treatment phases of their disease cancer patients often require increased protein and caloric levels, but achieving these levels is sometimes difficult because of food aversions, anorexia, the inability to participate in the normal functions of eating, or an altered perception of tastes and odors. This chapter provides a general description of four areas—staffing, menu planning, tray delivery systems, and cafeteria feeding—that are important to all food service facilities serving cancer patients.

## STAFFING LEVELS

All cancer patients are at risk nutritionally and therefore must be individually assessed and educated as to their specific nutrition needs. This individual assessment and education takes time and consequently requires a high staff-to-patient ratio. The ability of staff to devote an adequate amount of time to patients, however, has been constrained in recent years with the growing emphasis on outpatient care, which has been spurred largely by the attempt of health care institutions to conform to diagnosis-related groups. Consequently, the inpatient population has an increasing concentration of acutely ill

patients who require class III nursing care (i.e., those requiring seven nursing hours or more per day). From a nutritional standpoint, these patients also require additional assessment, monitoring, and education.

At the University of Texas M.D. Anderson Cancer Center an effort is made to assign a dietitian to every 35 to 55 patients. For the intensive care units the dietitian must be assigned an even smaller number of patients. Even when patients no longer require aggressive nutrition intervention from the dietary staff, their need for personal contact is still present. Dying patients need to feel that they are not abandoned by the health care providers.

Specific staffing levels for cancer patients have not been established at M.D. Anderson Cancer Center, nor have specific standards been established for class III patients by the American Dietetic Association. Multi-institution time studies would be helpful in establishing guidelines for staff levels by developing acceptable ranges of productivity standards. The Clinical Nutrition Management Dietetic Practice Group, in conjunction with 21 Chicago area hospitals, worked on a project for productivity studies for clinical dietitians; the results have not yet been published. At M.D. Anderson Cancer Center a study is in progress with the goal of establishing a range of time standards for specific clinical tasks. This is the start of developing staffing levels on the basis of actual rather than estimated work loads.

## MENUS

The menu for the cancer patient can be the same as that for any other patient population, with one significant difference: items must be made available on demand for the patient.

### Write-In List

The psychology of food likes and dislikes may become prominent during cancer treatment. Because many of the side effects of treatment change taste and odor preferences, patients have definite ideas about what they want to eat. This may change throughout their treatment course and may even change daily or hourly. To assist in providing for the nutrition needs of the patient who cannot find anything to choose from on the preprinted patient menu, a menu write-in list similar to the one shown in Exhibit 26-1 can be developed. The list is given to the patient by the dietetic technician on admittance. The patient is instructed to use the list when the daily menu is not acceptable. The patient keeps the list at the bedside for easy reference. When menu selection is made, the patient chooses write-in items from the list. If the patient receives the tray but finds that the choices are now unacceptable because of a recent change in medical condition, he or she may request a replacement food item from the dietary worker.

### Nourishments

Providing the cancer patient with more than adequate opportunities to meet nutrition requirements is essential in the care and treatment of this population. Therefore, the number and amounts of nourishments and supplements provided to cancer patients are much larger than those provided to most other groups of patients. An example of the selections available at M.D. Anderson Cancer Center for 10:00 a.m., 3:00 p.m., and 8:00 p.m. is shown in Exhibit 26-2.

The clinical dietitian or the dietetic technician can order items listed for the patient to fit personal preferences and disease treatments. In addition to a nourishment and supplement list and a menu write-in list, an evening nourishment menu is provided for all patients regardless of the specific diet order. Examples of menus that are provided for each specific diet type are shown in Exhibit 26-3. Patients choose from these menus when they choose their meals. The evening nourishment list is an attachment to each menu (some institutions may refer to it as a snack menu). The items to serve on the evening nourishment list are planned when the rest of the menu is planned on the basis of the same criteria used for menu planning. Past history of patient requests is considered important because at the end of a treatment day the need is different as a result of the stress of the treatments administered.

### Recipes

In developing items for the nourishment and supplement list, factors to consider (in addition to cost, availability, ease of serving, and acceptability) are ratios of calories to protein, calories to volume, and protein to volume and the use of homemade items. American society, all the modern conveniences notwithstanding, still places a high value on the homemade item. Patients perceive the homemade item as representing a caring attitude from the care giver. Using a homemade supplementary drink (Exhibit 26-4) is preferable to using a commercial one provided that resources are available to make and serve it. Many additional flavors can be offered to the patient that are not readily available commercially. The homemade items represent a uniqueness of the patient's nutrition support network that can assist in reducing negative comments regarding food service.

Patients undergoing treatment at times experience an aversion to the sweet foods that are given to increase caloric requirements. The development of tart drinks can aid in solving this problem. A recipe for Citrotein gelatin, one such item used for nourishment, is shown in Exhibit 26-5. Exhibits 26-6 and 26-7 provide

**Exhibit 26-1** Sample Menu Write-In List

THE UNIVERSITY OF TEXAS M.D. ANDERSON CANCER CENTER
DEPARTMENT OF NUTRITION AND FOOD SERVICE

### MENU WRITE-IN LIST

The following items are always available in addition to the items on the menu you receive each day. In order to receive these items, they must be ordered on your menu for the next day and turned in to your food service hostess by 10:00 a.m. on the day before service.

#### BREAKFAST ITEMS
(Available only at breakfast)

I.  *CEREALS*
Cheerios
Cream of Rice
40% Bran Flakes
Product 19

II. *EGGS*—Plain Omelet

III. *MISCELLANEOUS*
Beef Jerky          Italian Ice
Crackers            Lemon Wedges
Custard
Gelatin
Ice Cream—Chocolate, Vanilla, Strawberry

#### LUNCH AND DINNER ITEMS
(Available only at lunch and dinner)

I.  *MAIN COURSES* (Heated)
Burrito
Cheeseburger
Chicken—White meat only. Specify baked or oven-fried.
Chili
Eggs—Hard cooked, poached, or scrambled
Fish—Baked or breaded baked
Grilled Cheese Sandwich (Not recommended. This item will be soggy due to our heating system.)

Hamburger
Hot Dog
Hot Dog with Chili
Macaroni and Cheese
Omelet—Plain or Cheese
Roast Beef
Sliced Turkey

II. *COLD MAIN COURSES*
Salads: Chef Salad
Chicken Salad
Cottage Cheese and Canned Fruit Plate

Cottage Cheese and Fresh Fruit Plate
Egg Salad
Pimento Cheese Salad
Tuna Salad

*continues*

**Exhibit 26-1** continued

Sandwiches: Please circle mustard or mayonnaise in condiment section on menu.

Chicken Salad Sandwich

Egg Salad Sandwich

Ham Sandwich

Ham and Cheese Sandwich

Peanut Butter Sandwich

Pimento Cheese Sandwich

Roast Beef Sandwich

Sliced American Cheese
 Sandwich

Tuna Salad Sandwich

Turkey Sandwich

III.  *SOUPS*

Broth—Beef or Chicken

Chicken Rice Soup

Cream of Mushroom Soup

Cream of Pea Soup

Turkey Noodle Soup

Vegetable Beef Soup

*LOW SALT SOUPS*

LS Beef Broth

LS Chicken Broth

LS Cream of Mushroom Soup

LS Cream of Pea Soup

LS Cream of Tomato Soup

LS Turkey Noodle Soup

LS Vegetable Soup

IV.  *VEGETABLES*

Carrots

Corn

Green Beans

Green Peas

Potatoes—French fries or mashed
 (French fries not recommended.
 This item will be soggy due to our
 heating system.)

Rice

V.  *SALADS*

Canned Fruits—Peaches, Pears,
 Applesauce, Pineapple

Cottage Cheese

Celery and Carrot Sticks

Jell-O—Red

Lemon Wedges

Relish Cup

Sliced Tomato

Yogurt—Plain or fruit (Please *do not*
 specify flavor.)

VI.  *DESSERTS*

Custard

Graham Crackers

Ice Cream—Chocolate, Vanilla, Strawberry

Italian Ice

Popsicle

Pudding—Chocolate, Vanilla

Sherbet—Orange, Lime

VII.  *BEVERAGES*

Coke

Diet Coke

Eggnog

Gatorade—Orange, Lime

Lemonade

Milkshake—Chocolate, Vanilla,
 Strawberry

Punch

Sprite

Variety of Fruit and Vegetable
 Juices

VIII.  *MISCELLANEOUS*

Corn Chips

Potato Chips

*Source:* Courtesy of the Department of Nutrition and Food Service, The University of Texas M.D. Anderson Cancer Center.

**Exhibit 26-2** Sample of Selections Available for Write-In Menus

Week     I        II

M T W T F S S

**NOURISHMENT/MENU WRITE IN CODE LIST**

**NOURISHMENT: 10   3   HS**

Date: _____

***BEVERAGES, JUICES, SUPPLEMENTS***

| Code | | Item |
|---|---|---|
| (_) | 1 | Apple Juice (4 oz) M |
| (_) | 1PX | Apple Juice (4 oz) + Poly (2 Tbsp) M |
| (_) | 2 | Apricot Nectar (4 oz) M |
| (_) | 2PX | Apricot Nectar (4 oz) + Poly (2 Tbsp) M |
| (_) | 3 | Carbonated Beverage, Coke (8 oz) M |
| (_) | 4 | Carbonated Beverage, Sprite (8 oz) M |
| (_) | 5 | Carbonated Beverage, Diet Coke (8 oz) M |
| ( ) | 6 | Carbonated Beverage, Gingerale (12 oz) M |
| (_) | 7 | Cereal Cream (7 oz) M |
| (_) | 7-1/2 | Cereal Cream (4 oz) M |
| (_) | 8 | CIB, Vanilla + Whole Milk (7 oz) M |
| (_) | 8S | CIB, Vanilla + Skim Milk (7 oz) M |
| (_) | 8C | CIB, Vanilla + Cream (7 oz) M |
| (_) | 8DP | CIB, Vanilla, Dry Pack M |
| (_) | 9 | CIB, Chocolate + Whole Milk (7 oz) M |
| (_) | 9S | CIB, Chocolate + Skim Milk (7 oz) M |
| (_) | 9C | CIB, Chocolate + Cream (7 oz) M |
| (_) | 9DP | CIB, Chocolate, Dry Pack M |
| (_) | 10orX | Citrotein, Orange (7 oz) M |
| (_) | 10puX | Citrotein, Punch (7 oz) M |
| (_) | 10LX | Citrotein, Lemonade (7 oz) M |
| (_) | 10PX | Citrotein (7 oz) + Poly (4 Tbsp) M |
| (_) | 11 | Cranberry Juice (4 oz) M |
| (_) | 11PX | Cranberry Juice (4 oz) + Poly (2 Tbsp) M |
| (_) | 12VX | Ensure, Vanilla (8 oz) M |
| (_) | 12CX | Ensure, Chocolate (8 oz) M |
| (_) | 13SX | Ensure Plus, Strawberry (8 oz) M |
| (_) | 13VX | Ensure Plus, Vanilla (8 oz) M |
| (_) | 13CX | Ensure Plus, Chocolate (8 oz) M |
| (_) | 14 | Eggnog (7 oz) M |
| (_) | 14-1/2 | Eggnog (4 oz) M |
| (_) | 15or | Gatorade, Orange (7 oz) M |
| (_) | 15L | Gatorade, Lime (7 oz) M |
| (_) | 16or | Gatorade, Orange (qt) |
| (_) | 16L | Gatorade, Lime (qt) |
| (_) | 17 | Grape Juice (4 oz) M |
| (_) | 17PX | Grape Juice (4 oz) + Poly (2 Tbsp) M |
| (_) | 18 | Grapefruit Juice (4 oz) M |
| (_) | 18PX | Grapefruit Juice (4 oz) + Poly (2 Tbsp) M |
| (_) | 19X | Osmolite (8 oz) M |
| (_) | 20X | Isocal HCN (8 oz) M |
| (_) | 21 | Lemonade (7 oz) M |
| (_) | 22 | Milk, Whole (8 oz) M |
| (_) | 22-1/2 | Milk, Whole (4 oz) M |
| (_) | 23 | Milk, Whole (7 oz) + NFDM (4 Tbsp) M |
| (_) | 24 | Milk, Skim (8 oz) M |
| (_) | 24-1/2 | Milk, Skim (4 oz) M |
| (_) | 25 | Milk, Skim (7 oz) + NFDM (4 Tbsp) M |
| (_) | 26 | Milk, Chocolate (8 oz) M |
| (_) | 26-1/2 | Milk, Chocolate (4 oz) M |
| (_) | 27 | Milk, Butter (8 oz) M |
| (_) | 27-1/2 | Milk, Butter (4 oz) M |
| (_) | 28C | Diet Shake, Chocolate, Whole (7 oz) M |
| (_) | 28CL | Diet Shake, Chocolate, Lowfat (7 oz) M |
| (_) | 28V | Diet Shake, Vanilla, Whole (7 oz) M |
| (_) | 28S | Diet Shake, Strawberry, Whole (7 oz) M |
| (_) | 29V | Milkshake, Vanilla (8 oz) M |
| (_) | 29C | Milkshake, Chocolate (8 oz) M |
| (_) | 29S | Milkshake, Strawberry (6 oz) M |
| (_) | 30 | Milkshake, Peanut Butter with Milk (6 oz) M |
| (_) | 31 | Milkshake, Banana with Cream (6 oz) M |
| (_) | 32 | Milkshake, Vanilla House with Milk (6 oz) M |
| (_) | 33A | Milkshake, Chocolate Almond with Cream (6 oz) M |
| (_) | 33B | Milkshake, Chocolate House with Milk (6 oz) M |
| (_) | 34 | Non Dairy Creamer (8 oz) M |
| (_) | 34-1/2 | Non Dairy Creamer (4 oz) M |
| (_) | 35 | Orange Juice (4 oz) M |
| (_) | 35PX | Orange Juice (4 oz) + Poly (2 Tbsp) M |
| (_) | 36X | Pulmocare (8 oz) M |

*continues*

**Exhibit 26-2** continued

## Nourishment/Menu Write In Code List
## Page 2

| | | |
|---|---|---|
| (_) 37 | Orange Pineapple Fluff (6 oz) M |
| (_) 38 | Peach Nectar (4 oz) M |
| (_) 38PX | Peach Nectar (4 oz) + Poly (2 Tbsp) M |
| (_) 39 | Pear Nectar (4 oz) M |
| (_) 39PX | Pear Nectar (4 oz) + Poly (2 Tbsp) M |
| (_) 40 | Pineapple Juice (4 oz) M |
| (_) 40PX | Pineapple Juice (4 oz) + Poly (2 Tbsp) M |
| (_) 41X | Polycose (4 oz bottle) M |
| (_) 42X | Polycose (2 Tbsp) + Iced Tea (8 oz) M |
| (_) 43X | Polycose (2 Tbsp) + Coffee (8 oz) M |
| (_) 44X | Polycose (2 Tbsp) + Hot Chocolate (8 oz) M |
| (_) 45X | Polycose (2 Tbsp) + Hot Tea (8 oz) M |
| (_) 46 | Prune Juice (4 oz) M |
| (_) 46PX | Prune Juice (4 oz) + Poly (2 Tbsp) M |
| (_) 47 | Punch |
| (_) 48 | Raspberry Fluff with Cream (6 oz) M |
| (_) 49VX | Sustacal, Vanilla (8 oz) M |
| (_) 49CX | Sustacal, Chocolate (8 oz) M |
| (_) 50 | Tomato Juice (4 oz) M |
| (_) 50PX | Tomato Juice (4 oz) + Poly (2 Tbsp) M |
| (_) 50LS | LS Tomato Juice (4 oz) M |
| (_) 51X | Travasorb MCT (200 cc) M |
| (_) 52 | V-8 Juice (6 oz) M |
| (_) 52PX | V-8 Juice (6 oz) + Poly (2 Tbsp) M |
| (_) 53C-1/4X | Tolerex, Cranberry-or (210 cc) M |
| (_) 53C-1/2X | Tolerex, Cranberry-or (210 cc) M |
| (_) 53C-3/4X | Tolerex, Cranberry-or (210 cc) M |
| (_) 53CX-Full | Tolerex, Cranberry-or (210 cc) M |
| (_) 54G-1/4X | Tolerex, Grape (210 cc) M |
| (_) 54G-1/2X | Tolerex, Grape (210 cc) M |
| (_) 54G-3/4X | Tolerex, Grape (210 cc) M |
| (_) 54G-Full | Tolerex, Grape (210 cc) M |
| (_) 55or-1/4X | Tolerex, Orange (210 cc) M |
| (_) 55or-1/2X | Tolerex, Orange (210 cc) M |
| (_) 55or-3/4X | Tolerex, Orange (210 cc) M |
| (_) 55or-Full | Tolerex, Orange (210 cc) M |

### DESSERTS
| | |
|---|---|
| (_) 56 | Cake |
| (_) 57 | Cookies, Creme Sand, Choc |
| (_) 58 | Cookies, Creme Sand, Vanilla |
| (_) 59 | Cookies, Choc Chip |
| (_) 60 | Cookies, Fig Newton |

| | | |
|---|---|---|
| (_) 61 | Cookies, Vanilla Wafers (5) M |
| (_) 62 | Custard (4 oz) M |
| (_) 62D | Custard, Diet (4 oz) M |
| ( ) 63 | Fruit, Cnd Applesauce (1/2 c) M |
| ( ) 63D | Fruit, Cnd Diet Applesauce (1/2 c) M |
| ( ) 64 | Fruit, Cnd Apricot Halves (5) M |
| ( ) 64D | Fruit, Cnd Diet Apricot Halves (5) |
| ( ) 65 | Fruit, Cnd Peach Halves (2) M |
| ( ) 65D | Fruit, Cnd Diet Peach Halves (2) M |
| ( ) 66 | Fruit, Cnd Pear Halves (2) M |
| ( ) 66D | Fruit, Cnd Diet Pear Halves (2) |
| ( ) 67 | Fruit, Cnd, Rotation |
| (_) 68 | Fruit, Fresh Rotation M |
| (_) 69 | Fruit, Fresh Apple M |
| (_) 70 | Fruit, Fresh Orange M |
| (_) 71 | Fruit, Fresh Banana M |
| (_) 72 | Gelatin (4 oz) M |
| ( ) 72CX | Gelatin, Citrotein (4 oz) M |
| ( ) 72D | Gelatin, Diet (4 oz) M |
| ( ) 72PX | Gelatin, Poly (4 oz) M |
| (_) 73V | Ice Cream, Vanilla (4 oz) M |
| (_) 73C | Ice Cream, Chocolate (4 oz) M |
| (_) 73S | Ice Cream, Strawberry (4 oz) M |
| (_) 74C | Italian Ice, Cherry (4 oz) M |
| (_) 74L | Italian Ice, Lemon (4 oz) M |
| ( ) 75 | Pie, Cream M |
| ( ) 76 | Pie, Fruit M |
| (_) 77C | Popsicle, Cherry M |
| (_) 77or | Popsicle, Orange M |
| (_) 77G | Popsicle, Grape M |
| ( ) 78V | Pudding, Vanilla (4 oz) M |
| ( ) 78C | Pudding, Chocolate (4 oz) M |
| ( ) 79BX | Pudding, Sustacal Butterscotch (5 oz) M |
| (_) 79VX | Pudding, Sustacal Vanilla (5 oz) M |
| (_) 79CX | Pudding, Sustacal Chocolate (5 oz) M |
| (_) 80L | Sherbet, Lime M |
| (_) 80or | Sherbet, Orange M |
| (_) 81P | Yogurt, Plain (8 oz) M |
| (_) 81F | Yogurt, Fruited (8 oz) M |
| (_) 82X | Attain, 8 oz |
| (_) 83X | Enrich, Vanilla (8 oz) M |
| (_) 84 | Strawberry House Shake with Cream (6 oz) M |
| (_) 85A | Cheese, American (1 oz) M |
| (_) 85C | Cheese, Cheddar (3/4 oz) M |
| (_) 85LS | Cheese, LS (1 oz) M |
| (_) 86-1/4 | Cheese, Cottage (1/4 c) M |
| (_) 86-1/2 | Cheese, Cottage (1/2 c) M |
| (_) 86LFLS-1/4 | Cheese, Cottage (1/4 c) M |

**Exhibit 26-2** continued

## Nourishment/Menu Write In Code List
## Page 3

| | | | | | | |
|---|---|---|---|---|---|---|
| (_) | 86LFLS-1/2 | Cheese, Cottage (1/2 c) M | ( ) | 94-1/2 | Sandwich, Ham (1/2) M |
| (_) | 87 | Cheese (1 oz) + Crackers (4) M | ( ) | 95 | Sandwich, Ham and Cheese M |
| (_) | 88 | Peanut Butter (2 Tbsp) M | ( ) | 95-1/2 | Sandwich, Ham and Cheese (1/2) M |
| (_) | 89 | Peanut Butter Cracker Sand M | | | |
| (_) | 90PG | (10) 22-1/2 + Dry Cereal | ( ) | 96 | Sandwich, Pimiento Cheese M |
| | | (3) 85A + 112 | ( ) | 96-1/2 | Sandwich, Pimiento Cheese (1/2) M |
| | | (9) 86-1/2 + 65D | | | |
| ( ) | 91 | Sandwich, Am Cheese M | ( ) | 97 | Sandwich, Peanut Butter M |
| ( ) | 91-1/2 | Sandwich, Am Cheese (1/2) M | ( ) | 97-1/2 | Sandwich, Peanut Butter (1/2) M |
| ( ) | 92 | Sandwich, Chicken Salad M | (_) | 98 | Sandwich, Roast Beef M |
| ( ) | 92-1/2 | Sandwich, Chicken Salad (1/2) M | (_) | 98-1/2 | Sandwich, Roast Beef (1/2) M |
| ( ) | 93 | Sandwich, Egg Salad M* | ( ) | 99 | Sandwich, Tuna Salad M |
| ( ) | 93-1/2 | Sandwich, Egg Salad (1/2) M* | ( ) | 99-1/2 | Sandwich, Tuna (1/2) M |
| ( ) | 94 | Sandwich, Ham M | (_) | 100 | Sandwich, Turkey M |

---

| | | | | | | |
|---|---|---|---|---|---|---|
| (✔) | 100-1/2 | Sandwich, Turkey (1/2) M | (✔) | 110 | Chips, Cheese M |
| (✔) | ADD: | LS to Code for LS Bread M | (✔) | 111 | Crackers, Graham M |
| | | WW to code for Whole Wheat Bread M | (✔) | 112 | Crackers, Saltines M |
| | | R to Code for Rye Bread M | (✔) | 112LS | Crackers, Low Sodium M |
| | | RELISH for Sandwich M | (✔) | 112M | Crackers, Melba Toast M |
| (✔) | 101X | Resource, Choc Dry Pack M | (✔) | 112R | Crackers, Rye Twins M |
| (✔) | 102X | Resource, Vanilla Dry Pack M | (✔) | 112SE | Crackers, Sesame Twins M |
| (✔) | 103 | Relish Cup | (✔) | 113 | Cream Cheese M |
| (✔) | 104X | Ensure Flavor Pkt | (✔) | 114 | Peanuts M |
| | | | (✔) | 115 | Ketchup M |
| ***MISCELLANEOUS*** | | | (✔) | 116 | Mustard M |
| (✔) | 105 | Almonds | (✔) | 117 | Mayonnaise M |
| (✔) | 106 | Bread (Add LS, WW, or R to Code) | (✔) | 118 | Syrup, Chocolate M |
| | | | (✔) | 119 | Syrup, Strawberry M |
| (✔) | 107P | Candy, Peppermint M | (✔) | 120 | Taco Sauce M |
| (✔) | 107S | Candy, Sour M | (✔) | 121 | Beef Jerky M |
| (✔) | 108 | Chips, Potato M | (✔) | 122 | Jelly |
| (✔) | 109 | Chips, Corn M | (✔) | 123 | Honey |
| | | | (✔) | 124 | Dry Cereal |

✔  Item is available for late nourishments and menus.
X  Indicates patient is to be <u>charged</u> for item.
*  Available <u>only</u> when on menu.

*Source:* Courtesy of the Department of Nutrition and Food Service, The University of Texas M.D. Anderson Cancer Center.

**Exhibit 26-3** Sample Menus for Specific Diet Types

SUNDAY II
REGULAR

# Evening Nourishment

This is your evening nourishment menu for today. Please (circle) selections.
Limit of 3 please.

**SANDWICHES (1/2)**
Ham
Turkey
Roast Beef

**CHIPS**
Potato Chips
Fritos
Cheetos

**SNACKS, CRACKERS AND COOKIES**
Cheese and Crackers
Peanut Butter
Crackers
Chocolate Cream Filled Cookies

**FRUIT**
Canned Peaches
Canned Pears
Apple
Banana
Orange

**CONDIMENTS**
Ketchup
Mustard
Mayonnaise

**FROZEN DESSERTS**
Ice Cream (Vanilla, Chocolate)
Sherbet (Orange, Lime)

**BEVERAGES**
Whole Milk
2% Milk
Skim Milk
Chocolate Milk
Milkshake (Chocolate, Vanilla, Strawberry)
Eggnog
Cola
Lemon Lime

**COLD FOODS**
Gelatin
Custard
Cottage Cheese

**JUICES**
Orange    Apple
Grape

Name _____ Room _____

SUNDAY II
SOFT/MECHANICAL SOFT/PUREED

# Evening Nourishment

This is your evening nourishment menu for today. Please (circle) selections.
Limit of 3 please.

**SANDWICHES (1/2)**
Ham *
Turkey *
Roast Beef *
Pimento Cheese

**SNACKS, CRACKERS & COOKIES**
Cheese and Crackers *
Peanut Butter *
Crackers*
Chocolate Cream Filled Cookies*

**FRUIT**
Canned Peaches
Canned Pears
Banana

**CONDIMENTS**
Ketchup
Mustard
Mayonnaise

**FROZEN DESSERTS**
Ice Cream (Vanilla, Chocolate)
Sherbet (Orange, Lime)

**BEVERAGES**
Whole Milk
2% Milk
Skim Milk
Chocolate Milk
Milkshake (Chocolate, Vanilla, Strawberry)
Eggnog
Cola
Lemon Lime

**COLD FOODS**
Gelatin
Custard
Cottage Cheese

**JUICES**
Orange
Grape
Apple

*Not allowed on mechanical soft and pureed diets.

Name _____ Room _____

Exhibit 26-3 continued

SUNDAY II
CALORIE CONTROLLED

# Evening Nourishment

This is your evening nourishment menu for today. Please (circle) selections. Limit of 3 please.

**SANDWICHES (1/2)**
Ham
Turkey
Roast Beef

**SNACKS AND CRACKERS**
Cheese and Crackers
Peanut Butter
Graham Crackers
Crackers

**FRUIT**
Diet Canned Peaches
Diet Canned Pears
Apple
Banana (1/2)
Orange

**CONDIMENTS**
Ketchup
Mustard
Mayonnaise

**BEVERAGES**
Whole Milk
2% Milk
Skim Milk
Iced Tea

**COLD FOODS**
Diet Gelatin
Diet Custard
Cottage Cheese

**JUICES**
Orange
Grape
Apple

Name _____ Room _____

SUNDAY II
RESTRICTED FIBER

# Evening Nourishment

This is your evening nourishment menu for today. Please (circle) selections. Limit of 3 please.

**COLD FOODS**
Ham Roll-up
Turkey Roll-up
Hard Cooked Egg
Gelatin
Custard
Cottage Cheese

**SNACKS AND CRACKERS**
Cheese and Crackers
Crackers
Graham Crackers (2)
Chocolate Cream Filled Cookies
Vanilla Wafers
Hard Candy

**FRUIT**
Canned Peaches (L)
Canned Pears (L)

**CONDIMENTS**
Ketchup
Mustard
Mayonnaise

**FROZEN DESSERTS**
Ice Cream (Vanilla, Chocolate)
Sherbet (Orange, Lime)

**BEVERAGES**
Whole Milk
2% Milk
Skim Milk
Milkshake (Chocolate, Vanilla, Strawberry)
Eggnog
Cola
Lemon Lime

**JUICES**
Orange
Grape
Apple

Name _____ Room _____

*continues*

Exhibit 26-3 continued

SUNDAY II
BLAND

# Evening Nourishment

This is your evening nourishment menu
for today. Please (circle) selections.
Limit of 3 please.

**SANDWICHES** (1/2)
Ham
Turkey
Roast Beef

**CHIPS**
Potato Chips
Fritos
Cheetos

**SNACKS, CRACKERS & COOKIES**
Cheese and Crackers
Peanut Butter
Crackers
Vanilla Cream Filled Cookies

**FRUIT**
Canned Peaches
Canned Pears
Apple
Banana
Orange

**CONDIMENTS**
Ketchup
Mustard
Mayonnaise

**FROZEN DESSERTS**
Ice Cream (Vanilla)
Sherbet (Orange, Lime)

**BEVERAGES**
Whole Milk
2% Milk
Skim Milk
Milkshake (Vanilla, Strawberry)
Eggnog
Lemon Lime

**COLD FOODS**
Gelatin
Custard
Cottage Cheese

**JUICES**
Orange
Grape
Apple

Name _____ Room _____

SUNDAY II
RESTRICTED SODIUM

# Evening Nourishment

This is your evening nourishment menu
for today. Please (circle) selections.
Limit of 3 please.

**SANDWICHES** (1/2)
Roast Beef
Turkey

**CRACKERS**
Graham Crackers
LS Crackers

**FRUIT**
Canned Peaches
Canned Pears
Apple
Banana
Orange

**CONDIMENTS**
Ketchup
Mustard
Mayonnaise

**FROZEN DESSERTS**
Ice Cream (Vanilla, Chocolate)
Sherbet (Orange, Lime)

**BEVERAGES**
Whole Milk
2% Milk
Skim Milk
Cola
Lemon Lime

**COLD FOODS**
Gelatin
Custard
Cottage Cheese

**JUICES**
Orange
Grape
Apple

Name _____ Room _____

**Exhibit 26-3** continued

CLEAR LIQUID

# Evening Nourishment

This is your evening nourishment menu for today. Please (circle) selections. Limit of 3 please.

**JUICES**
Orange
Apple
Grape

**COLD FOODS**
Gelatin
Italian Ice
Popsicle

**BEVERAGES**
Cola
Lemon Lime
Gingerale

FULL LIQUID

# Evening Nourishment

This is your evening nourishment menu for today. Please (circle) selections. Limit of 3 please.

**COLD FOODS**
Plain Yogurt
Custard
Gelatin

**JUICES**
Orange
Apple
Grape

**BEVERAGES**
Whole Milk
2% Milk
Skim Milk
Chocolate Milk
Milkshake (Vanilla, Chocolate. Strawberry)
Eggnog
Cola
Lemon Lime
Gingerale

**FROZEN DESSERTS**
Ice Cream (Vanilla, Chocolate)
Sherbet (Orange, Lime)
Italian Ice

SUNDAY II
PEDIATRIC

# Evening Nourishment

This is your evening nourishment menu for today. Please (circle) selections. Limit of 3 please.

**SANDWICHES (1/2)**
Ham
Turkey
Roast Beef
**CHIPS**
Potato Chips
Fritos
Cheetos
**SNACKS, CRACKERS AND COOKIES**
Cheese and Crackers
Peanut Butter
Crackers
Chocolate Cream Filled Cookies
**FRUIT**
Canned Peaches
Canned Pears
Apple
Banana
Orange
**CONDIMENTS**
Ketchup
Mustard
Mayonnaise
**FROZEN DESSERTS**
Ice Cream (Vanilla, Chocolate)
Sherbet (Orange, Lime)
**BEVERAGES**
Whole Milk
2% Milk
Skim Milk
Chocolate Milk
Milkshake (Chocolate, Vanilla, Strawberry)
Eggnog
Cola
Lemon Lime
**COLD FOODS**
Gelatin
Custard
Cottage Cheese
**JUICES**
Orange    Apple
Grape

Name_____ Room_____ | Name_____ Room_____ | Name_____ Room_____

*Source:* Courtesy of the Department of Nutrition and Food Service, The University of Texas M.D. Anderson Cancer Center.

**Exhibit 26-4** Sample Recipes for Homemade Supplementary Drinks

---

### THE UNIVERSITY OF TEXAS M.D. ANDERSON CANCER CENTER
### DEPARTMENT OF NUTRITION AND FOOD SERVICE

## SUPPLEMENTARY DRINKS

### HIGH PROTEIN MILK

1 cup whole milk
4 tablespoons instant non-fat dry milk

Add non-fat dry milk; beat until dissolved.
Refrigerate.

Yield: 1 serving
270 calories/serving

### HIGH PROTEIN EGGNOG

1 cup High Protein Milk
1 or 2 raw eggs*
1 teaspoon sugar
1/2 teaspoon vanilla

Beat eggs well, add part of milk and instant non-fat dry milk,
dissolve. Add the rest of the milk, sugar, vanilla, and mix. Drink
immediately.

Yield: 1 serving
346 calories/serving

### HIGH PROTEIN MILKSHAKE

1 cup High Protein Milk
1/2 cup ice cream
1 raw egg*
Flavoring as desired

Add scoop of ice cream to milk. Mix well. Add flavoring as
desired. Refrigerate. (A raw egg may be added for extra
protein.)

Yield: 1 serving
530 calories/serving

### HIGH PROTEIN INSTANT BREAKFAST DRINK

1 cup whole milk
1 package instant breakfast drink

Yield: 1 serving
290 calories/serving

This may be taken as a routine supplement. If you are unable
to take solid food and must depend on liquids, the following
ingredients may be added to increase the nutritional and
caloric value of the above recipe:

1 raw egg*
1/2 cup ice cream

520 calories/serving

*To prevent Salmonella contamination, eggs should be 1) fresh, 2) not cracked,
3) thoroughly clean, 4) consumed immediately or within two hours when added to
supplementary drinks.

*Source:* Courtesy of the Department of Nutrition and Food Service, The University of Texas M.D. Anderson Cancer Center.

**Exhibit 26-5** Recipe for Citrotein Gelatin

---

### *Citrotein Gelatin*

1 cup boiling water
1 3-oz package flavored gelatin powder*
1 cup cold water
2/3 cup or 2 1.57-oz packets Citrotein powder

1. Dissolve gelatin in boiling water.
2. Add cold water to gelatin mixture.
3. Add Citrotein powder and stir vigorously.
4. Chill until set.

*Exciting flavor combinations: Use lemon, strawberry, orange, peach, mixed fruit or apricot flavored gelatin with Orange Citrotein, grape, black cherry, strawberry, raspberry, black raspberry or cherry flavored gelatin with Grape Citrotein and lemon, strawberry, mixed fruit, raspberry, cherry, or orange flavored gelatin with Punch Citrotein.

Yield: 2 10–fl oz servings
Analysis:   one serving: 13.6 g protein
68.7 g carbohydrate
0.4 g fat, 333 calories

*Source:* Courtesy of the Department of Nutrition and Food Service, The University of Texas M.D. Anderson Cancer Center.

---

additional suggested recipes. Others can be developed as needed.

Increasing the nutrient density of food items is a method to increase the nutrient intake of the cancer patient. Modular protein, carbohydrate, and lipid products that are commercially available can be added to food items to increase their nutrient content. Also, the addition of nonfat dry milk, syrup, sugar, butter, sauces, and gravies increases the nutrient density of foods.

### Food from Sources Other than the Institution

How to handle food from outside sources is a problem not unique to cancer patients. Each institution must set its own guidelines on the basis of local and state health codes. Many large, metropolitan health care institutions have a large percentage of foreign patients in their inpatient populations. The probability that such an institution's food service can meet the specific ethnic needs of a diverse foreign population is unlikely

given present cost-reduction and cost-containment efforts, so that being as flexible as possible with the patient and family members regarding food brought in from the outside is recommended.

### TRAY DELIVERY SYSTEMS

The selection of a tray delivery system is crucial. Criteria used to select a system must include food color and odor and temperature maintenance.

### Color

Colors used in tray delivery systems are more important with cancer patients than with other types of patients. Because of the treatment modalities used the cancer patient becomes sensitive to intense colors, which can sometimes trigger nausea. The colors must be subdued but also good for food presentations. Plain white or

**Exhibit 26-6** Recipes for Use with Citrotein

---

THE UNIVERSITY OF TEXAS M.D. ANDERSON CANCER CENTER
DEPARTMENT OF NUTRITION AND FOOD SERVICE

### CITROTEIN

Citrotein is a low residue, orange flavored protein supplement. It may be taken with meals or between meals. Citrotein powder is available in a 12 ounce bulk can or in a 14.1 ounce carton with individual 1.18 ounce serving packets. The 12 ounce can is most economical, but the individual serving packets are convenient. The following recipes use Citrotein:

#### Orange Soda

3/4 cup water
1/4 cup Citrotein powder or 1 1.18-oz packet Citrotein
1/2 cup orange soda

Mix all ingredients well. May be taken over ice or frozen.

#### Jell-O Punch

1 cup hot water
1 package Jell-O (tropical fruit, orange, etc.)
2 cups cold water
1/4 cup Citrotein powder or 1 1.18-oz packet Citrotein

Mix hot water and Jell-O well. Add 2 cups cold water and mix well. Combine 3/4 cup of the above Jell-O mixture with 1/4 cup Citrotein powder or 1 1.18-oz packet Citrotein. May be taken over ice or frozen.

#### Orange Float

1/4 cup Citrotein powder or 1 1.18-oz packet Citrotein
3/4 cup water
1 scoop orange sherbet
1/4 cup Sprite

Mix all above by hand or in blender. May be taken over ice or frozen.

*Source:* Courtesy of the Department of Nutrition and Food Service, The University of Texas M.D. Anderson Cancer Center.

---

off-white china is recommended. Tray-top items should use subdued shades of gray, mauve, gold, yellow, or green.

### Odor

During certain parts of treatment the cancer patient becomes extremely sensitive to odors that may be taken for granted by the general population. For example, the odor of plastic is described by some patients as unpleasant. The odor of the materials used in the tray, dishes, and supplies should be evaluated when the materials are chilled, at room temperature, and heated. The odor of covered foods when the cover or lid is removed should be considered. This can be managed if the person delivering the trays to the patient removes the cover or lid just before entering the patient's room.

**Exhibit 26-7** Tart Recipes for Use with Citrotein

---

THE UNIVERSITY OF TEXAS
M.D. ANDERSON CANCER CENTER
DEPARTMENT OF NUTRITION AND FOOD SERVICE

## TART DRINK RECIPES

### Orange Frappe

| | |
|---|---|
| 2 ounces lemonade | 440 calories |
| 2 ounces orange juice | 5 grams PRO |
| 4 ounces 1/2 and 1/2 | 69 grams CHO |
| 1/2 cup orange sherbet | 16 grams Fat |
| 1 jar strained apricots with tapioca | |

### Lemon Flip

| | |
|---|---|
| 4 ounces buttermilk | 320 calories |
| 4 ounces lemonade | 12 grams PRO |
| 3/4 cup vanilla ice cream | 45 grams CHO |
| | 12 grams Fat |

### Raspberry Fluff

| | |
|---|---|
| 8 ounces raspberry yogurt | 430 calories |
| 4 ounces 1/2 and 1/2 | 8 grams PRO |
| 2 ounces cranberry juice | 57 grams CHO |
| | 17 grams Fat |

### Pineapple-Orange Fluff

| | |
|---|---|
| 6 ounces pineapple yogurt | 330 calories |
| 1/2 cup orange sherbet | 8 grams PRO |
| | 61 grams CHO |
| | 6 grams Fat |

*Source:* Courtesy of the Department of Nutrition and Food Service, The University of Texas M.D. Anderson Cancer Center.

---

## Temperature Maintenance

The importance of keeping hot food hot is usually evident in quality control programs designed for patient service. With cancer patients, keeping cold foods cold is just as important. Many times cold foods are more easily tolerated during certain phases of treatment when food aromas are offensive. Hence keeping cold food cold is necessary not only for safety but also for patient satisfaction.

The actual temperature of the food served is key. Methods to maintain the recommended temperature range of 45° to 50°F vary with the type of tray delivery system. The system should allow for the shortest possible time from refrigeration to bedside for cold foods. A decentralized system that uses a floor pantry is recommended. There are several decentralized systems currently available for rethermalizing food. An added benefit of a decentralized system is the ease of serving patients who need an additional tray or snack between standard mealtimes. Because the food is on the patient's floor it can be rethermalized on demand by the food service worker or nursing staff rather than having to be brought from the main kitchen.

## CAFETERIA FEEDING

If a large outpatient population of cancer patients is fed in the cafeteria that is used by staff and visitors, special considerations in menu planning are necessary. A line of supplements and milk shakes should be offered for sale. The trend in public cafeterias is to market foods that are low in fat, sodium, and calories as defined by the dietary guidelines of the American Heart Association and the American Cancer Society. These guidelines were designed for the healthy population for prevention, however, not for treatment of a disease state. Thus the needs of healthy patrons can differ greatly from those of patients.

The dietitian must meet both kinds of needs in the cafeteria setting. Both populations must be educated regarding identification of appropriate choices so that their specific dietary needs are fulfilled. For example, patrons with cancer need nutrient-dense foods such as rich desserts, sauces and gravies, and fried foods. The disease-free patron should be directed to the low-fat, low-calorie items such as the salad bar, fruit bar, and plain meats. An ongoing dietary education program should be designed to distinguish between the prevention and the treatment of cancer. Too often patients and their family members believe that a prevention diet should be followed when a treatment diet is appropriate.

# The Nutrition Support Team

*Debbie Zibell-Frisk*

## HISTORY

The use of a nutrition support team is a relatively new approach to the clinical management of cancer patients. The concept evolved about 20 years ago, when the discovery was made that despite the advanced technology and sophistication of modern oncologic medicine cancer patients were dying of malnutrition and that, ironically, the malnutrition was often induced by hospitalization (Butterworth, 1974). The use of parenteral nutrition was introduced as a means to maintain adequate nutrition status and thus to prevent the effects of severe weight loss and protein deficits in patients who would otherwise continue to starve as a result of their surgery or disease process.

This therapy requires interested clinicians who are willing to learn a new technique to lessen the consequences of malnutrition and to prevent the mechanical, septic, and metabolic complications of the delivery of nutrition support. Representatives from the nutrition, nursing, and pharmacy departments are invited to participate in the development of a nutrition support team. These departments are the core of the team because of the professional expertise of the individual members. Dietitians provide knowledge about nutrition assessment and the application of clinical nutrition. Nurses have experience

working with the intravenous tubing, feeding bags, and pumps used in the delivery of tube feedings and intravenous solutions to patients. Pharmacists are needed for their expertise in compounding and monitoring parenteral nutrition prescriptions. Thus these three professions work together to form the traditional nutrition support team.

For the team to function effectively, two additional members are needed: an administrative director and a medical director. The administrator is usually from the department of pharmacy and helps establish a cost center to generate revenue. The revenue is usually derived from patient charges for parenteral and enteral solutions and helps offset the salaries of the team members. The ideal for team effectiveness is for all the members to be working on a full-time basis as one department. For nutrition support teams that are unable to establish their own department or cost center, however, members are either part-time clinicians or full-time team members who remain members of their individual departments as well.

Although the administrative director is not always involved in the clinical management of the patient, he or she is vital to the team's continued existence and success. In today's economic climate, department budgets are becoming tighter and are more closely scrutinized than before. Thus the administrator of the nutrition support team must be sincerely interested in the team's survival to justify its expense.

The medical director is responsible for the clinical management of the patient. The first nutrition support team medical directors were most often surgeons who were interested in the development of parenteral nutrition therapy and protocols for placement of catheters needed for delivery of formulas to patients. Other medical directors were physicians in the specialties of gastroenterology or pediatrics who saw nutrition support as a valuable tool in daily practice.

Much has been learned about this new specialty since the early days of nutrition support. The nutrition formulas and the hardware used to deliver them continue to be improved and revised. The goal is to provide regimens that are specific to individual patient needs in the safest and most cost-effective manner.

## ACTIVITIES OF THE NUTRITION SUPPORT TEAM

Today's nutrition support teams perform the following activities.

### Parenteral and Enteral Nutrition Management

It is the function of the nutrition support team to determine the most appropriate route of nutrition support. Consideration must be given to the functional capacity of the gastrointestinal tract, the patient's ability to eat, and the intended length of therapy. In addition, the team designs the nutrition regimen so that it meets the patient's individual requirements for calories, protein, vitamins, minerals, and water.

Once the regimen is initiated, the team is responsible for daily monitoring. This includes visiting the patient to determine how well the therapy is being tolerated and paying careful attention to subjective complaints as well as to physical signs and symptoms. The assessment of the patient's weight and protein status should be done on a routine basis according to the team's protocol. Other laboratory tests such as measurement of serum electrolytes, glucose, magne-

sium, phosphate, prothrombin time, and partial thromboplastin time are performed according to individual patient circumstances.

If the patient is able to resume an oral diet, the team will request calorie counts and document the adequacy of oral intake. This helps determine when nutrition support therapy can be safely terminated or when another modality such as oral supplements should be instituted. Similarly, if the nutrition support is needed on a long-term basis, the team devises the regimen so that it meets the patient's full nutrition requirements.

### Home Nutrition Support

If nutrition therapy is needed for the duration of the patient's life or for an extended period, the nutrition support team coordinates a home nutrition program. This involves ensuring that the patient's diagnosis mandates home enteral or parenteral therapy so that insurance coverage can be determined.

The team then instructs the patient and family or support person in clean and proper technique in the hospital so that the procedures can be carried out in a comfortable and safe manner in the home. The team performs periodic checks of the home patient to ensure that the regimen is being tolerated, to follow the course of the disease and its treatment, and to make changes in the nutrition prescription if needed.

### Cost Containment

In the day-to-day practice of the nutrition support team it is essential that cost-effective measures be employed. Examples are switching from the parenteral to the enteral route when the gastrointestinal tract is functional, using the most conservative approach to minimize potential complications, and developing formularies to limit inventory and cost.

### Research

The research activities of nutrition support teams vary. Small teams or those with part-time members may find it difficult to participate in ongoing research because of time constraints. Often patient care responsibilities are all that can be accomplished, and of course these take priority. Nevertheless, research should be a goal of all nutrition support teams so that information can be shared to enhance the practice of nutrition support.

### Education

The team conducts periodic inservice programs for the attending and resident physicians to present new products and techniques. Similar programs are also designed for the in-house staff of dietitians, nurses, and pharmacists. The team becomes the resource for nutrition-related information. In addition, the team may be asked to present seminars outside the hospital or may wish to conduct seminars to attract outside team members to the institution. Either activity could be a money-making venture for the team.

### Quality Assurance

The nutrition support team should conduct routine reviews of the efficacy and outcome of nutrition support therapy. This should be performed for both non–team managed patients as well as those patients for whom the team is responsible. Although nutrition support practice is not currently reviewed by the Joint Commission on the Accreditation of Hospitals, self and peer review help document effectiveness and target practice goals.

### STANDARDS OF PRACTICE

To delineate the roles of individual nutrition support team members and to promote a consistent level of care, the American Society for Parenteral and Enteral Nutrition (ASPEN) has published standards of practice. These standards are available as:

1. definitions of terms used in ASPEN guidelines and standards
2. standards for nutrition support for hospitalized patients
3. standards for nutrition support for home patients
4. standards for practice for the nutrition support dietitian
5. standards for practice for the nutrition support nurse
6. standards for practice for the nutrition support pharmacist
7. standards for practice for the nutrition support physician

A complete set of ASPEN guidelines and standards may be obtained from the national office (8605 Cameron Street, Suite 500, Silver Spring, Maryland 20910; telephone [301] 587-6315).

### GOALS OF AND INDICATIONS FOR NUTRITION INTERVENTIONS

The goal of a nutrition support team is to establish guidelines and protocols for clinical management intended to maximize benefits for patients receiving parenteral or enteral nutrition while minimizing the potential complications of the nutrition therapy chosen. This is best accomplished by a multidisciplinary team consisting of a physician, dietitian, nurse, and pharmacist, all of whom bring unique expertise and knowledge to ensure the most appropriate nutrition care of the patient.

Nutrition support is indicated when a patient is unable to meet his or her metabolic demands by the usual route of oral intake. The enteral route should be given first consideration because of its cost, safety, and physiologic benefits. Parenteral nutrition should be reserved for patients with nonfunctioning gastrointestinal tracts and for those whose trial of enteral nutrition was unsuccessful.

### Indications for Enteral Nutrition

#### Persistent Anorexia

Often as a result of prolonged illness or chemotherapy and radiation therapy, patients experience persistent poor appetite. When efforts to improve intake with the use of oral supplements fail, insertion of a small-bore feeding tube for providing enteral nutrition should be considered. This method utilizes a functional gastrointestinal tract and often results in improved appetite and oral intake after enteral nutrition therapy has been instituted.

### Head and Neck Cancer

Enteral nutrition should again be considered for patients with head and neck cancer or if surgery of the head and neck area impairs or prevents swallowing. If the impairment is permanent, then placement of a gastrostomy or jejunostomy feeding tube makes long-term enteral nutrition aesthetically acceptable to the patient and thus makes management easy, especially if self-care is intended. A tube exiting the stomach is much easier to handle than a nasogastric tube. Also, an ostomy tube eliminates the need for checking tube placement before feeding.

### Inadequate Oral Intake Resulting from Brain Metastases or Neurologic Injury

A patient who is not alert and thus incapable of oral intake but who has a functional gastrointestinal tract is also a candidate for enteral nutrition support. Efforts must be made to decrease the risk of aspiration, such as elevating the head of the bed 30° or more and infusing the formula at a rate that is well tolerated.

## Indications for Parenteral Nutrition

When parenteral nutrition is implemented, it is the duty of the nutrition support team to follow the patient's clinical course. If the gastrointestinal tract becomes viable, every effort should be made to convert to enteral nutrition support.

### Severe or Prolonged Gastrointestinal Side Effects of Chemotherapy or Radiation Therapy

When a patient experiences prolonged vomiting or severe diarrhea, parenteral nutrition provides replacement nutrition and fluids by bypassing the compromised gastrointestinal tract.

### Surgery Requiring Prolonged Periods without Oral Intake

Parenteral therapy should always be considered when the period without oral intake exceeds or is expected to exceed 5 to 7 days. At this point a deficit in visceral protein status is evident, and wound healing and immune function are likely to be impaired.

### Fistula

If a high-output fistula is present in the small bowel, parenteral nutrition may help decrease output and close the fistula by decreasing small bowel secretions. For this to be effective, no oral diet should be given.

### Obstruction Secondary to Abdominal Carcinomatosis

When metastases fill the abdominal or pelvic cavities, frequent bowel obstructions occur. Thus parenteral nutrition provides maintenance nutrition support and bypasses the gastrointestinal tract.

## ROLE OF THE TEAM AND INDIVIDUAL MEMBERS

The nutrition support team identifies patients who need nutrition support; determines the appropriate therapy, route, and regimen; and provides support in the safest and most effective manner.

The combined expertise of the individual team members makes the team unit clinically sound and efficient. As stated above, the traditional team consists of a physician, dietitian, nurse, and pharmacist. Other members may include representatives from physical therapy, the medical library, social work, infectious disease, and intravenous medicine. Some facilities have specialty nutrition support teams in the areas of oncology, pediatrics, surgery, and the like.

The nutrition support team can thus be composed of various health care professionals. Regardless of the team's size the members work together to provide optimal nutrition support, and all members share the common goal of promoting the patient's well-being. Initially nutrition support teams were often considered a part-time service, with representatives from needed departments reviewing the charts of a handful of patients each week. Many teams today comprise full-time members who are responsible for the nutrition management of 20 to 30 patients per day or more, although the numbers are variable.

### Physician

The physician usually serves as the medical director of the team and oversees the team's daily operations. He or she is responsible for the development and implementation of guidelines for parenteral and enteral nutrition procedures. The director confirms the team's recommendations for nutrition support therapy and helps monitor the patient's clinical response. He or she contributes information regarding diagnosis and disease processes. Other duties can include supervising the nutrition regimens of home patients, initiating research projects, and periodic review of statistical data for quality control.

Thus the physician needs a strong knowledge base in biochemistry and nutrition in health and disease. He or she must also know the technical aspects of nutrition therapy. The physician's expertise enables him or her to identify coexisting diseases and to understand how they will affect the nutrition support therapy as well as to evaluate organ function, such as cardiac, hepatic, or renal failure, and sepsis.

### Dietitian

The dietitian brings to the team the unique contribution of training and practice that is specifically nutrition based. This expertise is invaluable when the nutrition history of new patients is being taken. The interview is directed toward gathering important details of weight loss, usual intake, bowel patterns, and the effects of recent radiation therapy or chemotherapy. The nutrition assessment follows to determine the patient's weight and protein status so that the nutrition support therapy is appropriate for individual needs.

With parenteral therapy the dietitian's primary role is to ensure that all the patient's nutrition requirements are being met. More patient contact occurs during weaning from the parenteral formula. At this time nutrition supplements are introduced and calorie counts begun in an effort to keep calorie intake close to estimated needs. During this transitional period the dietitian observes the patient for tolerance of oral intake and modifies the diet according to chewing, swallowing, or absorption limitations. The dietitian thus helps determine when parenteral support can safely be discontinued.

The dietitian also assesses patients who are receiving enteral nutrition support. The primary purpose is to select a formula appropriate for the patient's nutrition needs and absorptive function. It is also necessary for the dietitian to monitor the patient for adequate intake and gastrointestinal tolerance. Once a suitable regimen has been established, the dietitian reviews the patient's medical record periodically to ensure that routine assessments of weight and protein status are being performed. If a patient is to continue enteral support at home, the dietitian coordinates the home nutrition prescription and participates in teaching the patient and family about how to administer the tube feeding.

### Nurse

The nurse also contributes knowledge about the patient who is receiving nutrition therapy. The nurse's information includes fluid balance, bowel sounds and stool elimination, fever, presence of respiratory distress, status of the catheter and feeding tube site, and changes in mental status. He or she also serves as patient advocate, interpreting goals for the patient and giving emotional and psychologic support as needed. This is especially important when patients are being considered for home nutrition support. The nurse has an active role in teaching home patients how to administer parenteral nutrition, including care of the catheter, and maintains frequent contact with the patient after discharge.

It is also a responsibility of the team nurse to ensure that protocols regarding administration of parenteral and enteral nutrition are being followed by other nurses. The team nurse is a liaison between the team and the nursing staff, providing inservice education regarding new procedures and orienting new graduate nurses.

## Pharmacist

The pharmacist brings to the team an interest in the clinical application of pharmacology. He or she has expertise in compounding principles that safeguards the parenteral nutrition formula against contamination. He or she also contributes information regarding drug-nutrient interactions as well as the best way to administer a drug through a feeding tube.

Daily monitoring of patients receiving parenteral nutrition is performed by the pharmacist to ensure correct formulation of orders and to provide the most cost-effective regimen. The pharmacist serves as a liaison to the pharmacy department to assist in the development of protocols and quality control guidelines for the admixture and administration of parenteral nutrition formulas.

The pharmacist also participates in the teaching of home parenteral nutrition patients. After the patient's hospital discharge the pharmacist, together with the team physician, monitors blood chemistries and the clinical course to make any necessary changes in the home nutrition prescription.

## Optional Team Members

### Physical Therapist

Although a physical therapist is not considered part of the traditional nutrition support team, his or her services should be considered part of routine care. Regular exercise benefits the malnourished patient by enhancing the utilization of nutrients and promoting synthesis of lean body mass. Aggressive provision of calories and protein will not replace lost muscle mass until active muscular movement and work is being performed (Grant, 1980). Otherwise, increased fat deposition is likely to occur.

Other benefits of exercise include maintaining circulatory and respiratory systems, minimizing thrombophlebitis and pneumonia, increasing physical strength for return of independent care, and promoting appetite. Thus physical therapy should be incorporated into the care plan, especially for patients requiring long-term nutrition support.

### Librarian

A willing and dedicated librarian can help the team by scanning medical journals for articles related to nutrition support and assisting with research efforts. Without the librarian's professional expertise, the wealth of information available makes this an almost impossible task to perform.

### Social Worker

Assistance from the social work department is valuable in psychologic assessment and counseling of patients requiring long-term nutrition support to help them adjust to extended hospitalization and artificial feeding. If patients are to be considered for continued nutrition support at home, the social worker can assist in determining insurance coverage, assessing the home environment, and identifying appropriate family members or friends to participate in the patient's nutrition care at home. The social worker can also identify the need for additional assistance in the home, such as home health aides, and can make the arrangements for this.

### Infectious Disease Specialist

An infectious disease specialist assists in data collection relating to infection incidence and reports catheter-related infections. This not only helps identify problem situations but also provides data on infection rates for comparison with other data reported in the literature. The attempt is to reduce in-house catheter infection rates. If a reduction in this rate compared to rates from previous years can be documented, or if the rate is less than published data from other institutions, then cost savings may be evident. Such information is extremely important when attempting to justify the team's existence in today's climate of budgetary restraints.

*Intravenous Medicine Specialist*

If a hospital has an established team of intravenous specialists, these individuals can be utilized to perform central line dressing changes to ensure consistent technique and adherence to protocol. Such specialists can also assist in catheter placement.

## IMPACT OF NUTRITION SUPPORT TEAMS

Studies have indicated that the use of nutrition support teams results in safe and cost-effective delivery of nutrition support (Nehme, 1980; Schneider & Ruberg, 1983). These studies suggested a reduction in the catheter sepsis rate and metabolic complications in patients who were supervised by nutrition support teams compared to those who were not.

The cost can be reduced by making use of skilled prescription writers, which results in a decreased rate of discarded formula, restricted use of albumin, decreased numbers of laboratory tests, and conversion to home nutrition support when appropriate to decrease the patient's hospital stay. In addition, cost is curtailed by the continued assessment of the route of nutrition administration. This means that requests for the initiation of parenteral nutrition may be denied if it is not indicated or if a functional gastrointestinal tract is present. Similarly, regimens should be converted from parenteral to enteral formulas as soon as it is feasible to do so.

## THE NUTRITION SUPPORT TEAM IN CANCER THERAPY

Patients with malignant diseases, particularly tumors of the gastrointestinal tract, often develop significant weight loss and malnutrition before oncologic therapy. Cancer treatments can increase the degree of malnutrition, and the combined effects of aggressive therapy and progressive malnutrition may lead to irreversible nutrition deficits. Effective nutrition support promotes weight gain, positive nitrogen balance, and better tolerance of antineoplastic therapy.

Controversy still exists regarding the efficacy of nutrition support during cancer therapy. Until more conclusive data are available, the decision to provide nutrition support should be made by the patient and his or her physician. The members of the nutrition support team can offer their experienced opinions but probably should not make the ultimate decision.

Once a patient has made the decision to undergo treatment for his or her disease, he or she is entitled to full nutrition support. The provision of adequate nutrition helps lessen the gastrointestinal side effects of therapy, and improved nutrition status helps achieve the maximum benefits of therapy. Nutrition support also helps promote the psychologic well-being of the patient by at least temporarily removing the struggle of eating. Nevertheless, issues of cost effectiveness, risk to the patient, length of therapy, and gastrointestinal function must be addressed to determine the most appropriate route of therapy. It should be mentioned that if a cancer patient is not malnourished aggressive nutrition support is not expected to have any measurable effect on the results of antineoplastic therapy (MacFayden, Copeland, & Dudrick, 1983). Nutrition support alone will not cure cancer.

A major challenge in providing nutrition support in cancer therapy is finding the route that is most acceptable to the patient, which may not be the team's route of choice. Often the team meets the patient for the first time after many months of ongoing cancer therapy. The patient may have already been subjected to disfiguring surgery, hair loss from chemotherapy, or burn marks from radiation therapy. As a result of this, many patients have a poor self-image and feel a lack of control. The introduction of a nutrition support team encouraging the use of a feeding tube as the answer to the patient's nutrition problems is likely to be seen as another blow to the patient's self-esteem.

The team members should spend time with the patient and allow him or her to verbalize feelings, but they should also explain the intended nutrition therapy and why it was chosen as the best one for the patient. It is not easy to convince every patient, and often modalities of therapy must be changed temporarily to meet the psychologic needs of a patient. Thus, even though enteral tube feedings may be the most appropriate choice, the team may have to appease the patient and provide short-term peripheral parenteral nutrition support until the team members achieve a trusting relationship with the patient and until the patient recognizes the need for long-term therapy. Allowing the patient to meet other patients who are using feeding tubes and to hear of their successes can also be helpful.

Once an oncology patient reaches the point at which nutrition support becomes necessary, therapy is usually needed for the duration of his or her life. If the medical condition is stable, home nutrition support may be initiated. As the team members become familiar with the patient's physical and emotional needs by arranging frequent contact and follow-up, they can determine whether and when nutrition prescriptions should be changed on the basis of the changing medical condition.

The following case examples illustrate the role of the nutrition support team in cancer therapy.

1. A.E. was a 59-year-old man who was diagnosed in 1983 with cancer of the rectum. At the time of surgical resection it was found that the patient had significant metastases, and he was further diagnosed as having abdominal carcinomatosis. Parenteral nutrition was initiated after surgery.

   Attempts to increase oral intake were not successful because the patient developed frequent bowel obstructions and required placement of a nasogastric tube for decompression suctioning.

   Although the patient was given a prognosis of less than 3 months' life expectancy, he was strongly in favor of continuing chemotherapy and parenteral nutrition support. A permanent infusion catheter was placed, and his wife was instructed about how to administer parenteral nutrition so that the therapy could be continued at home.

   The patient improved his weight and was able to regain enough strength to resume his watch and jewelry repair work

from his home. He enjoyed a good quality of life for another 2 years before he died.

2. C.F. was 70 years old when he was diagnosed with cancer of the larynx in June 1986. Initial radiation therapy was unsuccessful, and a laryngectomy was performed 5 months later. A tracheoesophageal fistula developed postoperatively, and the nutrition team was consulted about home enteral nutrition per small-bore nasogastric tube. The patient's wife was anxious and could not be trained in the home feeding procedure. Thus the patient performed self-care and proved to be quite able to do so. Home therapy was needed for only 2 months because the fistula closed and oral intake was resumed.

   A year later the patient was rehospitalized, and the team was consulted again. The patient now reported decreased swallowing ability and nausea and vomiting from chemotherapy. A percutaneous endoscopic gastrostomy (PEG) feeding tube was placed for long-term nutrition support. The gastrointestinal tract was deemed functional because the nausea and vomiting were transient and controlled with medication. The patient and family were able to accept the need for PEG feeding because of the previous successful home enteral therapy. The patient was unable to return home before his death, but supportive enteral therapy was maintained until that time.

3. D.T. was a 64-year-old man with metastatic cancer of the kidney. The nutrition support team was consulted because the patient experienced persistent anorexia from chemotherapy. Enteral nutrition per small-bore nasogastric tube was initiated because the therapy was expected to be short term. The patient was never able to regain his appetite or desire to eat, however. The patient, his wife, and his daughter were trained to continue the therapy at home.

   This patient received home enteral nutrition for 14 months. His family was supportive and helped make it a successful therapy. The patient had been approached regarding placement of a PEG but refused this procedure. When the nasogastric tube needed to be replaced, he performed self-intubation for more comfortable insertion.

D.T. tolerated his regimen well. About 3 months before his death he became volume intolerant and required a change to a formula containing 2.0 kcal/mL to maintain his cyclic schedule. He was able to maintain his weight and outlived his original prognosis of 6 months' life expectancy.

## CONCLUSION

The development of nutrition support over the past 20 years has enabled clinicians to become more adept in identifying and treating malnutrition. Parenteral and enteral nutrition support benefits patients in various clinical settings, including oncology.

The team approach has resulted in fewer catheter-related infections, insertion complications, and metabolic complications in patients managed by a nutrition support team compared to those who have not received such management. The team can determine which patients are at risk for malnutrition, perform ongoing assessment of the effectiveness of nutrition support regimens, and perform quality control through audits and should be viewed as a necessary cost-containing measure for acute care. Because cancer patients often exhibit nutrition problems with extended hospitalization, the nutrition support team can provide invaluable assistance in their treatment.

## REFERENCES

Butterworth, C.E. (1974). The skeleton in the hospital closet. *Nutrition Today, 2*, 4–8.

Grant, J.P. (1980). A team approach. In *Handbook of total parenteral nutrition* (pp. 4–7). Philadelphia: Saunders.

MacFayden, B.V. Jr., Copeland, E.M. III, & Dudrick, S.J. (1983). Surgery and oncology. In A.H. Schneider, C.A. Anderson, & D.B. Cousins (Eds.), *Nutritional support of medical practice* (pp. 622–624). Philadelphia: Harper & Row.

Nehme, A.E. (1980). Nutritional support of the hospitalized patient: The team concept. *Journal of the American Medical Association, 243*, 1906–1908.

Schneider, P.J., & Ruberg, R.L. (1983). Cost containment of nutritional support. Paper presented at the 18th annual American Association of Hospital Pharmacists Midyear Clinical Meeting, Atlanta, GA.

# Chapter 28

# Management Options: Clinical Nutrition Management in a Cancer Treatment Setting

*Carol Frankmann*

Clinical nutrition management has emerged as a management specialty in today's health care environment. As resources have become more limited and as patient acuity has increased, the clinical focus has moved from "Are we giving the best care?" to "Are we giving the care essential to optimum outcome in each medical condition?" The latter question has proved to be even more challenging to address than the former and requires critical determination of the nutrition care most beneficial in specific medical situations as well as managerial accountability and innovation in the utilization of resources. This challenge is intensified for the clinical nutrition manager in a cancer treatment setting because of the prevalence of nutrition problems in patients with malignancy and the complex interrelationship of nutrition, disease, and efficacy of antineoplastic therapy.

## PREVALENCE OF NUTRITION PROBLEMS

General acute tertiary care facilities report that their screening procedures refer approximately one-third of the patient population to a dietitian for evaluation of potential nutrition problems (DeHoog, 1985; Hedberg et al., 1988). At the University of Texas M.D. Anderson Cancer Center, screening tools indicate that about 80%

of patients require referral to a dietitian for evaluation at the time of hospital admission (Abdalla, Bradford, & Stepinoff, 1989). These reports seem to substantiate the presence of a high incidence of nutrition problems in cancer patient populations. Consequently, it appears that the ratio of clinical nutrition staff to patients needs to be higher in a cancer treatment setting than in a general acute care setting.

## CLINICAL STAFFING LEVELS

To date, no models have been published that identify the clinical staffing levels required to provide nutrition care for patients undergoing treatment for cancer. Several inquiries have been made to M.D. Anderson Cancer Center for such information; the time per task and patient acuity data needed to complete a staffing model are still being collected at this institution, however. Efforts to obtain similar information from other cancer centers have been unsuccessful.

Because of the lack of a model, there has been some interest in actual staffing levels at a cancer center. As a point of reference, information about staffing levels at M.D. Anderson Cancer Center is outlined in Table 28-1. Nevertheless, the information in this table is of limited value as a guide to appropriate staffing levels. For example, the protected environment dietitian manages

**Table 28-1** M.D. Anderson Cancer Center: 1989 Clinical Nutrition Staffing Levels

| Position | Hospital Beds | Clinic Visits | FTEs* |
|---|---|---|---|
| Clinical nutrition manager | | | 1.0 |
| Outpatient staff | | 375,890 | |
| Dietitian | | | 2.0 |
| Inpatient staff | 487 | | |
| Dietitian | | | 11.0 |
| Dietetic technician | | | 4.0 |
| Protected environment manager | 20 | | 1.0 |
| TOTAL | 507 | 375,890 | 19.0 |

*Full-time equivalent positions.

germ-free food preparation and service in addition to providing clinical care and nutrition research support in that specialized area. The table does not include positions for two research dietitians, both of whom provide some nutrition care while obtaining clinical research data. It also is important to recognize that recent increases in patient visits in the clinic setting have not yet been accompanied by increases in nutrition care staff. Before changes in staff are recommended, however, it is necessary that patient acuity levels and commensurate nutrition care requirements be defined, that appropriate personnel to perform each task be identified, and that the time required for completion of tasks be determined. This information, along with the number of hospital days or clinic visits for identified levels of patient acuity, can be used to determine the required nutrition care services and personnel. The target date for completion of such a staffing model at M.D. Anderson Cancer Center is late 1990.

## CLINICAL STAFF STRUCTURE

At M.D. Anderson Cancer Center, all dietetic technicians are assigned to the inpatient area and are responsible for daily nutrient intake analysis, menu correction, and screening. The minimum requirement for the position is completion of an American Dietetic Association–approved dietetic technician program. On-the-job training requires 3 to 4 months.

Dietitians are required to be registered by the Commission on Dietetic Registration at the time of employment and to obtain licensure by the Texas State Board of Examiners of Dietitians. Both credentials must be maintained throughout their employment. Previous experience with aggressive nutrition support or with oncology patients (or both) is preferred, as is an advanced degree in a nutrition-related field.

Provision of nutrition care for patients with cancer requires an integration of nutrition expertise with knowledge of the disease process and antineoplastic therapy. Although this can be acquired with training and self-education, mastery requires clinical practice in oncology. Dietitians at M.D. Anderson Cancer Center report that it takes approximately 6 months in the clinical setting to achieve this initially and an additional 1 to 3 months to achieve it when changing to a new oncology subspecialty area.

In a cancer center, the diversity of the disease is apparent. The inherent medical specialization creates subspecialty areas of practice and knowledge in the field of oncology for dietitians as well as oncologists. At M.D. Anderson Cancer Center, positions for dietitians include one or two oncology subspecialty areas. The combinations of oncology services for each position are developed by the clinical staff and approved by the clinical nutrition manager. From their experience, the dietitians seek to balance the workload of positions by combining subspecialty services that have different levels of patient acuity, different lengths of stay, and different prognoses as well as similar treatment and convenient geographic location. Because these characteristics change over time, position assignments have been revised every 2 to 3 years. Current staff assignments are as follows:

1. Inpatient clinical dietitian assignments
   - leukemia service and pediatric service
   - gastrointestinal oncology service, teaching service, and clinical immunology service
   - genitourinary oncology service
   - medical oncology breast service and melanoma and sarcoma service
   - bone marrow transplantation service and lymphoma service
   - urology service
   - head and neck surgery service, head and neck medical oncology service, and leukemia service
   - general surgery service
   - thoracic oncology service
   - gynecology service
   - critical care areas and nutrition support service
2. Outpatient dietitian assignments
   - ambulatory treatment center, chemotherapy, immunotherapy, surgery
   - radiotherapy

When it becomes available, the utilization of a staffing model will make patient care assignments less rigid than those outlined above because staff power allocation will then be dictated by patient need for nutrition services. Although such a system will result in a more efficient distribution of staff resources, it will require each dietitian to acquire expertise in a greater number of disease and treatment parameters. Thus the time required for a new staff member to become fully productive will increase.

## PROVISION OF CARE

Traditionally, screening tools have identified all patients with cancer to be at nutrition risk. For this reason, dietitians at M.D. Anderson Cancer Center had long sought to assess the nutrition status of all patients within 72 hours of their admission to the hospital. Shortened hospital stays resulted in a marked increase in the number of hospital admissions, however. Without comparable increases in staff power, it became necessary to evaluate the need for a comprehensive nutrition assessment of every patient at the time of hospital admission.

A pilot nutrition screening program was developed to determine the usefulness of the screening process in a cancer population. Separate nutrition screening forms were developed and implemented for pediatric and adult patients (Richardson & Garcia, 1989) (Exhibit 28-1). A review of the completed nutrition screening forms indicated that only 80% of patients required further evaluation of nutrition status at the time of admission (Abdalla et al., 1989). Hence it became apparent that a screening tool would be as useful in targeting patients requiring nutrition care in a cancer treatment setting as in any other setting.

Moreover, the screening process can be completed within 24 hours of admission. This shortened time frame is beneficial for detecting problems in patients who are admitted for only 24 to 48 hours. In the past, attempts to provide nutrition assessment within 72 hours would have resulted in many of those patients not being evaluated for nutrition problems before discharge. The screening process is of particular value in an oncology population because treatment may require a series of short hospital stays.

Because patient status changes during hospitalization, patients who do not require nutrition intervention at the time of screening are rescreened every 7 days during their stay (Exhibit 28-2). Again, the screening process permits timely identification of patients with potential nutrition problems.

Among patients who require nutrition intervention, there is a need to prioritize the delivery of that care. For some time, nursing has used a classification system that identifies the level of care required for each patient (Georgette, 1970). A similar system is needed to classify patients according to the urgency and complexity of nutrition intervention. Efforts to develop a nutrition patient acuity classification system are under way at M.D. Anderson Cancer Center.

**Exhibit 28-1** Pediatric Initial Nutrition Screen Form

THE UNIVERSITY OF TEXAS
M.D. ANDERSON CANCER CENTER
DEPARTMENT OF NUTRITION AND FOOD SERVICE

Patient Data

### PEDIATRIC NUTRITION SCREEN

Admitting Date:_____

Name: _____          Room No.

Please answer the following questions so that we can provide your child with the appropriate nutrition care.

1. Is your child experiencing nausea and/or vomiting which continues
   between treatments?                                                Yes      No

2. Is your child experiencing mouth sores which are affecting his/her
   ability to eat?                                                    Yes      No

3. Is your child experiencing changes in his/her appetite which are affecting
   the amount he/she eats?                                            Yes      No

4. Is your child having diarrhea?                                     Yes      No
   If yes, how many bowel movements is he/she having day?      _____

5. Is your child constipated?                                        Yes      No

6. What is your child's current weight?                              _____ lbs

7. Has your child ever weighed more than he/she does now?            Yes      No
   If yes, what is the most he/she has ever weighed?          _____ lbs

8. Does your child have any food allergies or intolerances?          Yes      No
   If yes, please specify _____

---

**OFFICE USE ONLY**

Diet Order_____          Diagnosis:_____

Ser Alb/Date: _____      Age: _____      Highest Wt: _____

Height: _____ Cm         Ht/Age %ile: _____      %Wt Loss: _____

Weight: _____ Kg         Wt/Age %ile: _____      Wt/Ht: %: _____

                                   _____    _____
                                        Dietetic Technician          Date

Nutrition Care Level     I   or   >I

CR/aal
2/89

*Source:* Courtesy of the Department of Nutrition and Food Service, M.D. Anderson Cancer Center.

**Exhibit 28-2** Pediatric Follow-Up Nutrition Screen Form

---

THE UNIVERSITY OF TEXAS
M.D. ANDERSON CANCER CENTER
DEPARTMENT OF NUTRITION AND FOOD SERVICE

Patient Data

## PEDIATRIC NUTRITION SCREEN

Admitting Date:_____

Name: _____

Room No.

---

Please answer the following questions so that we can provide your child with the appropriate nutrition care.

1.  Has your child's nutrient intake decreased significantly since his/her admission?                                                                    Yes          No

    If yes, what do you think is causing this decrease?     Nausea/vomiting    _____
                                                            Mouth sores        _____
                                                            Decreased appetite _____

4.  Is your child having diarrhea?                                                                    Yes          No
    If yes, how many bowel movements is he/she having day?                           _____

5.  Is your child constipated?                                                                        Yes          No

---

OFFICE USE ONLY

Diet Order:_____

Height: _____ Cm          % Wt Loss: _____

Weight: _____ Kg          Wt/Ht %: _____


_____          _____
Dietetic Technician                      Date


Nutrition Care Level     I    or    >I

CR/aal
2/89

*Source:* Courtesy of the Department of Nutrition and Food Service, M.D. Anderson Cancer Center.

While that system is being developed, patient care by the dietitian is prioritized as follows:

- *Priority 1:* patients receiving enteral tube or parenteral nutrition support; patients who have had nothing by mouth and have been without nutrition support for 5 days; physician orders for nutrition care
- *Priority 2:* patients receiving oral supplements; patients with potential problems identified through nutrition screening; patients receiving modified diets

To track the nutrition care required by and given daily to each patient, the clinical staff has developed a form for recording that information. These forms are maintained on a weekly basis and are kept in the patient care area. The forms help the dietitian organize his or her daily activities and communicate essential information to the dietitian who is providing relief coverage.

To maximize the professional time spent in nutrition education for the patient, dietitians participate in multidisciplinary classes designed to provide the patient and significant others with general information. Classes are offered regularly to clinic patients on nutrition and chemotherapy and to hospital patients' families on caring for the patient at home. Flip charts and video tapes are incorporated into the presentations to reduce preparation time, to provide consistency in content, and to enhance interest. The video tape about nutrition and chemotherapy is used by the inpatient dietitian to reduce the time required for individual instruction of patients. This is accomplished by suggesting that the patient watch the video on the hospital television channel. Education by the dietitian can then focus on individual patient needs. Moreover, the patient and significant others can watch the video as often as needed to reinforce learning about chemotherapy and nutrition.

### ENTERAL FORMULARY

The enteral formulary at M.D. Anderson Cancer Center is generic and is determined by means of a collaborative process that involves clinical and management staff. It, of course, reflects the nutrition needs of the patient population that it serves. It includes more than 30 product categories; moreover, it allows duplication of products within the categories for some oral supplements. This duplication is necessary because of the importance of taste acceptance for the success of an oral regimen, the well-documented taste changes that occur in cancer patients (DeWys & Walters, 1975; Settle, Quinn, & Kare, 1978; Mossman & Henkin, 1978; Trant, Serin, & Douglass, 1982), and the development of taste fatigue. The last of these often occurs with the long-term use of supplements, which is generally associated with prolonged treatment.

Palatability is a key factor in selecting products for formulary categories that require oral administration. For this reason, palatability is determined by means of a blind taste evaluation of oral supplements available in the marketplace. Because cancer patients may rank the taste of nutrition products differently than healthy subjects (DeWys & Herbst, 1977), the palatability evaluation process includes both clinical staff and a panel of patients who are undergoing treatment from a cross-section of regimens. The results of these evaluations are used in determining which products are acceptable for consideration as oral formulary products.

### STAFF DEVELOPMENT

The need to develop expertise in oncology and to stay abreast of changes in nutrition is a challenge to the dietitian in this specialty setting. For this reason, members of the clinical staff at M.D. Anderson Cancer Center have developed and implemented a clinical practice conference. It includes a monthly journal club, presentations by medical and administrative staff, and presentations by clinical dietitians on their specialty expertise. Although participation is voluntary, these activities are consistently well attended.

Clinical staff members are also encouraged to present original work at national meetings; preparation of the presentations for these meetings undergoes peer review, a group process that improves the quality of the presentations and allows all staff members to participate in and to learn from the preparation process. Every 2 to 3 years, the department sponsors a symposium on nutrition and cancer. This also provides an opportunity for staff development because all members prepare presentations or participate in the planning and implementation of a professional conference.

Work with chronically ill, and sometimes terminally ill, patients can be stressful. This fact is openly accepted and discussed among professional clinical staff, and support is obtained from peers and other health care team members. This creates a positive, caring environment, and staff derive a wholesome sense of accomplishment from the difference that professional efforts make in achieving realistic, meaningful goals for patients with cancer.

## OPTIMUM OUTCOME

Just as many clinical nutrition managers are interested in studies of the cost benefit of nutrition services, a major focus for clinical managers in oncology continues to be whether the nutrition care essential to optimum outcome in the treatment of malignancy is being provided. In the mid 1970s Lanzotti, Copeland, George, Dudrick, and Samuels (1975) reported an improved response to treatment of lung cancer in patients with a weight loss of more than 6% who received total parenteral nutrition compared to those who did not. This retrospective study led to speculation that total parenteral nutrition may improve treatment outcome for all cancer patients. To assess the efficacy of total parenteral nutrition as an adjunct to therapy, a series of prospective, randomized trials was performed (Popp, Fisher, Wesley, Aamodt, & Brennan, 1981; Jordan et al., 1981; Nixon et al., 1981; Samuels, Selig, Ogden, Grant, & Brown, 1981; Ghavimi, Shils, Scott, Brown, & Tamaroff, 1982).

The results of these studies, as well as others, were reviewed recently in a position paper issued by the American College of Physicians (1989). In developing the paper, a statistical technique was used to pool the results of 12 randomized controlled trials and to arrive at the best estimates for the effect of parenteral nutrition support on patient survival and tumor response rates. This analysis indicated that, overall, patients receiving nutrition support were less likely to achieve partial or complete response to treatment or to survive as long compared to control

patients. It also found that any effect on hematologic or gastrointestinal toxicity was small and not likely to be clinically significant. More important, the use of parenteral nutrition was associated with a fourfold increased risk of significant infection. On the basis of these findings, the college recommended that the routine use of parenteral nutrition for patients undergoing chemotherapy should be strongly discouraged and that, in deciding whether to use such therapy in individual patients whose malnutrition is judged to be life threatening, physicians should take into account the possible exposure to increased risk.

It is essential that this position paper's findings and recommendations not be interpreted as evidence that all modes of nutrition support are without benefit to cancer patients whose nutrition status mandates intervention. It is important to remember that the thrust of these studies was to assess the efficacy of total parenteral nutrition as an adjunct to therapy, not to determine the efficacy of optimum nutrition support for each individual. Consequently, total parenteral nutrition was delivered to patients whose nutrition status was good as well as to those who were malnourished. When the data were analyzed on the basis of patient nutrition status, there was evidence that nutrition support may not be detrimental in the malnourished patient. Hence it was concluded that the net effect of parenteral nutrition support in malnourished patients is unknown and that trials to determine conclusively the direction of its effect (i.e., beneficial or detrimental) may be justified.

In addition, because total parenteral nutrition was viewed as therapy, a number of studies were designed to provide a standard volume of total parenteral nutrition for all patients rather than to adjust the level of support to individual nutrition needs. In view of the current understanding of the hazards associated with overfeeding, it is feasible that the level of total parenteral nutrition given may have been a factor in the negative outcome observed in these studies.

The major risk associated with total parenteral nutrition was an increased infection rate. Certainly, this warrants the recommendation that physicians consider the risk in recommending total parenteral nutrition. It also reinforces the need to use enteral nutrition support whenever the gut permits because no similar risk of significant infection is associated with enteral nutrition support. Clearly, future studies to assess the benefit of nutrition support in cancer patients should utilize the mode of support that is most appropriate given the patient's condition and involves the least risk.

In conclusion, the American College of Physicians (1989) noted that the total number of patients studied was small and that subgroups of patients or conditions of treatment may exist for which total parenteral nutrition support is beneficial. Similar studies have yet to be done in reference to bone marrow transplantation and radiation therapy. It was also acknowledged that basic scientific investigation into the poorly understood determinants of malnutrition in patients with cancer and the effects of total parenteral nutrition support on metabolism in these patients is also essential. Thus the nutrition care essential to optimum outcome in the treatment of malignancies has yet to be determined.

## FUTURE CHALLENGES

Challenges for the clinical nutrition manager in a cancer treatment setting abound. The need to determine the cost benefit of nutrition services is essential and yet complicated by the complex interrelationship of nutrition, cancer, and efficacy of treatment. Nevertheless, its elucidation is a key to effective use of nutrition care resources rather than just efficient use achieved by means of sophisticated staffing models and productivity indicators. More important, the real reward in meeting this challenge is that its accomplishment will enable each cancer patient to receive the nutrition care essential for optimum outcome.

## REFERENCES

Abdalla, C.M., Bradford, K.B., & Stepinoff, J. (1989). Maximum utilization of hospital stay via implementation of a nutrition screen in a cancer center. *Journal of the American Dietetic Association, 89*(Suppl.), A-71.

American College of Physicians. (1989). Position paper: Parenteral nutrition in patients receiving cancer chemotherapy. *Annals of Internal Medicine, 110*, 734–736.

DeHoog, S. (1985). Identifying patients at nutritional risk and determining clinical productivity: Essentials for an effective nutrition care program. *Journal of the American Dietetic Association, 12*, 1620–1622.

DeWys, W.D., & Herbst, S. (1977). Oral feeding in the nutritional management of the cancer patient. *Cancer Research, 37*, 2429–2431.

DeWys, W.D., & Walters, K. (1975). Abnormalities of taste sensation in cancer patients. *Cancer, 36*, 1888–1896.

Georgette, J.K. (1970). Staffing by patient classification. *Nursing Clinics of North America, 5*, 329–339.

Ghavimi, F., Shils, M.E., Scott, B.F., Brown, M., & Tamaroff, M. (1982). Comparison of morbidity in children requiring abdominal radiation and chemotherapy, with and without total parenteral nutrition. *Journal of Pediatrics, 101*, 530–537.

Hedberg, A., Garcia, N., Trejus, I.J., Weinmann-Winkler, S., Gabriel, M.L., & Lutz, A.L. (1988). Nutritional risk screening: Development of a standardized protocol using dietetic technicians. *Journal of the American Dietetic Association, 88*, 1553–1556.

Jordan, W.M., Valdivieso, M., Frankmann, C., Gillespie, M., Issell, B.F., Bodey, G.P., & Freireich, E.J. (1981). Treatment of advanced adenocarcinoma of the lung with ftorafur, doxorubicin, cyclophosphamide, and cisplatin (FACP) and intensive IV hyperalimentation. *Cancer Treatment Reports, 65*, 197–205.

Lanzotti, V.J., Copeland, E.M. III, George, S.L., Dudrick, S.J., & Samuels, M.L. (1975). Cancer chemotherapeutic response and intravenous hyperalimentation. *Cancer Chemotherapy Reports, 59*, 437–439.

Mossman, K.L., & Henkin, R.I. (1978). Radiation-induced changes in taste acuity in cancer patients. *International Journal of Radiation Oncology/Biology/Physics, 4*, 663–670.

Nixon, D.W., Moffitt, S., Lawson, D.H., Ansley, J., Lynn, M.J., Kutner, M.H., Heymsfield, S.B., Wesley, M., Chawla, R., & Rudman, D. (1981). Total parenteral nutrition as an adjunct to chemotherapy in metastatic colorectal cancer. *Cancer Treatment Reports, 65*(Suppl. 5), 121–128.

Popp, M.B., Fisher, R.I., Wesley, R., Aamodt, R., & Brennan, M.F. (1981). A prospective randomized study of adjuvant parenteral nutrition in the treatment of advanced diffuse lymphoma: Influence on survival. *Surgery, 90*, 195–203.

Richardson, C.A., & Garcia, M.E. (1989). Development of a screening tool for pediatric patients at a cancer center. *Journal of the American Dietetic Association, 89*(Suppl.), A-77.

Samuels, M.L., Selig, D.E., Ogden, S., Grant, C., & Brown, B. (1981). IV hyperalimentation and chemotherapy for stage III testicular cancer: A randomized study. *Cancer Treatment Reports, 65*, 615–627.

Settle, R.G., Quinn, M.R., & Kare, M.R. (1978). *Taste evaluation of cancer patients: Report to National Institutes of Health, Bethesda, MD* (Contract NO1-CP-65791). Paper presented at the meeting on gustatory evaluation of cancer patients, 4 August 1989, Bethesda, MD.

Trant, A.S., Serin, J., & Douglass, H.O. (1982). Is taste related to anorexia in cancer patients? *American Journal of Clinical Nutrition, 36*, 45–58.

# Part V

# Other Concerns

# Chapter 29

# Home Care Training and Management Options

*Abby S. Bloch and*
*Rachel Barcia-Morse*

Cancer patients are now spending less time in the hospital and more time at home or in non–acute care settings. Methods of providing for their nutrition needs must be adapted to the outpatient setting so that feedings are appropriate for the patient's condition and requirements.

Improved methods of feeding, such as the use of soft, comfortable nasogastric tubes, have made it possible for many patients to be successfully nourished with tube feedings at home. Percutaneous endoscopic gastrostomy (PEG) and jejunostomy (PEJ) tubes offer nonsurgical alternatives to nasoenteric feeding when appropriate. Other factors that have contributed to successful home feedings are the development of efficient delivery systems; small, inexpensive enteral feeding pumps and administration sets; and improved techniques for the delivery of tube feedings such as the use of prefilled, semirigid formula containers. Patients can be managed at home safely and efficiently with the use of these new systems (Adams & Wirching, 1984; American Society for Parenteral and Enteral Nutrition [ASPEN], 1987, 1988).

The nutritionist, social worker, nurse, and physician should all become involved in planning the discharge and successful home care of the patient receiving enteral feedings. This chapter presents the steps that must be implemented, from initiation of tube feeding up to and including discharge planning, to ensure successful

management of the patient receiving nutrition support at home.

## PREDISCHARGE MANAGEMENT

Within 72 hours of a patient's admission to the hospital, a nutrition assessment or screening should be completed by the clinical dietitian. Patients who have experienced a 10% to 20% weight loss in reference to their usual body weight and are unable orally to ingest adequate amounts of food because of mucositis, tumor obstruction, nausea, vomiting, or anorexia are candidates for tube feeding if poor oral intake will continue, thereby placing the patient at nutrition risk. Other indications for tube feeding include fistulas caused by radiation enteritis in the esophageal area, a blockage in the head or neck area, and rapid transit of the gastrointestinal tract (Bloch, 1989). In some cases in which radiation enteritis, partial obstruction, or esophageal surgery affects intake enough to compromise the patient's nutrition status, a PEG or surgical gastrostomy may be selected. If a patient has a partial or total gastrectomy or tumor growth in the stomach region, a PEJ or surgical jejunostomy may be indicated.

Many patients are tube fed throughout the period of hospitalization and are identified as candidates for home nutrition support during this time. If enteral feeding has not been given during most of the period of hospitalization, the patient should be started on such feedings at least 4 or 5 days before discharge. This allows the clinicians time to establish tolerance and to resolve any problems related to the feeding process that may develop. Feedings should be increased gradually in volume, starting at 50 mL/hour of a full-strength, nutritionally complete liquid formula or specialized formula as determined by the patient's clinical condition. The patient progresses by 10 to 25 mL/hour/day as tolerated until adequate nutrition is achieved. If volume becomes a problem, then the formula may be concentrated or the rate adjusted to accommodate the patient's tolerance.

## DISCHARGE PLANNING

The managing physician initiates home tube feeding orders as soon as the patient is identified as an appropriate candidate for home enteral management. In addition to adjusting the formula rate and concentration to meet the patient's caloric needs, the physician adjusts the feeding schedule to reflect the hours during which the patient will be on feedings at home. If the volume that is needed to meet the patient's goals is not consistent with the hours during which the feeding will run, then the formula concentration must be manipulated. In this way the transition from hospital management to home management will be well organized and smooth (Jeejeebhoy & Meguid, 1986).

If the patient is ambulatory but needs to be fed continuously with a pump, nighttime feeding is suggested. This allows the patient to fulfill his or her nutrition needs while asleep so that he or she is free of the tube during waking hours. Not all patients can tolerate this regimen, however. The patient should be tested while he or she is still in the hospital to determine the feasibility of this schedule. If the patient can be fed by bolus, this is performed three to six times during the day to meet nutrition needs.

In spite of assessment efforts, however, candidates for home nutrition support are frequently identified as they are walking out the door or shortly before discharge. The dietitian may not always have the time for an extended training or adjustment period with the patient. Under such circumstances telephone communication often is the only realistic means of management available to the nutritionist. By close and constant telephone contact with the patient and family, the nutritionist can explain the steps of the feeding procedure and review the rate increase schedule as well as reinforce the need to keep the head and shoulders above the chest, to flush the line, to monitor for symptoms of intolerance, and so forth.

Outpatients start tube feedings almost immediately after the PEG procedure is completed. While the patient rests in the hospital after the procedure, he or she as well as family members are instructed about the care of the PEG, tube feeding procedures, the rate increase schedule, potential complications, and pump management.

Intake of 35 to 40 calories and 1.0 to 1.5 g of protein per kilogram body weight is a general guide to determine the patient's energy and protein needs. There are numerous commercial formulas available for tube feedings that can meet these needs. Each formula differs in caloric density and content of calories, protein, fat, electrolytes, and lactose (Bloch, 1987a, 1989; Chory & Mullen, 1986; Letsou, 1987). The cost of the formula varies from product to product. Therefore, selection of the appropriate formula to meet the individual's needs should be done with care (Appendix 29-A).

## THE NUTRITION SUPPORT TEAM

### Social Worker

The social worker plays an important role in organizing the patient's home care. He or she interacts with the family well in advance of the patient's discharge and assesses the psychologic, financial, and clinical status of the patient and the logistics of providing home nutrition support (Case, 1986).

A patient who is ambulatory may be able to cope with his or her own tube feeding management at home. If not, the patient may need a visiting nurse or round-the-clock nursing services. The social worker helps determine whether a patient's spouse and family members are capable emotionally and physically of caring for the patient at home. In some instances, a nursing home or extended care facility may be a more realistic solution for the long-term management of an individual who needs more care than can be provided at home.

If a tube feeding has been ordered, the social worker may be the liaison among the hospital, nutritionist, family, and home care provider. He or she prepares the family for home management of the patient and may order special equipment, if needed, from a local pharmacy, a distribution center, a home care company, the hospital, or other sources.

The social worker discusses reimbursement options with the family. In some instances, the patient may be covered only by Medicare or Medicaid. If supplies or services are being obtained from a commercial company, the social worker discusses further billing options with the patient if full coverage is not provided by third-party payors.

## Coordinator

A discharge information form should be devised so that necessary information can be recorded from the patient's chart (Exhibit 29-1). This record is then transmitted to the home care company or other supplier of home nutrition support services. The company checks the information for insurance coverage purposes and contacts the family members to schedule a convenient delivery date for supplies (preferably before the patient's discharge). The discharge information, along with clinical notes and other relevant information, is also available for the nutritionist to refer to as needed for follow-up.

The person responsible for coordinating these arrangements—frequently a secretary, unit clerk, or coordinator—confers with the nutritionist who is managing the patient. The coordinator then notifies the company about supply and equipment needs and that the patient has been trained in feeding procedures. Diet orders and the discharge date can be verified at this time. In some instances, a nurse employed by the home

care company may be required to visit the patient on the day of discharge. The coordinator must alert the home care company if this service is needed during the first several days at home.

## Nurse

Families are often apprehensive about having the responsibility of managing the tube-fed patient at home. The nurse is the one professional who has interacted with the patient daily over an extended period of time and has established a good rapport with the patient and family (Englert & Patterson, 1986).

If the patient has been maintained on bolus feedings during hospitalization, the nurse may have instructed him or her in this technique. The nurse should also work with the patient and family members each time the patient is fed to reinforce their training in tube feeding techniques. Comprehension of instructions may be limited initially by intelligence level or a language barrier, so that it is important for the nurse to reinforce during hospitalization the steps needed for the patient to manipulate successfully the feeding system. Reinforcement of techniques and procedures before discharge ensures that the patient has full understanding of the methods. This gives patients a sense of security because they know that they can manage their tube feeding successfully before they are faced with attempting the task at home (Lum & Gallagher-Allred, 1984).

## Nutritionist

The nutritionist is responsible for setting up the time and place for initial training of the patient and family members and the nurse or home health aide in home tube feeding management. The nutritionist must have an understanding of the medical, nursing, psychologic, and social problems of the patient whom he or she is about to train (Gilbert, 1986).

The patient's name, diagnosis, and managing physician, the name of the company (if any) that will be managing the feeding and providing the formula or supplements, and the kind of tube and

**Exhibit 29-1** Sample Patient Discharge Information Form

MEMORIAL SLOAN-KETTERING CANCER CENTER
PATIENT DISCHARGE INFORMATION


NAME:_____Birthdate:_____

ADDRESS:_____SOC. SEC. #_____

_____SPOUSE:_____

Telephone: HOME:_____BUS:_____

BUS. ADDRESS:_____

EMERGENCY CONTACT:_____

  DIAGNOSIS:_____

  PHYSICIAN:_____  EXT.# _____ROOM# _____

INSURANCE CARRIER:_____POLICY #_____

INSURANCE CARRIER:_____POLICY #_____

INSURANCE CARRIER:_____POLICY #_____

PUMP MODEL:_____FEEDING TUBE:_____

FORMULA:_____RATE/HR X HRS:_____

AMT. FORMULA DAILY:_____CAN. SIZE:_____

OTHER ADDITIVES:_____

SUPPLIES/MONTH:___TUBES:_____BAGS:_____OTHER:_____

DATE TRAINED:_____SUPPLIES SENT:_____AMT._____

DISCHARGE DATE:_____PROGNOSIS:_____

  HEIGHT:_____

  PRESENT WEIGHT:_____

  ALLERGIES:_____

*Source:* Courtesy of Memorial Sloan-Kettering Cancer Center.

its placement should be documented. It is important to keep records up-to-date for follow-up home management as well as for the yearly census for administrative purposes (Exhibit 29-2).

A file should be established that includes the information that the coordinator obtained and transmitted to the home care company for delivery of supplies. Together with relevant clinical information and a copy of the tube feeding instructions given to the patient, this file enables the nutritionist to have complete information about the patient at all times.

## PATIENT TRAINING

The patient's family members usually have had a few days to familiarize themselves with methods of tube feeding. They may have had an opportunity to observe the nurse setting up the equipment. In some cases the patient may have started working with the nurse in self-feeding techniques.

The nutritionist who is managing the patient's feedings usually provides this training as soon as the patient and family have overcome their apprehensions about managing the feedings themselves. During the first training session both oral and written instructions plus a demonstration of the care of the feeding tube, formula preparation, and the operation of the pump are given to the patient and family members. The manipulation of the system is verbally taught to patients, and a checklist is given to them for referral. A card with the nutritionist's name and telephone number is also attached for the patient's referral if questions or problems arise at home. Patient training is documented on a training summary form that is kept with the patient's file (Exhibit 29-3).

Training is divided into three areas: tube care, feeding management, and feeding modalities.

### Tube Care

The patient must be trained to flush his or her nasoenteric or PEG tube before and after each feeding with approximately 50 mL of tap water delivered through a 50-mL syringe. He or she

may be encouraged to flush the line with water once or twice during the day to obtain extra fluid. The amount of water used depends on the patient's hydration status; 100 mL six to eight times per day is usually sufficient to hydrate the patient. If dehydration is a concern, then the patient is encouraged to use more water for flushing. If fluid restrictions are necessary, then only a minimal amount of water is recommended. If the patient is using enteral feeding as the sole source of nutrition, then additional fluids such as juice, milk if tolerated, or other beverages are recommended between feedings. Fluid status is a crucial area of concern with these patients and must be monitored conscientiously by the managing dietitian.

The chances of the nasoenteric tube's clogging increase tremendously if the tube is not rinsed after each use. When medication is given through the tube, the same rinsing procedure is required. If the patient's tube should become clogged, he or she should flush it with 10 mL and then with 1 mL of warm water. If this is not successful, the patient must inform his or her managing physician of the situation.

The patient is made aware of the importance of not having bacteria form in the tube by careless handling or exposure to contaminants. Good hygiene, both personally (such as hand washing) and in the form of good bag and formula handling such as refrigeration of opened formula and thorough washing of the bag and containers used for formula storage, should be reviewed and reinforced.

Reusable freezer packs are recommended to keep the formula chilled so that bacteria do not form in the feeding bag while it is in use. The feeding should also start out cold. Although many health care professionals believe that the formulas for tube feedings should be at room temperature or warmed, the cold, slow-drip feeding method has no adverse effect on the patient's tolerance, and using a chilled formula decreases the risk of introducing airborne contaminants during continuous feeding.

Patients can use the same feeding bag for 1 week or longer. They are instructed to wash the bag thoroughly each day with warm, soapy water, to rinse it well with warm water, and to let it drain dry between feedings. After about

**Exhibit 29-2** Sample Clinical Information Form

MEMORIAL SLOAN-KETTERING CANCER CENTER
HOME ENTERAL FORM

CLINICAL INFORMATION        DATE_____

NAME_____PHONE: HOME_____WORK_____

ADDRESS_____CHART #_____

SEX_____ AGE_____ HEIGHT_____ WT_____ USUAL WT_____ DX_____

DISCHARGE MEDS_____KARNOFSKY INDEX_____

REASON FOR TUBE FEEDING_____WT, START TF_____DATE_____

M.D._____PHONE EXT._____ROOM #_____TEAM\_\_\_NONTEAM\_\_\_

_____

_____

CARE PLAN

TUBE TYPE/SIZE_____DRESSING TYPE/CARE_____

DELIVERY METHOD: BOLUS/GRAVITY/PUMP    PUMP TYPE_____

GOAL KCAL/VOLUME_____USE OF TUBE: FEEDING/FLUID/MEDS

_____

_____

D/C DATE_____FORMULA_____RATE_____VOLUME_____

_____

_____

PATIENT FOLLOW-UP

| DATE | WT | RATE | KCAL | COMMENTS |
|------|----|------|------|----------|
|      |    |      |      |          |
|      |    |      |      |          |
|      |    |      |      |          |
|      |    |      |      |          |
|      |    |      |      |          |

DATES OF HOSPITALIZATION_____

SUMMARY OF CARE

END DATE_____ REASON FOR STOPPING TF_____

*Source:* Courtesy of Memorial Sloan-Kettering Cancer Center, Department of Clinical Nutrition Support.

**Exhibit 29-3** Sample Patient Training Summary Form

MEMORIAL SLOAN-KETTERING CANCER CENTER
TRAINING SUMMARY

PATIENT_____

MSKCC LIAISON_____

PRIMARY CARE GIVER: PATIENT/FAMILY/NURSING/OTHER_____

CAREGIVER NAME_____ RELATIONSHIP_____

AVAILABILITY_____

LANGUAGE SPOKEN BY: PATIENT_____ PRIMARY CAREGIVER_____

| | DATE COMPLETED | COMMENTS |
|---|---|---|
| TUBE INSERTION BY PATIENT/FAMILY | | |
| TUBE CARE/FLUSHING | | |
| FORMULA PREPARATION AND HANDLING | | |
| FEEDING RATE/SCHEDULE | | |
| PUMP OPERATION/ALARMS | | |
| GRAVITY/BOLUS TECHNIQUES | | |
| MONITORING: WT, STOOL, URINE, FLUID STATUS | | |

INTERVENTIONS REVIEWED FOR THE FOLLOWING COMPLICATIONS:

PUMP FAILURE_____ TUBE BLOCKAGE_____ TUBE DISPLACEMENT_____
DIARRHEA_____ CONSTIPATION_____ ABDOM. DISTENTION_____
NAUSEA_____ VOMITING_____ ASPIRATION_____
FEVER_____ INFECTION_____ OTHER_____

_____

_____

QUALITY CONTROL SUMMARY

| | DATE | INITIALS |
|---|---|---|
| INSTRUCTION ENTERED INTO HOME FEEDING LOG | _____ | _____ |
| HOME CARE PROGRAM OFFICE NOTIFIED | _____ | _____ |
| SUPPLY NEEDS CALCULATED & DOCUMENTED | _____ | _____ |
| WRITTEN INSTRUCTIONS PROVIDED & REVIEWED | _____ | _____ |
| TELEPHONE FOLLOW-UP PROCEDURE EXPLAINED | _____ | _____ |
| CLINIC FOLLOW-UP EXPLAINED | _____ | _____ |

*Source:* Courtesy of Memorial Sloan-Kettering Cancer Center, Department of Clinical Nutrition Support.

1 week the tubing begins to fatigue (stretch), so that the patient may not receive an accurate drop rate or the pump may signal the need for a bag replacement.

The patient is asked to make an indelible black mark or to place a piece of tape at the tip of the tube where it protrudes from the nostril or, in the case of a PEG, just past the puncture site. This allows patients to be aware of any movement of the tube of more than 1 in, which indicates slippage or altered placement. They are told to call the physician and to report this change immediately if it occurs.

The patient is also asked to monitor any changes in clinical status such as fever, infection, nausea, vomiting, constipation or diarrhea (the patient should report the kind, amount, color, and number of bowel movements), abdominal distention, and gas. The patient also must check for equipment failure and must report aspiration. If any of the above occurs, the patient is advised to stop the tube feeding for 2 to 3 hours and to restart it at a slower rate. If the patient experiences no further discomfort, he or she may slowly increase the rate back to normal as tolerated. If any symptoms arise again the tube feeding is stopped immediately, and the managing physician and dietitian are called.

The patient is taught to keep his or her head elevated to at least 30° or to use two pillows while receiving the tube feeding day or night to prevent aspiration. If the patient is sitting up in a chair or walking around, naturally the risk for aspiration is decreased. The patient should not lie in a supine position for at least 30 minutes after the feeding ends.

There are, of course, the little "housekeeping techniques" of which the patient must be made aware. For example, the house may not have three-pronged electric outlets, so that a two-way or three-way adaptor may be needed to accommodate the pump's electric plug.

### Feeding Management

The patient is usually given a schedule to increase the rate of the tube feeding and to decrease the number of hours of the tube feeding. The final goal is usually 150 to 160 mL for 12 to 14 hours as tolerated.

The best method for gaining weight is for the patient to use a formula containing 1.5 kcal/mL at night. The patient can then eat and drink as tolerated during the day for extra calories. This of course is dependent on the patient's physical condition as well as on the family's lifestyle and schedule (Bloch, 1987b). If the patient is bedridden and if the family is available for daytime feeding, this may work better than nighttime management. Patients who are ambulatory but homebound may prefer to feed themselves while they are awake during the day. The advantage of the home enteral program is that it is flexible and can be tailored to suit whatever schedule best fits the individual needs of the patient and family.

When two formulas are used together, they should be mixed in a large pitcher and refrigerated. The mixture can then be used as needed. Refrigerated formula that has been open for more than 48 hours should not be used.

The patient must weigh himself or herself on the first day at home and then every 5 to 6 days thereafter. The patient and the nutritionist can then determine whether the patient is receiving enough calories and adequate nutrition intake to meet present needs. If a rapid weight gain occurs, edema or spontaneous tumor growth should be considered.

### Feeding Modalities

Many patients require pumps for their home formula delivery system (Exhibit 29-4). The pump may or may not have its own delivery system. Most pumps have bags that are specifically designed for use with the system. There are also universal bags that can be used for several types of pumps (Barcia-Morse, 1983; Chory & Mullen, 1986).

Most pumps deliver from 5 to 300 mL/hour and accommodate adjustments of 5 to 25 mL/hour. Many pumps need to be attached to intravenous line poles or placed close to the patient's bed, and others are free standing. Pumps can be disconnected from the electric outlet and run by battery for many hours if desired. Should the patient have any problems with the pump, formula, feeding bag, or supplies, he or she is instructed to call the home care company that is providing these items.

For patients who have a normal gastrointestinal tract, such as those with head and neck cancer, gravity bolus feeding is encouraged (Exhibit 29-5). Some patients feel more confident using a feeding bag rather than a pump or syringe. The patient is instructed to place 250 to 300 mL of formula in the feeding bag and to regulate the flow by adjusting the clamp on the tubing. The patient is encouraged to take this volume slowly (over 20 to 60 minutes depending on tolerance) and to administer it at least three to five times a day. Gradually the patient may increase the volume to 400 mL per feeding for five feedings. As he or she becomes more stable, the time needed to administer each feeding can be decreased if tolerated. The goal usually is 500 mL in each of four feedings of 2,000 to 2,500 calories depending on the calorie level of the formula per milliliter and the requirements of the patient.

The last type of feeding modality is the syringe bolus method (Exhibit 29-6). This has been especially successful with patients who have a PEG. Syringe bolus feedings are faster and less expensive than pump or gravity bolus feedings and should be encouraged if the patient can tolerate them.

The patient takes the first 240 mL of formula with the use of a 60-mL syringe and waits 30 to 45 minutes. If bloating or abdominal discomfort develops, the patient is encouraged to wait a little longer and then to repeat the same procedure with the second can or the remainder of formula allocated for that feeding.

If the patient is taking six cans (1,440 mL at 1.5 calories/mL for a total of 2,160 calories), he or she can perform self-feeding in three sessions by slowly administering one-third the total volume (two cans) by bolus each time. If more calories are needed or if the volume is not tolerated, adjustments in the rate and number of sessions can be made to meet the patient's needs.

After the patient has been thoroughly trained in the appropriate feeding modality, a discharge planning form is inserted into the patient's file (Exhibit 29-7).

## SERVICES AVAILABLE AT HOME

A comforting aspect of home tube feeding management is that a nurse from the home care company that provides the supplies to the patient's home is available to come to the patient's house on discharge. If requested, the home care nurse arrives on the patient's first postdischarge day. Nurses may visit the patient on subsequent days as required on the basis of the patient's condition or home environment and needs.

If there is a question regarding the patient's home tube feeding, the nurse is instructed to call the nutritionist or clinician. For example, how medications are to be incorporated into the feeding may need clarification. If the medication is solid, then emphasis may be required on careful pulverizing or thorough dissolving of the medication before administration so that it does not clog the small-diameter tube and exit ports. Feeding schedules and nutrient goals may also need to be clarified so that the visiting nurse and the clinical managers are approaching the home care of the patient in consistent fashion.

If needed, a visiting nurse or aide is available to make daily visits. He or she works with the family in monitoring the progress of the tube feeding regimen and the patient's tolerance and assists with tube feeding management when needed. In some instances, round-the-clock nurses may be appropriate depending on the seriousness of the patient's illness and the need for other nursing services such as surgical dressing or ostomy management.

The nutritionist usually calls the patient on his or her first day home. The nutritionist notes the patient's baseline weight as measured by the scale in the home and asks the patient how he or she is tolerating the tube feeding. The nutritionist advises the patient to increase the rate of the tube feeding as indicated by the rate schedule that was given to the patient before discharge and also inquires about the patient's bowel movements (volume, color, and consistency). The nutritionist checks to make sure that the patient made an appointment to see his or her physician in the outpatient clinic approximately 2 weeks after discharge for clinical follow-up care.

If the patient has had a PEG placed, the nutritionist usually asks whether the site is raised or red or if any oozing is present. The patient also reports any changes in temperature. The nutritionist also periodically reviews the medications that the patient is taking at home and notes any

**Exhibit 29-4** Sample Patient Instructions for Pump Use

## MEMORIAL SLOAN-KETTERING CANCER CENTER
### DAILY ASSEMBLY AND CHECKLIST

1) _____ inches of tubing remain outside. Before using the tube daily, confirm its placement. Inject water via syringe to clean tubing just prior to feeding.

2) DIRECTIONS: 1. Close control clamp completely. 2. Fill with desired amount of formula. 3. Close top. 4. Slowly open clamp and fill entire line with fluid. 5. Close clamp. 6. Hang bag. 7. Insert bottom of drip chamber into pump set positioning bar. 8. Squeeze drip chamber and insert between alarm sensors. NOTE:

AVOID FILLING THE DRIP CHAMBER MORE THAN HALF FULL.

9. Grasp silicone tubing and gently stretch around rollers. Insert retainer into pump set positioning bar. Thread tubing around tubing guide. 10. *Open control clamp.* 11. Set desired flow rate in ml/hr. Attach plastic tip to patient's tube. 12. Press start/stop switch. 13. Proceed with feeding.

3) The pump has a battery which recharges when the pump is plugged in. The pump should be plugged in whenever possible to prevent temporary drainage of the battery power. Kinking of the tubing will prevent flow.

4) Head and shoulders are elevated at least 30° during feeding and for 30 minutes after.

5) Flush tubing with a syringe and warm water before and after each feeding.

6) Wash the bag and tubing with warm soapy water and rinse thoroughly. Allow the bag to drip dry with all clamps and caps open. The system may be reused until leakage or fatigue of silicone tubing occurs.

COMMENTS: _____

_____

_____

_____

ADDITIONAL ITEMS TO BE SUPPLIED BY PATIENT:
3 prong/2 prong adaptor
Freezer pack (blue ice)

## PROGRESS CHECK

1) Record weight as often as possible—note swelling of feet or hands.

2) Report changes in stool or urine color, consistency or frequency and volume.

3) Report abdominal discomfort, nausea, vomiting, or other problems which might relate to the feeding.

4) Telephone the Nutrition Support Kitchen dietitian weekly between clinic visits until further notice.

5) Food or fluids taken in addition to the tube feeding should be reviewed periodically with the dietitian.

6) If admitted to the hospital, please telephone the Nutrition Support Kitchen as soon as possible.

Pertinent Data: _____

| Date | Pump Set At: | Feeding Hours | Total Volume/ml | Total Volume Cups/Oz. |
|---|---|---|---|---|
| | | | | |
| | | | | |
| | | | | |
| | | | | |
| | | | | |

**CLINICAL NUTRITION SUPPORT KITCHEN**
Room C-1161, Old Memorial
Memorial Sloan-Kettering Cancer Center
1275 York Avenue, New York, NY 10021

*Source:* Courtesy of Memorial Sloan-Kettering Cancer Center, Department of Clinical Nutrition Support.

**Exhibit 29-5** Sample Patient Instructions for Gravity Bolus Feeding

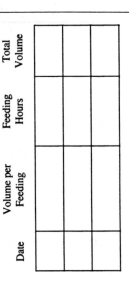

MEMORIAL SLOAN-KETTERING CANCER CENTER
DAILY ASSEMBLY AND CHECKLIST

1) _____ inches of tubing remain outside. Before using the tube daily, confirm its placement by injecting water via syringe.

2) Close tubing clamps before filling the Kangaroo bag. Ice the formula in the bag and refrigerate open unused formula.

3) Clear the air out of the system by opening the tubing control clamp and allowing the formula to fill the tubing.

4) To set the feeding rate, pour _____ of formula into the bag; adjust the control clamp so that _____ flows in _____. Once the drip rate is established, larger volumes can be added as needed.

5) Hang the bag above the head to ensure gravity flow; shifts in bag elevation will cause erratic flow. Kinking of the tubing will prevent flow.

6) Head and shoulders are elevated at least 30° during feeding and for 30 minutes after.

7) Flush the tubing with a syringe at the end of the feeding.

8) Wash the bag and tubing with warm soapy water and rinse thoroughly. Allow the bag to drip dry with all clamps and caps open. The system may be reused until leakage occurs.

| Date | Volume per Feeding | Feeding Hours | Total Volume |
|------|--------------------|----------------|--------------|
|      |                    |                |              |
|      |                    |                |              |
|      |                    |                |              |

*Source:* Courtesy of Memorial Sloan-Kettering Cancer Center, Department of Clinical Nutrition Support.

**Exhibit 29-6** Sample Patient Instructions for Syringe Bolus Feeding

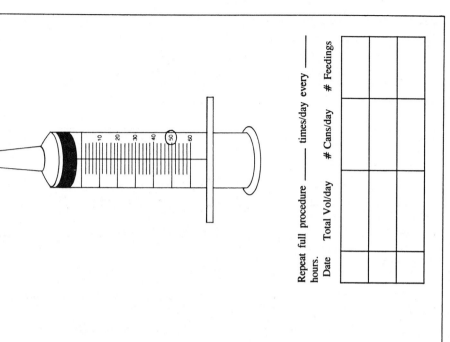

## MEMORIAL SLOAN-KETTERING CANCER CENTER
### BOLUS FEEDING PROCEDURE

1) Flush tubing with 30-50 cc tap water.

2) Fill 60 cc syringe with formula.

3) Attach tip of syringe to end of tubing or adapter. Be sure tip of syringe is snugly inserted.

4) Slowly push plunger down. Refill syringe until contents of can are finished (about 4 feedings).

5) Flush tubing and syringe.

6) Wait 15-30 minutes or until comfortably able to tolerate second can.

7) Repeat steps 1-5 with second can.

Head and shoulders should be elevated at least 30° during feeding and for 30 minutes after.

Flush the tubing with a syringe of 50 cc of water at beginning and end of each feeding.

Wash syringe and tubing with warm water after each feeding.

Repeat full procedure _____ times/day every _____ hours.

| Date | Total Vol/day | # Cans/day | # Feedings |
|---|---|---|---|
|  |  |  |  |
|  |  |  |  |
|  |  |  |  |

Make an appointment to see Dr. _____ in the Nutrition Clinic in 2 weeks after discharge.

*Source:* Courtesy of Memorial Sloan-Kettering Cancer Center, Department of Clinical Nutrition Support.

**Exhibit 29-7** Sample Discharge Planning Form

MEMORIAL SLOAN-KETTERING CANCER CENTER
DISCHARGE PLANNING: CLINICAL NUTRITION SUPPORT

Patient: _____ Chart No.: _____

|  | Date |  | Date |
|---|---|---|---|
| Pt identified as a potential candidate for HTF |  | Written instructions provided and reviewed |  |
| Pt/family trained in formula preparation |  | Tube feeding precautions and potential complications discussed with pt/family |  |
| Pt/family trained in pump management |  | Supplies ordered |  |
| Tube feeding rate schedule established |  |  |  |

_____
Date        Signature

*Source:* Courtesy of Memorial Sloan-Kettering Cancer Center, Department of Clinical Nutrition Support.

changes in type or dosage. He or she questions the patient about chemotherapy or radiation therapy and also asks about therapy that the patient may be contemplating for the future, such as physical rehabilitation or learning how to swallow saliva so that oral intake can resume.

If the patient complains that he or she is gaining too much weight and asks whether formula intake should be reduced, the nutritionist refers the patient to his or her physician and then encourages the patient to call back with the physician's decision. If the rate of the tube feeding cannot be tolerated, the nutritionist explains to the patient that he or she should take the total volume of formula over more hours at a slower rate. Some patients who are unable to take the tube feeding as prescribed lose weight and become dehydrated. The patient may have to be hospitalized in such a case.

Sometimes patients are too weak to be weighed on their home scale or to visit their physician as an outpatient. The nutritionist can only monitor the formula that is given daily to the patient in these instances. A patient in this state may also become constipated, in which case the nutritionist encourages him or her to ask the physician about increasing fluid volume, using stool softeners, or increasing the fiber content of the feeding formula. If the patient can swallow, increased oral intake of fiber may be encouraged. The choice of formula may need to be altered to allow additional fiber in the feeding if requested by the physician.

It is desirable to be in touch with patients every 10 days to 2 weeks. In the interim periods patients are instructed to call if they have any questions or problems regarding the tube feeding method or formula. It is difficult to reach some patients every 2 weeks for evaluation, but attempts to do so must be made nonetheless because otherwise they may become lost to follow-up.

## ROLE OF THE PHYSICIAN IN THE OUTPATIENT NUTRITION CLINIC

The physician usually sees the patient in the clinic 2 to 3 weeks after discharge. At that time the medical history is reviewed, and a physical examination and laboratory tests are done for follow-up monitoring. Should the patient lose a pound or two while at home, an increase in calorie content, rate, or volume of the feeding may be considered. The patient may request a shorter feeding time to aid his return to a more normal lifestyle. In such cases the physician may switch the patient to a more concentrated, high-calorie formula and decrease the number of hours for the tube feeding. The nutritionist must pay attention to the need for free water and the hydration status of the patient if the new formula is more concentrated than the one previously used. Likewise, if the patient's oral intake and weight increase the physician may decrease the volume and calorie content of the formula.

Patients may become constipated during the weeks at home on tube feeding as well as develop abdominal distention as the rate of the tube feeding is increased. The physician may need to prescribe a stool softener or a combination of formulas or change the formula to one with a high fiber content. To alleviate the problem of abdominal distention the rate of tube feeding may be decreased while the length of time during which it is given is extended. If the distention subsides, the feeding rate is gradually increased to the original goal and patient response determined.

Over the next few weeks or months the patient may need to return periodically to the outpatient clinic for monitoring by the physician. As mentioned above the nutritionist or designated liaison should be in telephone contact with the patient every 10 days to 2 weeks and should send a memo to the managing physician regarding the patient's tolerance of and response to the tube feeding.

A patient who has successfully gained weight on the tube feeding at home with a pump may wish to advance to bolus feedings with a syringe. Others may want to continue tube feedings only on certain days of the week as their oral intake increases. Eventually the physician and patient may agree to discontinue the tube feeding once the patient successfully demonstrates that he or she can maintain a desired weight. Periodic 3-day calorie counts from oral and formula intake give the physician and nutritionist an idea as to whether the patient is meeting nutrition needs while maintaining his or her weight.

## CONCLUSION

Clinical experience in managing patients at home on tube feeding has shown that patients and family members can and do manage tube feedings well with the support of the team efforts of the physician, nurse, nutritionist, social worker, and home care company (Appendix 29-B). By providing the technologic means, the psychologic support, and the logistic methods successfully to meet nutrition needs in the home environment, home feedings give patients the opportunity to return to their own surroundings and to those whose love and concern for them can provide the best medicine.

### REFERENCES

Adams, M., & Wirching, R.G. (1984). Guidelines for planning home enteral feedings. *Journal of the American Dietetic Association, 84,* 68.

American Society for Parenteral and Enteral Nutrition Board of Directors. (1987). Guidelines for the use of enteral nutrition in the adult patient. *Journal of Parenteral and Enteral Nutrition, 11,* 435.

American Society for Parenteral and Enteral Nutrition. (1988). ASPEN standards for home nutrition support—Home patients. *Nutrition in Clinical Practice, 3,* 202–205.

Barcia-Morse, R. (1983). Selection of enteral equipment. *Nutrition Support Services, 3,* 15–23.

Bloch, A.S. (1987a). Enteral formulas. *Nutrition Support Services, 7,* 23–24.

Bloch, A.S. (1987b). Nocturnal tube feedings. *Dysphagia, 2,* 3–7.

Bloch, A.S. (1989). Preparing the patient for home enteral management. In M. Hermann-Zaidins & R. Touger-Decker (Eds.), *Nutrition support in home health* (pp. 89–100). Rockville, MD: Aspen.

Case, M.R. (1986). The role of the hospital social worker in nutritional support services. *Nutrition Support Services, 6,* 26.

Chory, E.T., & Mullen, J.L. (1986). Nutritional support of the cancer patient: Delivery systems and formulations. *Surgical Clinics of North America, 66,* 1105–1120.

Englert, D.M., & Patterson, R.S. (1986). Nursing procedures and delivery equipment. *Nutrition Support Services, 6,* 23.

Gilbert, K.A. (1986). Needs theory and health education: A psychological approach to teaching home nutritional therapy. *Nutrition Support Services, 6,* 23–24.

Jeejeebhoy, K.N., & Meguid, M.M. (1986). Assessment of nutritional status in the oncology patient. *Surgical Clinics of North America, 66,* 1077–1090.

Letsou, A. (1987). Nutritional product chart #2: Enteral formulas. *Nutrition Support Services, 7,* 12–21.

Lum, L.L.Q., & Gallagher-Allred, C.R. (1984). Nutrition and the cancer patient: A cooperative effort by nursing and dietetics to overcome problems. *Cancer Nursing, 7,* 469–474.

# Appendix 29-A

# Comparison Charts Available from Vendors

*Enteral Nutrition Ready Reference,* by Ross Laboratories, Columbus, OH, September 1988.

*Enteral Formula Comparison Chart,* by Sherwood Medical, St. Louis, MO, 1988.

*Your Source Chart,* by Sandoz Nutrition, Minneapolis, MN, 1989.

*Enteral Nutrition Product Advisor,* by Mead Johnson, Evansville, IN, 1986.

Local representatives from each company will be able to provide copies of these materials.

# Appendix 29-B

# Instructional Materials Available from Vendors

*Your Personal Guide to Home Tube Feeding,* by Norwich Eaton, Norwich, NY.

*The Patient's Guide to Tube Feeding at Home,* by Sandoz Nutrition, Minneapolis, MN.

*Topics in Enteral Nutrition for Long Term Care,* by Sandoz Nutrition, Minneapolis, MN.

*Long-Term Tube Feeding,* by Sandoz Nutrition, Minneapolis, MN.

*The Prevention and Management of Tube Feeding Complications, Study Guide,* by Sandoz Nutrition, Minneapolis, MN.

*PEG/PEJ—What are They?* by Ross Laboratories, Columbus, OH.

*Mastering the Technique of Tube Feeding at Home by Nasogastric, Nasoduodenal, or Nasojejunal Tube,* by Ross Laboratories, Columbus, OH.

*Mastering the Technique of Tube Feeding at Home by Gastrostomy or Jejunostomy,* by Ross Laboratories, Columbus, OH.

*Home Tube Feeding Instruction Kit,* by Ross Laboratories, Columbus, OH.

*Tube Feeding at Home—A Manual of Instruction for Home Tube Feeding Care,* by Mead Johnson, Evansville, IN.

Local representatives from each company will be able to provide copies of these materials.

# Chapter 30

# Ethical and Psychologic Issues Relating to the Cancer Patient

*Julie O'Sullivan Maillet*

Cancer is a physical illness that affects the patient and family in multiple ways at different points in the disease process. This chapter identifies some of the psychologic and ethical issues facing the cancer patient at different periods of his or her illness to assist the dietitian in the application of the science of nutrition to human needs.

Although the dietitian does not treat the psychologic issues that the patient and family face, he or she must understand their attitude toward death and their fears of impending treatment. The dietitian must understand infirmities that the patient is likely to experience and how the patient's self-image and place in the family structure may change. The dietitian must be concerned about these issues when working with the patient and family.

Inherent in the code of ethics for registered dietitians (American Dietetic Association [ADA], *Code*, 1988) is consideration of the opinion of the patient with regard to the above issues. Patients' values and beliefs are as diversified as the number of cancers and the number of treatments available, and the dietitian needs to respect and understand these beliefs.

## DIAGNOSIS

The National Cancer Institute has appropriately sensitized Americans to link diet and cancer. At the time of cancer diagnosis, then, a common reaction is guilt. The patient may think

"I could have eaten better—it was the high fat, the smoked foods, the caffeine, and the insufficient fiber."

The dietitian has a number of options in such cases. First of all, he or she needs to determine whether diet is related to the specific cancer. Numerous cancers such as Hodgkin's disease, leukemias, or sarcomas do not correlate at all with diet. If the cancer is not related to diet, the dietitian needs to explain this to the patient. Even if the cancer is one that does correlate with diet (e.g., colon, prostate, or breast cancer), it may not correlate with the patient's diet; for example, consumption of fatty smoked foods has been shown to correlate with stomach cancer but not with colon cancer. Even if the cancer risk and diet do correlate, the patient must understand that diet is but one factor in the development of cancer. In addition the link between diet and cancer is new information, so that the patient could not have followed dietary recommendations for his or her lifetime. The dietitian may need to explain thoroughly to the patient and family that, although nutrition is associated with the development of certain kinds of cancer, a causal relationship has not been shown.

## TREATMENT

### Minimal Nutrition Impact

The point of the dietitian's initial consultations is to minimize guilt and instead to start focusing on the current diet and what may need to be changed about it. Therapeutic management of nutrition needs is the major goal during active treatment; preventive nutrition as a goal may come later. The patient's high motivation to maintain his or her health provides an excellent opportunity for nutrition education. The value of proper nutrition in promoting overall good health and physical well-being should be emphasized, but the patient must understand that diet cannot cure cancer and that, regardless of diet, cancer can recur.

Nutrition quackery is tempting to patients at this point. Patients are often willing to try almost any diet. The dietitian has a number of responsibilities. The first is, obviously, not to make claims for the role of nutrition in cancer treatment beyond what has been scientifically shown. The second is to promote optimal nutrition. The third is to provide the patient with information about the controversies regarding nutrition and cancer. Finally, the dietitian needs to know the research that has been done on nutrition and cancer and the credibility of that research. The dietitian needs to be clear about the facts: what is known, what research is based on findings in humans and what is based on animal models, and the conclusiveness of the findings. Only then can the patient be in a position to have confidence in the dietitian's recommendations.

The dietitian needs to keep an open mind about alternate therapies. Cancer patients may decide to try controversial therapies with full understanding of their limited scientific bases. The dietitian's responsibility is to provide the facts without being judgmental and to advise the patient if the contemplated therapy is potentially injurious to his or her health. An example is megavitamin therapy. The dietitian needs to explain what is known about this type of therapy, to give a professional recommendation, and to educate the patient about recommended daily allowances, vitamin and mineral needs during stress, specific features of different vitamins, and the risks of ingesting toxic levels of vitamins and minerals. Taking vitamins in nontoxic amounts that have not been shown to be beneficial is an example of a therapy that is not injurious but also not scientifically grounded. The key is to work with the patient's specific

intake of dietary supplements and to try to optimize that intake. As with any counseling, however, the patient makes the final decision and the decision should be respected even if the dietitian disagrees with it.

All diets need to be evaluated in terms of a continuum of benefit and no harm, no benefit and no harm, and no benefit and harm. A diet or therapy that is harmful because it eliminates other needed therapies needs much more serious discussion with the health care team and patient than a diet with no benefit but no harm. Besides physical harm, financial and psychologic harm must be considered.

## Moderate Nutrition Impact

During chemotherapy, radiation therapy, and gastrointestinal surgery diet is focused on meeting the immediate needs for calories, protein and other macronutrients, and micronutrients, not on cancer prevention. Patients sometimes have trouble understanding why the concentrated-calorie diet is so different from a prevention diet. The importance of explaining the purpose of such a diet cannot be overemphasized. The patient may be experiencing guilt about past eating habits and a desire to rectify the diet now and may be confused about the dietitian's recommending a calorie-dense diet. Fear that the dietitian is trying to cause injury may develop.

The difference in nutrition requirements at various stages of illness also needs explanation. Throughout moderate to intensive therapy, nutrition is aimed at promoting healing and strength. Although a 10- to 20-lb weight loss may seem to the patient to be a move in the right direction, the dietitian must make it clear that the point of nutrition management is maintenance of weight, especially if high-dose radiation therapy or chemotherapy is planned.

Patients need understanding and support during radiation therapy and chemotherapy. Nutrition is often one of the only areas over which the patient has control. The ability to manipulate intake to consume sufficient calories is a momentous success for the patient. Nausea, vomiting, a sore mouth, esophageal reflux, taste aversions, and anorexia are major obstacles to eating. Success in this area, both major and minor, should be acknowledged and rewarded. Reasonable goals need to be articulated; for example, minimizing weight loss may be a more realistic goal than gaining or maintaining weight. The importance of maximizing intake whenever possible should be encouraged. Emphasis should be placed on the patient's helping himself or herself, not on guilt associated with the inability to eat. For example, encouragement to eat can be given in the form of placing snack foods by the patient's chair so that the patient can eat when he or she decides.

### Critical Nutrition Need

If intake and nutritional status are approaching a critical point, nutrition consequences need to be discussed with the patient. The patient must understand the impact of limited intake and the options available to compensate for it, such as the use of nutrition supplements, tube feeding, and parenteral feeding. The health care team, with a united voice, must explain the benefits and consequences of each option and the time frame—short or long term—that may be involved.

Because it is the patient's life that is being discussed, the patient is the appropriate person to make decisions regarding nutrition interventions. Facilitating informed decision making is the ethical responsibility of the dietitian or health care team member who presents the options to the patient, but the health care team must accept the patient's decision and do the best they can for him or her. The ADA's position paper on feeding terminally ill patients (ADA, 1989) reviews decision making regarding enteral and parenteral feeding.

The cooperation of the family is also needed. The psychologic effect of the patient's illness on the family may need the attention of the health care team. The dietitian needs to help the family establish realistic expectations. Families need to understand the difficulties that the patient may experience with intake and rapid alterations of food preferences resulting from the disease. Families and friends need to encourage the patient to eat, but they must not force food. The

idiosyncrasies of intake must be viewed as being beyond the patient's control; families must realize that rejection of favorite foods is not rejection of the provider of the food. Families need to know appropriate foods to provide as well as when and how to encourage the patient to eat. The patient and family may disagree about the best treatment. The health care team needs to assist the family in understanding the reasons for the patient's wishes.

### CESSATION OF TREATMENT

Once therapy is stopped, the patient needs to understand the potential importance of nutrition in promoting the return of physical strength. Weight goals need to be set, possibly with a margin of safety for future therapy. The merits of diet in secondary prevention need to be considered.

The patient must not be made to feel abandoned. Cessation of treatment should not equate with cessation of care. If the end stages of disease have started, treatment options from feeding desired foods to providing parenteral nutrition should be discussed. If, on the other hand, reentry into the workplace or other social function is a possibility, questions about long-term nutrition support can be addressed, such as whether nasogastric feeding should be changed to gastrostomy feeding.

Remission may never occur, or it may last for years. Throughout this period the patient may still be looking for alternative treatment options. The dietitian must maintain his or her credibility by understanding and keeping up-to-date with trends presented in the media and by discussing new treatment modalities with the patient.

### COURSE OF DISEASE

During a cancer patient's course of disease, remissions and therapy may continue periodically. The impact on the patient's hopes and fears must be considered. Chronic disease can cause psychologic stress, financial stress, and depression. Factual information must be balanced with empathy and realism. Most patients appreciate being told the options in straight-forward but sympathetic terms.

## END-STAGE DISEASE

When conventional treatment is deemed no longer useful or appropriate, the patient may decide to accept this or try experimental treatment if available. Aggressive medical therapy deserves aggressive nutrition support to optimize outcome if the patient agrees. In any case, the cessation of medical therapy does not preclude the provision of nutrition therapy.

Nutrition has not been definitively linked to prolonged survival, but it can have a positive psychologic impact. Cancer cachexia can be particularly disturbing to the patient and family. Weight maintenance may boost the patient's self-image, and the favorable response of others serves as positive reinforcement. It should be remembered, however, that the patient's ability to eat does not necessarily mandate feeding. If the patient does not wish to eat, he or she should not be forced to do so. The dietitian's personal beliefs may differ from the patient's on this point, but they are not better (or worse) than the patient's.

The dietitian needs to understand the level at which the patient is dealing with his or her impending death and to consider the family's acceptance of the terminal stages of the disease. Kubler-Ross (1969) provided classic descriptions of the feelings that cancer patients may have as death approaches and outlined five stages in the process of dealing with death: denial and isolation, anger, bargaining, depression, and acceptance. The patient may vacillate among the different stages during the course of the disease and the final stages of the illness.

For the health care provider, consideration of these stages may assist in patient care. During denial and isolation there may be unreliability with respect to food intake. The nutrition provider needs to reinforce the importance of eating but must respect the patient's immediate need to deny his or her illness. When the patient is angry, food and eating-related issues may become the target of the anger. Disagreement with the dietitian regarding the diet and complaints about food are common at this time. The client may refuse to eat to exercise control. Anger at the lack of medical and nutrition research may surface. The nutrition provider needs to continue to communicate with and encourage the patient regarding areas in which the patient can control the diet.

Bargaining may be the point at which the client looks to nutrition quackery as a solution. Emphasis needs to be placed on the facts and realistic expectations of nutrition. During the period of depression, the nutrition provider needs to respect the patient's sense of loss and to continue to be supportive. At the point of acceptance the patient may be detaching himself or herself from the world, and the nutrition provider needs to respect this as well.

## CONCLUSION

Working with cancer patients is a rewarding endeavor. Maintenance of nutrition status can help patients feel better physically and better about themselves. The dietitian needs to be aware of patients' attitudes toward their illness and nutrition. With this information, the dietitian can fully address patients' needs.

**REFERENCES**

American Dietitic Association. (1988). Code of ethics for the profession of dietetics. *Journal of the American Dietetic Association, 88,* 1592–1593.

American Dietetic Association. (1989). Position of the American Dietetic Association: Issues in feeding the terminally ill. *Dietitians in Nutrition Support Newsletter, 11,* 2–9.

Kubler-Ross, E. (1969). *On death and dying.* New York: Macmillan.

# Chapter 31

# Cancer Quackery

*Mindy Hermann-Zaidins and Ira Milner*

An estimated $4 billion is spent annually by Americans on cancer quackery (House Select Committee, 1984). Unproven* treatment methods, many of which are nutrition related, are widely sought by cancer patients and their families. Of great concern is the fact that more than 40% of patients begin these treatments when they are symptom free or in early disease stages, when conventional treatments would probably cure them of their disease (Cassileth, Lusk, Strouse, & Bodenheimer, 1984).

Dietitians frequently are called on to render an opinion or analysis of a particular program and to guide patients toward a medically acceptable treatment approach. For this reason, it is important for dietitians to familiarize themselves not only with the unproven methods but also with the patient's rationale for seeking treatment not approved by the medical community and with tips and methods for advising patients.

The American Cancer Society (1987) defines unproven methods as diagnostic tests or therapeutic modalities that are promoted for general use in cancer prevention, diagnosis, or treatment but are not recommended for use on the basis of clinical judgment. These methods have not been objectively, reliably, responsibly, and reproducibly demonstrated in the peer-reviewed literature to be more effective than suggestion or doing nothing (Herbert, 1986).

When evaluating a therapy, the dietitian must answer four basic questions:

1. Has the therapy been proven to be more effective than doing nothing?
2. Is it as safe as doing nothing?
3. Does the potential for benefit exceed the potential for harm to the patient and family?
4. Have proponents of the therapy borne the responsibility for demonstrating efficacy and safety in an acceptable manner?

More often than not, questionable cancer treatments do not withstand scientific scrutiny.

## WHY PEOPLE TURN TO UNSCIENTIFIC THERAPIES

A major reason why cancer patients and their families turn to unscientific therapies is to gain control over the treatment and course of the disease. When considering the relationship between nutrition and cancer, patients may believe, or may be led to believe, that cancer is only a symptom of poor diet, stress, and environmental toxicities. Applying logic to this percep-

---

*The terms unproven, unproved, unconventional, unscientific, unorthodox, questionable, and alternative are used interchangeably throughout this chapter.

tion, the patient deduces that if a "bad" diet causes symptoms then a "good" diet can relieve them and that it is possible to build biologic and mental defenses against cancer (Gillick, 1985). Therefore, a dietary approach appears to make more sense to some patients than conventional therapy.

Several factors explain in part why patients turn to unconventional cancer therapies.

- Patients are looking for hope and magic. Cancer is a disease with major morbidity and mortality; many types of cancer have relatively low cure rates (American Cancer Society, 1988).
- In their search for another chance, patients may turn to unproven approaches that offer promises and testimonials of an easy, "natural," and harmless cure (Holland, 1982; Subcommittee, 1983).
- Patients tend to overestimate and overanticipate the pain and side effects of standard therapies. Traditional cancer treatments can be physically uncomfortable when accompanied by pain, nausea and vomiting, and other side effects, a point that is heavily stressed by questionable practitioners in their referrals to chemotherapy, radiation therapy, and surgery as "poisoning, burning, and butchering." Therefore, seemingly harmless dietary approaches are appealing as an alternative.
- Many patients turn to unorthodox methods out of discouragement and despair concerning the realities of standard treatment (Cassileth & Brown, 1988) over which they have little control. They fear being abandoned by their physician once all standard medical options have been exhausted and there is no treatment modality left for the physician to offer (Holland, 1982).
- Patients and their families often "research" treatment options but uncritically accept misinformation without appropriate scrutiny (Monaco & Renner, 1985). Much of the misinformation is promulgated by quacks through the media, a source that the public perceives as presenting the truth.
- Patients and their families desire a better relationship with physicians and other health care providers. Many feel that they are unable to communicate with their own physicians and that they do not receive enough time and attention. In contrast, the quack practitioner appears to be extremely attentive to the needs of patients and provides the patient with a feeling of comfort and security (Hewer, 1983). The proponent of questionable therapies also may inflate his or her experience or credentials to improve credibility (Monaco & Renner, 1985).
- Unproven therapies are widely and readily available in spite of efforts by the Food and Drug Administration (FDA), States' Attorneys General, United States Post Office, American Cancer Society, National Council Against Health Fraud, and health professionals to control quackery. It seems that, whenever one unorthodox therapy is cut off, two new ones pop up to replace it (Brigden, 1987).

## CHARACTERISTICS OF UNCONVENTIONAL THERAPIES

A number of basic characteristics are common to unconventional therapies, although specific treatment modalities are quite varied. Unproved approaches may be comprehensive, offering treatment, support groups, and newsletters. They tend to encompass lifestyle-oriented activities of daily living that are easy for the patient to understand and to which they can relate (Cassileth & Brown, 1988). In contrast, conventional medical approaches may be perceived as overly scientific, almost mystical, and destructive.

The following features of unproven approaches are fairly consistent (Subcommittee, 1983):

- No treatments are based on theories proved in widely accepted, peer-reviewed medical publications. Some proponents seize on and espouse theories that are under aggressive investigation by the scientific community (e.g., the use of β-carotene in cancer prevention) and try to apply them to treatment. Another common practice is to use medically accepted diet recommendations for reducing cancer risk, such as lowering fat intake and increasing fiber, as justification for an unproven diet that is restricted in fat and high in fiber.

- Unproved treatments usually are not administered in established medical or scientific centers. The best-known treatment centers offering bogus cures tend to be outside the United States in Mexico or the Caribbean.

- Proponents state that a "special" diet must be followed for their particular therapy to work. The diet often is administered in addition to other treatments.

- Only specially trained persons are said to be able to produce results with the treatment. This explanation is used to justify the fact that medical investigators have not been able to duplicate the results obtained by proponents of unproved therapies.

- The "toxicity" of conventional therapies is overstated by using words such as burning, poisoning, and butchering, whereas unscientific treatments are called painless and nontoxic.

- Claims of cure are published in the media rather than in responsible peer-reviewed journals and often are in the form of testimonials. Treatments are pitched as miraculous breakthroughs. Some practitioners may argue that they are too busy helping patients to spend time conducting controlled trials and publishing their results.

- Claims are excessive and promise dramatic benefits, such as the cure or prevention of cancer (Herbert, 1984b).

- Claims of benefit often can be explained by the placebo effect. Treatment failures, deaths, and misdiagnoses never are mentioned in promotion, information, or testimonial literature (Herbert, 1984a).

- Some practitioners have specious credentials that are not recognized in the scientific community (Jarvis, 1966), including degrees with no relationship to standard medical credentials (e.g., ND, Doctor of Naturopathy) and degrees from unaccredited institutions. Many others hold the MD or osteopathic degrees. One study showed that more than 60% of unorthodox practitioners held the MD (Cassileth et al., 1984).

- Major proponents are not recognized as responsible experts in cancer treatment and decry responsible methods of treatment.

- The promoters demand that patients have "freedom of choice" in selecting their anticancer treatment.

Proponents employ several explanations regarding cancer causation, treatment, and prevention. They claim that patients have metabolic abnormalities, anaerobic tumor metabolism, and deficiencies of cellular oxidation (Vissing & Petersen, 1981) and that tumors are merely symptoms of an underlying metabolic disturbance. This approach often gives patients the feeling that proper supplements and lifestyle changes that are promised to "correct the metabolism" will restore normalcy (Ross, 1985) and eliminate the tumor.

## DIETARY APPROACHES

Specific unproved or disproved dietary approaches to the treatment of cancer vary from practitioner to practitioner. Patients who travel to a well-known clinic or center are likely to be exposed to that center's established treatment philosophy and program. Those who undergo unscientific therapy locally may receive a conglomeration of treatment methods that represent the components of several programs. The most common treatments can be grouped into three main categories: metabolic therapy, megavitamins, and diet.

### Metabolic Therapy

Metabolic therapy is based on the disproved theory that toxins and wastes accumulate in the human body and are the basic cause of all degenerative disease. Therefore, the metabolic approach centers on "detoxification" and "rejuvenation" with juice fasts, enemas, dietary supplements, enzymes, organic foods, and animal organ extracts (Lowell, 1987). The Gerson program, which is currently available in Baja California, includes a rigorous juice fast. Patients receive four types of pressed juices—orange, apple-carrot, green leaf, and raw liver-carrot—rotated on an hourly basis. The only foods permitted in the early stages of the program are fruits and vegetables, potatoes, oatmeal, and special soups and breads.

Dietary regimens usually limit or exclude animal protein under the unproved premise that tumors develop as a result of a pancreatic enzyme deficiency. A low-protein diet purportedly spares pancreatic enzymes, allowing them to digest the tumor.

## Megavitamins and Other Dietary Supplements

Administration of vitamin megadoses is one aspect of metabolic therapy. Megavitamins were popularized in the 1970s, when the Laetrile regimen was widely used, and currently are administered either alone or in conjunction with other treatment modalities. One advocate of megavitamin therapy, Linus Pauling, has claimed that mortality due to cancer could be decreased by 75% by the proper use of vitamin C alone (Bosco, 1979).

Vitamins are recommended for a number of unproven effects, including "tumor cell respiration," "free radical scavenging," and "antioxidation" (Kittler, 1978; Moertel et al., 1982). The B-complex vitamins, zinc, selenium, cadmium, vanadium, and vitamins C, E, and A are most commonly prescribed along with the pseudovitamins $B_{13}$ (orotic acid), $B_{15}$ (pangamic acid), and $B_{17}$ (Laetrile).

## Modified Diets

Dubious approaches to cancer treatment frequently include dietary modifications. The diets prescribed often are extremely unbalanced, but the imbalance is "justified" by one or more unproven theories.

### Vegetarian Diet

Many of the vegetarian-type diets are low in protein and limit or exclude animal products.

The Gerson diet introduces small amounts of meat, fish, and dairy products only after 4 to 6 weeks. Other diets may be based solely on raw fruits and vegetables, whole grains, and cereals. Little attention is paid to meeting protein requirements with nonanimal sources.

One questionable theory implicates a high-protein diet as the cause of cancer (Kelley, 1969). Dietary protein is said to "deplete" pancreatic enzymes necessary for tumor digestion; for this reason, patients are encouraged to limit protein intake, thereby "conserving" enzymes. The same program, however, encourages consumption of raw liver, uncooked eggs, and unpasteurized milk products, a source of protein but also of potentially toxic bacteria.

### Macrobiotic Diet

The macrobiotic philosophy dictates that illness develops from an imbalance of *yin* and *yang,* the purported opposing forces of the universe. Likewise, tumors themselves are classified as either *yin* or *yang* and are said to be caused by a diet that is dominated by one of the two forces. Therefore, the macrobiotic approach calls for a diet that will correct the body's imbalance.

Food selection in the macrobiotic diet is based on proportionate volumes of five food groups. Although specific foods and proportions are adapted to the type of tumor, the diet generally is 50% to 60% grains, 20% to 30% vegetables, 5% to 10% dried beans and seaweeds, and 5% to 10% soups. Small amounts of fish are included in some macrobiotic diets. Within each category, foods may be recommended for regular or occasional use. Consumption of other foods, such as meat, poultry, eggs, dairy products, sugar, and vegetables not indigenous to the patient's geographic region, is discouraged. The macrobiotic diets popularized in the 1980s by Michio Kushi are less restrictive than the Zen macrobiotic diet of previous decades that was promoted by George Ohsawa and based primarily on brown rice.

Some macrobiotic literature recommends that seriously ill cancer patients be monitored closely by the appropriate medical profession. Other patients may be encouraged to work with the macrobiotic therapist while continuing medically acceptable therapy.

## Other Therapies

### Laetrile

The Laetrile programs center on the administration of Laetrile, also known as amygdalin or vitamin $B_{17}$, which is a popularized name for a compound that is synthesized from apricot and other fruit seeds. It was a popular unproved treatment modality in the 1970s and early 1980s until its ineffectiveness in treating cancer was verified in clinical trials conducted at major cancer treatment centers (Moertel et al., 1982). In spite of this conclusive evidence, however, Laetrile still is widely available. Other components of the Laetrile regimen are megavitamins, pancreatic enzymes, and a vegetarian-type diet.

### Organ Extracts

Organ extracts or desiccated organs from animals are said to revitalize their counterparts in the human body. Desiccated liver powder is among the most widely used extracts.

### Enemas

Enemas are a common component of unproved programs and are administered purportedly to aid in "detoxification." One regimen includes a standard enema containing castor oil, a caffeine–potassium citrate solution, defatted ox bile powder, and soapy water. Others may be made from chamomile tea, green vegetable juices, "ozone," or Epsom salts with coffee. Coffee enemas, a common component of many regimens, originally were said to promote a "healing crisis" characterized by nausea, vomiting, intestinal spasms, gas, lack of appetite, weight loss, fever, cramping, and dehydration (Gerson, no date).

## IMMUNOAUGMENTATIVE THERAPY

Immunoaugmentative therapy (IAT), which is thought by its founder, Lawrence Burton, to correct a cancer patient's faulty immune system, could become as explosive a political issue in the 1990s as was Laetrile in the 1970s. Burton, a zoologist, established a clinic in Freeport, Bahamas in 1977 after failing to comply with

Food and Drug Administration procedures in conducting human research trials in the United States (Curt, Katterhagen, & Mahaney, 1986). An immune therapy clinic recently opened in Tijuana, Mexico.

Immunoaugmentative therapy is purportedly effective in the prevention, treatment, and even detection of all types of cancer (Burton, no date). Injections of a serum consisting of combinations of four supposedly naturally occurring blood components are the principal means of treatment. These components, derived from necrotic tumor tissue and the blood from persons with cancer and healthy donors, are referred to as "tumor antibody," which is said to attack and destroy cancer cells; "tumor complement," which activates the tumor antibody; "blocking protein," which is responsible for inhibiting the action of the tumor antibody; and "deblocking protein," which neutralizes the effect of the blocking protein (Immunology Researching Centre, no date). Burton theorizes that, when these substances are in balance and when the immune mechanism is functioning normally, the tumor antibody fulfills its cancer-destroying function. When tumor cells produce amounts of the blocking protein in excess of the tumor antibody, however, the immune system is overwhelmed, and cancer cells proliferate (Immunology Researching Centre, no date). Dietary supplements are prescribed as an adjunct to IAT.

Thousands of dollars are spent by IAT patients for a cycle of treatment lasting a minimum of 6 to 8 weeks (Burton, no date). IAT also is offered to patients with acquired immunodeficiency syndrome (AIDS).

## HARM DONE BY QUACKERY

The proliferation of quackery is damaging to patients, their families, and the community. This harm can be broken down into four major categories: physical, psychologic, financial, and societal.

### Physical

Many of the unproved diets cause nutrition deficiencies or toxicities or overall malnutrition.

Although the macrobiotic diet has been "liber-alized" in recent years, it still is deficient in niacin, riboflavin, vitamin $B_{12}$, and vitamin D and may also be low in bioavailable calcium, iron, and zinc (Hermann-Zaidins, 1986). Because it is not calorically dense, the mac-robiotic diet may not provide adequate overall nutrition for anorectic cancer patients who are unable to consume adequate quantities of food. Patients with intestinal impairments, including malabsorption, radiation enteritis, AIDS- or chemotherapy-induced diarrhea, or narrowing of the bowel, should be extremely wary of this diet because, in addition to other shortcomings, it is high in fiber.

Juice fast "detoxification" may cause severe diarrhea that worsens if laxatives such as castor oil, Epsom salts, or other forms of magnesium have been added to the regimen. Raw liver juice, eggs, and milk may be bacterially contaminated.

Megavitamin supplements, particularly fat-soluble vitamins, can be toxic to the patient. Pseudovitamins such as $B_{13}$, $B_{15}$, and $B_{17}$ are ineffective and potentially harmful. Laetrile, which is 6% cyanide by weight, has been associ-ated with numerous deaths (Herbert, 1984a).

Commonly utilized dietary supplements are of questionable benefit. One program calls for the ingestion of linseed and castor oils, potassium and iodine solutions, and digestive enzymes (Gerson, 1977). These additives can be expected to cause diarrhea and fluid and electrolyte losses. Under the rubric of "detoxification," the patient is told that the side effects are evidence of the body's efforts to rid itself of accumulated toxins.

Length and quality of life can deteriorate, rather than improve, for patients who undergo unorthodox treatments and abandon conven-tional modalities. The patient may be physically less comfortable because of the rigors of unproved treatments and the usual omission of pain medications. An improper or inadequate diagnosis by an unorthodox practitioner leading to neglect of the underlying disease may cause a deterioration of the patient's medical status. A tumor whose proliferation could have been con-trolled by chemotherapy may grow rapidly if treatment is not continued. The greatest tragedy occurs when patients with tumors that are in early or curable stages opt to forgo effective

medical treatments in favor of unproven dietary approaches.

Among the potential side effects of enemas are diarrhea, diminished peristalsis (Use of enemas, 1984), dehydration, colonic fistula development, amoebic enteritis (Istre, 1982) and other colonic infections (Case against colonic irrigation, 1985), mucosal damage, and fluid and electrolyte imbalance. The addition of known cathartics, such as castor oil or Epsom salts, may compound the patient's discomfort by causing additional diarrhea. Coffee enemas have been shown to cause fluid and electrolyte imbalances and possibly death (Eisele & Reay, 1980).

Although IAT is promoted as being "safe" and "nontoxic" (Literature, 1981), it presents serious health hazards (Curt et al., 1986). Numerous samples of IAT blood serum were found to be contaminated with organisms that cause hepatitis B and with the AIDS virus (Isola-tion, 1985). Indeed, several cases of hepatitis B have been documented (Isolation, 1985). The Centers for Disease Control isolated active AIDS virus from one sample and reported 16 cases of abscess formation at IAT injection sites (Cutaneous, 1984).

As a result of political pressure exerted by Congressman Guy Molinari (R–NY), Congress' Office of Technology Assessment (OTA) has undertaken a comprehensive and exhaustive investigation of IAT and many other question-able cancer treatment methods. Completion of OTA's findings is expected in early 1990 (Julia Ostrowsky, personal communication).

## Psychologic

The psychologic harm in unscientific therapies affects the patient and family in a number of ways. Many proponents offer false hope for a cancer cure; worse, they often blame the patient if their prescribed therapy does not work. This approach instills feelings of guilt and anxiety in patients over having chosen medically accepted therapy rather than consultation with an unscientific practitioner (Jungi, 1986) or having committed errors in following the unproved reg-imen. Patients and their families may be told that "detoxification" will now be more difficult because conventional therapy was initiated first. The psychologic effects on family members endure long after the patient has died.

Unproved regimens distort the patient's perspective of good and bad. For example, responsible chemotherapies may be called poisons or toxins, whereas the useless and potentially deadly Laetrile is promoted as safe and effective. Excessive trust is placed in the unconventional practitioner, who may encourage rejection of the medical establishment.

### Financial

A patient's financial resources may be drained rapidly by unproved regimens. The cost of supplies, diagnostic tests, and travel often adds up to several thousand dollars per month. One patient spent several hundred dollars on mail-order vitamins that did not arrive until several months after she died. It is common for clinics and mail-order houses to require payment up front to ensure that they receive their money independent of the patient's insurance coverage. A typical 3-week stay in a Tijuana clinic costs approximately $7,000.

### Societal

Unscientific approaches adversely affect faith in the medical system. A commonly promoted perception is that the medical profession is filled with inappropriate practice and greed and offers little compassion and caring for the patient's well-being. The passage of legislation sanctioning unorthodox regimens has further undermined trust and belief in standard medical practice.

The proliferation of unproved therapies diverts funding and attention from legitimate research and treatment. Cleverly contrived bills for treatment at quack centers may be covered by some insurance carriers; this practice ultimately raises the overall cost of insurance coverage. The amount of money spent annually by Americans on ineffective cancer treatments exceeds the budget for the National Cancer Institute.

Physicians and other health care professionals who spend time fighting quackery have less time to address worthwhile medical issues.

### WHAT YOU CAN DO

The Laetrile hoax provided health professionals with a valuable lesson: it is crucial to take an active role in combatting cancer quackery. An important factor contributing to Laetrile's success was the meagerness and lateness of the medical community's response to the Laetrile movement (Lerner, 1984).

Although Laetrile was first promoted by Ernst Krebs, Sr., and his son during the early 1950s, it gained most of its popularity in the 1970s (Wilson, 1988). By the latter part of that decade it had become a household word and had been used by approximately 70,000 Americans (Lerner, 1984), despite the fact that it lacked FDA approval and that most medical and scientific experts considered it ineffective. Yet consumer and legislative interest remained intense for several years. Ultimately, legalization of Laetrile occurred in 27 states (Wilson, 1988).

How could the most studied failure in the history of medicine achieve such success? What its promoters lacked in the way of scientific evidence demonstrating its effectiveness they made up for in political savvy, rallying to the cry of "freedom of choice." They also employed sophisticated marketing and propaganda techniques to influence a vulnerable public and to manipulate the political and regulatory process.

As Herbert (1981) warned, a real danger exists that legitimate nutrition science will be overwhelmed by pseudoscience and quackery. To allow unorthodox, fringe practitioners to continue promoting their nostrums unchallenged undermines the legitimacy of true science. Indeed, the propaganda efforts of organizations and individuals who promote questionable cancer remedies have been successful, resulting in their widespread attraction and use. Cassileth et al. (1984) have demonstrated this point: 40% of conventionally treated cancer patients whom they questioned discontinued conventional care once unorthodox treatment began.

Many physicians unwittingly refer patients to quack practitioners by default (Holohan, 1987); in fact, there is a significant inverse relation between the quality of a patient's experience with conventional medicine and his or her use of unproven methods (Cassileth & Brown, 1988). Although the relationship between the patient and physician is a crucial factor in determining whether a patient will seek unorthodox treatments, the relationship between the patient and other members of the orthodox cancer treatment team also is important. Nutritionists and other allied health professionals may at times be better able than the physician to meet the information and emotional needs of cancer patients and their families. For this reason, and because most unorthodox methods include a nutrition component, dietitians and nutritionists can play a valuable role in the fight against cancer quackery.

## Be Informed

Knowledge is one of the most effective weapons to deploy against quackery (Sampson, 1988). It is essential to be familiar with and conversant in the various questionable cancer treatment approaches, their rationales, and the misconceptions that cancer quacks use to promote them. Jarvis (1983) reviews the more common of these misconceptions and provides the facts necessary to dispel them. Appendixes 31-A and 31-B list credible resources for health care professionals. Another resource is the American Cancer Society's Committee on Unproven Methods, which regularly publishes program reviews in the journal *CA*.

Dietitians especially need to get the facts about the nutrition aspects of questionable treatment methods not only intelligently to address patient queries but also to share this information with other members of the health care team. Information can be obtained in various ways: by visiting local health food stores and alternative bookstores; by obtaining copies of free literature and perusing popular books to see what patients are reading; and by soliciting information from the major "alternative" treatment and education centers, information services, and support groups through telephone calls and letters

(Appendixes 31-C and 31-D). One underground cancer resource guide lists addresses, telephone numbers, and other pertinent information about these centers, services, and groups in North America and worldwide (Fink, 1988). Nutritionists should encourage patients to discuss their unorthodox treatments and to provide diets and other written information about those treatments. A vitamin history should be included in the patient assessment.

Patients expect critical, informed responses to their questions in clear, nontechnical terms (Monaco & Renner, 1985). Mentioning the absence of peer-reviewed journal articles or double-blind studies is ineffective and probably counterproductive (Monaco, 1986). Patients want to know whether a questionable approach has been disproven, and, if not, what the chances are of its being efficacious. Many people who turn to unproven methods are highly educated and have read extensively about conventional and unorthodox treatment modalities (Cassileth et al., 1984) and have made an informed choice to commit time and resources to unorthodox treatment (Cassileth & Brown, 1988).

Brigden (1987) emphasizes the necessity of attacking the underlying rationale for a particular treatment. Patients involved with cancer quackery are given what appears even to the educated layperson to be common-sense explanations that, in reality, make no sense when critically reviewed. Promoters of unproven methods frequently lead cancer patients to believe that poor dietary habits are the underlying cause of their disease and that proper diet can therefore reverse the malignancy. Thus a discussion of the cancer process, its legitimate treatment, and the true role that diet plays in the disease often is useful.

## Communicate Effectively, and Have the Proper Attitude

The pros and cons of a particular method should be discussed in an objective, nonjudgmental manner. This indicates to the patient a willingness to listen; an angry or authoritarian response undermines the practitioner's ability to convince the patient to remain in conventional care (Holland, 1982).

The nutritionist should try not to make the patient feel foolish by rejecting outright any unproven method that he or she may be considering. Rather, the nutritionist should be tolerant of the patient's need to explore unconventional methods and maintain an open, receptive attitude to new ideas, encouraging the patient to raise questions about unscientific methods without fear of being ridiculed and abandoned. Some unproven therapies (e.g., the Simonton method of mental imagery) may not be detrimental to patients if used as an adjunct and not as a replacement for conventional treatment (Kill, 1988). Battles must be chosen wisely, with attention focused on those products and services that are potentially harmful.

Patients are more likely to trust and respect legitimate practitioners and less likely to seek unproven methods when emotional support and hope are provided and genuine concern and interest in the patient's well-being are displayed (Holland, 1982). Danielson, Stewart, and Lippert (1988) suggest that a sensitive and empathetic approach that gives patients realistic hope and control is of primary importance and that patients should be reassured that pain will be controlled and that they will not be abandoned.

## Give Patients a Sense of Control

Cassileth and Brown (1988) recommend giving patients a role in their care by suggesting reasonable dietary guidelines that will diffuse the attraction of alternative dietary therapies. Cancer patients need to exhibit control over their illness as an antidote for their sense of helplessness (Holland, 1982); they need to feel that they are fighting back against the disease. Jarvis (1983) also recommends incorporating a healthful dietary regimen into the treatment program; he warns, however, that the patient should not be led to believe that this dietary program is curative.

The nutrition professional should serve as a facilitator, assisting the patient in making wise food choices within established guidelines and making specific suggestions when necessary. Referral of the patient to legitimate support groups, including those offered by the American Cancer Society, also is beneficial.

## Network with Other Professionals

Nutritionists can network with other nutrition and health professionals to identify and combat quackery at the grass-roots level. Coalitions can be formed to gather information, to critique questionable products and services, and to establish local information repositories for professional and consumer use. Plans can be developed to monitor the media for inaccurate health information and to respond when deceptive or misleading material is published or aired. Because public libraries are a common source of medical and health information, reliable sources can be suggested to librarians.

## Support Legislation and Enforcement Efforts

Both individually and through coalitions, nutrition professionals can support legislation and public and voluntary agencies that protect health consumers from worthless and potentially harmful products and services. Legislators can be influenced through provisions of testimony, letter writing, and telephone calls. Questionable products and services should be reported to appropriate agencies and organizations (Appendix 31-E). Patients who have been involved with cancer quackery should be encouraged to file lawsuits against the practitioners.

A major problem in combatting quackery is the patients' reluctance to complain to enforcement agencies and to pursue legal action. Some are embarrassed at having been fooled, whereas others experience difficulty obtaining help through the courts. The National Council Against Health Fraud (NCAHF) Task Force on Victim Redress, formed in 1988, is a potentially powerful legal antiquackery tool. It was created to help patients involved with quackery obtain competent legal assistance and to provide their attorneys with useful, up-to-date information and expert witnesses. It is hoped that this legal recourse will send a clear message to quacks that robbing consumers of their money and their health will not be tolerated and will bring national attention to the scope of the health fraud problem.

## Dealing with the Media

Because the media is a major vehicle used for the dissemination of questionable cancer treatments, it is important that it be dealt with effectively. When objectionable advertising, broadcasts, or newspaper or magazine articles are printed or aired, nutrition professionals should complain through letters and telephone calls to advertising managers, editors, publishers, producers, or station managers. If resistance is encountered, colleagues, friends, and family members should be encouraged to write and call (Barrett, 1987).

Nutrition professionals can establish a relationship with the local media by praising them when reporting is accurate and offering to be interviewed or to share reliable information to correct previous misinformation.

## CONCLUSION

The nature of cancer is such that some patients will turn to unconventional therapies regardless of guidance from dietitians and other health care professionals. Recognizing this, the dietitian should strive to develop a rapport with the patient and family, to educate them about the pros and cons of their chosen regimen, and to try, at minimum, to improve the quality and balance of their diet. The dietitian should not feel that counseling efforts were unsuccessful because the patient refuses to give up an unscientific regimen. Instead, counseling offers the opportunity to guide the patient toward a more balanced program.

It is important to have a comprehensive understanding of cancer quackery to be effective in educating patients. By recognizing the rationale behind the patient's decision-making process, the dietitian will better understand the patient's motivations and can be more influential. The dietary and other characteristics of specific programs fall under a handful of basic categories, all of which have nutrition-related consequences that the dietitian can address. The programs themselves as well as credible medical authorities and organizations are excellent resources for information.

The NCAHF newsletter (1989, p. 5) offers an important message about the responsibility of physicians and other health care professionals to deal with quackery:

> Quackery's inevitability is like that of disease and death, and just as physicians do not give up on these human problems, neither should they surrender to quackery without a fight. The realistic goal is not to eliminate quackery, but to minimize its negative impact upon society.

## REFERENCES

American Cancer Society. (1987). *Fact book for health professionals*. New York: Author.

American Cancer Society. (1988). *Cancer facts and figures—1988*. New York: Author.

Barrett, S. (1987). Fighting quackery: Tips for activists. *Nutrition Forum Newsletter, 4,* 49–51.

Bosco, D. (1979, July). Vitamin C and cancer: An interview with Dr. Ewan Cameron. *Prevention, 31*(7), 48.

Brigden, M.L. (1987). Unorthodox therapy and your cancer patient. *Postgraduate Medicine, 81,* 271–280.

Burton, L. (No date). *Immuno-augmentative approach to cancer control* (Form 7332). Freeport, Grand Bahama Island: Immunology Researching Centre.

The case against colonic irrigation. (1985, September 27). *California Morbidity.*

Cassileth, B.R., & Brown, H. (1988). Unorthodox cancer medicine. *CA—A Cancer Journal for Clinicians, 38,* 176–185.

Cassileth, B.R., Lusk, E.J., Strouse, T.B., & Bodenheimer, B.J. (1984). Contemporary unorthodox treatments in cancer medicine. *Annals of Internal Medicine, 101,* 105.

Curt, G., Katterhagen, G., & Mahaney, F. Jr. (1986). Immunoaugmentative therapy: A primer on the perils of unproved treatments. *Journal of the American Medical Association, 255,* 505–507.

Cutaneous nocardiosis in cancer patients receiving immunotherapy—Bahamas. (1984). *Morbidity and Mortality Weekly Report, 33,* 471–447.

Danielson, K., Stewart, D., & Lippert, G. (1988). Unconventional cancer remedies. *Canadian Medical Association Journal, 138,* 1005–1011.

Eisele, J.W., & Reay, D.T. (1980). Deaths related to coffee enemas. *Journal of the American Medical Association, 244,* 1608.

Fink, J.M. (1988). *Third opinion: An international directory to alternative therapy centers for the treatment and prevention of cancer.* Garden City Park, NY: Avery Publishing Group.

Gerson, M. (1977). *A cancer therapy: Results of fifty cases* (3rd ed.). Del Mar, CA: Totality Books.

Gerson, A. (No date). *The Gerson primer, a patient information pamphlet.*

Gillick, M.R. (1985). Common-sense models of health and disease. *New England Journal of Medicine, 313,* 700–703.

Herbert, V. (1981). Will questionable nutrition overwhelm nutrition science? *American Journal of Clinical Nutrition, 34,* 2848–2853.

Herbert, V. (1984a). Faddism and quackery in cancer nutrition. *Nutrition and Cancer, 6,* 196.

Herbert, V. (1984b). Nine ways to spot a quack. *Health, 1,* 39.

Herbert, V. (1986). Unproven (questionable) dietary and nutritional methods in cancer prevention and treatment. *Cancer, 58,* 1930–1941.

Hermann-Zaidins, M.G. (1986). Questionable dietary anticancer therapies. *Current Concepts and Perspectives in Nutrition, 5,* 1–12.

Hewer, W. (1983). The relationship between the alternative practitioner and his patient. *Psychotherapy and Psychosomatics, 40,* 172–180.

Holland, J.C. (1982). Why patients seek unproven cancer remedies: A psychological perspective. *CA—A Cancer Journal for Clinicians, 32,* 20.

Holohan, T. (1987). Referral by default: The medical community and unorthodox therapy. *Journal of the American Medical Association, 257,* 1641–1642.

House Select Committee on Aging. (1984, May 31). *Quackery: A $10 billion scandal.* Washington, DC: Government Printing Office.

Immunology Researching Centre. (No date). *Informational brochure.* Freeport, Grand Bahama Island: Author.

Isolation of human T-lymphotropic virus type III/lymphadenopathy-associated virus from serum proteins given to cancer patients—Bahamas. (1985). *Morbidity and Mortality Weekly Report, 34,* 489–491.

Istre, G.R. (1982). An outbreak of amebiasis spread by colonic irrigation at a chiropractic clinic. *New England Journal of Medicine, 307,* 339–342.

Jarvis, W.T. (1966). Elements of quackery. Reprinted from *Unproved methods of cancer treatment.* New York: American Cancer Society.

Jarvis, W.T. (1983). Cancer: Boon for quackery. In M.N. Currie (Ed.), *Patient education in the primary care setting, proceedings of the sixth annual conference.* Kansas City, MO: The Project for Patient Education in Family Practice.

Jungi, W.F. (1986). Risks of alternative cancer treatment. *Onkologie, 9,* 231–234.

Kelley, W.D. (1969). *An answer to cancer.* Wintrop, WA: Kelley Research Foundation.

Kill, K.A. (1988). Unproven cancer therapies. *American Pharmacist, 28,* 18–22.

Kittler, B. (1978). *Laetrile: Nutritional control of cancer with vitamin $B_{17}$.* Denver: Royal.

Lerner, I.J. (1984). The whys of cancer quackery. *Cancer, 53,* 815–819.

Literature distributed to the Florida Legislature, 1981.

Lowell, J. (1987). Questionable cancer treatments and regimens. In J. Lowell (Ed.), *Health hoaxes and hazards.* Tucson: Nutrition Information Center.

Moertel, C.G., Fleming, T.P., Rubin, J., Kvols, L.K., Sarna, G., Koch, R., Currie, V.E., Young, C.W., Jones, S.E., & Darignon, J.P. (1982). A clinical trial of amygdalin (Laetrile) in the treatment of human cancer. *New England Journal of Medicine, 306,* 201.

Monaco, G.P. (1986). The primary care physician: The first line of defense in the battle against health fraud. *Medical Times, 114,* 43–48.

Monaco, G.P., & Renner, J.H. (1985). Teaching patients and the public how to discern health fraud and abuse. *Patient Education Proceedings, 8,* 157–165.

National Council Against Health Fraud. (1989, May/June). Physicians group releases position paper on quackery. *National Council Against Health Fraud Newsletter, 12,* 5.

Ross, W.E. (1985). Unconventional cancer therapy. *Comprehensive Therapy, 11,* 37–43.

Sampson, W.J. (1988). Why quacks befuddle physicians. *California Physician,* 16–18.

Subcommittee on Unorthodox Therapies, American Society of Clinical Oncology. (1983). Ineffective cancer therapy: A guide for the layperson. *Journal of Clinical Oncology, 1,* 154–164.

Use of enemas is limited. (1984). *FDA Consumer, 18,* 33.

Vissing, Y.M., & Petersen, J.C. (1981). Taking Laetrile: Conversion to medical deviance. *CA—A Cancer Journal for Clinicians, 31,* 365.

Wilson, B. (1988). The rise and fall of Laetrile. *Nutrition Forum Newsletter, 5,* 33–40.

# Appendix 31-A

# Antiquackery Books and Booklets

American Medical Association. (1988). *Alternative therapies, unproven methods and health fraud: A selected annotated bibliography*. Chicago: American Medical Association.

Barrett, S. (1980). *The health robbers: How to protect your money and your life* (2nd ed). Philadelphia: Stickley.

California Medical Association. (1987). *The professional's guide to health and nutrition fraud*. San Francisco: Sutter.

Cornacchia, H.J., & Barrett, S. (1989). *Consumer health: A guide to intelligent decisions* (4th ed.). St. Louis: Mosby.

Fried, J. (1984). *Vitamin politics*. Buffalo, NY: Prometheus Books.

Herbert, V. (1981). *Nutrition cultism: Facts and fictions*. Philadelphia: Stickley.

Herbert, V., & Barrett, S. (1981). *Vitamins and "health" foods: The great American hustle*. Philadelphia: Stickley.

Jarvis, W. (1983). *Quackery and you*. Washington, DC: Review & Herald.

Jarvis, W. (1985). *Food: Facts and fallacies A–Z*. Washington, DC: Review & Herald.

Lowell, J.A. (1987). *Health hoaxes and hazards*. Tucson: Nutrition Information Center.

Marshall, C.W. (1985). *Vitamins and minerals: Help or harm?* Philadelphia: Stickley.

San Bernardino County Department of Public Health, Nutrition Program. (1988). *Nutrition and cancer patient kit*. San Bernardino: Author.

Stalker, D., & Glymour, C. (1985). *Examining holistic medicine*. Buffalo, NY: Prometheus Books.

Subcommittee on Health and Long-Term Care, Select Committee on Aging. (1984). *Quackery: A $10 billion scandal* (Comm. Publ. No. 98-435). Washington, DC: Government Printing Office.

Tyler, V.E. (1987). *The new honest herbal: A sensible guide to herbs and related remedies*. Philadelphia: Stickley.

Yetiv, J.Z. (1986). *Popular nutritional practices: A scientific appraisal*. Toledo, OH: Popular Medicine.

# Appendix 31-B

# Antiquackery Periodicals

*Consumer Reports*
  PO Box 53029
  Boulder, CO 80322

*Environmental Nutrition Newsletter*
  2112 Broadway, Suite 200
  New York, NY 10023

*FDA Consumer*
  Superintendent of Documents
  Government Printing Office
  Washington, DC 20402

*National Council Against Health Fraud
  Newsletter*
  National Council Against Health Fraud, Inc.
  PO Box 1276
  Loma Linda, CA 92354

*Nutrition Forum Newsletter*
  J.B. Lippincott Company
  East Washington Square
  Philadelphia, PA 19105

*Priorities*
  American Council on Science and Health
  1995 Broadway, 16th Floor
  New York, NY 10023

# Appendix 31-C

# Major Unorthodox Treatment Centers in North America

| Center | Address and Telephone Number(s) | Primary Therapies |
|---|---|---|
| American Biologics–Mexico S.A. Medical Center | 1180 Walnut Avenue<br>Chula Vista, CA 92011<br>(619) 429-8200 | Supplements, Laetrile, detoxification, metabolic therapy |
| Center for Holistic and Natural Medicine | 920 Judson Place<br>Stratford, CT 06497<br>(203) 377-7606 | Metabolic therapy, supplements, macrobiotics |
| Clinica Manner, Tijuana, Mexico | PO Box 4290<br>San Ysidro, CA 92073<br>(706) 680-4222 | Metabolic therapy, supplements, enemas, Laetrile |
| Gerson Institute, Hospital De Baja California Tijuana, Mexico | PO Box 430<br>Bonita, CA 92002<br>(619) 267-1150 | Juice fasts, detoxification, enemas, supplements, Laetrile |
| Hospital Ernesto Contreras, Tijuana, Mexico | 190 Calle Primera<br>San Ysidro, CA 92073<br>(800) 523-8795<br>(800) 262-0212 (California) | Laetrile, metabolic therapy, supplements, detoxification, spiritual counseling |
| Hospital Santa Monica/Agua Caliente Spa and Resort | 424 Calle Primera, number 102<br>San Ysidro, CA 92073<br>(619) 428-1146 | Hydrogen peroxide, intravenous nutrients, colonics |
| Immune Therapy Clinic | 416 W. San Ysidro Boulevard<br>Suite L-702<br>San Ysidro, CA 92073<br>(619) 428-2211 | Immunoaugmentative therapy |
| Kushi Institute | PO Box 1100<br>Brookline Village, MA 02147<br>(617) 738-0045 | Macrobiotics |
| Saint Jude International Clinic | 911 Television Street<br>Tijuana, Mexico<br>(706) 684-7333 | Vegetarian diets, organic foods |

# Appendix 31-D

# Information Sources for Unproven Therapies

| Source | Address and Telephone Number | Services |
|---|---|---|
| Arlin J. Brown Information Center, Inc. | PO Box 251<br>Fort Belvoir, VA 22060<br>(703) 451-8638 | Information, newsletters |
| Cancer Control Society | 2043 North Berendo Street<br>Los Angeles, CA 90027<br>(213) 663-7801 | Information, clinic tours, resource lists, publications |
| Coalition for Alternatives in Nutrition and Healthcare, Inc. (CANAH) | PO Box B-12<br>Richlandtown, PA 18955<br>(215) 346-8461 | Information |
| Committee for Freedom of Choice in Medicine, Inc. | 1180 Walnut Avenue<br>Chula Vista, CA 92011<br>(619) 429-8200 | Newsletters |
| Foundation for Alternative Cancer Therapies (FACT) | PO Box HH<br>Old Chelsea Station<br>New York, NY 10011<br>(212) 741-2790 | Information, resource lists |
| International Association of Cancer Victors and Friends | 7740 Manchester Avenue, number 110<br>Playa del Rey, CA 90293<br>(213) 822-5032 | Information, publications |
| National Health Foundation | 212 West Foothill Boulevard<br>PO Box 688<br>Monrovia, CA 91016<br>(818) 357-2181 | Information |

# Appendix 31-E

# Where To Complain or Seek Help about Cancer Quackery

| Problem | Agency To Contact |
|---|---|
| False advertising | • Bureau of Consumer Protection, Federal Trade Commission, Washington, DC 20580<br>• Regional Federal Trade Commission Office<br>• National Advertising Division, National Council of Better Business Bureaus, 845 Third Avenue, New York, NY 10022<br>• Editor or station manager of media outlet where ad appeared |
| Product marketed with false or exaggerated claims | • Health Fraud Branch, Food and Drug Administration, 5600 Fishers Lane, Rockville, MD 20857<br>• Regional Food and Drug Administration Office<br>• State's Attorney General<br>• Congressional representatives<br>• Local Better Business Bureau<br>• State Health Department |
| Phony mail-order promotion | • Chief Postal Inspector, U.S. Postal Service, Washington, DC 20260<br>• Editor or station manager of media outlet where ad appeared |
| Improper treatment by licensed practitioner | • Local medical society, if practitioner belongs<br>• Local hospital, if practitioner is on staff<br>• State licensing board<br>• Private attorney for possible lawsuit |
| Improper treatment by unlicensed practitioner | • Local district attorney<br>• State's Attorney General<br>• Local newspaper or television station<br>• Private attorney for possible lawsuit<br>• National Council Against Health Fraud Task Force on Victim Redress |
| Advice needed about questionable product or service | • National Council Against Health Fraud, Inc., PO Box 1276, Loma Linda, CA 92354 |

*Source:* From ''Where To Complain'' by S. Barrett, 1987, *Nutrition Forum Newsletter,* now published by J.B. Lippincott, Philadelphia. Reprinted by permission.

# Frequently Requested Telephone Numbers for Information Services

**International Cancer Information Center**
International Cancer Research Data Bank ..................... (301) 496-7403
   PDQ Service Desk ......................................... (301) 496-7403
   PDQ News Editor ......................................... (301) 496-4907
Marketing Office ........................................... (301) 496-2794
Publications Branch ....................................... (301) 496-1997
   Manuscript Submissions (Journal of the National Cancer Institute
   and NCI Monographs) ................................. (301) 496-6975

Government Printing Office
Publications Subscription Information ....................... (202) 783-3238

National Library of Medicine
   MEDLARS Management (Database Subscription
   Information) ............................................. (301) 496-6193
.......................................... (800) 638-8480

**Office of Cancer Communications**
Press Inquiry ............................................. (301) 496-6641
Public or Patient Inquiry .................................... (301) 496-5583
Public and Patient Education Programs ...................... (301) 496-6792
Slides, Photographs, Audiovisuals .......................... (301) 496-4394

Cancer Information Service .................................. 1-800-4-CANCER
(1-800-422-6237)

Cancer Training Branch ..................................... (301) 427-8898
   (Extramural Research Training Fellowships)

Centers and Community Oncology Program (CCOP) .............. (301) 427-8708

Office of Grants Inquiries (NIH) .................................     (301) 496-7441

Office of International Affairs
  (Scientific Exchanges/Bilateral Agreements) ..................     (301) 496-4761

Personnel Locator
  NCI ......................................................     (301) 496-9221
  NIH ......................................................     (301) 496-2351

Surveillance, Epidemiology and End Results (SEER) Reporting ....     (301) 427-8829

Bulk Orders of Government Publications .......................     1-800-638-6694

# Resources and References

**HEALTHFINDER** lists and describes toll-free numbers of organizations that provide health-related information. These organizations do not diagnose or recommend treatment for any disease. Some offer recorded information; others provide personalized counseling, referrals, or written materials. Unless otherwise stated, numbers can be dialed within the continental United States and operate Monday through Friday. The following is a selected list taken from HEALTHFINDER.

Acquired Immunodeficiency Syndrome (AIDS)
Public Health Service AIDS Information Hotline
(800) 342-AIDS
(800) 342-SIDA for Spanish-speaking callers
Provides recorded information to the public about the prevention and spread of AIDS. 24 hours per day, 7 days per week.

National AIDS Information Clearinghouse
(800) 458-5231
Distributes a number of publications about AIDS, including the Surgeon General's report and American Red Cross publications. Refers callers to local information numbers for specific information about AIDS and treatment sources. A service of the Public Health Service, 9 a.m. to 7 p.m. eastern standard time.

AMC Cancer Information
(800) 525-3777
Provides information about causes of cancer, prevention, methods of detection and diagnosis, treatment and treatment facilities, rehabilitation, and counseling services. A service of AMC Cancer Research Center, Denver, CO, 8 a.m. to 5 p.m. mountain time.

Cancer Care, National Cancer Foundation
(212) 302-2400
Provides professional counseling, planning, and some home care assistance to patients and families. Distributes materials about the impact of catastrophic illness on families and on the mental health of children.

National Library Service for the Blind and Physically Handicapped
    (202) 287-5100
        Works through local and regional libraries to provide free library service to persons unable
        to read or use standard printed materials because of visual or physical impairment.
        Provides information about blindness and physical handicaps on request. A list of par-
        ticipating libraries is available.

Cancer Information Service (CIS)
    (800) 4-CANCER
    (800) 524-1234 in Oahu, HI
    (800) 638-6070 in Arkansas
    (301) 427-8656 in Maryland
        Answers cancer-related questions from the public, cancer patients and families, and health
        professionals. No diagnosis is made or treatment recommended. Spanish-speaking staff
        members are available to callers from the following areas: California, Florida, Georgia,
        Illinois, northern New Jersey, New York City, and Texas. A service of the National
        Cancer Institute, 9 a.m. to 10 p.m. eastern standard time daily, 10 a.m. to 6 p.m.
        Saturday.

Y-Me Breast Cancer Support Group
    (800) 221-2141
    (312) 799-8228 in Illinois
        Provides breast cancer patients with presurgery counseling, treatment information, and
        patient literature; also makes referrals according to guidelines from its medical advisory
        board. 9 a.m. to 5 p.m. central time. Local number, 24 hours per day, 7 days per week.

Clearinghouse on the Handicapped
    (202) 732-1244
        Responds to inquiries by referral to organizations that supply information to handicapped
        individuals relating to their own disabilities. Provides information about federal benefits,
        funding, and legislation for the handicapped.

Children's Hospice International
    (800) 242-4453
    (703) 684-0330 in Virginia
        Provides support system and resource bank–sharing expertise and information with health
        care professionals, families, and the network of organizations within a community that
        offer hospice care to terminally ill children. Distributes educational materials. 9 a.m. to
        5 p.m. eastern standard time.

Hospice Education Institute Hospicelink
    (800) 331-1620
    (203) 767-1620 in Connecticut
        Offers general information about hospice care and makes referrals to local programs. Does
        not offer medical advice or personal counseling. 9 a.m. to 5 p.m. eastern standard time.

ODPHP National Health Information Center
    (301) 565-4167
        Helps the public locate health information through identification of health information
        resources and an inquiry and referral system. The center, formerly the National Health

Information Clearinghouse, refers questions to appropriate resources that in turn respond directly to inquiries. Prepares and distributes publications and directories about health promotion and disease prevention topics.

National Rehabilitation Information Center
 (301) 588-9284 in Maryland
 (800) 342-2742 (voice and TDD)
  Provides information about disability-related research, resources, and products for independent living. Provides fact sheets, resource guides, and research and technical publications.

Second Surgical Opinion Hotline
 (800) 638-6833
 (800) 492-6603 in Maryland
  Helps consumers locate a specialist near them for a second opinion in nonemergency surgery. A service of the Health Care Financing Administration. Department of Health and Human Services. 8 a.m. to 12 a.m. daily.

National Second Surgical Opinion Program
 (800) 638-6833
 (800) 492-6603 in Maryland
  Provides information for people faced with the possibility of nonemergency surgery. Sponsors a toll-free telephone number to assist the public in locating a surgeon or other specialist.

# Community Clinical Oncology Program

The National Cancer Institute (NCI) launched a large-scale Community Clinical Oncology Program (CCOP) with the awarding of funds in fiscal year 1983 to community hospitals or groups of community cancer specialists across the country. As of January 1988 there were 52 CCOPs in 31 states.

The program is designed to combine the expertise of community physicians with ongoing research projects and to introduce the newest clinical research findings into community settings. Evaluation results to date show that the CCOP has been effective in accruing patients to clinical research protocols. More than 13,600 patients were entered in research studies through CCOPs in the program's first 3 years. There has been a notable increase in the number of community physicians and hospitals participating in clinical research since the inception of the CCOP.

Qualified community physicians participate in clinical trials by affiliating with NCI-supported treatment study programs at research bases—major medical centers and national and regional clinical cooperative groups—that conduct large treatment studies. Each community program is expected to enter evaluable patients on approved clinical research protocols being conducted in the centers or cooperative groups that have been selected for inclusion among the program's research affiliations. Currently there are 17 such research bases.

A clinical trial evaluates the newest treatments for cancer patients. The research therapies used in a clinical trial are designed to answer specific questions to find new and better ways to help cancer patients. By increasing the number of patients in treatment studies, the program reduces the time needed to find answers to important questions about new therapies. All patients involved in research studies must provide informed consent.

What follows is a list of the 52 currently funded CCOPs, their principal investigators, and their locations. The currently funded research bases are also listed. Some of the individual community programs are single clinics, groups of practicing oncologists, or single hospitals. Others are consortia of physicians, clinics, and hospitals. NCI funding goes to each local program through a community hospital or health care organization associated with that program, and treatment of patients is directed by the local physicians.

A second request for applications for the CCOP issued in July 1986 resulted in 133 applications. The program requirements have been expanded to include participation in cancer control research in addition to clinical treatment research. Additional cancer control research responsibilities will provide a basis for involving a wider segment of the community (including minority groups and underserved populations) in cancer control research and for investigating the impact of cancer therapy and control advances on community medical practices. This will also increase the involvement of primary health care providers and other specialists (e.g., surgeons, urologists, and gynecologists) as well as state health departments with the CCOP investigators in treatment and cancer control research, providing an opportunity for education and exchange of information.

For additional information about cancer, write to the Office of Cancer Communications, National Cancer Institute, Bethesda, MD 20892 or call the toll-free telephone number of the Cancer Information Service: 1-800-4-CANCER. In Alaska, call 1-800-638-6070; in Hawaii, on Oahu call 524-1234 (neighbor islands call collect). Spanish-speaking staff members are available to callers from the following areas (daytime hours only): California, Florida, Georgia, Illinois, New Jersey (area code 201), New York, and Texas.

## Community Clinical Oncology Programs (CCOPs)

### Principal Investigators and Components

When a component does not have a city with its title, it is located in the CCOP office city.

**ARIZONA**
Phoenix:

GREATER PHOENIX CCOP
1117 Willeta Ave.
Phoenix, AZ 85006

David K. King, MD
(602)239-2413

Hospitals

Good Samaritan Medical Center
John C. Lincoln Hospital and
   Health Center
Maricopa Medical Center
Maryvale Samaritan Hospital
St. Joseph's Hospital and Medical Center
Phoenix Children's Hospital
Thunderbird Samaritan Hospital,
   Glendale

**CALIFORNIA**
Fresno:

SAN JOAQUIN VALLEY CCOP
Fresno Community Hospital
PO Box 1232
Fresno, CA 93715

Phyllis Ager Mowry, MD
(209)442-3959

### Hospitals

Fresno Community Hospital/
  Medical Center
Veterans Administration Hospital
Valley Medical Center
Saint Agnes Hospital

Bakersfield:
Greater Bakersfield Memorial Hospital
Kern Medical Center
Mercy Hospital
San Joaquin Community Hospital

### Outpatient Cancer Center

Regional Cancer and
  Blood Disease Center
  of Kern

Los Angeles:
CENTRAL LOS ANGELES CCOP
Los Angeles Oncologic Institute
St. Vincent Medical Center
2131 West Third Street
Los Angeles, CA 90057

Cary A. Presant, MD
(818)960-5581

### Hospital

St. Vincent Medical Center

Sacramento:
SACRAMENTO CCOP
Sutter Community Hospitals
Sutter Cancer Center
5275 F Street
Sacramento, CA 95819

Vincent Caggiano, MD
(916)733-1098

### Hospitals

Sutter Community Hospitals
Mercy Hospital of Sacramento

## DELAWARE
Wilmington:
THE MEDICAL CENTER OF
  DELAWARE COMMUNITY CLINICAL
  ONCOLOGY PROGRAM
ATTN: Pauline Lauer, Rm 406
PO Box 1668
Wilmington, DE 19899

Irving M. Berkowitz, MD
(302)731-8116

### Hospitals

Medical Center of Delaware, Inc
Wilmington Hospital, Wilmington
Christiana Hospital, Newark

**FLORIDA**
Gainesville:    FLORIDA PEDIATRIC CCOP                James L. Talbert, MD
                Florida Association of Pediatric Tumor   (904)375-6848
                   Programs
                PO Box 13372, University Station
                Gainesville, FL 32604

                Hospitals

                All Children's Hospital, St. Petersburg
                Jacksonville Wolfson Children's Hospital
                Orlando Regional Medical Center
                Sacred Heart Children's Hospital,
                   Pensacola
                Pediatric University Hospital, San Juan,
                   Puerto Rico
                Auxilio Mutuo Hospital, Hato Rey,
                   Puerto Rico


Miami Beach:    MT. SINAI COMMUNITY ONCOLOGY         Mark C. Wallack, MD
                   PROGRAM                            (305)674-2760
                Mt. Sinai Medical Center, Department of
                   Surgery
                4300 Alton Road
                Miami Beach, FL 33140

                Hospital

                Mt. Sinai Medical Center


**GEORGIA**
Atlanta:        ATLANTA REGIONAL CCOP                Colleen S. Austin, MD
                St. Joseph's Hospital                 (404)851-6615
                5665 Peachtree Dunwoody Rd, NE
                Atlanta, GA 30342-1701

                Hospital

                St. Joseph's Hospital of Atlanta


Augusta:        UNIVERSITY HOSPITAL CCOP             Stephen M. Shlaer, MD
                University Hospital                   (404)722-4245
                1350 Walton Way
                Augusta, GA 30910

                Hospitals

                University Hospital
                Medical College of Georgia

**ILLINOIS**

| | | |
|---|---|---|
| Evanston: | COMMUNITY CLINICAL ONCOLOGY<br>   PROGRAM<br>KELLOGG CANCER CENTER<br>EVANSTON HOSPITAL<br>2650 Ridge Avenue<br>Evanston, IL 60201 | J.D. Khandekar, MD<br>(312)492-2000 |

Hospital

Evanston Hospital

| | | |
|---|---|---|
| Peoria: | ILLINOIS ONCOLOGY RESEARCH<br>   ASSOCIATION<br>COMMUNITY CLINICAL ONCOLOGY<br>   PROGRAM<br>Methodist Medical Center of Illinois<br>214 NE Glen Oak Avenue, Suite 605<br>Peoria, IL 61603 | Stephen A. Cullinan,<br>   MD<br>(309)672-5780 |

Hospitals

The Methodist Medical Center of Illinois
St. Francis Medical Center

Offices

Oncology-Hematology
   Associates of Illinois
Midwest Radiation
   Therapy Consultants,
   Ltd

| | | |
|---|---|---|
| Springfield: | CENTRAL ILLINOIS CCOP<br>Voluntary Hospitals of America–IL<br>520 North 4th Street<br>Springfield, IL 62702 | J. Gale Katterhagen,<br>   MD<br>(217)788-4959 |

Hospitals

Memorial Medical Center
Decatur Memorial Hospital

Health System

Voluntary Hospitals of
   America–Illinois

| | | |
|---|---|---|
| Urbana: | CARLE CANCER CENTER CCOP<br>Carle Clinic Association<br>602 West University Avenue<br>Urbana, IL 61801 | Alan Kramer Hatfield,<br>   MD<br>(217)337-3010 |

Hospital

Carle Foundation Hospital

**IOWA**

Des Moines:    IOWA ONCOLOGY RESEARCH          Roscoe Morton, MD
               ASSOCIATION                     (515)244-7586
               Community Clinical Oncology Program
               1048 Fourth Avenue
               Des Moines, IA 50314

               Hospitals

               Iowa Methodist Medical Center
               Iowa Lutheran Hospital
               Mercy Hospital Medical Center
               Des Moines General Hospital
               Charter Community Hospital

**KANSAS**

Wichita:       WICHITA CCOP                    Henry E. Hynes, MD
               St. Francis Regional Medical Center    (316)262-4467
               929 N St. Francis
               Box 1358
               Wichita, KS 67201

               Hospitals

               St. Francis Regional Medical Center
               St. Joseph Medical Center
               Wesley Medical Center

**LOUISIANA**

New Orleans:   OCHSNER CCOP                    Carl G. Kardinal, MD
               Ochsner Clinic                  (504)838-3910
               1514 Jefferson Highway
               New Orleans, LA 70121

               Hospitals                       Group Practices

               Ochsner Foundation Hospital     Radiation Oncology
               Children's Hospital                Center, Baton Rouge
               Forrest General Hospital, Hattiesburg,    General
                  MS                           Mary Bird Perkins
               Methodist Hospital, Hattiesburg, MS    Radiation Center
               Medical Center of Baton Rouge   Ochsner Clinic, New
                                                  Orleans
                                               Hattiesburg Clinic, MS
                                               Intercommunity Cancer
                                                  Center
                                               Ochsner Clinic, Baton
                                                  Rouge

**MAINE**

Bangor:

EASTERN MAINE MEDICAL CENTER
Cancer Control Program
c/o EMMC Tumor Clinic
489 State Street
Bangor, ME 04401-6674

Alan W. Boone, MD
(207)945-7481

Hospital

Eastern Maine Medical Center

Portland:

SOUTHERN MAINE CCOP
Oncology Hematology Associates
180 Park Avenue
Portland, ME 04102

Ronald J. Carroll, MD
(207)773-1754

Hospitals

Maine Medical Center
Mercy Hospital
Southern Maine Medical Center,
  Biddeford
St. Mary's Hospital, Lewiston
Central Maine Medical Center, Lewiston

Offices

Oncology/Hematology
  Associates
Stephen Blattner, MD

**MICHIGAN**

Grand
Rapids:

GRAND RAPIDS CCOP
Butterworth Hospital
100 Michigan NE
Grand Rapids, MI 49503

James Borst, MD
(616)774-1230

Hospitals

Blodgett Memorial Medical Center
Butterworth Hospital
Ferguson Hospital
Saint Mary's Hospital
Metropolitan Hospital
Holland Community Hospital

Kalamazoo:

KALAMAZOO CCOP
Borgess Medical Center
1521 Gull Road
Kalamazoo, MI 49001

Phillip Stott, MD
(616)383-7007

Hospitals

Borgess Medical Center
Bronson Methodist Hospital

**MINNESOTA**
Duluth:

COMMUNITY CLINICAL ONCOLOGY
   PROGRAM
THE DULUTH CLINIC, LTD
400 East Third Street
Duluth, MN 55805

James E. Krook, MD
(218)722-8364,
   extension 311

Hospital

St. Mary's Medical Center

Group/Office Practice

The Duluth Clinic, Ltd
Miller-Dwan Radiation
   Therapy Department

St. Louis
Park:

W. METRO–MINNEAPOLIS CCOP
Park-Nicollet Medical Foundation
5000 West 39th Street
St. Louis Park, MN 55416

Patrick J. Flynn, MD
(612)927-3491
Ann Deshler, RN
(612)927-3491 or
   927-3301

Hospitals

Methodist Hospital
Abbott-Northwestern Hospital,
   Minneapolis
Metropolitan Medical Center, Minneapolis
North Memorial Medical Center,
   Robbinsdale
Fairview-Southdale Hospital, Edina
Mercy Medical Center, Coon Rapids
Unity Medical Center, Fridley

Group Practice

Park-Nicollet Medical
Center

**MISSISSIPPI**
Tupelo:

NORTH MISSISSIPPI CCOP
North Mississippi Medical Center
830 South Gloster Street
Tupelo, MS 38801

Julian B. Hill, MD
(601)844-9166

Hospital

North Mississippi Medical Center

**MISSOURI**
Columbia:

COMMUNITY CLINICAL ONCOLOGY
   PROGRAM
ELLIS FISCHEL STATE CANCER
   CENTER
115 Business Loop 70 West
Columbia, MO 65203

Ronald Vincent, MD
(314)875-2100

Hospital

Ellis Fischel State Cancer Center

Kansas City:      KANSAS CITY CLINICAL ONCOLOGY        Robert J. Belt, MD
                      PROGRAM                          (816)276-7834
                  Baptist Memorial Hospital
                  6601 Rockhill Road
                  Kansas City, MO 64131

                  Hospitals

                  Baptist Medical Hospital
                  Menorah Medical Center
                  Research Medical Center
                  St. Mary's Hospital
                  Trinity Lutheran Hospital
                  Shawnee Mission Medical Center,
                      Shawnee Mission


Springfield:      OZARK REGIONAL CCOP                  John W. Goodwin, MD
                  621 East Elm                         (417)883-7422
                  Springfield, MO 65806

                  Hospitals

                  St. John's Regional Health Center
                  Lester E. Cox Medical Centers


St. Louis:        ST. LOUIS CCOP                       Patrick H. Henry, MD
                  Suite 3018                           (314)569-6959
                  St. John's Mercy Medical Center
                  621 South New Ballas Road
                  St. Louis, MO 63141

                  Hospitals

                  Christian Hospital NE/NW
                  Missouri Baptist Hospital
                  St. John's Mercy Medical Center
                  St. Joseph's Hospital, Kirkwood
                  DePaul Health Center, Bridgeton


**NEVADA**
  Las Vegas:      SOUTHERN NEVADA CANCER               John A. Ellerton, MD
                      RESEARCH FOUNDATION CCOP         (702)384-0013
                  501 South Rancho Drive
                  Suite C-14
                  Las Vegas, NV 89106

                  Hospitals

                  University Medical Center of Southern
                      Nevada
                  Valley Hospital Medical Center

**NEW JERSEY**

Hackensack:  BERGEN-PASSAIC CCOP
Hackensack Medical Center
30 Prospect Avenue
Hackensack, NJ 07601

Richard Rosenbluth,
MD
(201)441-2363

Hospitals

Hackensack Medical Center
Holy Name Hospital, Teaneck

**NEW YORK**

Binghamton:  TWIN TIERS CCOP
Our Lady of Lourdes Hospital
169 Riverside Drive
Binghamton, NY 13905

Bruce D. Boselli, MD
(717)888-5858,
  extension 2141

Hospitals

Our Lady of Lourdes Memorial Hospital
Robert Packer Hospital, Sayre, PA

Manhasset:  NORTH SHORE UNIVERSITY
  HOSPITAL CCOP
Don Monti Division of Oncology
300 Community Drive
Manhasset, NY 11030

Vincent P. Vinciguerra,
MD
(516)562-4160

Hospitals

North Shore University Hospital–
  Division of Oncology
North Shore University
  Hospital–Pediatrics
The New York Hospital, New York City
University of Connecticut Health Center,
  Farmington
State University Hospital, Brooklyn
Brookdale Hospital Medical Center,
  Brooklyn
Montefiore Medical Center, Bronx

Offices

Robert Weiner, MD
Ezriel Diamond, MD
Joseph Pipala, MD
Michael Dosik, MD
Mark Lipshutz, MD
Francis Arena, MD
Hal Gerstein, MD
Reed Phillips, MD
Klaus Dittmar, MD
Frank Tomao, MD
Francis X. Moore, MD
Robert Levy, MD
Jakow Diener, MD
Farida Chaudhri, MD

New York:  ST. VINCENT'S CCOP OF NEW YORK
St. Vincent's Hospital and Medical Center
153 West 11th Street, Cronin 812
New York, NY 10011

Mary M. Kemeny, MD
(212)790-8368

Hospital

St. Vincent's Hospital and Medical Center

Rochester:          IROQUOIS CCOP                                    Kishan J. Pandya, MD
                    St. Mary's Hospital Medical Oncology            (716)464-3591
                    89 Genesee Street
                    Rochester, NY 14611

                    Hospitals

                    St. Mary's Hospital
                    Mary Imogene Bassett Hospital,
                        Cooperstown


Syracuse:           HEMATOLOGY-ONCOLOGY                              Santo M. DiFino, MD
                        ASSOCIATES OF CENTRAL NEW                    (315)474-6391
                        YORK
                    COMMUNITY CLINICAL ONCOLOGY
                        PROGRAM
                    101 Union Avenue, Suite 611
                    Syracuse, NY 13203

                    Hospitals                                        Offices

                    St. Joseph's Hospital Health Center             Hematology-Oncology
                    Crouse Irving Memorial Hospital                     Associates of Central
                    Community General Hospital                          New York


**NORTH**
**CAROLINA**
    Winston-        SOUTHEAST CANCER CONTROL                         Charles L. Spurr, MD
    Salem:              CONSORTIUM                                   (919)748-3142
                    COMMUNITY CLINICAL ONCOLOGY
                        PROGRAM
                    1940 Beech Street
                    Winston-Salem, NC 27103-2643

                    Hospitals                                        Group Practices

                    Forsyth Memorial Hospital                        Brodkin, Slatkoff &
                    Medical Park Hospital                                Hopkins, Winston-
                    Memorial Mission Hospital, Asheville                 Salem
                    St. Joseph's Hospital, Asheville                 Asheville Hematology &
                    Veterans Administration Medical Center,              Oncology Associates
                        Asheville                                    Wilmington Health
                    Presbyterian Hospital, Charlotte                     Associates
                    The Moses H. Cone Memorial Hospital,             Department of
                        Greensboro                                       Radiation Therapy,
                                                                         New Hanover
                                                                         Memorial, Hospital,
                                                                         Wilmington
                                                                     James F. Wortman,
                                                                         MD, Wilmington

Southeast Cancer Control Consortium, **SOUTH CAROLINA**
       Richland Memorial Hospital, Columbia    Carolina Health
       Baptist Medical Center, Columbia          Care–Companion
       W.J.B./Dorn V.A. Hospital, Columbia     HMO, Florence
       Self Memorial Hospital, Greenwood      Piedmont Internal
       McLeod Regional Medical Center,         Medicine, Greenwood
          Florence


Southeast Cancer Control Consortium, **TENNESSEE**
       Holston Valley Hospital & Medical Center,   Ervin A. Hire, MD,
          Kingsport                        Kingsport
                                         Ruth T. Young, MD,
                                         Kingsport
                                         Talton Brooks, MD,
                                         Kingsport


Southeast Cancer Control Consortium, **VIRGINIA**
       Memorial Hospital, Danville            David C. Caldwell, MD
       Memorial Hospital of Martinsville and
          Henry County


**NORTH DAKOTA**
    Fargo:        ST. LUKE'S HOSPITALS CCOP     Greg McCormack, MD
               5th Street at Mills Avenue          (701)237-2397
               Fargo, ND 58122

               Hospital                        Group Practice

               St. Luke's Hospitals             Fargo Clinic Ltd, Merit
                                            Care


**OHIO**
    Columbus:     COLUMBUS CCOP             Jerry T. Guy, MD
               Grant Medical Center           (614)461-3295
               111 South Grant Avenue
               Columbus, OH 43215

               Hospitals

               Mt. Carmel Health
               Grant Medical Center
               St. Anthony Medical Center
               Doctors Hospital (North and West)
               Community Hospital (Springfield and
                 Clark County), Springfield
               Mercy Medical Center, Springfield

| | | |
|---|---|---|
| Dayton-<br>Kettering: | DAYTON CCOP<br>Kettering Medical Center<br>3525 Southern Boulevard<br>Kettering, OH 45429 | James S. Ungerleider,<br>MD<br>(513)299-7204 |

Hospitals

Good Samaritan Hospital
Grandview Hospital
Kettering Medical Center, Kettering
Miami Valley Hospital
St. Elizabeth Medical Center
Veterans Administration Medical Center

| | | |
|---|---|---|
| Toledo: | TOLEDO CCOP<br>Toledo Community Hospital Oncology<br>    Program<br>3314 Collingwood, Suite 502<br>Toledo, OH 43610 | Charles D. Cobau, MD<br>(419)255-5433 |

Hospitals                                          Group Practice

The Toledo Hospital                                The Toledo Clinic
Riverside Hospital
Flower Memorial Hospital, Sylvania
St. Charles Hospital, Oregon, OH
Fremont Memorial Hospital, Fremont, OH
Firelands Community Hospital, Sandusky,
    OH
Emma L. Bixby Hospital, Adrian, MI
St. Joseph Mercy Hospital, Ann Arbor, MI

**OKLAHOMA**

| | | |
|---|---|---|
| Tulsa: | NATALIE WARREN BRYANT CCOP<br>Saint Francis Hospital/NWBCC<br>6161 South Yale<br>Tulsa, OK 74136 | Alan M. Keller, MD<br>(918)494-1530 |

Hospital

Natalie Warren Bryant Cancer Center

**OREGON**

| | | |
|---|---|---|
| Portland: | COLUMBIA RIVER CCOP<br>Providence Medical Center<br>4805 NE Glisan<br>Portland, OR 97213 | Gordon L. Doty, MD<br>(503)239-7767 |

Hospitals

Emanuel Hospital
Good Samaritan Hospital and Medical
    Center
Providence Medical Center
St. Vincent Hospital and Medical Center
Southwest Washington Hospitals,
    Vancouver, WA


**PENNSYLVANIA**
Danville:       GEISINGER CLINIC ONCOLOGY          Albert M. Bernath, MD
                    PROGRAM                         (717)271-6413
                Department of Hematology/Oncology
                Geisinger Medical Center
                North Academy Avenue
                Danville, PA 17822

                Hospital

                Geisinger Clinic and Medical Center


Pittsburgh:     ALLEGHENY CCOP                      Reginald P. Pugh, MD
                Division of Medical Oncology        (412)359-3630
                Allegheny General Hospital
                320 East North Avenue
                Pittsburgh, PA 15212-9986

                Hospitals

                Allegheny General Hospital
                Sewickley Valley Hospital
                YHA, Inc Western Reserve Care System
                The Washington Hospital, Washington
                Frick Community Health Center,
                    Mt. Pleasant
                Jameson Memorial Hospital, New Castle


Scranton:       MERCY HOSPITAL CCOP                 William J. Heim, MD
                Mercy Hospital                      (717)342-3675
                746 Jefferson Avenue
                Scranton, PA 18501

                Hospital                            Group Practice

                Mercy Hospital                      Hematology and
                                                        Oncology Associates
                                                        of Northeast
                                                        Pennsylvania

**SOUTH CAROLINA** (See also above listings under **North Carolina**, Southeast Cancer Control Consortium)

Spartanburg: SPARTANBURG CCOP
Oncology Research Department
Spartanburg Regional Medical Center
101 East Wood Street
Spartanburg, SC 29303

John H. McCulloch, MD
(803)585-8343

Hospitals

Spartanburg Regional Medical Center
Mary Black Memorial Hospital
Doctors Memorial Hospital

**SOUTH DAKOTA**

Sioux Falls: SIOUX FALLS COMMUNITY CANCER
CONSORTIUM
Central Plains Clinic, Ltd
1301 South 9th Avenue, Suite 501
Sioux Falls, SD 57105

Loren K. Tschetter, MD
(605)331-3160

Hospitals

McKennan Hospital
Veterans Administration Hospital
Sioux Valley Hospital

Offices

Medical Oncology
Associates
Central Plains Clinic,
Ltd
Medical X-Ray Center

**TENNESSEE** See above, Southeast Cancer Control Consortium, **TENNESSEE**

**VERMONT**

Rutland: GREEN MOUNTAIN ONCOLOGY
GROUP
Cancer Program Office
160 Allen Street
Rutland, VT 05701

H. James Wallace, Jr.,
MD
(802)775-7111,
extension 184

Hospitals

Rutland Regional Medical Center
Central Vermont Hospital, Barre
Fanny Allen Hospital, Winooski

**VIRGINIA** (See also above listings for Virginia under **NORTH CAROLINA** Southeast Cancer Control Consortium)

Roanoke:   CCOP OF ROANOKE
Roanoke Hospital Association
PO Box 13367
Roanoke, VA 24033

Stephen H. Rosenoff, MD
(703)981-7424

Hospitals

Roanoke Memorial Hospitals
Community Hospital of Roanoke Valley
Lewis-Gale Hospital, Salem
Veterans Administration Medical Center, Salem
Bluefield Community Hospital, WV

Group Practices

Oncology and Hematology Associates of Southwest Virginia
Lewis-Gale Clinic, Salem

**WASHINGTON**

Seattle:   CCOP–VIRGINIA MASON RESEARCH CENTER
The Mason Clinic
1000 Seneca Street, RI-RC
Seattle, WA 98101

Albert B. Einstein, Jr., MD
(206)223-6942

Hospitals

Virginia Mason Medical Center
Valley Medical Center, Renton
Evergreen Hospital Medical Center, Kirkland
Kadlec Medical Center, Richland

Office Practices

Valley Internal Medicine, Renton
The Richland Clinic, Richland

Tacoma:   NORTHWEST COMMUNITY CCOP
314 South K Street, Suite 108
Tacoma, WA 98405

Ronald Goldberg, MD
(206)597-7461

Hospitals

Multicare Medical Center (Tacoma General)
St. Joseph Hospital
Humana Hospital
Lakewood Hospital
St. Joseph Hospital, Aberdeen
Grays Harbor Community Hospital, Aberdeen
St. Peter Hospital, Olympia
Black Hills Community Hospital, Olympia
Good Samaritan Hospital, Puyallup
Kaiser Permanente, Portland, OR

**WEST VIRGINIA**

Charleston:     WEST VIRGINIA COMMUNITY          Steven J. Jubelirer, MD
                ONCOLOGY PROGRAM                 (304)348-9541
                Charleston Area Medical Center
                Memorial Division
                3200 MacCorkle Avenue, SE
                Charleston, WV 25304

Hospitals

Charleston Area Medical Center
Raleigh General Hospital, Beckley
St. Mary's Hospital, Huntington
Cabell Huntington Hospital, Huntington
Veterans Administration Medical Center,
     Huntington
St. Joseph's Hospital, Parkersburg
Wheeling Hospital, Wheeling

**WISCONSIN**

Marshfield:     COMMUNITY CLINICAL ONCOLOGY      Tarit K. Banerjee, MD
                PROGRAM                          (715)387-5134
                Marshfield Medical Research Foundation
                1000 North Oak Avenue
                Marshfield, WI 54449

Hospital                                         Group/Office Practice

St. Joseph's Hospital                            Marshfield Clinic

**Research Bases and Principal Investigators**

Clinical Trials Groups

ECOG     *Eastern Cooperative Oncology Group*
         Chair: Paul Carbone, MD, University of Wisconsin Clinical Cancer Center,
         Madison, WI

SWOG     *Southwest Oncology Group*
         Chair: Charles Coltman, Jr., MD, Cancer Therapy and Research Center, San
         Antonio, TX

NCCTG    *North Central Cancer Treatment Group*
         Chair: Charles Moertel, MD, Mayo Foundation, Rochester, MN

RTOG     *Radiation Therapy Oncology Group*
         Chair: James Cox, MD, American College of Radiology, Philadelphia, PA

**CALGB**   *Cancer and Leukemia Group B*
Chief of Staff: W. Bradford Patterson, MD, Dana-Farber Cancer Institute, Boston, MA

**NSABP**   *National Surgical Adjuvant Project for Breast and Bowel Cancers*
Chair: Bernard Fisher, MD, University of Pittsburgh, Pittsburgh, PA

**CCSG**   *Children's Cancer Study Group*
Chair: Denman Hammond, MD, University of Southern California, Los Angeles, CA

**POG**   *Pediatric Oncology Group*
Jeffrey Krischer, PhD, Statistical Office, University of Florida, Gainesville, FL

## NCI-Supported Cancer Centers

*Dana-Farber Cancer Institute*
W. Bradford Patterson, MD, Boston, MA

*Memorial Sloan-Kettering Cancer Center*
David Kelsen, MD, New York, NY

*Oncology Research Center, Bowman Gray School of Medicine of Wake Forest University*
Robert L. Capizzi, MD, Winston-Salem, NC

*Fox Chase Cancer Center*
John R. Durant, MD, Philadelphia, PA

*Northern California Cancer Center*
Theodore L. Phillips, MD, Belmont, CA

*University of Rochester Cancer Center*
John M. Bennett, MD, Rochester, NY

*Illinois Cancer Council*
Nancy Cairns, PhD, Chicago, IL

*M.D. Anderson Hospital and Tumor Institute*
Rodger J. Winn, MD, Houston, TX

## State Health Department

*Minnesota Department of Health*
Donald B. Bishop, PhD, Minneapolis, MN

# Comprehensive\* and Clinical\*\* Cancer Centers Supported by the National Cancer Institute

The National Cancer Institute supports a number of cancer centers throughout the country that develop and investigate new methods of cancer diagnosis and treatment. Information about referral procedures, treatment costs, and services available to patients can be obtained from the individual cancer centers listed below.

ALABAMA

**University of Alabama Comprehensive Cancer Center\***
1918 University Boulevard
Basic Health Sciences Building, Room 108
Birmingham, AL 35294
(205)934-6612

ARIZONA

**University of Arizona Cancer Center\*\***
1501 North Campbell Avenue
Tucson, AZ 85724
(602)626-6372

CALIFORNIA

**The Kenneth Norris Jr. Comprehensive Cancer Center\* and**
**The Kenneth Norris Jr. Hospital and Research Institute\*\***
University of Southern California
1441 Eastlake Avenue
Los Angeles, CA 90033-0804
(213)226-2370

**Jonsson Comprehensive Cancer Center (UCLA)\***
10-247 Factor Building
10833 Le Conte Avenue
Los Angeles, CA 90024-1781
(213)825-8727

**City of Hope National Medical Center\*\***
Beckman Research Institute
1500 East Duarte Road
Duarte, CA 91010
(818)359-8111, extension 2292

**University of California at San Diego Cancer Center\*\***
225 Dickinson Street
San Diego, CA 92103
(619)543-6178

**Charles R. Drew University of Medicine and Science**
(consortium)
12714 South Avalon Boulevard, Suite 301
Los Angeles, CA 90061
(213)603-3120

**Northern California Cancer Center** (consortium)
1301 Shoreway Road
Belmont, CA 94002
(415)591-4484

COLORADO                **University of Colorado Cancer Center\*\***
4200 East 9th Avenue, Box B190
Denver, CO 80262
(303)270-3019

CONNECTICUT             **Yale University Comprehensive Cancer Center\***
333 Cedar Street
New Haven, CT 06510
(203)785-6338

DISTRICT OF COLUMBIA    **Howard University Cancer Research Center\***
2041 Georgia Avenue, NW
Washington, DC 20060
(202)636-7610 or 636-5665

**Vincent T. Lombardi Cancer Research Center\***
Georgetown University Medical Center
3800 Reservoir Road, NW
Washington, DC 20007
(202)687-2110

FLORIDA

**Sylvester Comprehensive Cancer Center***
University of Miami Medical School
1475 Northwest 12th Avenue
Miami, FL 33136
(305)548-4850

ILLINOIS

**Illinois Cancer Council*** (includes institutions listed and several
other organizations)
Illinois Cancer Council
36 South Wabash Avenue
Chicago, IL 60603
(312)226-2371

University of Chicago Cancer Research Center
5841 South Maryland Avenue
Chicago, IL 60637
(312)702-9200

KENTUCKY

**Lucille Parker Markey Cancer Center****
University of Kentucky Medical Center
800 Rose Street
Lexington, KY 40536-0093
(606)257-4447

MARYLAND

**The Johns Hopkins Oncology Center***
600 North Wolfe Street
Baltimore, MD 21205
(301)955-8638

MASSACHUSETTS

**Dana-Farber Cancer Institute***
44 Binney Street
Boston, MA 02115
(617)732-3214

MICHIGAN

**Meyer L. Prentis Comprehensive Cancer Center of
Metropolitan Detroit***
110 East Warren Avenue
Detroit, MI 48201
(313)745-4329

**University of Michigan Cancer Center****
101 Simpson Drive
Ann Arbor, MI 48109-0752
(313)936-2516

MINNESOTA

**Mayo Comprehensive Cancer Center***
200 First Street Southwest
Rochester, MN 55905
(507)284-3413


NEW HAMPSHIRE

**Morris Cotton Cancer Center****
Dartmouth-Hitchcock Medical Center
2 Maynard Street
Hanover, NH 03756
(603)646-5505


NEW YORK

**Memorial Sloan-Kettering Cancer Center***
1275 York Avenue
New York, NY 10021
1-800-525-2225

**Columbia University Cancer Center***
College of Physicians and Surgeons
630 West 168th Street
New York, NY 10032
(212)305-6730

**Roswell Park Memorial Institute***
Elm and Carlton Streets
Buffalo, NY 14263
(716)845-4400

**Mt. Sinai School of Medicine****
One Gustave L. Levy Place
New York, NY 10029
(212)241-8617

**Albert Einstein College of Medicine****
1300 Morris Park Avenue
Bronx, NY 10461
(212)920-4826

**New York University Cancer Center****
462 First Avenue
New York, NY 10016-9103
(212)340-6485

**University of Rochester Cancer Center****
601 Elmwood Avenue, Box 704
Rochester, NY 14642
(716)275-4911

NORTH CAROLINA

**Duke University Comprehensive Cancer Center***
PO Box 3843
Durham, NC 27710
(919)286-5515

**Lineberger Cancer Research Center****
University of North Carolina School of Medicine
Chapel Hill, NC 27599
(919)966-4431

**Bowman Gray School of Medicine****
Wake Forest University
300 South Hawthorne Road
Winston-Salem, NC 27103
(919)748-4354

OHIO

**Ohio State University Comprehensive Cancer Center***
410 West 12th Avenue
Columbus, OH 43210
(614)293-8619

**Case Western Reserve University****
University Hospitals of Cleveland
Ireland Cancer Center
2074 Abington Road
Cleveland, OH 44106
(216)844-8453

PENNSYLVANIA

**Fox Chase Cancer Center***
7701 Burholme Avenue
Philadelphia, PA 19111
(215)728-2570

**University of Pennsylvania Cancer Center***
3400 Spruce Street
Philadelphia, PA 19104
(215)662-6364

**Pittsburgh Cancer Institute****
230 Lothrop Street
Pittsburgh, PA 15213-2592
1-800-537-4063

RHODE ISLAND

**Roger Williams General Hospital****
825 Chalkstone Avenue
Providence, RI 02908
(401)456-2070

TENNESSEE

**St. Jude Children's Research Hospital\*\***
332 North Lauderdale Street
Memphis, TN 38101
(901)522-0694

TEXAS

**The University of Texas M.D. Anderson Cancer Center\***
1515 Holcombe Boulevard
Houston, TX 77030
(713)792-6161 (Physicians)
(713)792-3245 (Patients)

UTAH

**Utah Regional Cancer Center\*\***
University of Utah Medical Center
50 North Medical Drive, Room 2C10
Salt Lake City, UT 84132
(801)581-4048

VERMONT

**Vermont Regional Cancer Center\*\***
University of Vermont
1 South Prospect Street
Burlington, VT 05401
(802)656-4580

VIRGINIA

**Massey Cancer Center\*\***
Medical College of Virginia
Virginia Commonwealth University
1200 East Broad Street
Richmond, VA 23298
(804)786-9641

**University of Virginia Medical Center\*\***
Box 334
Primary Care Center, Room 4520
Lee Street
Charlottesville, VA 22908
(804)924-2562

WASHINGTON

**Fred Hutchinson Cancer Research Center\***
1124 Columbia Street
Seattle, WA 98104
(206)467-4675

WISCONSIN

**Wisconsin Clinical Cancer Center***
University of Wisconsin
600 Highland Avenue
Madison, WI 53792
(608)263-6872

For additional information about cancer, write to the Office of Cancer Communications, National Cancer Institute, Bethesda, MD 20892 or call the toll-free telephone number of the Cancer Information Service: 1-800-4-CANCER. In Hawaii, on Oahu call 524-1234 (neighbor islands call collect). Spanish-speaking staff members are available to callers from the following areas (daytime hours only): California, Florida, Georgia, Illinois, New Jersey (area code 201), New York, and Texas.

*Source:* From "Community Clinical Oncology Program" in *Cancer Facts*, Bethesda, MD.: The Office of Cancer Communications, National Cancer Institute, January 1988.

# Chartered Divisions of the American Cancer Society, Inc.

**Alabama Division, Inc.**
402 Office Park Drive
Suite 300
Birmingham, Alabama 35223
(205) 879-2242

**Alaska Division, Inc.**
406 West Fireweed Lane
Suite 204
Anchorage, Alaska 99503
(907) 277-8696

**Arizona Division, Inc.**
2929 East Thomas Road
Phoenix, Arizona 85016
(602) 224-0524

**Arkansas Division, Inc.**
P.O. Box 3822
Little Rock, Arkansas 72203
(501) 664-3480-1-2

**California Division, Inc.**
1710 Webster Street
P.O. Box 2061
Oakland, California 94612
(415) 893-7900

**Colorado Division, Inc.**
2255 South Oneida
P.O. Box 24669
Denver, Colorado 80224
(303) 758-2030

**Connecticut Division, Inc.**
Barnes Park South
14 Village Lane
Wallingford, Connecticut 06492
(203) 265-7161

**Delaware Division, Inc.**
1708 Lovering Avenue
Suite 202
Wilmington, Delaware 19806
(302) 654-6267

**District of Columbia Division, Inc.**
Universal Building, South
1825 Connecticut Avenue, N.W.
Suite 315
Washington, D.C. 20009
(202) 483-2600

**Florida Division, Inc.**
1001 South MacDill Avenue
Tampa, Florida 33629
(813) 253-0541

**Georgia Division, Inc.**
46 Fifth Street, NE
Atlanta, Georgia 30308
(404) 892-0026

**Hawaii Pacific Division, Inc.**
Community Services Center Bldg.
200 North Vineyard Boulevard
Honolulu, Hawaii 96817
(808) 531-1662-3-4-5

**Idaho Division, Inc.**
1609 Abbs Street
P.O. Box 5386
Boise, Idaho 83705
(208) 343-4609

**Illinois Division, Inc.**
37 South Wabash Avenue
Chicago, Illinois 60603
(312) 372-0472

**Indiana Division, Inc.**
9575 N. Valparaiso Ct.
Indianapolis, Indiana 46268
(317) 872-4432

**Iowa Division, Inc.**
8364 Hickman Road, Suite D
Des Moines, Iowa 50322
(515) 253-0147

**Kansas Division, Inc.**
3003 Van Buren Street
Topeka, Kansas 66611
(913) 267-0131

**Kentucky Division, Inc.**
Medical Arts Bldg.
1169 Eastern Parkway
Louisville, Kentucky 40217
(502) 459-1867

**Louisiana Division, Inc.**
Fidelity Homestead Bldg.
837 Gravier Street
Suite 700
New Orleans, Louisiana 70112-1509
(504) 523-2029

**Maine Division, Inc.**
52 Federal Street
Brunswick, Maine 04011
(207) 729-3339

**Maryland Division, Inc.***
8219 Town Center Drive
P.O. Box 82
White Marsh, Maryland 21162-0082
(301)529-7272

**Massachusetts Division, Inc.**
Carhart Memorial Bldg.
247 Commonwealth Avenue
Boston, Massachusetts 02116
(617) 267-2650

**Michigan Division, Inc.**
1205 East Saginaw Street
Lansing, Michigan 48906
(517) 371-2920

**Minnesota Division, Inc.**
3316 West 66th Street
Minneapolis, Minnesota 55435
(612) 925-2772

**Mississippi Division, Inc.**
1380 Livingston Lane
Lakeover Office Park
Jackson, Mississippi 39213
(601) 362-8874

**Missouri Division, Inc.**
3322 American Avenue
Jefferson City, Missouri 65102
(314) 893-4800

**Montana Division, Inc.**
313 N. 32nd Street
Suite #1
Billings, Montana 59101
(406) 252-7111

**Nebraska Division, Inc.**
8502 West Center Road
Omaha, Nebraska 68124-5255
(402) 393-5800

**Nevada Division, Inc.**
1325 East Harmon
Las Vegas, Nevada 89119
(702) 798-6877

**New Hampshire Division, Inc.†**
360 Route 101, Unit 501
Bedford, New Hampshire 03102-6821
(603) 669-3270

**New Jersey Division, Inc.**
2600 Route 1, CNN 2201
North Brunswick, New Jersey 08902
(201) 297-8000

**New Mexico Division, Inc.**
5800 Lomas Blvd., N.E.
Albuquerque, New Mexico 87110
(505) 262-2336

**New York State Division, Inc.**
6725 Lyons Street, P.O. Box 7
East Syracuse, New York 13057
(315) 437-7025

☐ **Long Island Division, Inc.**
145 Pidgeon Hill Road
Huntington Station, New York 11746
(516) 385-9100

☐ **New York City Division, Inc.**
19 West 56th Street
New York, New York 10019
(212) 586-8700

☐ **Queens Division, Inc.**
112-25 Queens Boulevard
Forest Hills, New York 11375
(718) 263-2224

☐ **Westchester Division, Inc.**
30 Glenn St.
White Plains, New York 10603
(914) 949-4800

**North Carolina Division, Inc.**
11 South Boylan Avenue
Suite 221
Raleigh, North Carolina 27603
(919) 834-8463

**North Dakota Division, Inc.**
Hotel Graver Annex Bldg.
115 Roberts Street
P.O. Box 426
Fargo, North Dakota 58107
(701) 232-1385

**Ohio Division, Inc.**
5555 Frantz Road
Dublin, Ohio 43017
(614) 889-9565

**Oklahoma Division, Inc.**
300 United Founders Blvd.
Suite 136
Oklahoma City, Oklahoma 73112
(405) 946-5000

**Oregon Division, Inc.**
0330 S.W. Curry
Portland, Oregon 97201
(503) 295-6422

**Pennsylvania Division, Inc.**
Route 422 & Sipe Avenue
Hershey, Pennsylvania 17033-0897
(717) 533-6144

☐ **Philadelphia Division, Inc.**
1422 Chestnut Street
Philadelphia, Pennsylvania 19102
(215) 665-2900

**Puerto Rico Division, Inc.**
Calle Alverio #577,
Esquina Sargento Medina,
Hato Rey, Puerto Rico 00936
(809) 764-2295

**Rhode Island Division, Inc.**
400 Main Street
Pawtucket, Rhode Island 02860
(401) 722-8480

**South Carolina Division, Inc.**
2214 Devine Street
Columbia, South Carolina 29205
(803) 256-0245

**South Dakota Division, Inc.**
4101 Carnegie Circle
Sioux Falls, South Dakota 57106-2322
(605) 336-0897

**Tennessee Division, Inc.**
1315 Eighth Avenue, South
Nashville, Tennessee 37203
(615) 255-1ACS

**Texas Division, Inc.**
P.O. Box 140435
Austin, Texas 78714-0435
(512) 928-2262

**Utah Division, Inc.**
610 East South Temple
Salt Lake City, Utah 84102
(801) 322-0431

**Vermont Division, Inc.**
13 Loomis Street, Drawer C
Montpelier, Vermont 05602
(802) 223-2348

**Virginia Division, Inc.**
4240 Park Place Court
Glen Allen, Virginia 23060
(804) 270-0142/(800) 552-7996

**Washington Division, Inc.**
2120 First Avenue North
Seattle, Washington 98109-1140
(206) 283-1152

**West Virginia Division, Inc.**
2428 Kanawha Boulevard
East Charleston, West Virginia 25311
(304) 344-3611

**Wisconsin Division, Inc.**
615 North Sherman Avenue
Madison, Wisconsin 53704
(608) 249-0487

**Wyoming Division, Inc.**
3109 Boxelder Drive
Cheyenne, Wyoming 82001
(307) 638-3331

# National Headquarters: American Cancer Society, Inc., 1599 Clifton Road N.E., Atlanta, GA 30329

*New address effective March 1, 1989

†New address effective April 15, 1989

*Source:* Reprinted by permission of the American Cancer Society, Inc.

*Source:* From "Comprehensive and Clinical Cancer Centers Supported by the National Cancer Institute" in *Cancer Facts*, Bethesda, MD.: The Office of Cancer Communications, National Cancer Institute, April 1989.

# Services and Programs

The American Cancer Society (ACS) provides numerous national and local services, including the following national services and rehabilitation programs. These programs are designed to help patients learn more about their disease and its treatment and to provide psychologic and social support. I Can Cope, Reach to Recovery, CanSurmount, "Look Good . . . Feel Better," and the Cancer Adjustment Program are open to any interested persons. Information about these programs is available from state chapters of the ACS.

The **I Can Cope** program is a patient and family education program available in large clinics and hospitals. This program provides information about cancer therapy, treatment, side effects, nutrition, resource availability, and other topics of interest.

**Reach to Recovery** is a breast cancer rehabilitation program designed to assist the woman who has or has had breast cancer in the physical, emotional, and cosmetic needs related to her disease and its treatment. In addition, literature and services are available to help the husband or significant other, children, and friends of the breast cancer patient.

**CanSurmount** is a program run by cancer patients who are trained to help other cancer patients adjust to the physical, psychologic, and social problems brought on by their condition.

CanSurmount is a basic patient visitor program designed as a short-term program for patients with many types of cancer and for the families of such patients. It does not include those patients eligible for the Reach to Recovery, Laryngectomy, or Ostomy programs. It involves a one-to-one visit by a person who has experienced the same type of cancer as the patient and who offers the patient functional, emotional, and social support.

The **Cancer Adjustment Program** is a flexible service of group counseling and individual crisis intervention that focuses primarily on emotional and social problems.

**Laryngectomy** is a service designed to promote and support the total rehabilitation of the individual who has had a laryngectomy (surgical removal of the larynx). Divisions are encouraged to cooperate with the International Association of Laryngectomees.

The **"Look Good . . . Feel Better"** program is designed to help chemotherapy and radiation therapy patients alleviate the side effects of their treatments through the use of cosmetic and beauty techniques that help the patient maintain a positive self-image.

**Ostomy** is a program designed to provide mutual aid, emotional support, and education to individuals with an ostomy resulting from intestinal or urinary cancers so that they may enjoy optimal physical and social function. Divisions are encouraged to cooperate with the United Ostomy Association.

**Childhood Cancer** is a service for both the child with cancer and members of the family. It acquaints parents with the special problems that they may encounter in caring for the child with cancer. Divisions are encouraged to cooperate with Candlelighters, an organization that works to identify and develop solutions to the problems of living with and treating childhood cancer.

In 1988, more than half a million people with cancer participated in the various ACS rehabilitation programs. These patients were helped in the adjustment to laryngectomy, mastectomy, and ostomy rehabilitation.

Local ACS units are involved in basic service programs, including resources, information, and guidance. ACS programs may include more expensive services such as home care programs, blood programs, and childhood cancer programs.

The ACS provides professional education publications for the medical and allied health professional. For a complete listing of the publications available, contact your local ACS unit. Most of the publications are free of charge.

The national headquarters provides assistance to all cancer patients as well as to professionals. The address is 1599 Clifton Road NE, Atlanta, GA 30329.

Numerous publications are available from the National Cancer Institute (NCI) ranging from nutrition to all aspects of cancer. A complete list of NCI publications can be obtained by writing or calling

The National Cancer Institute
Cancer Information Service (CIS)
Building 31, Room 10A18
Bethesda, MD 20892
(800)4-CANCER

Some of the services or publications available to the professional from the National Institutes of Health are as follows.

**Physician Data Query (PDQ)**

This service provides both doctors and patients with access to up-to-date cancer treatment information. Through the PDQ, you can learn about cancer staging, appropriate options at any given stage of cancer, and your prognosis for survival. You can also receive information about the closest treatment center and find out which physicians in your area are offering the most current state-of-the-art treatment.

**Publications**

The National Cancer Institute publishes a series of booklets. This series, titled *What You Need to Know. . .*, discusses almost every type of cancer. When requesting one of these booklets, be sure to specify the exact type of cancer.

The following is a partial listing of some of the excellent booklets provided by NCI:

*Advanced Cancer: Living Each Day*
*Answers to Your Questions About Metastatic Cancer*
*Chemotherapy and You: A Guide to Self-Help During Treatment*
*Control of Cancer Pain Fact Sheet*
*Eating Hints: Recipes and Tips for Better Nutrition During Cancer Treatment*
*Radiation Therapy and You: A Guide to Self-Help During Treatment*
*Radiation Therapy: A Treatment for Early-Stage Breast Cancer*
*Taking Time: Support for People with Cancer and the People Who Care About Them*
*When Cancer Recurs: Meeting the Challenge Again*

Also of interest to professionals is *Fighting Cancer in America: Achieving the "Year 2000 Goal,"* which presents the findings and recommendations of the 1987 to 1988 public participation hearings of the National Cancer Advisory Board on cancer prevention and early detection.

## Other Helping Organizations

What follows is a list of other organizations designed to help cancer patients and their families. If you think that any of these organizations could help you, don't hesitate to call or write to the organization at the telephone number or address provided.

### Cancer Management Center

This program utilizes a multidisciplinary professional panel to give second opinions about an individual's cancer treatment free of charge.

> Cancer Management Center
> 4410 Main Street
> Kansas City, MO 64111
> (816)932-8453

### Cancer Hotline

This service provides "phone mates" for people when they are diagnosed. The phone mate is another cancer patient who has recovered from a similar type of cancer and is able to offer information and support.

> Cancer Hotline
> Kansas City, MO
> (816)932-8453

### Leukemia Society of America (LSA)

This organization supplies information about medical, psychologic, and financial help for leukemia patients and in some cases provides financial help of up to $750 for outpatient costs not covered by other sources. LSA publishes a quarterly newsletter and *Update*, which is a regular series of reports on leukemia research programs and treatment advances.

> Leukemia Society of America
> 733 Third Avenue
> New York, NY 10017
> (212)573-8484

### Make Today Count

Make Today Count is a peer support network with more than 200 local chapters around the world. These groups offer emotional support to people with all types of life-threatening illnesses and are not limited to cancer alone. This self-help organization often depends on the buddy system to assist people in improving the quality of their lives despite chronic illness.

> Make Today Count
> PO Box 22
> Osage Beach, MO 65065
> (314)348-1619

### National Coalition for Cancer Survivorship

This is a network of independent organizations and individuals who work in the area of cancer support and survivorship. They serve as a clearinghouse for information and material about survivorship.

> National Coalition for Cancer Survivorship
> 323 Eighth Street SW
> Albuquerque, NM 87102
> (505)764-9956

### United Ostomy Association

This group arranges for new ostomy patients to receive hospital and home visits from individuals who have recovered from ostomy. The visitors assist in rehabilitation through moral support and education. The organization publishes *Ostomy Quarterly* for members and supports efforts for improved equipment, supplies, and management techniques.

> United Ostomy Association
> 2001 West Beverly Boulevard
> Los Angeles, CA 90057
> (213)413-5510

# Pain Control Referral Groups

Committee on Pain Therapy and Acupuncture
American Society of Anesthesiologists
515 Busse Highway
Park Ridge, IL 60068
(312)825-5586


International Association for the Study of Pain
Department of Anesthesiology
Room RN-10
University of Washington School of Medicine
Seattle, WA 98195
(206)292-7521


National Hospice Organization
1311-A Dolley Madison Boulevard
McLean, VA 22101
(703)356-6770

**Appendix H**

# Pain Clinics

This is only a partial listing. A more comprehensive listing may be found in American Pain Society, American Academy of Pain Medicine. (1989). *Directory of Pain Management Facilities*. Washington, DC: Author.

Pain Treatment Center
King/Drew Medical Center
Los Angeles, CA 90059
William Delgardo, Medical Director


UCLA Pain Management Center
Los Angeles, CA 90024-6909
Theresa Ferrer, Medical Director


USCF Pain Management Center
San Francisco, CA 94117
Warren McKay, Medical Director


Arthur Taub, MD, PhD, PC
New Haven, CT 06510
Arthur Taub, Medical Director


University of Miami Comprehensive Pain &
  Rehabilitation Center
Miami Beach, FL 33139
Hubert Rosomoff, Medical Director

Department of Anesthesia—Pain Control
  Service
Northwestern University
Chicago, IL 60611
James Erickson, Medical Director


NIDR/NIH Pain Clinic
National Institutes of Health
Bethesda, MD 20892
John Decker, Medical Director


Massachusetts General Hospital
Cancer Pain Center
Boston, MA 02114
Raymond Maciewicz, Medical Director


Pain Treatment Service Brigham & Women's
  Hospital
Boston, MA 02115
Angelo Rocco, Medical Director


Boston Pain Center
Brockton, MA 02401
Gerald M. Aronoff, Medical Director


Pain Control Center
University of Massachusetts Medical Center
Worcester, MA 06155
W. Thomas Edwards, Medical Director

Mayo Medical Center
Rochester, MN 55905
Lee Nauss, Medical Director

The Chronic Pain Center of Southern New
    Jersey
Haddon Heights, NJ 08035
John Stambaugh, Medical Director

Pain Management Center of University of
    Medicine and Dentistry of New Jersey
Newark, NJ 07103-2757
Wen-hsien Wu, Medical Director

Unified Pain Service
Montefeore Medical Center
Bronx, NY 10467
Ronald Kanner, Medical Director

Lenox Hill Hospital
Pain Evaluation & Treatment Service
New York, NY 10021
Norman Marcus, Medical Director

Anesthesiology Pain Service, New York
    Hospital
New York, NY 10021
Joseph Artusio, Medical Director

Pain Clinic
Memorial Sloan-Kettering Cancer Center
New York, NY 10021
Kathleen Foley, Medical Director

New York University Comprehensive Pain
    Center
New York University Medical Center
New York, NY 10016
Arthur Battista, Medical Director

Duke Pain Clinic
Durham, NC
Bruno Urban, Medical Director

University of Cincinnati
Pain Control Center
Cincinnati, OH 45267
Richard Gregg, Medical Director

Mercy Pain Team
Oklahoma City, OK
Carol Wenzl, Administrative Director

Hahnemann Pain Treatment Program
% Department of Neurosurgery
Philadelphia, PA 19102-1192
Perry Black, Medical Director

Temple Pain Control Center
Temple Hospital
Philadelphia, PA
Edward Resnick, Medical Director

Pain Control Center
Presbyterian University Hospital
Pittsburgh, PA
Ruben Tenicela, Medical Director

Pain Evaluation & Treatment Institute
Pittsburgh, PA
Richard Stieg, Medical Director

Texas Pain & Stress Center
Houston, Texas
A. David Axelrod, Medical Director

University of Texas Health Science Center
Pain Management Clinic
San Antonio, Texas
Somayaji Ramamurthy, Medical Director

Fred Hutchinson Cancer Research Center
Seattle, WA
Costantino Benedetti, Medical Director

University of Washington Multidisciplinary
    Pain Center
Seattle, WA
John Loeser, Medical Director

University Of Texas M.D. Anderson Cancer
    Center
Houston, Texas
Stratton Hill, Medical Director

# Index

steroid treatment, 208
symptoms, 206
gastrointestinal, diet progression, 207
Granulocytopenia
microbial colonization, 126
physiology, 125-126
Gravity bolus feeding, 345
patient instructions, sample, 348
Growth, children, 141, 142
Guilt, cancer patient, 355, 356-357
Gut atrophy, 42

# H

Harris-Benedict equation, basal energy expenditure, 230
Head and neck cancer
alcoholism, 54
chemotherapy, side effects, 58
chyle fistula, 60
complications, 63
dysphagia, 65-71
enteral nutrition, 320
epidemiology, 53
etiology, 53
nutrition assessment, 53-55, 67-68
nutrition care, 60-63
nutrition problems, 175-176
nutrition support, 185
psychologic impact, 54-55
radiation therapy, side effects, 57-58
surgery, side effects, 55-57
swallowing disorders, 58-59
Healthfinder, resources, 377-379
Hepatic dysfunction, alcoholism, 62
High-calorie, high-protein diet, 21
Home care, 337-351
coordinator, 339
delivery system, 344-345
nurse, 339
nutrition support team, 318, 339
nutritionist, 339, 341
social worker, 338-339
parenteral feeding, 147
Hormonal abnormality, appetite-suppressing, 43
Hormonal therapy, breast cancer, metastatic, 156
Hypercalcemia, 103
Hypermetabolism, anorexia, 5-6
Hypertension, nutrition management, 103
Hypertrophy, ileal, 112
Hypoalbuminemia, 6, 202, 282

Hypogeusia, radiation-related, 211
suggested intervention, 193
Hypoglossal nerve, 67

# I

Ileum, resection, 112
Ileus, parenteral feeding, 278
Immunoaugmentative therapy, 363
Immunocompromise, 125
Immunosuppressed patient, infection prevention, 126-127
Immunotherapy, head and neck cancer, side effects, 58
Infection
alimentary, 165
bone marrow transplantation–caused, 204
oral
marrow transplant–related, 209-210
radiation therapy–related, 175
risk factors, 125
role of food, 127-133
Infection prevention, immunosuppressed patient, 126-127
Information services, telephone number, 375-376
Informed consent, 357
Instructional materials, tube feeding, home, 354
Insulin, hydrazine sulfate, 4
Intestinal absorption, chemotherapy effect, 167
Intestinal fistula, radiation-induced, suggested intervention, 197
Intestinal hypomotility, parenteral feeding, 278
Intestinal obstruction, parenteral nutrition, 278
Intestine
radiation-induced injury, surgical resection, 188
radiation therapy, 187
Intravenous medicine specialist, nutrition support team, 323
Intubation, nasal, 279
short-term nutrition support, 279
Isolation
standard reverse, 127
total reverse, 126-127

# J

Jaundice, pancreatic cancer, 88
Jejunal interposition, 56
Jejunostomy, 279
needle catheter, 270-271
percutaneous, 271

Pancreatectomy, total, 92-93
  drawing, 98
Pancreatic cancer
  anorexia, 88
  chemotherapy, 93, 95
  clinical features, 87-89
  enteral formula, 90
  incidence, 87-89
  jaundice, 88
  nutrition therapy, 89
  palliative management, 93
  presurgical considerations, 89
  radiation therapy, 95
  symptoms, 88
Pancreatic enzyme, 120
  replacement, 92
Pancreaticoduodenectomy, partial, 89-92
Pancreatin, dosage, 93
Pancreatitis, 169
Parenteral nutrition, 163. *See also* Total parenteral
  nutrition
  access site, 27
  bowel cancer, 120-121
  cancer treatment outcome, 333-334
  home, pediatric, 147
  indication, 320
  long-term, transitional support, 278
  management, nutrition support team, 318
  peripheral, 62
Patient interview, nutrition assessment, 229-231
Pediatric patient. *See* Children
Peripheral neuritis, 169
Physical examination, nutrition assessment, 32
Physician
  nutrition support team, 321
  outpatient clinic, 350-351
Physician data query, 412
Polyuria, 104
Postgastrectomy diet, 97
  gastric pull-up, 57
Potassium content, food, 106-107
Potassium restriction, renal failure, acute, 105
Protein absorption, bowel cancer, 117
Protein intake, enhancing, 264
Protein metabolism, derangement, 12
Protein requirements, 20
  measurement, 19-20
Protein restriction, renal failure, acute, 107
Protein supplement, Citrotein, 314
Protein synthesis, hepatic, 97
Psychologic issues
  alternate therapy, 356

  cessation of treatment, 357
  diagnosis, guilt, 355
  end-stage disease, 358
  family cooperation, 357
  quackery, 356
Psychologic status, 26
  stress, 4
Pulmonary aspiration, stomach contents, 270
Pulmonary edema, weight gain, 205
Pump
  enteral feeding, 273
  patient instructions, sample, 346-347

## Q

Quackery, 356, 359-368
  books refuting, 370
  characteristics, 360-361
  complaint directory, 374
  enemas, 363
  enforcement, 367
  evaluation, 359
  financial harm, 365
  immunoaugmentative therapy, 363
  information sources, 373
  Laetrile, 363
  legislation, 367
  macrobiotic diet, 362
  media involvement, 368
  megavitamins, 362
  metabolic therapy, 361-362
  organ extracts, 363
  patient rationale, 359-360
  periodicals refuting, 371
  physical harm, 363-364
  psychologic harm, 364-365
  role of health professional, 365-368
  societal harm, 365
  treatment centers, 372
  vegetarian diet, 362
Quality assurance, nutrition support team, 319

## R

Radiation therapy
  abdomen
    complications, 187-190
    nutrition problems, 177-178
  ageusia, 47
  breast cancer
    metastatic, 156
    nutrition management, 155-156